GERONTOLOGICAL NURSING & HEALTHY AGING

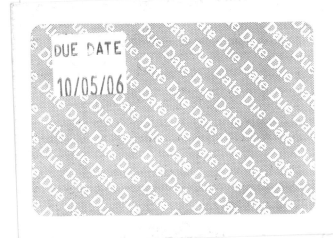

GERONTOLOGICAL NURSING & HEALTHY AGING

Second Edition

PRISCILLA EBERSOLE, PhD, RN, FAAN
Professor Emerita
San Francisco State University
San Francisco, California

PATRICIA HESS, PhD, APRN, BC, NAP
Professor of Nursing
San Francisco State University
San Francisco, California

THERIS TOUHY, ND, APRN, BC
Associate Professor, Christine E. Lynn College of Nursing
Assistant Dean, Undergraduate Programs
Florida Atlantic University
Boca Raton, Florida

KATHLEEN JETT, PhD, APRN, GNP, BC
Assistant Professor, Christine E. Lynn College of Nursing
Florida Atlantic University
Boca Raton, Florida

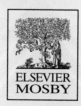

ELSEVIER
MOSBY

ELSEVIER
MOSBY

11830 Westline Industrial Drive
St. Louis, Missouri 63146

GERONTOLOGICAL NURSING & HEALTHY AGING, SECOND EDITION
Copyright © 2005, Mosby, Inc.

Notice

Nursing is an ever-changing field. Standard safety precautions must be followed, but as new research and clinical experience broaden our knowledge, changes in treatment and drug therapy may become necessary or appropriate. Readers are advised to check the most current product information provided by the manufacturer of each drug to be administered to verify the recommended dose, the method and duration of administration, and contraindications. It is the responsibility of the licensed prescriber, relying on experience and knowledge of the patient, to determine dosages and the best treatment for each individual patient. Neither the publisher nor the author assumes any liability for any injury and/or damage to persons or property arising from this publication.

Previous edition copyrighted 2001 by Mosby, Inc.

Library of Congress Cataloging-in-Publication Data

Geriatric nursing & healthy aging / Priscilla Ebersole . . . [et al.].–2nd ed.
   p. ; cm.
  Rev. ed. of: Geriatric nursing and healthy aging / Priscilla Ebersole. 1st ed. 2001.
  Includes bibliographical references and index.
  ISBN 13: 978-0-323-03165-3 ISBN 10: 0-323-03165-X
  1. Geriatric nursing. 2. Aging. 3. Aged–Health and hygiene. I. Title: Geriatric nursing and healthy aging. II. Ebersole, Priscilla. III. Ebersole, Priscilla. Geriatric nursing and healthy aging.
  [DNLM: 1. Geriatric Nursing. 2. Aging. 3. Health Promotion–Aged. 4. Holistic Nursing–Aged. WY 152 G36964 2005]
  RC954.G455 2005
  618.97'0231–dc22

2005041517

Publisher: Michael S. Ledbetter
Senior Developmental Editor: Laurie K. Gower
Publishing Services Manager: Jeff Patterson
Senior Project Manager: Anne Konopka
Designer: Jyotika Shroff

ISBN 13: 978-0-323-03165-3
ISBN 10: 0-323-03165-X

Printed in the United States of America.

Last digit is the print number: 9 8 7 6 5 4 3 2

Reviewers

Jean Benzel-Lindley, PhD(c), RN
Assistant Professor of Nursing
University of Nevada
Reno, Nevada

Joyce Syatauw Tanaka, MSN, RN, BC
Assistant Professor
Ohlone College
Fremont, California

Preface

This second edition of *Gerontological Nursing & Healthy Aging* has been prepared by Theris Touhy and Kathleen Jett. We are delighted to have such capable professionals, both gerontological nurse practitioners, willing to take on this intense and arduous task with such devotion and competence. It is always difficult to let go of something as demanding and stimulating as the geriatric nursing textbooks that we have invested in so heavily over several decades. This "letting go" has been much easier than we expected because Drs. Touhy and Jett have done such a superb job. Just as with aging, one passes on the torch to those of the next generation of geriatric nurse professionals, who will continue to advocate for the health of older adults in their practice and their writing.

Their achievement in producing such a superior text reflects their commitment to providing the most current thinking in gerontological nursing. They have closely collaborated with each other and with us to maintain the principles of healthy aging and wellness that are fundamental to our philosophy. Their own approach is unique to them but combines the best of our thoughts and of theirs. We are extremely gratified and know that the future of our gerontological nursing text is in expert hands.

Priscilla Ebersole
Patricia Hess

This text is about health, wellness, and aging. It is designed to provide nurses, faculty, and students with the most current information about best practice gerontological nursing, an area often neglected in basic nursing education and nursing texts. In Section I, the topics of communication and healthy aging are explored, from the origins of gerontological nursing and the impact of culture and health disparities, to the importance of skillful documentation. In Section II, the many changes associated with normal aging are presented, along with specific implications for nursing and working with the older adult to respond and adapt to the changes with the goal of maintaining or restoring optimal wellness. Section III focuses on common health problems seen in older adults and what nurses can do to help elders living with chronic illness. This section does not provide the in-depth coverage of the topics that one would find in a medical-surgical nursing textbook, but highlights the key aspects of the problems as they relate specifically to older adults. In Section IV, we reach out beyond the elder to the family and the health care system. Here we provide basic information that every nurse working with older adults needs to know. Finally, in Section V we present discussions of the global topics that affect all elders: coping with grief, dying and death, the impact of the environment on safety and security, and living options across the continuum of care.

The text is organized for optimal student learning experiences. Each chapter begins with the phenomenological consideration of the lived experience of an elder. Key concepts, glossaries, learning activities, and discussion questions summarize the important points presented and relate directly to the objectives of the chapter. Resources, including teaching materials, films, and websites, are provided at the end of each chapter for the reader who may wish to seek additional information or referral sources.

New to this edition is the Evolve Learning System, an online supplement for instructors. Accessible at http://evolve.elsevier.com/Ebersole/gerontological/, this ancillary includes many resources designed to help the instructor present the content of this book. Resources include:

- Instructor's Resource Manual with Chapter Summaries
- Suggested Classroom and Clinical Activities
- Review/Critical Thinking Activities
- ExamView Test Bank with 250+ questions in the latest NCLEX examination format

Nurses with competence in the care of older people will be in great demand as the population ages. Gerontological nurses have always assumed a leadership role in improving care for elders, ensuring fulfillment of all levels on Maslow's Hierarchy of Needs, and promoting healthy aging. Through their expertise, commitment, dedication, advocacy, and compassion, gerontological nurses who work with older adults in all settings will continue to be leaders in creating models that truly change the culture of existing systems. Nurses play an essential role in creating environments of care in which older adults can reach their full potential, thriving, not merely surviving, in the latter part of life. Our hope is that the nursing practice of those who read this book will be enriched, just as ours has been, by sharing the wisdom and beauty of older adults.

We would like to thank Priscilla Ebersole and Patricia Hess for the opportunity to write this new edition and to share their beautiful words and passion for gerontological nursing. We hope that our work honors them and the specialty we all love. It has been a real privilege for us to be a part of the work of two gerontological nurses from whom we have learned how to care for older people.

Theris Touhy
Kathleen Jett

Contents

Introduction to Healthy Aging

GLOSSARY

Cohort Group where members share some common experience.

Holistic health care That which considers the whole person and the interaction with and between the parts.

Resilience The ability to continue despite challenges.

THE LIVED EXPERIENCE

I believe a human life is like a river, meandering through its course, rushing through rapids, flowing placidly over the plains, twisting and turning through countless bends until it spends itself. It is the same river; yet it looks very different from one place to another. So it is with our lives; circumstances vary from one time to another in the course of a life, but I think each stage has its own value.

Georgia, a 35-year-old

It is so strange! I only realize I'm considered old when I'm automatically given a senior discount without even asking. Sometimes I will catch a glance from someone who seems as if he or she is afraid I may need help, and of course my children notice if I forget something and are kind enough to not mention it. As if they never forget anything!! But the strangest is when I catch a glimpse of a wrinkled old lady and realize it is my own reflection. How can that be?

Reba, a 75-year-old

*P*roviding nursing care to older persons is a rewarding, life-affirming vocation. Through this textbook we hope to provide students with the basics to begin a career as a gerontological nurse or simply care for older adults with more skills and sensitivity. We present an overview of aging, the health care needs of older adults, and the vital and exciting role of the nurse in facilitating healthy aging.

AGING

Although all of us begin aging at birth, both the meaning of aging and who is recognized as the aged are determined by society and culture and influenced by history and gender. In the early American Puritan community of the 1600s, the process of aging was considered a sacred pilgrimage to God, and as such, the aged were revered. By the late 1800s the aged were devalued as youth became the symbol of growth and expansion. In 1935 the time when one became old or aged was set at 65, the age of retirement, when one became eligible for the new benefit of Social Security. Since then the age of retirement is slowly increasing (see Chapter 24). Psychologists have divided the "old" into three groups: the young-old, roughly 65 to 74 years old; the middle-old, 75 to 84 years old; and the old-old, or those over 85. A fourth group is rapidly growing in numbers, centenarians. According to a study at Boston University there were approximately 40,000 persons in the United States over the age of 100 in 2002. By the early part of the 2020s this number may reach 3 million (Boston University, 2002).

Groups of people, usually born within the same decade, may share a common historical context. The term *cohort* is usually applied to such a group. For example, men born between 1920 and 1930 were very likely to have been active participants in World War II and the Korean War. In comparison, men born between 1940 and 1950 were likely to have been involved in the Vietnam conflict, an entirely different experience. It is not surprising that these two groups of men have different perspectives and different health problems. Likewise, most women born between 1920 and 1930 were raised with what are known as traditional values and roles and may have either never worked outside the home or been limited to lower-paying "women's work," such as housekeeping, teaching, and nursing. In contrast, women born between 1930 and 1940 had pressure to work outside the home and also had considerably more opportunities, partially as a result of the feminist revolution of the 1960s.

Gender can have a significant effect on various aspects of aging. Women usually live longer than men and are much more likely to live alone after widowhood. Men who survive their wives often remarry and live alone significantly less often than women. However, women usually have larger social networks outside the work environment than men, which could potentially reduce social isolation after the death of a spouse or companion. And gender-related health problems emerge: women increasingly confront osteoporosis and breast and uterine cancer, whereas men are vulnerable to prostate enlargement and cancer. Cardiac problems affect both genders about equally, but women are treated less aggressively than are men.

Finally, we have an increasing influence of ethnicity on aging. The United States is experiencing a "gerontological explosion" of ethnically diverse older adults, primarily those persons of color. Persons comprising groups that have been considered statistical minorities in the late 1900s can now be considered an emerging majority as the relative percentage of their numbers rises rapidly. See Figure 1-1 for the projected changes in the demographics of older adults by the year 2050. The growing number of new elders of color may challenge the nurse to understand a different set of expectations and traditions. Nursing programs may need to evolve to include working with interpreters or learning another language as a part of their requirements (see Chapter 4).

HEALTH, WELLNESS, AND AGING

This text is about health, wellness, and aging. The focus of health is a reflection of the goals of the nation and the call for health professionals as set forth in the document *Healthy People 2000* and the updated *Healthy People 2010* (USDHHS, 2000). The revised goals of 2010 are to (1) increase the span of healthy life for Americans and (2) reduce health

Percent

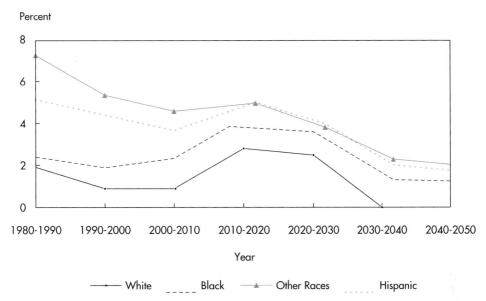

Figure 1-1 Annual rate of increase in elderly population by race and ethnicity: 1980 to 2050. (Modified from Angel JL, Hogan DP: The demography of minority aging populations. In The Gerontological Society of America: *Minority aging,* Washington, DC, 1994, The Society.)

disparity among Americans (Box 1-1). It must be noted that the first goal is to increase both the life span and the time that persons remain healthy or the quality of life lived. As health professionals, gerontological nurses have a special responsibility for helping the nation achieve these goals.

Health and wellness may take on different meanings in later life compared with earlier life. With age there is usually an accumulation of disease states. For persons living in nursing homes it is not uncommon for one person to have six or more diagnoses on the medical record, and the nurse may be participating in the treatment of all of these. One may ask, "Is a goal toward wellness possible? Can the idea of wellness be applied to someone who is dealing with chronic illnesses?" We answer with a resounding "Yes!"

The definitions of health vary greatly and are influenced by culture and where one is on the life span. The strong emergence of the holistic health movement has resulted in even broader definitions of health, to include wellness. Wellness involves one's whole being—physical, emotional, mental, and spiritual—all of which are vital components (Figure 1-2). Dunn (1961) defined the holistic approach to health as "an integrated

method of functioning which is oriented toward maximizing the potential of which the individual is capable within the environment where he is functioning." The holistic definition does not limit health to just its physical or mental or even social aspects but, rather, incorporates all these facets into the total picture. Wellness involves achieving a balance between one's internal and external environment and one's emotional, spiritual, social, cultural, and physical processes.

Wellness is a state of being and feeling that one strives to achieve through motivation and positive health practices. An individual must work hard to achieve wellness just as he or she must work hard to perform competently at a job. In working toward wellness, an individual may reach plateaus in his or her ascension to higher-level wellness. The person may also regress because of an illness event or simply the various cycles of life, but these events can be a stimulus for growth potential and a return to moving along the wellness continuum (Figure 1-3).

Consistent with Dunn (1961), health in later life is often thought of in terms of functional ability rather that the absence of disease, that is, the ability to do what is important to that person.

Box 1-1   Healthy People 2010

Goals
Goal #1: Increase the Span of Healthy Life:
To help individuals of all ages increase life
expectancy *and* improve their quality of life.
Goal #2: Reduce Health Disparities: To
eliminate health disparities among different
segments of the population.

Focus Areas and Objectives
The nation's progress in achieving the two overar-
ching goals of *Healthy People 2010* will be monitored through 467 objectives in 28 focus areas.
Many objectives focus on interventions designed
to reduce or eliminate illness, disability, and
premature death among individuals and communities. Others focus on broader issues, such as
improving access to quality health care, strengthening public health services, and improving the
availability and dissemination of health-related
information. Each objective has a target for specific
improvements to be achieved by the year 2010.

Healthy People 2010 Focus Areas
- Access to quality health services
- Arthritis, osteoporosis, and chronic back
  conditions
- Cancer
- Chronic kidney disease
- Diabetes
- Disability and secondary conditions
- Educational and community-based programs
- Environmental health
- Family planning
- Food safety
- Health communication
- Heart disease and stroke
- Human immunodeficiency virus (HIV)
- Immunization and infectious diseases
- Injury and violence prevention
- Maternal, infant, and child health
- Medical product safety
- Mental health and mental disorders
- Nutrition and overweight
- Occupational safety and health
- Oral health
- Physical activity and fitness
- Public health infrastructure
- Respiratory diseases
- Sexually transmitted diseases
- Substance abuse
- Tobacco use
- Vision and hearing

Source: U.S. Department of Health and Human Services (USDHHS): *Healthy people 2010*, Washington, DC, 2000, US
Government Printing Office, USDHHS.
http://www.health.gov/healthypeople.

This may mean the ability to live independently
or the ability to enjoy the great-grandchildren
when they visit at the nursing home, but it is
always individually determined. Well-being for
those older than 60 years is strongly related to
health but is affected also by socioeconomic
factors, degree of social interaction, marital
status, and aspects of one's living situation and
environment.

A positive approach to health emphasizes
strengths, resilience, resources, and capabilities
rather than focusing on existing pathological conditions. A wellness perspective is based on the
belief that every person has an optimal level of
function regardless of his or her situation. Even
with chronic illness or with multiple disabilities or

while dying, movement toward higher wellness is
possible if the emphasis of care is placed on the
promotion of function in the least restrictive environment, with support and encouragement for the
individual to find meaning in the situation, whatever it is.

The wellness continuum picks up where the
traditional medical model leaves off. Instead of a
downward negative trajectory for the health of the
aged, focused on deterioration, the wellness model
rises and moves in a positive direction (Figure
1-4). When one considers the wellness or holistic
approach as an appropriate model for working
with older adults, one regards the illness and wellness continuum from a positive direction and the
role of the individual as active.

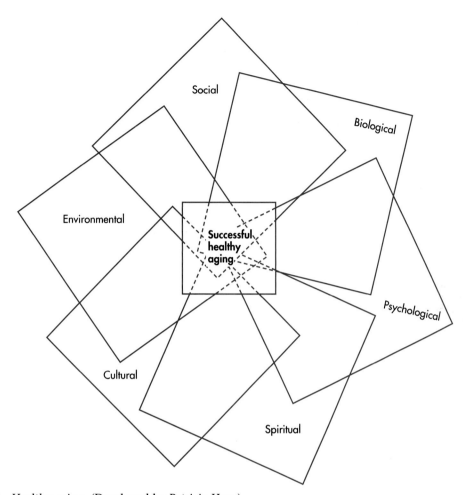

Figure 1-2   Healthy aging. (Developed by Patricia Hess.)

ALTERNATIVE HEALTH CARE

As persons strive for wellness they use treatments and techniques that they have found helpful in the past. These will include what are known as biomedical approaches as well as those referred to as complementary and alternative medicine (CAM). CAM has been used extensively and effectively for centuries, particularly in Asian countries. Although there have always been home gardens with medicinal herbs, the types of CAM available have increased significantly in recent years.

Because of public interest and citizen involvement, the National Institutes of Health (NIH) established in 1992 the National Center for Complementary and Alternative Medicine. Recent estimates are that almost one half of U.S. residents use some form of complementary medicine—often because they are dissatisfied with conventional medical approaches (Lorenzi, 1999). These strategies include focusing or transferring of positive energies through meditation, visualization, touch, massage, acupressure, acupuncture, magnets, crystals, aromas, and colors. Also, numerous nutritional supplements and herbs are popular. Some of these are legitimate, and some are fads. Nutritionists, nurses, physicians, acupuncturists, and chiropractors are only a few of the providers that offer services to the public.

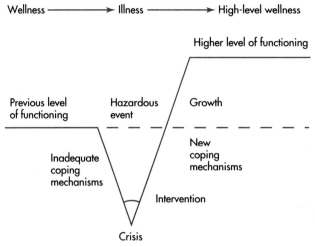

Figure 1-3   Growth potential: crisis as a challenge.

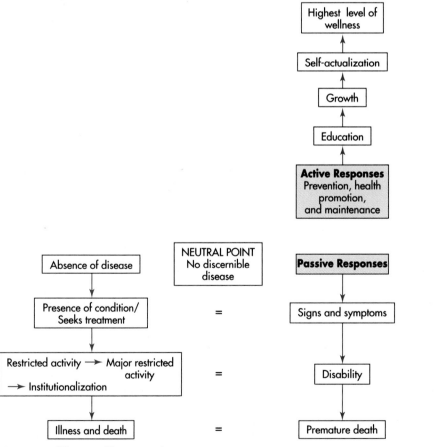

Figure 1-4   Illness-wellness continuum.

Some types of CAM have been recognized to the extent that the associated costs are covered by Medicaid, Medicare, and some insurance companies. The research related to both the risks and benefits of each of these approaches is currently underway. Several of the most commonly seen approaches are described in Chapter 16.

MASLOW'S HIERARCHY OF HUMAN NEEDS

Maslow's theories of the hierarchy of human needs provide an organizing framework for this text and for understanding individuals and their concerns at any particular time and in any particular situation (Figure 1-5). It also can serve as a guide for prioritizing nursing interventions to promote healthy aging. The hierarchy ranks needs from the most basic, related to the maintenance of biological integrity, to the most complex, associated with self-actualization. According to this theory the higher levels cannot be met without first meeting the lower level needs. In other words, moving toward healthy aging is an evolving and developing process. As basic level needs are met, the satisfaction of higher level needs is possible, with ever deepening richness to life, regardless of one's age. The nurse will prioritize care from the most essential to those things we think of as quality of life.

As far back as Hippocrates and Galen the basic needs of all living people were recognized as the need for air, fluids, nutrition, hygiene, elimination, activity, and skin integrity. More recently these needs are identified as self-care requirements (Box 1-2). Along with these is the basic need for comfort or relief from suffering. The gerontological nurse works to ensure that these needs are met for older adults and realizes that as these are met, higher levels of wellness are possible. The person with dementia may begin to wander or become agitated because of the need to find a toilet and not knowing where to look. Until the toileting needs are met, the nurse's attempt to comfort or redirect is likely to be ineffective and frustrating. The person who lives alone but is unable to shop or cook will be distressed and perhaps irritable until arrangements can be made for home-delivered meals, either commercially or through a friend or family member.

As people's basic needs are met they will feel safe and secure. They will likely sleep better and feel more comfortable interacting with others. While interacting with others, people often begin to meet their needs of belonging. Maslow sees people as social beings with a need to belong to something outside of themselves. These needs are met through memberships in churches, synagogues, mosques, and civic or social organizations and through ties to family and friends. After retirement a member of a work organization may replace the belonging need with special interest groups. If it is not replaced there is a risk for isolation and depression. When a person moves to live with a child in a distant city or into an assisted living facility or nursing home, meeting belonging needs can be especially challenging and the nurse may work with the elder to form new alliances and associations. The nurse works to create environments in which meaningful relationships and activities can remain a part of the elder's life.

A person whose basic needs are met, who feels safe and secure, and who has a sense of belonging will also have self-esteem and self-efficacy. In other words, people will accept and honor who they are and feel that they have some personal power and self-confidence; they will know that they are important as people and that they inherently have value. Self-esteem is not something someone can give to anyone else. It is, however, something that others can negatively influence through ageist attitudes and behavior. For example, anytime the nurse assumes that a patient cannot do something based solely on the person's age, one is being ageist and is actually belittling the individual. Unfortunately this is commonly seen but can be challenged by the knowledgeable and sensitive gerontological nurse.

Finally, some people reach Maslow's highest level of wellness, that of self-actualization. Self-actualization is seen as people reaching out beyond themselves and finding meaning in their lives and a sense of fulfillment. This may not seem possible for all, but the nurse can foster this in unique and important ways. One of the authors (KJ) was asked to speak to a group in a nursing

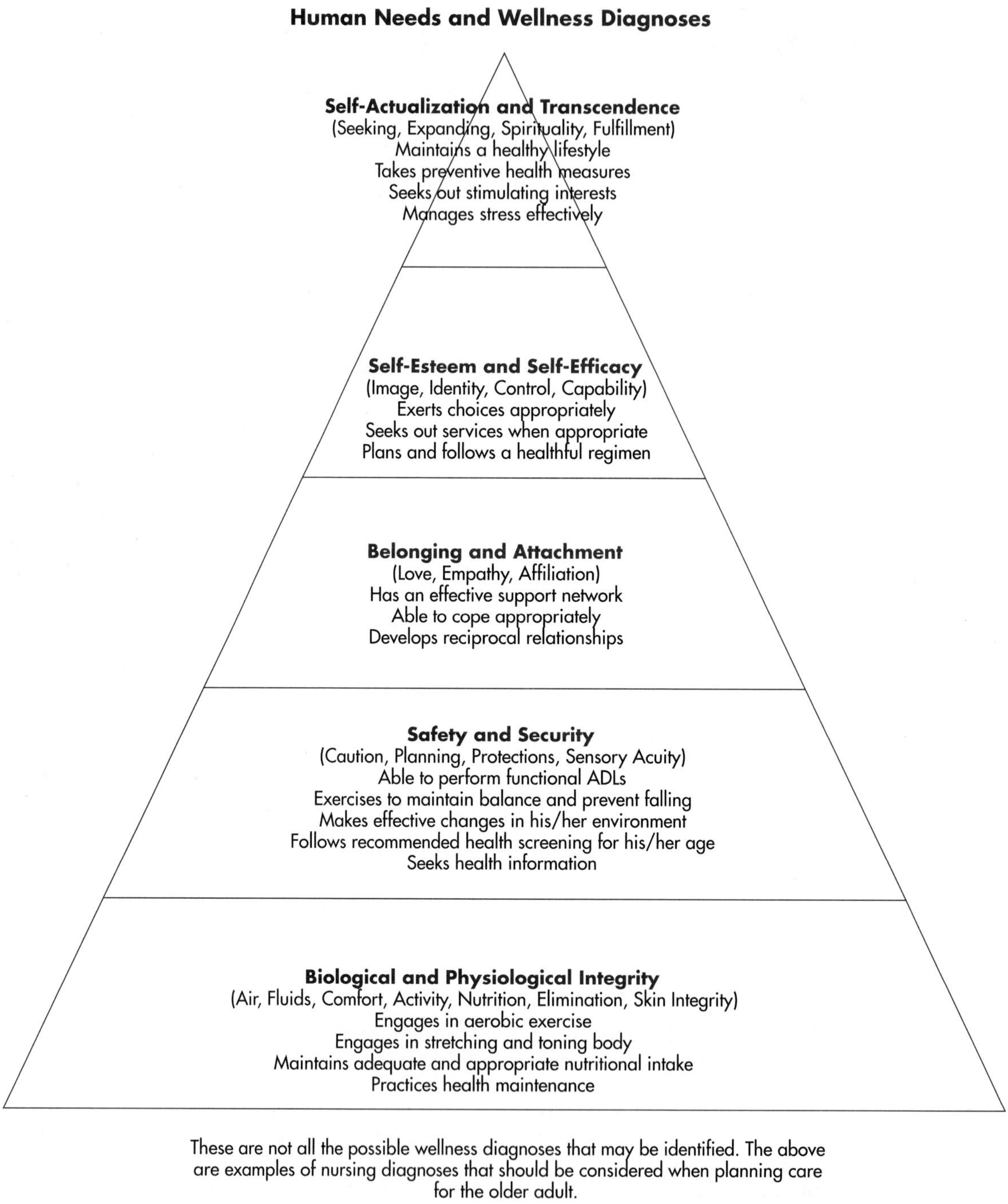

Human Needs and Wellness Diagnoses

Self-Actualization and Transcendence
(Seeking, Expanding, Spirituality, Fulfillment)
Maintains a healthy lifestyle
Takes preventive health measures
Seeks out stimulating interests
Manages stress effectively

Self-Esteem and Self-Efficacy
(Image, Identity, Control, Capability)
Exerts choices appropriately
Seeks out services when appropriate
Plans and follows a healthful regimen

Belonging and Attachment
(Love, Empathy, Affiliation)
Has an effective support network
Able to cope appropriately
Develops reciprocal relationships

Safety and Security
(Caution, Planning, Protections, Sensory Acuity)
Able to perform functional ADLs
Exercises to maintain balance and prevent falling
Makes effective changes in his/her environment
Follows recommended health screening for his/her age
Seeks health information

Biological and Physiological Integrity
(Air, Fluids, Comfort, Activity, Nutrition, Elimination, Skin Integrity)
Engages in aerobic exercise
Engages in stretching and toning body
Maintains adequate and appropriate nutritional intake
Practices health maintenance

These are not all the possible wellness diagnoses that may be identified. The above are examples of nursing diagnoses that should be considered when planning care for the older adult.

Figure 1-5   Human needs and wellness diagnoses. *ADLs,* Activities of daily living.

Box 1-2	Universal Self-Care Requirements

1. Maintaining sufficient intake of air, water, food
   a. Taking in that quantity required for normal functioning with adjustments for internal and external factors that can affect the requirement, or, under conditions of scarcity, adjusting consumption to bring the most advantageous return to integrated functioning
   b. Preserving the integrity of associated anatomic structures and physiologic processes
   c. Enjoying the pleasurable experiences of breathing, drinking, and eating without abuses
2. Provision of care associated with eliminative processes and excrements
   a. Bringing about and maintaining internal and external conditions necessary for the regulation of eliminative processes
   b. Managing the processes of elimination (including protection of the structures and processes involved) and disposal of excrement
   c. Providing subsequent hygienic care of body surfaces and parts
   d. Caring for the environment as needed to maintain sanitary conditions
3. Maintenance of body temperature and personal hygiene
   a. Bringing about and/or maintaining internal and external conditions necessary for regulating body temperature processes
   b. Using personal capabilities and values as well as culturally prescribed norms as bases for maintaining personal hygiene
   c. Caring for the environment to maintain a healthy living condition
4. Maintenance of a balance between activity and rest
   a. Selecting activities that stimulate, engage, and keep in balance physical movement, affective responses, intellectual effort, and social interaction
   b. Recognizing and attending to manifestations of needs for rest and activity
   c. Using personal capabilities, interests, and values as well as culturally prescribed norms as bases for development of a rest-activity pattern
5. Maintenance of a balance between solitude and social interaction
   a. Maintaining that quality and balance necessary for the development of personal autonomy and enduring social relations that foster effective functioning of individuals
   b. Fostering bonds of affection, love, and friendship; effectively managing impulses to use others for selfish purposes, disregarding their individuality, integrity, and rights
   c. Providing conditions of social warmth and closeness essential for continuing development and adjustment
   d. Promoting individual autonomy as well as group membership

From U.S. Department of Health and Human Services: *Toward a plan for the chronically mentally ill. Report to the Secretary of Health and Human Services*, Washington, DC, 1980, USDHHS.

home about death and dying. To her surprise the room was not filled with staff, as she had expected, but with the frailest of elders confined to wheelchairs. Instead of the usual lecture, she talked about legacies and asked the silent audience, "What do you want people to remember about you? What made your life worthwhile?" Without exception each member of the audience had something to say, from "I had a beautiful garden" to "I was a good mother" to "I helped design a bridge." Meaning can be found for life everywhere—you just have to ask.

IMPLICATIONS FOR GERONTOLOGICAL NURSING

The unique practice of gerontological nursing has been recognized since 1904, when the *American Journal of Nursing* published an article on old age, disease, and nursing. Nurses attracted to this specialized field recognize that expertise in caring for older adults can make a significant difference in the quality of life of the persons served. Nursing is a vital aspect of the health care of aging persons. In times of illness and rehabilitation, the outcomes for the person, including survival, more often than not depend on the nursing care received.

Although much of the nursing care of the aged is provided in nursing homes, gerontological nurses today practice in settings across the continuum of care, including acute care hospitals, rehabilitation centers, nursing homes, and assisted living facilities. Gerontological nursing also occurs in the community, in persons' homes through home health and hospice, and in senior centers and adult day health and fitness or wellness centers. Gerontological nurses have opportunities anywhere along the continuum of aging services from caring for the most ill and frail to those who are active and independent. In most situations the nurse functions as the key member of the health care team and, in many cases, functions autonomously. Terry Fulmer, co-director of the John A. Hartford Foundation Institute for Geriatric Nursing, says, "Long ago I realized that, in the arena of caring for the aged, I could have an autonomous nursing practice that would make a real difference in medical outcomes. I could practice the full scope of nursing. It gave me a great sense of freedom and accomplishment" (Ebersole, 1999).

It is the responsibility of the nurse to assist elders to achieve the highest level of wellness in relation to whatever situation exists. The nurse can, through knowledge and affirmation, empower, enhance, and support the person's movement toward the highest level of wellness possible. The nurse assesses and can help explore the underlying situation that may be interfering with the achievement of wellness, and work with the person and significant others to develop affirming and appropriate plans of care. The nurse and the elder collaboratively implement interventions to achieve individual goals and evaluate their effectiveness. The goals of the nurse are to care and comfort always, to cure sometimes, to help persons improve or maintain their quality of lives, and to prevent that which can be prevented.

KEY CONCEPTS

- Gerontological nursing is an opportunity to make a significant difference in the lives of older adults.

- The meaning of aging is influenced by many factors.
- Nurses have a responsibility to contribute to the nation's goals of increasing the quality of life lived and to reduce health disparities.
- Health, history, and gender are among the major factors influencing the aging experience.
- Each cohort is in some ways distinctly different from others, and individual persons become more unique the longer they live. Thus one must be cautious in attributing of older adults any specific characteristics to "old age."
- All persons, regardless of age or life/health situation, can be helped to achieve a higher level of wellness, which is uniquely defined by each person.
- Complementary and alternative approaches to medicine and health care have the potential of helping a large number of people. However, as Americans increase their use of complementary and alternative medicine, caution must be used to ensure the quality and safety of the practices.
- Maslow's Hierarchy of Needs can be used as an organizing framework for health promotion, regardless of age or situation.
- Gerontological nurses have key roles in the provision of the highest quality of care to older adults in a wide range of settings and situations.

Activities and Discussion Questions

1. Discuss the ways in which elders contribute to society today.
2. Interview an older person, and ask how he or she has changed since being 25 years old.
3. Discuss health and wellness with your peers. Develop a definition applicable to an aged person.
4. Discuss the dimensions of wellness and which you think may be most important.
5. Explain wellness in the context of chronic illness.
6. Discuss how you seek wellness in your own life.
7. Discuss what you can do to enhance the quality of life for the persons to whom they provide care.
8. Draw a picture of yourself at 80.

9. Discuss how older adults are portrayed in a popular T.V. show or movie.

RESOURCES

Websites

Administration on Aging
website: www.aoa.gov

Gerontological Society of America
website: www.geron.org

Hartford Institute for Geriatric Nursing
website: www.hartfordign.org

Healthy People 2010
website: www.healthypeople.gov

Long Term Care Nurse Leadership
website: http://ltcnurseleader.umn.edu

National Gerontological Nurses Association
website: www.ngna.org

Nurse Competency in Aging Project
website: www.geronurseonline.org

Photography of Chester Higgins ("Eldergrace")
website: www.miradoremagazine.com/eldergrace

REFERENCES

Boston University: A *look at centenarians: a report of the New England centenarian study*, 2002. Available at www.bumc.bu.edu. Accessed 8/26/04.

Dunn HL: *High-level wellness,* Arlington, Va, 1961, Beatty.

Ebersole P: Leaders in geriatric nursing: the dynamic duo: Mathy Mezey and Terry Fulmer, *Geriatr Nurs* 20(2):106-107, 1999.

Lorenzi EA: Complementary/alternative therapies: so many choices, *Geriatr Nurs* 20(3):125-133, 1999.

U.S. Department of Health and Human Services (USDHHS): *Healthy people 2010*, Washington, DC, 2000, US Government Printing Office, USDHHS.

Gerontological Nursing History, Education, and Roles

2

LEARNING OBJECTIVES

Upon completion of this chapter, the reader will be able to:

- Discuss the history of gerontological nursing and the factors influencing the development of the specialty practice.
- Describe several gerontological nursing roles and educational preparation for practice.
- Identify elements of the American Nurses Association (ANA) Scope and Standards of Practice for Gerontological Nursing.
- Recognize and discuss the importance of certification.
- Discuss formal gerontological organizations and their significance to the gerontological nurse.
- Understand the importance of staff development and support for all levels of caregivers to increase satisfaction and effective gerontological practice.

▶ **THE LIVED EXPERIENCE**

I don't think I will work in gerontological nursing; it seems depressing. I don't know many older people, but they are all sick without much hope to get better. I'll probably go into labor and delivery or the emergency room where I can really make a difference.

Student nurse, age 24

To know that I have made them feel they are human, that they're loved . . . that someone still cares about them. I believe that lots of times they feel ignored and as if they have no value. It's very important to me that they feel valued and they know that they still contribute not only to society but to the personal growth of everyone that comes into interaction with them.

Gerontological nurse, age 35, working in a nursing home

*T*his chapter examines the foundations of the specialty practice of gerontological nursing, education, roles, organizations, and communication attributes that contribute to competent and satisfying practice in the care of older adults.

GERONTOLOGICAL NURSING: DEVELOPMENT OF A SPECIALTY

Geriatric nursing, the first name given to the nursing specialty, was replaced by *gerontological*

nursing in 1976 to reflect nursing's emphasis on health rather than disease. Burnside (1988) noted that there is ambivalence about the choice of the terminology because both terms are in common usage in nursing. *Gerontic nursing* was another term coined by Laurie Gunter and Carmen Estes (1979) to describe the specialty, but it is rarely seen in the literature today. Gerontological nursing will be used throughout this book, reflecting the newer terminology and broader scope of the specialty.

In all areas of practice, nurses complain about the lack of professional supports, inadequate time, and fragmentation of care. Nurses must consciously seek appropriate education and practice settings that allow them to find satisfaction in nursing. Many have found their place in long-term care and community settings where contact with clients and residents is ongoing. Increasing numbers of students are choosing to specialize in the care of older adults because of the possibility of sustained and meaningful relationships and the opportunity to practice within a nursing model of care. Although interest in the specialty and numbers of nurses prepared academically are increasing, there remains a critical need for gerontological nurses. With estimates that the U.S. population of older adults aged 65 and over will double by 2030, nurses with expertise in gerontological nursing will be in great demand. The projected need for gerontological nurses in all settings is expected to reach 1.1 million by 2030 (Klein, 1997). "Whether in the home, hospital, or various community and long-term care agencies, the older adult requires comprehensive care that focuses on individualized health promotion and disease prevention, ongoing assessment of functional and cognitive status, rapid identification of acute problems, rehabilitation and restorative care, ongoing education, and appropriate referrals" (ANA, 2001, pp. 7-8). Historically, nurses have always been in the frontlines caring for the aged. They have provided hands-on care, supervision, administration, program development, teaching, and research and are, to a great extent, responsible for the rapid advance of gerontology as a profession. Nurses have been, and continue to be, the mainstay of care of older adults (Wykle, McDonald, 1997; Mezey, Fulmer, 2002).

The origins of gerontological nursing began when Florence Nightingale, the founder of modern nursing, accepted a position as superintendent in an institution comparable to today's nursing home, the Institution for the Care of Sick Gentlewomen in Distressed Circumstances. Patients at this institution were primarily governesses and ladies' maids from wealthy English families (Wykle, McDonald, 1997). Awareness of the need for education in gerontological nursing, as well as the need for improvement in care for institutionalized older adults, was first noted in the American nursing literature in the early 1900s. In 1908, Lavinia Dock, editor of the *American Journal of Nursing* (Dock, 1908), discussed the findings of a report of scathing conditions in almshouses (early nursing homes) and supported the need for trained nurses to work in these institutions and for student education in almshouses. Another editorial in the *American Journal of Nursing* in 1925 called for nurses to consider a specialty in nursing care of the aged. Again, in 1943, an article describing nursing care of the aged recommended that nurses with special aptitude care for the aged and that nursing and medical schools include geriatric education (Geldbach, 1943). The first book on gerontological nursing was written by Newton and Anderson in 1950 (Newton, Anderson, 1950), and in 1966, the Division of Geriatric Nursing Practice was established within the ANA, giving nursing care of the aged specialty status along with maternal/child, medical-surgical, psychiatric, and community health.

Considered nursing's newest and youngest specialty, gerontological nursing emerged as a circumscribed area of practice only within the last 5 decades. Before 1950, gerontological nursing care was seen as the application of general principles of nursing to the older client with little recognition of this area of nursing as a specialty similar to obstetric, pediatric, or surgical nursing. Whereas most specialties in nursing practice developed from those identified in medicine, this was not the case with the specialty of gerontological nursing since health care of the elderly was traditionally considered within the domain of nursing (Davis, 1985). In examining the history of gerontological nursing, one must marvel at the advocacy and perseverance of nurses who have remained deeply committed to the care of older adults despite struggling against insurmountable odds over the years. We are proud to be the standard-bearers of excellence in care of the aged (Box 2-1).

Gerontological nurse educators, scholars, and clinicians continue their commitment to and advocacy for older people. Gerontological nurses have made substantial contributions to the body of knowledge guiding best practices in the care of older people. Nursing research has provided a solid knowledge base for important clinical issues, such as restraint reduction, incontinence, care of people with Alzheimer's disease, informal caregiving, nutrition, health promotion, care environments, physical and emotional health, and reminiscence therapy (Fitzpatrick, Fulmer, 2000).

Box 2-1 **Professionalization of Gerontological Nursing**

1906 First article published in *American Journal of Nursing (AJN)* on care of the aged

1925 *AJN* considers geriatric nursing as a possible specialty in nursing

1950 Newton and Anderson publish first geriatric nursing textbook
  Geriatrics becomes a specialization in nursing

1962 American Nurses Association (ANA) forms a national geriatric nursing group

1966 ANA creates the Division of Geriatric Nursing
  First master's program for clinical nurse specialists in geriatric nursing developed by Virginia Stone at Duke University

1970 ANA establishes Standards of Practice for Geriatric Nursing committee, chaired by Dorothy Moses; included Lois Knowles and Mary Shaunnessey

1973 ANA defined Standards of Practice for Geriatric Nursing

1974 Certification in geriatric nursing practice offered through ANA; process implemented by Laurie Gunter and Virginia Stone

1975 *Journal of Gerontological Nursing* published by Slack; first editor, Edna Stilwell

1976 ANA renames Geriatric Division "Gerontological" to reflect a health promotion emphasis
  ANA publishes Standards for Gerontological Nursing Practice; committee chaired by Barbara Allen Davis
  ANA begins certifying geriatric nurse practitioners
  Nursing and the Aged edited by Burnside and published by McGraw-Hill

1977 First gerontological nursing track funded by Division of Nursing and established by Sr. Rose Therese Bahr at University of Kansas School of Nursing

1979 *Education for Gerontic Nursing* written by Gunter and Estes; suggested curricula for all levels of nursing education
  ANA Council of Long Term Care Nurses established; group first chaired by Ella Kick

1980 *Geriatric Nursing* first published by *AJN*; Cynthia Kelly, editor

1981 ANA Division of Gerontological Nursing issues statement regarding scope of practice

1983 Florence Cellar Endowed Gerontological Nursing Chair established at Case Western Reserve University, first in the nation; Doreen Norton, first scholar to occupy chair
  National Conference of Gerontological Nurse Practitioners established

1984 National Gerontological Nurses Association established

Division of Gerontological Nursing Practice becomes Council on Gerontological Nursing (councils established for all practice specialties)

1986 ANA publishes survey of gerontological nurses in clinical practice

1987 ANA revises and issues Scope and Standards of Gerontological Nursing Practice

1989 ANA certifies gerontological clinical nurse specialists

1990 ANA establishes a Division of Long-Term Care within the Council of Gerontological Nursing

1992 ANA redefines long-term care to include life-span approach
  John A. Hartford Foundation funds a major initiative to improve care of hospitalized older patients: Nurses Improving Care to Hospitalized Elderly (NICHE)

1993 National Institute of Nursing Research established as separate entity

1994 ANA redefines Scope and Standards of Gerontological Nursing Practice

1996 John A. Hartford Foundation establishes the Institute for Geriatric Nursing at New York University under the direction of Mathy Mezey

2000 Recommended baccalaureate competencies and curricular guidelines for geriatric nursing care published by the American Association of Colleges of Nursing and the John A. Hartford Foundation Institute for Geriatric Nursing

2001 ANA, in collaboration with the National Gerontological Nursing Association, National Association of Directors of Nursing Administration in Long Term Care, and the National Conference of Gerontological Nurse Practitioners, publishes revised Scope and Standards of Gerontological Nursing Practice and reaffirms the need for competent gerontological nursing

2003 Nurse Competence in Aging (funded by the Atlantic Philanthropies Inc.) initiative to improve the quality of health care to older adults by enhancing the geriatric competence of nurses who are members of specialty nursing associations (ANA, ANCC, John A. Hartford Foundation Institute for Geriatric Nursing)

2004 Nurse Practitioner and Clinical Nurse Specialist Competencies for Older Adult Care published by the American Association of Colleges of Nursing and the Hartford Geriatric Nursing Initiative
  ANA Scope and Standards of Practice for all registered nurses referenced to include care of older adults

Gerontological nursing research has gained wide acceptance in the scientific community and has made significant contributions to improved patient care and to policy decisions that influence care outcomes, particularly in the long-term care setting. Gerontological nurses have taken their place as vital members of the interdisciplinary community of gerontological professionals. Advanced-practice gerontological nurses have demonstrated positive outcomes as well as cost-effectiveness across a variety of settings. Research has shown that better care for older adults is possible and should be expected. The task before us now is to communicate the knowledge to all nurses who care for older adults in all settings (Mezey, Fulmer, 2002). There remains an urgent need for increased funding for gerontological nursing research, particularly in the areas of new health care delivery models for older adults; clinical care concerns; and home, nursing home, assisted living, and community based health care (Wykle, McDonald, 1997).

ANA and the Scope and Standards of Gerontological Nursing Practice

To develop accurate and informed attitudes, gerontological nursing organizations have established standards, legitimized the specialty, upgraded the knowledge base, enhanced the image of gerontological nurses, and identified the benefits of working with older adults. Nursing is the first of the professions to develop standards of gerontological care and the first to provide a certification mechanism to ensure specific professional expertise through credentialing. In 1973 the ANA first defined standards of geriatric care, and geriatric nursing was the first specialty to establish standards of practice within the ANA. In 1976 and 1987 these were redefined as standards and scope of gerontological nursing practice.

In 1995 and again in 2001 the ANA updated the scope and standards of gerontological nursing practice. The 2001 edition was published jointly with the National Gerontological Nursing Association, the National Conference of Gerontological Nurse Practitioners, and the National Association of Directors of Nursing Administration in Long Term Care. The 2001 document emphasizes the need for competence in care of older adults so that

professional nurses will be prepared to "meet the special needs of the increasing numbers of older adults, particularly those over 85 years of age, minorities, and those with decreased financial and social resources" (ANA, 2001, p. 7). The scope of practice for gerontological nursing, levels of gerontological nursing practice (basic and advanced), standards of clinical gerontological nursing care, and gerontological nursing performance are discussed in the document. Knowledge and skills necessary for the practice of basic gerontological nursing are listed in Box 2-2. The 2004 ANA Scope and Standards of Practice for all registered nurses now also includes specific reference to care of older adults.

Certification is a means of ensuring the public that the certified individual has pursued some specialized study in a given area, has successfully demonstrated requisite knowledge, and has been awarded recognition of this achievement. ANA certification in gerontological nursing is one evidence of professional competency and a sign to health care administrators and the public of a commitment by nurses to the care of older adults (Gaines, 1994). The certification program for gerontological nurses began in 1975 and was the first certification program offered by ANA (Moses, 1979). The original protocol has since been expanded to include nurse practitioners, clinical specialists, gerontological consultants, researchers, administrators, and educators. In October 1989 the first ANA examination for certification of gerontological clinical nurse specialists was given. This was a major step toward recognition of this specialized practice arena. Approximately 13,000 gerontological nurse generalists, 3422 gerontological nurse practitioners, and 736 gerontological clinical nurse specialists are certified. For additional information on certification and specialty practice, see Resources at the end of this chapter.

Graduate nursing programs in gerontology prepare nurses to be credentialed as the following:
1. Gerontological nurse practitioners
2. Gerontological clinical nurse specialists
3. Gerontological case managers for acute and long-term care
4. Nurse administrators in acute and long-term care
5. Gerontological faculty and staff development roles
6. Geropsychiatric nursing specialists

Box 2-2	Knowledge and Skills for Basic Gerontological Nursing

- Recognize the right of competent older adults to make their own care decisions and assist them in making informed choices.
- Establish a therapeutic relationship with the older adult to facilitate development of the plan of care, which may include family participation as needed.
- Use current gerontological standards to initiate, develop, and adapt the older adult's plan of care while involving the patient, family, and other providers as needed.
- Recognize age-related changes based on an understanding of physiological, emotional, cultural, social, psychological, economic, and spiritual functioning.
- Collect data to determine health status and functional abilities to plan, implement, and evaluate care.
- Participate and collaborate with members of the interdisciplinary team.
- Participate with older adults, their families if needed, and other health professionals in ethical decision making that is centered on the older adult, empathetic, and humane.
- Serve as an advocate for older adults and their families.
- Teach older adults and families about measures that promote, maintain, and restore health and functional performance; promote comfort; foster independence; and preserve dignity.
- Refer older adults to other professionals or community resources for assistance as necessary.
- Identify common chronic/acute physical and mental health processes and problems that affect older adults.
- Apply the existing body of knowledge in gerontology to nursing practice and intervention.
- Exercise accountability to older adults by protecting their rights and autonomy, recognizing and respecting their decisions about advance directives.
- Facilitate palliative care and comfort during the dying process to preserve dignity.
- Support the surviving spouse and family members, providing strength, comfort, and hope.
- Use the standards of gerontological nursing practice and collaborate with other health care professionals to improve the quality of care and quality of life of older adults.
- Engage in professional development through participation in continuing education, involvement in state and national professional organizations, and certification.

From American Nurses Association: *Scope and standards of gerontological nursing practice*, Washington, DC, 2001, ANA, pp 8-9.

GERONTOLOGICAL NURSING ORGANIZATIONS

Canadian Gerontologic Nurses Association

Our neighbors, the Canadian Gerontologic Nurses Association (CGNA), have grown enormously in strength and purpose in recent years. In addition, more than one half of the members of CGNA are certified by the Canadian Nurses Association. Although the percentage of elders in most provinces in Canada is somewhat less than ours, the social services and functional aids available (at no cost to those over 65 years of age) are a model toward which we may strive.

The domains of nursing practice and the seven practice standards of CGNA describe the appropriate therapeutic interventions or activities of the registered nurse that facilitate client health behavior directed toward promotion, prevention, maintenance, rehabilitation, or palliation. According to the CGNA, the goal of gerontological nursing is to optimize client function throughout his or her life span by reinforcing, supporting, and nurturing his or her ability to do the following:

1. Achieve optimal functional health status
2. Maintain homeostatic regulation
3. Facilitate psychological functioning, maintenance of lifestyle, and optimal quality of life
4. Preserve or develop meaningful relationships, including family and social support networks

5. Facilitate suitable access to and benefit of the health care and other systems
6. Identify safety risks and possible alternatives and advocate for the right of the client to live at personal risk without endangering others

National Gerontological Nursing Association

The National Gerontological Nursing Association (NGNA) promotes gerontological nursing in order to influence the clinical care of older adults. NGNA, organized in 1984, is the first and only national association created specifically for all levels of nursing personnel specializing in the delivery of health care to the elderly. This non-profit association comprises registered nurses (RNs), licensed practical nurses/licensed vocational nurses (LPNs/LVNs), and certified nurse assistants (CNAs). However, the great majority of the nearly 2000 members are RNs. The goals of NGNA are listed in Box 2-3.

National Conference of Gerontological Nurse Practitioners

The National Conference of Gerontological Nurse Practitioners (NCGNP), founded in 1981 by a small group of GNPs, is an organization devoted solely to the promotion of high standards of health care for older persons through advanced gerontological nursing practice, education, and research. NCGNP represents nearly 3500 gerontological nurse practitioners and many family and adult nurse practitioners in gerontological practice. Goals of the organization are to advocate for quality care for all older adults; promote the professional development of advanced-practice nursing; provide continuing gerontological education for advanced-practice nurses; promote communication and professional collaboration among health care providers; and support research related to care of older adults.

National Association of Directors of Nursing Administration in Long-Term Care

The National Association of Directors of Nursing Administration in Long-Term Care (NADONA/

Box 2-3	Goals of NGNA

- Provide a forum in which gerontological nursing issues are identified and explored
- Promote the specialty of gerontological nursing
- Conduct educational programs
- Promote research in gerontological nursing
- Support the professional development of nurses whose practice includes older adults
- Engage in programs designed to demonstrate innovative techniques and approaches in gerontological health care to better meet the needs of America's aging population
- Advocate for legislation that enhances the care of older adults and the role of gerontological nursing in the care of older adults
- Provide grants to conduct activities that further the goals and purposes of NGNA
- Disseminate information related to gerontological nursing

NGNA, National Gerontological Nursing Association.

LTC), begun in 1986, is a nonprofit association serving directors and assistant directors of nursing in long-term care (DONs/ADONs). NADONA/LTC offers services, including legislative and professional networking and continuing education and training courses. NADONA/LTC has established standards of practice for DONs in long-term care and provides a certification system for DONs. The association has approximately 5000 members with 40 chapters in the United States and Canada. Their mission is to build a strong network of DONs and assistant DONs through education, communication, and service to the members.

Gerontological Society of America and American Society on Aging

The Gerontological Society of America (GSA) and the American Society on Aging (ASA) are interdisciplinary organizations devoted to the development and promotion of progress in research and service to the aged. Both these organizations have large contingents of nurse members. Nurses form the largest group of professionals belonging to GSA, and in 2004, Dr. Terry Fulmer was the first nurse to hold the position of president of the organization.

American Medical Directors Association and the American Geriatrics Society

The American Medical Directors Association is a professional association of medical directors, physicians, and nurse practitioners practicing in the long-term care continuum, dedicated to excellence in patient care by providing education, advocacy, information, and professional development. The American Geriatrics Society is a professional organization of health care providers dedicated to improving the health and well-being of older adults. Both these organizations have monthly journals and practice protocols for care of older adults. These excellent evidence-based practice protocols are available on their websites.

Long-term care nurses are particularly active in two other national organizations, the American Association of Homes and Services for the Aging (AAHSA) and the American Health Care Association (AHCA) (see Organizations at the end of this chapter for addresses). These organizations are highly visible in promoting legislation to strengthen the stature and practice opportunities in long-term care in numerous venues.

Certified Nursing Assistants and Nurse Aides

Although it is important to promote professional nursing care for all elders, most of the care and quality of life for institutionalized elders directly depend on certified nursing assistants (CNAs) or nurse aides. Gerontological nursing, to be satisfying for the professional and adequate for the patient, must begin at the bottom of the status ladder and work upward. When the aides are satisfied and feel truly appreciated, it is reflected in the professionalism of the entire service milieu, but who is their advocate? Who is concerned about the quality of their lives? Who listens to the aide's story? Who provides a time and place for mourning the loss of loved residents? Who provides health care for those aides as they give health care services to elders? Until we health care

professionals and our society make a real commitment to providing adequate wages and individual supports, both psychological and material, these neglected workers cannot be expected to have the energy or incentive to extend to elders in their care. Regardless of our credentials, our success as professionals in gerontological nursing will depend largely on how effectively we interact with, appreciate, and educate these frontline workers.

An important organization for nursing assistants in nursing homes is the National Association of Geriatric Nursing Assistants (NAGNA). NAGNA was established in 1995 as a professional association of CNAs for CNAs. The purpose of NAGNA is to ensure that the highest quality of care is provided to our elders living in nursing homes, achieved by elevating the professional standing and performance of the caregivers. Membership is open to nursing assistants and all long-term care staff. With a membership of more than 30,000 CNAs representing more than 500 nursing homes, the organization provides recognition for outstanding achievements, development training for CNAs, mentoring programs to reduce CNA turnover, and advocacy for issues important to long-term care and CNAs.

Another organization, the National Clearinghouse on the Direct Care Workforce, supports efforts to improve the quality of jobs for frontline workers who assist people who are elderly and/or living with disabilities. This organization provides information resources needed to effect change in industry practice, public policy, and public opinion. The Clearinghouse is also working with the Paraprofessional Healthcare Institute to improve understanding for the direct care workforce crisis through research and analysis funded by the U.S. Department of Health and Human Services and the Center for Medicare and Medicaid Services.

STAFF DEVELOPMENT

Staff development is an increasingly important part of the responsibility of every professional nurse. Equipment requirements, regulations, acuity level of clients, and expectations from the public change daily. Each health care organization should form a "vision statement" (philosophy and mission) that becomes the framework to guide leadership and management in their particular setting. With the increasing cultural diversity of both patients and staff in health care organizations, vision and mission statements need to address cultural competency. An example of a mission statement addressing cultural diversity in a nursing home is presented in Box 2-4. Within the parameters of the vision statement, specific objectives and programs should be written, prioritized, and periodically evaluated. Orientation, continued educational development, improvement of performance and clinical care, and support of staff are essential functions in any health care organization. These functions are often implemented by directors of staff development and clinical nurse specialists.

Two excellent resources for the education and development of nursing assistants are the textbook *Being a Long-Term Care Nursing Assistant* (Will-Black, Eighmy, 2002), and *CNA Career Ladder Made Easy: Everything You Need to Run a Successful Career Ladder Program* (Pillemer et al, 2001). Another highly recommended resource is the videotape *Heart Work*, produced by the Paraprofessional Healthcare Institute in collaboration with HomeCare Associates. *Heart Work* is created and performed by women who work as home health and nursing home aides. Through music, dance, storytelling, and interviews, the video provides a real, moving, and often honest account of what it means to be a paraprofessional caregiver. The *NGNA Core Curriculum for Gerontological Nursing* (Luggen, Meiner, 2000) and *NGNA Core Curriculum for Gerontological Advanced Practice Nurses* (Luggen et al, 1998) are also excellent resources for education and development of practitioners and educators.

Staff Support Groups

In stressful and busy health care work environments, group support activities are another way to enhance performance and satisfaction of staff. An example of a group support activity might be a gathering to share feelings about the death of a resident in a nursing home. In a recently completed research study on spiritual care of dying nursing home residents, nursing assistant participants discussed their feeling of intense grief on the death of a resident (Touhy, 2004). One of the aides

---

Box 2-4	**Sample Nursing Home Mission Statement Addressing Cultural Diversity**

We, the family and staff, strive to create an environment that respects every individual's uniqueness. We pride ourselves on providing caring service that will ensure client satisfaction and improve health care outcomes. Cultural competence and trust are the basis for any healing relationship and we pledge that we will care for each resident as we would for any of our loved ones, regardless of race, color, or religious background. Prejudices are not tolerated nor condoned at our facility. We may not all look alike or sound alike, but we are all here for one primary purpose and that is to make sure that the needs of the residents come first and foremost. We would like family members and the community to know that we work in a culturally diverse setting mindful of everyone's cultural values, beliefs, and behaviors. We ask that you join us in creating a harmonious place for our residents that is sensitive to cultural differences. Again, we believe that cultural competence requires awareness and most of all, RESPECT, in order for us to meet a common ground.

Developed by N Nestor, RN, MS, 2004.

---

said: "You get so close. I came in one day and they told me she had passed away. I was sad all day long, you wouldn't believe it. I was sad for a couple of days. I tried to make it go away, but you get so close to them it's like family." In the study, the only support provided for grieving was "informal" among workers. The majority of nursing homes do not provide any form of bereavement counseling or referrals for bereavement support after the death of a resident (Murphy et al, 1997). The following discussion offers some practical suggestions for the development and implementation of group support activities.

We advise organizing staff groups to meet needs at any level of Maslow's hierarchy. Even though most groups meet multiple needs, a primary focus should be established. Using the assessment of human needs as a basic guide, one can begin to determine the type of group most suitable in a given situation. What is the primary need in the particular work environment at that particular time? First, on the most basic level, the survival needs of staff, such as health and child care, must be adequately met. Problem solving around these issues may be the major goal, in which each member shares methods he or she uses to meet survival needs. Some facilities, because of purchasing in large quantities, pass savings on to personnel, allowing them to purchase food and other items at cost. Many facilities now offer some assistance with child care, and with the increasing cultural diversity of health care staff, English classes (ESL [English as a second language]) are also offered on site for employees.

At the second level, job security is fundamental. Informal or legal contracts should be supplied for every worker, regardless of status in the hierarchy of the organization. The contract should go beyond the standard job description to include the goals and expectations of the employee as well as the organization. The activity of negotiating these contracts not only provides a sense of security but also simultaneously raises the employees' self-esteem and sense of autonomy. Groups can be formed to discuss ways the organization can better meet the needs of staff for job security.

On the third level of the hierarchy, the sense of belonging can be cultivated in any group in which the leader focuses on commonalities rather than differences. What are the common concerns of the group? What are the satisfactions experienced in the work environment? In a recent project conducted by one of the authors of this book (TT), nursing home staff members were asked to describe a situation that best represented caring in their work. After qualitative analysis of the data, five major themes emerged (Box 2-5). The deep dedication and caring of staff in nursing homes are reflected beautifully in these themes. When we shared these themes with the staff, families, and residents, it not only validated their work but also became a source of pride. We too often focus on the negative aspects of care and rarely praise and encourage the positive.

Self-esteem, the fourth level of Maslow's hierarchy, is built when specific contributions of an employee are recognized by the group and when each feels his or her participation is recognized and deemed as important. The pinnacle of Maslow's hierarchy of needs is in reaching for self-

---

Box 2-5   How We Care: Voices of Nursing Home Staff

Responding to What Matters
Taking time to do the little things, competence, cleanliness, meeting basic needs, safe administration of medications, kindness and consideration

Caring as a Way of Expressing Spiritual Commitment
Spiritual beliefs led staff to long-term care and continue to motivate and guide the special care they give to residents; they reflect a spiritual commitment to caring for residents as expressed in the golden rule: "Do unto others as you would like done to you"

Devotion Inspired by Love for Others
Deep connection between staff and residents described as like family, caring for residents as you would for your own mother or father, sharing of good and bad times, going out on a limb to be an advocate, listening and staying with residents when others had given up

Commitment to Creating a Home Environment
Nursing home is the resident's home, staff are guests in the home; the importance of cleanliness, privacy, good food, and feeling part of a family

Coming to Know and Respect Person as Person
Treating residents, families, and one another with respect and dignity, being recognized for the person you are, intimate knowing of likes and dislikes, and individualized care

---

actualization and transcendence. This is a lifelong pursuit and one each individual identifies in his or her own creative manner. It is often enlightening to ask members to share experiences of deep personal significance that have occurred in the care of a resident. The example in the above section illustrates this.

This brief discussion of possible groups and effects shows the versatility of group work with employees and the potential it holds for strengthening bonds in the work environment.

Mentoring for Professional Growth and Development

In gerontological nursing, mentoring has played a predominant role. The field is comparatively new, and many nursing programs do not have strong courses in gerontologocial nursing or faculty educated in the specialty. Many individuals entered the field of aging without any particular professional preparation but have been individually guided toward professional competence by the efforts and inspiration of a dedicated mentor. The numerous needs of older adults and the special nature of their care require the most devoted and sophisticated nurses.

ROLES IN GERONTOLOGICAL NURSING

A gerontological nurse may be a generalist or a specialist. The generalist functions in a variety of settings—hospital, home, nursing home, community—providing nursing care to individuals and their families. The generalist works in various models of care provision and draws on the expertise of the specialist in planning and evaluating care.

The gerontological nursing specialist has advanced preparation at the master's level and performs all of the functions of the generalist but has developed clinical expertise, as well as an understanding of health and social policy and proficiency in planning, implementing, and evaluating health programs. To understand the variations of these categories and the progression of specialization see Figure 2-1. Table 2-1 shows the organization of nursing relating to care of the elderly.

One of the most important roles emerging in the past few decades is that of the gerontological nurse practitioner. Originally the development of the gerontological or geriatric nurse practitioner (GNP) emerged to meet the need for consistent, accessible, quality primary care for persons in underserved areas, such as nursing homes or remote rural areas. Today, with increasingly strong federal legislation to support advanced nursing practice, genontological nurse practitioners and gerontological nursing clinical specialists are involved in nursing homes, acute care and suba-

cute care facilities, assisted living and retirement complexes, health maintenance organizations (HMOs), day care settings, community clinics, physicians' offices, independent practices, and any situation requiring expert nursing in combination with midlevel medical practitioner skills. GNPs are prepared at the master's level, and there is presently a full range of opportunities and roles to be filled.

GERONTOLOGICAL NURSING EDUCATION

As we enter the twenty-first century, projections are that by 2030, 20% of the American population will be over the age of 65, with those over 85 showing the greatest increase in numbers. Older people are healthier, better educated, and more affluent, and they expect a much higher quality of life as they age than did their elders. Most nurses will care for older people during the course of their careers, and yet schools of nursing have only recently begun to include gerontological nursing content in their curricula, and most still do not have freestanding courses in the specialty similar to courses in maternal/child or psychiatric nursing. Content issues that are sorely neglected and need to be included are health promotion, mental health, elder abuse, atypical presentation of illness, acute care of older adults, long-term and palliative care, and minority and rural aging.

We believe those in the field of nursing education must seriously consider specific minimum requirements in care of older adults at each level of education to fulfill the responsibility of nurses to the public and the profession. One is not limited in gerontological nursing education to the acute care setting or the nursing home for clinical practice sites. Creative faculty members consider sites such as retirement homes, assisted living facilities, private practice with families, nutrition centers, home care agencies, adult day health programs, and housing complexes. Learning in these sites to understand the living situations and truly communicate with elders is the first step to providing appropriate care. Acute care hospitals and nursing homes are integral to the total picture but might be included later in the students' learning experience after they have worked with elders who

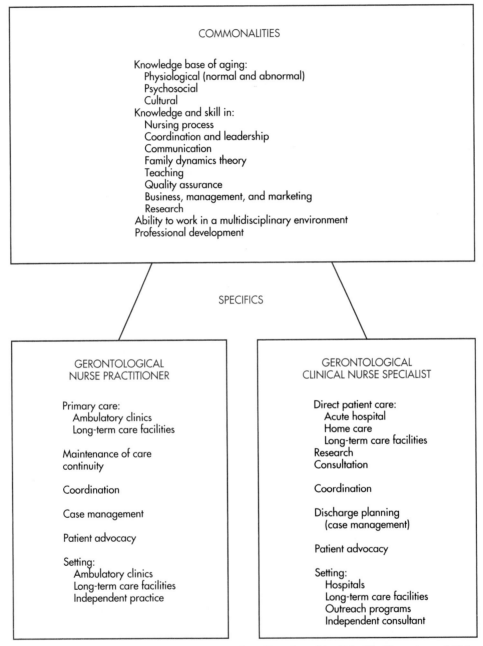

Figure 2-1   Established roles: commonalities and specifics. (Developed by Priscilla Ebersole and Helen Monea.)

Table 2-1 Organization of Nursing Relating to Care of the Elderly

Title	No. Years Education	Degree	Responsibilities Related to Care of Elderly
Professors of gerontological nursing	8 plus	PhD, EdD, or DNS	Research Teaching
Gerontological nurse practitioners	6	MS	Both medical and nursing functions in ambulatory and institutional settings Case managers
Gerontological nurse specialists	6	MS	Specialized nursing care of elderly clients Teachers and role models Case managers
Registered nurse—baccalaureate level	4-5	BS	Community health, hospital, home health agencies, nursing homes Case managers
Registered nurse—associate level	2-3	ADN	Hospital, home and nursing home staff nurses
Licensed practical nurses	1-1½		Nursing home staff Home nursing staff
Nursing aides and orderlies	0-6 mo		Nursing home staff Hospital staff

Sources: Mezey MD, Fulmer TT: Nursing. In Maddox GL, editor: *The encyclopedia of aging,* ed 2, New York, 1995, Springer; U.S. Bureau of the Census: *Statistical abstract of the United States,* ed 118, Washington, DC, 1998, U.S. Government Printing Office; American Nurses Association: *Facts about nursing,* Kansas City, Mo, 1992-1993, ANA, pp. 1-4.

have less acute or complex conditions. Nursing homes provide special opportunities for leadership training, nursing management of complex problems, and research application for more advanced students.

Ensuring gerontological nursing competency in all students graduating from a nursing program is imperative for improvement of health care to older adults. The Hartford Institute for Geriatric Nursing and the American Association of Colleges of Nursing (AACN) developed gerontological nursing competencies and curriculum materials for baccalaureate programs (http://www.aacn.nche.edu/Education/gercomp.htm). Continued support for gerontological nursing education from the Hartford Foundation is provided through grants and awards for innovative curricula and models, faculty development, research, and lead-ership activities. Nationally recognized competencies in gerontological nursing have also been developed for graduate programs preparing advanced-practice nurses in specialties other than gerontological nursing who will work with older adults, (http://www.aacn.nche.edu/Education/Hartford/OlderAdultCare.htm).

Recognizing the critical need for a nursing workforce prepared to deliver quality health care to the nation's aging population, and in light of the fact that few of the nation's 2.2 million practicing registered nurses have received any preparation in gerontological nursing, either in their educational programs or on the job, the ANA will be awarding grants in the Nurse Competence in Aging initiative. This 5-year program, funded by the Atlantic Philanthropies and representing a strategic alliance among

ANA, ANCC, and the John A. Hartford Institute for Geriatric Nursing, is designed to improve the quality of health care to older adults by enhancing the gerontological competence—the attitudes, knowledge, and skills—of nurses who are members of specialty organizations. The Nurse Competence in Aging initiative will provide grant and technical assistance to national specialty nursing associations, conduct a national gerontological nursing certification outreach, and develop a web-based comprehensive gerontological nursing resource center (www.hartfordign.org/nca).

GERONTOLOGICAL NURSES CARING FOR ONE ANOTHER

Nurses derive their interpersonal satisfactions from co-workers, clients, and professional organizations. Ongoing knowledge should be readily available and is integral to an encouraging work milieu. Throughout this chapter our intent is to convey the importance of nurses working together and caring for one another as we care for the aged. We have the special privilege to share the wisdom of older people as we journey with them through some of the most moving and profound life events. This cannot be taken lightly or held quietly and comfortably inside. In these situations, the close ties with co-workers and elders become especially significant. Opportunities to recognize and share the significance of these connections should be conscientiously developed. Only as nurses value and care for one another and feel valued can we reach out wholeheartedly and fully appreciate the elders in our care.

▶ KEY CONCEPTS

- Certification assures the public of nurses' commitment to specialized education and qualification for the care of the aged.
- All students graduating from nursing programs and all practicing nurses working with older adults should have competencies in gerontological nursing.
- The major changes in health care delivery and the increasing numbers of older adults have resulted in numerous revised, refined, and

emergent roles for nurses in the field of gerontological nursing. There is a critical shortage of competent and compassionate gerontological nurses.
- Advanced-practice nurses may have either nurse practitioner qualifications or clinical nurse specialist education or a combination of both.
- Advanced-practice role opportunities for nurses are numerous and offer more independence, are cost effective, and facilitate more holistic health care and improved outcomes for patients.
- Gerontological nursing at its best requires specialized education, maturity, commitment, and sensitivity.

▶ Activities and Discussion Questions

1. Identify factors that have influenced the progress of gerontological nursing as a specialty practice.
2. Consider and discuss with classmates the various gerontological nursing roles that you find most interesting and stimulating.
3. Discuss what you consider the most important elements of the 2001 American Nurses Association Scope and Standards of Practice for Gerontological Nursing.
4. Discuss the formal gerontological organizations and their significance to the practicing nurse.
5. Why do you think more students do not choose gerontological nursing as a specialty? What would increase interest in this area of nursing?
6. What do you think are the most important issues in gerontological nursing education at this time?

RESOURCES

Books and Publications

Heart Work. Available from the National Clearinghouse on the Direct Care Workforce, 349 E. 149th Street, Suite 401, Bronx, NY 10451 (866-402-4138) (www.directcareclearinghouse.org).

Scope and standards of gerontological nursing practice, ed 2, 2001, Washington, DC.: American Nurses Publishing.

Organizations

American Association of Colleges of Nursing
One Dupont Circle NW, Suite 530
Washington, DC 20036
(202) 463-6930; (202) 785-8300
website: http://www.aacn.nche.edu/

American Association of Homes and Services for the
 Aging
901 E Street NW, Suite 500
Washington, DC 20004-2037
(301) 490-0677
website: http://www2.aahsa.org/

American Geriatrics Society
The Empire State Building
350 Fifth Avenue, Suite 801
New York, NY 10118
(212) 308-1414
website: http://www.americangeriatrics.org

American Health Care Association
1201 L Street NW
Washington, DC 20005
(202) 842-8444
website: http://www.ahca.org/

American Medical Directors Association
10480 Little Patuxent Parkway, Suite 760
Columbia, MD 21044
(800) 876-2632
website: http://:www.amda.com

American Nurses Association (ANA)
Accreditation Board
600 Maryland Avenue SW, Suite 100 W
Washington, DC 20024-2571
(202) 554-4444
website: http://www.nursingworld.org/

American Nurses' Credentialing Center
600 Maryland Avenue SW, Suite 100 W
Washington, DC 20024-2571
(800) 284-CERT
website: http://www.nursingworld.org/ancc/

American Society on Aging
833 Market Street, Suite 511
San Francisco, CA 94103-1824
(415) 974-9600
website: http://www.asaging.org/

Canadian Gerontological Nursing Association
PO Box 368, Postal Station K
Toronto, Ontario M4P 2GT
website: http://www.cgna.net

Gerontological Society of America
1275 K Street NW, Suite 350

Washington, DC 20005-4006
(202) 842-1275
website: http://www.geron.org/

Hartford Institute for Geriatric Nursing
New York University, Steinhardt School of Education
Division of Nursing, John A. Hartford Foundation
 Institute for Geriatric Nursing
246 Greene Street
New York, NY 10003
(212) 998-9018; (212) 995-4561 (fax)
website: http://www.hartfordign.org

National Association of Directors of Nursing
 Administration in Long-Term Care
10101 Alliance Road, #40
Cincinnati, OH 45242
(513) 791-3679
website: http://www.nadona.org

National Association of Geriatric Nursing Assistants
2709 West 13th Street
Joplin, MO 64801
(800) 784-6049
website: http://www.nagna.org

National Clearinghouse on the Direct Care
 Workforce
349 East 149th Street, Suite 401
Bronx, NY 10451
(866) 402-4138
website: http://www.directcareclearinghouse.org

National Conference of Gerontological Nurse
 Practitioners
PO Box 232230
Centreville, VA 20120-2230
(703) 802-0088; (703) 802-1436 (fax)
website: http://www.ncgnp.org

National Gerontological Nursing Association
 (NGNA)
7794 Grow Drive
Pensacola, FL 32514-7072
(800) 723-0560; (850) 484-8762 (fax)
website: http://www.ngna.org

National League for Nursing (NLN) Accreditation
 Board
10 Columbus Circle
New York, NY 10019
website: http://www.nln.org/

REFERENCES

American Nurses Association: *Scope and standards of gerontological nursing practice,* Washington, DC, 2001, ANA.

Burnside IM: *Nursing and the aged*, New York, 1988, McGraw-Hill.

Davis B: Nursing care of the aged: historical evolution, *Am Assoc Hist Nurs* 47, 1985.

Dock L: The crusade for almshouse nursing, *Am J Nurs* 8, 1908.

Fitzpatrick JJ, Fulmer T, editors: *Geriatric nursing research digest*, New York, 2000, Springer.

Gaines JE: Here comes everybody in APN, *Adv Pract Nurse*, Spring/Summer, p. 42, 1994.

Geldbach S: Nursing care of the aged, *Am J Nurs* 43(12), 1943.

Gunter L, Estes C: *Education for gerontic nursing*, New York, 1979, Springer.

Klein S: *A national agenda for geriatric education: white papers*, Washington, DC, 1997, U.S. Department of Health and Human Services, Public Health Service, Health Resources and Services Administration, Bureau of Health Professions.

Luggen AS, Meiner SE: *NGNA core curriculum for gerontological nursing*, St Louis, 2000, Mosby.

Luggen AS, Travis S, Meiner SE: *NGNA core curriculum for gerontological advanced practice nurses*, Thousand Oaks, Calif, 1998, Sage.

Mezey MD, Fulmer TT: The future history of gerontological nursing, *J Gerontol* 57A(7), 2002.

Moses D: The nurse's role as advocate with the elderly. In Reinhardt A, Quinn M, editors: *Current practice in gerontological nursing*, St Louis, 1979, Mosby.

Murphy K, Hanrahan P, Luchins D: A survey of grief and bereavement in nursing homes: the importance of hospice grief and bereavement for the end-stage Alzheimer's disease patient and family, *J Am Geriatr Soc* 45(9):1104-1107, 1997.

Nestor N: Personal communication, 2004.

Newton K, Anderson H: *Geriatric nursing*, St Louis, 1950, Mosby.

Pillemer K, Meador R, Hoffman R, Schumacher M: *CNA career ladder made easy: everything you need to know to run a successful career ladder program*, Stamford, Ct, 2001, International Thomson Publishing.

Touhy T: Spiritual caring at the end-of-life in nursing homes. Unpublished manuscript, 2004.

Will-Black C, Eighmy J: *Being a long-term care nursing assistant*, ed 4, Washington, DC, 2002, Prentice Hall Health.

Wykle M, McDonald P: The past, present, and future of gerontological nursing. In Dimond M et al, editors: *A national agenda for geriatric education*, New York, 1997, Springer.

Communicating with Elders

3

LEARNING OBJECTIVES

Upon completion of this chapter, the reader will be able to:

- Discuss language disorders associated with neurological disruptions.
- Describe communication strategies for elders with language disruptions.
- Discuss the effect of Alzheimer's disease and related dementias on communication.
- Identify effective communication strategies that nurture personhood in elders with Alzheimer's disease and related dementias.
- Describe nursing assessment and interventions to help elders experiencing language and cognitive changes.
- Relate interventions that facilitate communication individually and in groups.
- Specify several teaching/learning strategies to facilitate elders' understanding and goal accomplishment.

GLOSSARY

Apraxia An impairment in the ability to manipulate objects or perform purposeful acts, including speech.

Cerebral vascular accident (CVA) (stroke) More recently, the term *brain attack* has been used to describe a CVA and to stress the importance of immediate emergency treatment. Stroke is defined as an interruption in the blood supply to the brain.

Idiom Language peculiar to a particular person, group, or class of people.

Infarction A localized area of tissue death resulting from an interruption of the blood supply.

Prosody The meter and rhythm of speech.

THE LIVED EXPERIENCE

Listen to the aged for they will tell you about living and dying.

Listen to the aged for they will enlighten you about problem-solving, sexuality, grief, sensory deprivation, and survival.

Listen to the aged for they will teach you how to be courageous, loving, and generous.

They are a distinguished faculty without formal classrooms, tenure, sabbaticals. They teach not from books but from long experience in living.

From Burnside IM: Listen to the aged, Am J Nurs 75(10):1801, 1975.

COMMUNICATION WITH ELDERS

Communication is the single most important capacity of human beings, the ability that gives us a special place in the animal kingdom. Little is more dehumanizing than the inability to reach out to others verbally. The need to communicate, to be listened to, and to be heard does not change with age or impairment. Communication with older adults provides the nurse with the opportunity to share in their wisdom and gain insight on life, both the elder's and the nurse's. Stephanie Nagley (1988) says, "Nursing care of the aged brings one in touch with the most basic and profound questions of human existence: the meanings of life and death; sources of strength and survival skills; and beginnings, endings, and reasons for being. It is a commitment to discovery of the self, and of the self I am becoming as I age." The very old are acutely aware of their limited time and, given the opportunity, generally are willing to talk about it and the problems they experience as well as their satisfactions.

Communicating effectively is an important skill in nursing. Good communication skills are the basis for accurate assessment, care planning, and the development of therapeutic relationships between the nurse and patient (Miller, 2002). Basic communication strategies that apply to all situations in nursing, such as attending, listening, clarifying, giving information, seeking validation of understanding, keeping focus, and using open-ended questions, are all applicable in communicating with older adults. Some situational modifications must be considered as well as some special circumstances. A discussion of the common problems, disorders, and impediments to communication that older adults often experience as a result of neurological or cognitive impairments and the implications for gerontological nursing and healthy aging is the focus of this chapter. Basic principles of group work with older adults and learning in later life are also discussed. Sensory changes accompanying aging and implications for communication are addressed in Chapter 9. Communication with those experiencing mental health disorders is addressed in Chapter 25.

Basically, elders may need more time to give information or answer questions, simply because they have a larger life experience to draw from. Sorting through thoughts requires intervals of silence, and therefore listening carefully without rushing the elder is very important. Word retrieval may be slower, particularly for nouns and names. Thoughts unstated are often as important as those that are verbalized. You may ask, "What are you thinking about right now?" Clarification is essential to ensure that you and the elder have the same framework of understanding. Many generational, cultural, and regional differences in speech patterns and idioms exist. Frequently seek validation of whatever you think you heard.

Open-ended questions are useful but difficult for some elders. Those who wish to please, especially when feeling vulnerable or somewhat dependent, may wonder what it is you want to hear rather than what it is they would like to say. When using closed questioning to obtain specific information, be aware that the elder may feel on the spot and the appropriate information may not be immediately forthcoming. This is especially true when asking questions to determine mental status. The elder may develop a mental block because of anxiety or feel threatened if questions are asked in a quizzing or demeaning manner. Some elders may want to share past memories with you. Listen carefully so that you can really come to know the person and how he or she has coped throughout life. And, finally, communicate with the elder as with a potential friend; share a bit of your own perceptions, thoughts, and experience when it will facilitate mutual understanding and increase rapport.

Communication that is most productive will initially focus on the issue of major concern to the elder, regardless of the priority of the nursing assessment. Nursing interventions should include verbal anticipatory rehearsal of any event expected to be stressful. The identification of a reliable and ongoing support system that will be available to the individual before and after any especially demanding event is essential.

The following sections of this chapter address neurological and cognitive disorders that impair the ability to communicate.

LANGUAGE ASSOCIATED WITH NEUROLOGICAL DISRUPTIONS

Three major categories of impaired verbal communication arise from neurological disturbances:

(1) reception, (2) perception, and (3) articulation. Reception is impaired by anxiety or related to a specific disorder, hearing deficits, and altered levels of consciousness. Perception is distorted by stroke, dementia, and delirium. Articulation is hampered by mechanical difficulties, such as dysarthria, respiratory disease, destruction of the larynx, and cerebral infarction with neuromuscular effects. Specific difficulties include the following:

1. *Anomia.* Word retrieval difficulties during spontaneous speech and naming tasks.
2. *Aphasia.* A communication disorder that can affect a person's ability to use and understand spoken or written words. It results from damage to the side of the brain dominant for language. For most people, this is the left side. Aphasia usually occurs suddenly and often results from a stroke or head injury, but it can also develop slowly because of a brain tumor, an infection, or dementia.
3. *Dysarthria.* Impairment in the ability to articulate words as the result of damage to the central or peripheral nervous system that affects the speech mechanism.

Aphasia

The most common language disorder after a cerebral vascular accident is aphasia. Aphasia, in varying degrees, affects a person's ability to communicate in one or more ways, including speaking, understanding, reading, writing, and gesturing. Depending on the type and severity of the aphasia, there may be little or no speech, speech that is fragmented or broken, or speech that is fluent but empty in content. When a cerebral vascular accident damages the dominant half of the brain (left side in right-handed people), some disruption will occur in the "word factory." Broca's area and Wernicke's area of the left cerebral cortex are integral to the expression and understanding of language. The National Aphasia Association categorizes the two major types of aphasia as fluent and nonfluent. Following is a description of several types of aphasia that the nurse may encounter with older adults:

- *Fluent aphasia* is the result of a lesion in the superior temporal gyrus, an area adjacent to the primary auditory cortex (Wernicke's area). This type is also known as sensory, posterior, or Wernicke's aphasia. Persons with fluent aphasia speak easily with many long runs of words, but the content does not make sense. There are word-finding problems and errors of word and sound substitution. Often the speech of persons with fluent aphasia sounds like "jabberwocky." Unrelated words may be strung together or syllables repeated. These persons also have difficulty understanding spoken language and may be unaware of their speech difficulties; it is as if they are in a foreign land.
- *Nonfluent aphasia* typically involves damage to the posteroinferior portions of the dominant frontal lobe (Broca's area). This type is also called motor, anterior, or Broca's aphasia. Persons with nonfluent aphasia usually understand others but speak very slowly and use minimal words. They often struggle to articulate a word and seem to have lost the ability to voluntarily control the movements of speech. Difficulties are experienced in communicating orally and in writing.
- *Verbal apraxia* or *apraxia of speech* is a motor speech disorder that affects the ability to plan and sequence voluntary muscle movements. The muscles of speech are not paralyzed; instead there is a disruption in the brain's transmission of signals to the muscles. When thinking about what to say, the person may be unable to speak at all or may struggle to say words. In contrast, the person may be able to say many words or sentences correctly when not thinking about the words. Apraxia frequently occurs with aphasia.
- *Anomic aphasia* is associated with lesions of the dominant temporoparietal regions of the brain, although no single locus has been identified. Persons with anomic aphasia understand and speak readily but may have severe word-finding difficulty. They may be unable to remember crucial content words. This is a frequent form of aphasia characterized by the inability to name objects. The individual struggles to come forth with the correct noun and often becomes frustrated at his or her inability to do so.
- *Global aphasia* is the result of large left hemisphere lesions and affects most of the language areas of the brain. Persons with global aphasia cannot understand words or speak intelligibly. They may use meaningless syllables repetitiously.

A speech language pathologist (SLP) should be consulted for each type of aphasia to develop appropriate rehabilitative plans as soon as the individual is physiologically stabilized. The speech pathologist can identify the areas of language that remain relatively unimpaired and can capitalize on the remaining strengths. Much can be done in aggressive speech-retraining programs to regain intelligible conversational ability. For those who do not regain meaningful speech, assistive and augmentative communication devices can be most helpful.

Implications for Gerontological Nursing and Healthy Aging

Nurses are responsible for accurately observing and recording the speech and word recognition patterns of the client and for consistently implementing the recommendations of the speech pathologist. Communication with the older adult experiencing aphasia can be frustrating for both the person and the nurse as both struggle to understand each other. It is important to remember that in most cases of aphasia the person retains normal intellectual ability. Therefore communication must always occur at an adult level but with special modifications. Hearing and vision losses can further contribute to communication difficulties for older adults with aphasia. Sensitivity and patience are essential to promote effective communication. It is most helpful if staff caring for the person remain consistent so that they can come to know and understand the needs of the person and communicate these to others. It is exhausting for the person to have to continually try to communicate needs and desires to an array of different people. Plans of care should have specific communication strategies that are helpful for the individual person so that all staff, as well as families and significant others, know the most effective way to enhance communication. See suggestions for communicating with aphasic patients in Box 3-1.

Alternative or augmentative systems are frequently used, and communication tools exist for every imaginable type of language disability. These can be low tech or high tech. An example of a low-tech system would be an alphabet or picture board that the individual uses to point to letters to spell out messages or point to pictures of common objects and situations. High-tech systems include electronic boards and computers. Studies have shown that computer-assisted therapy can help people with aphasia improve speech. An example is speech therapy software that displays a word or picture, speaks the word (using prerecorded human speech), records the user speaking, and plays back the user's speech. For individuals with hemiplegic or paraplegic conditions, electronic devices and computers can be voice activated or have specially designed switches that can be activated by just one finger or by slight contact with the ear, nose, or chin. Pharmacotherapy is a new, experimental approach to treating aphasia, and some studies indicate that drugs may help improve aphasia in acute stroke and assist in postacute and chronic aphasia.

Dysarthria

Dysarthria is a speech disorder caused by a weakness or incoordination of the speech muscles. It occurs as a result of central or peripheral neuromuscular disorders that interfere with the clarity of speech and pronunciation. Dysarthria is second only to aphasia as a communication disorder of older adults and may be the result of stroke, head injury, Parkinson's disease, multiple sclerosis, and other neurological conditions. Dysarthria is characterized by weakness, slow movement, and a lack of coordination of the muscles associated with speech. Speech may be slow, jerky, slurred, quiet, lacking in expression, and difficult to understand. It may involve several mechanisms of speech, such as respiration, phonation, resonance, articulation, and prosody (the meter, rhythm of speech). A weakness or lack of coordination in any one of the systems can result in dysarthria. If the respiratory system is weak, then speech may be too quiet and produced one word at a time. If the laryngeal system is weak, speech may be breathy, quiet, and slow. If the articulatory system is affected, speech may sound slurred and be slow and labored.

Treatment depends on the cause, type, and severity of the symptoms. An SLP works with the individual to improve communication abilities. Therapy for dysarthria focuses on maximizing the function of all systems. To attain or maintain the highest practicable level of speech articulation after an acute episode, such as stroke or surgery, a comprehensive treatment program must be developed by a speech pathologist, neurologist, and

Box 3-1	Communicating with Individuals Experiencing Aphasia

- Explain situations, treatments, and anything else that is pertinent to the person. Treat the person as an adult, and avoid patronizing and childish phrases. Talk as if the person understands.
- Be patient, and allow plenty of time to communicate in a quiet environment.
- Speak slowly, ask one question at a time, and wait for a response. Repeat and rephrase as needed.
- Create an environment in which the person is encouraged to make decisions, offer comments, and communicate thoughts and desires.
- Ask questions in a way that can be answered with a nod or the blink of an eye; if the person cannot verbally respond, instruct him or her in nonverbal responses.
- Be honest with the person. Let him or her know if you cannot quite understand what he or she is telling you but that you will keep trying.
- When you have not understood what the person said, it helps to repeat the part that you did not understand as a question so that the person only has to repeat the part that you did not understand. For example, if you hear "I would like a XX," rather than saying pardon and getting a repetition that may sound the same, try asking "You would like a ...?"
- Speak of things familiar and of interest to the person.
- Use visual cues, objects, pictures, gestures, and touch as well as words. Have paper and pencil available so you can write down key words or even sketch a picture.
- If the person has fluent aphasia, listen and watch for the bits of information that emerge from the words, facial expressions, and gestures. Ignore the nonwords.
- Encourage all speech. Allow the person to try to complete his or her thoughts, to struggle with words. Avoid being too quick to guess what the person is trying to express.
- Use augmentative communication devices, such as a picture board. These are useful to "fill in" answers to requests such as "I need" or "I want." The person merely points to the appropriate picture.

physical medicine/rehabilitation therapist. In progressive neurological disease it is important to begin treatment early and continue throughout the course of the disease with the goal of maintaining speech as long as possible.

Implications for Gerontological Nursing and Healthy Aging

The nurse needs to be familiar with techniques that facilitate communication with persons with dysarthria as well as strategies that can be taught to the person to improve communication. Boxes 3-2 and 3-3 present suggestions for the listener and the speaker to improve the effectiveness of communication with persons experiencing dysarthria. The nurse may encounter older people in the acute or long-term phase of an illness affecting communication. Although intensive rehabilitation efforts early are the most effective, all older adults with communication deficits should have access to state of the art techniques and devices that enhance communication, a basic human need. In addition to being knowledgeable about appropriate communication techniques, it is important for the nurse to be aware of equipment and resources available to the person with aphasia or dysarthria so that hope can be offered. Teaching families and significant others effective communication strategies is also an important nursing role. Several resources for people with aphasia and dysarthria are presented at the end of the chapter.

COMMUNICATING WITH INDIVIDUALS WITH COGNITIVE IMPAIRMENT

The experience of losing cognitive and expressive abilities is both frightening and frustrating. Memory impairments and communication disorders such as aphasia, apraxia, and agnosia can mean that people experiencing cognitive impairment have difficulty expressing their personhood

Box 3-2	**Tips for the Person with Dysarthria**

Explain to people that you have difficulty with your speech.

Try to limit conversations when you feel tired.

Speak slowly and loudly and in a quiet place.

Pace out one word at a time while speaking.

Take a deep breath before speaking so that there is enough breath for speech.

Speak out as soon as you breathe out to make full use of the breaths.

Open the mouth more when speaking; exaggerate tongue movements.

Make sure you are sitting or standing in an upright posture. This will improve your breathing and speech.

If you become frustrated, try to use other methods, such as pointing, gesturing, or writing, or take a rest and try again later.

Practice facial exercises (blowing kisses, frowning, smiling), and massage your facial muscles.

Adapted from Dysarthria and Coping with dysarthria. Accessed 7/3/04 from http:www.rcslt.org and www.asha.org.

Box 3-3	**Tips for Communicating with Individuals Experiencing Dysarthria**

Pay attention to the speaker; watch the speaker as he or she talks.

Allow more time for conversation, and conduct conversations in a quiet place.

Be honest, and let the speaker know when you have difficulty understanding.

If speech is very difficult to understand, repeat back what the person has said to make sure you understand.

Repeat the part of the message you did not understand so that the speaker does not have to repeat the entire message.

Allow more time for conversations.

Remember that dysarthria does not affect a person's intelligence.

Check with the person for ways in which you can help, such as guessing or finishing sentences or writing.

Adapted from Dysarthria and Coping with dysarthria. Accessed 7/3/04 from http:www.rcslt.org and www.asha.org.

in ways easily understood by others. However, the need to communicate and the need to be treated as a person remain despite memory and communication impairments. No group of patients is more in need of supportive relationships with skilled, caring health care providers. People with cognitive and communication impairments "depend on their relationship with and trust of others to provide emotional support, solve problems, and coordinate complex activities" (Buckwalter et al, 1995, p. 15). Our care must look beyond the disease and its effects to the person within. This makes it essential that nurses approach communication with cognitively impaired elders from a belief that the person is still a whole person, someone who can think, feel, learn, grow, and be in a relationship (Tappen et al, 1997; Touhy, 2004). "The person with dementia is not an object, not a vegetable, not an empty body, not a child, but an adult, who, given support, might exercise choices and respond to a respectful approach" (Woods, 1999, p 35). Communication

with the elder experiencing cognitive impairment requires special skills and patience.

Kitwood (1999) provided a simple way to learn techniques that keep the conversation open and encourage the person with cognitive impairment to respond. Envision a tennis game: the caregiver is like the tennis coach, and whenever the coach plays the ball, he or she seems to be able to put the ball where the person on the other side of the net can return it. The coach also returns the ball in such a way as to keep the rally going; he or she does not return it in order to score a point or win the match, but rather returns the ball so that the other player is able to reach it and, with encouragement, is able to hit it back over the net again. Similarly, in our communication with people with cognitive impairment, our conversations and words must be put into play in a way that the person can respond effectively and share thoughts and feelings. The best thing we can do is to treat everything that the person with cognitive impairment says, however jumbled it may seem, as important and an attempt to tell us something. It is our responsibility as skilled professionals to know how to understand and respond.

Much of the literature on communication with persons with cognitive impairment describes a person's attempt at speech in the later stages as nonsensical and devoid of meaning or insight, contributing to the impression of a diminishing self and inability to enter into therapeutic and meaningful relationships (Tappen et al, 1999). If nurses practice from this framework, then custodial and task-oriented care is all that can be offered and there is little purpose in initiating conversation in order to understand the individual. The word *dementia* often conjures up images of mute people sitting in wheelchairs in nursing homes condemned to a life of nothingness or, even worse, images of aggressive persons who are feared and often restrained. Despite a growing body of literature on the importance of person-centered care, therapeutic communication techniques, and therapeutic work with people with dementia, the emphasis in the literature and in practice continues to be on care of the body (bathing, feeding) and the management of aggressive and problematic behavior. Discussions of how to prevent catastrophic reactions and handle aggressive behavior are far more common than discussions of how to nurture personhood and quality of life.

Research conducted by Ruth Tappen of Florida Atlantic University and her colleagues provided insight into communication strategies that were helpful in creating and maintaining a therapeutic relationship with people in the moderate to later stages of dementia. The research challenged some of the commonly held beliefs about communication with persons with cognitive impairment, such as avoiding the use of open-ended questions and keeping communication focused only on simple topics, task-oriented topics, and questions that can be answered with yes or no. Further research findings provided suggestions for specific communication strategies as well as hope for nurses to establish meaningful relationships that nurture the personhood of people with cognitive impairments. In the Tappen et al studies (1997; 1999) more than 80% of subjects' responses were found to be relevant in the context of the conversation. It is essential to believe that the person is trying to communicate something and just as essential for the nurse to believe that what the person is trying to communicate is important enough to make the effort to understand. Because people with cognitive impairment cannot always tell us their stories, the nurse needs to come to know as much as possible about the person and his or her life so that communication and care can be individualized. It is important to involve families and significant others in our plans of care so that they can tell the story of the person. Box 3-4 presents suggestions for communication with persons experiencing cognitive impairment.

Implications for Gerontological Nursing and Healthy Aging

Nurses must understand and appreciate that every time they communicate with someone they affect the relationship with that person in either positive or negative ways depending on their attitudes and skills (Buckwalter et al, 1995). Care and communication that respect and value the dignity and worth of every person nursed, including those with cognitive impairment, and use of research-based communication techniques will enhance not only communication but also personhood. "Gerontological nurses who are sensitive to communication and interaction patterns can assist both formal and informal caregivers in using more personal verbal and nonverbal communication strategies which are humanizing and show respect for the person. Similarly, they can monitor and try to change object-oriented communication approaches, which are not only insensitive and dehumanizing, but also often lead to diminished self-image and angry, agitated responses on the part of the patient with cognitive impairment" (Buckwalter et al, 1995, p 15).

Assessment and evaluation of interactions and communication patterns, use of therapeutic communication techniques, and teaching others effective communication are other important roles for gerontological nurses. A story (Figure 3-1) describes a nursing situation that one nurse experienced in caring for a patient with dementia who was being admitted to a nursing home. Written from the perspective of the nurse and his knowing the patient, the story provides insight into impor-

---

Box 3-4	Four Useful Strategies for Communicating with Individuals Experiencing Cognitive Impairment

Simplification Strategies (useful with ADL)
- Give one-step directions.
- Speak slowly.
- Allow time for response.
- Reduce distractions.
- Interact with one person at a time.
- Give clues and cues as to what you want the person to do. Use gestures or pantomime to demonstrate what it is you want the person to do—for example, put the chair in front of the person, point to it, pat the seat, and say "Sit here."

Facilitation Strategies (useful in encouraging expression of thoughts and feelings)
- Establish commonalities.
- Share self.
- Allow the person to choose subjects to discuss. as if to an equal.
- Use broad openings, such as "How are you today?"
- Employ appropriate use of humor.
- Follow the person's lead.

Comprehension Strategies (useful in assisting in understanding of communication)
- Identify time confusion (in what time frame is the person operating at the moment?).
- Find the theme (what connection is there between apparently disparate topics?). Recognize an important theme, such as fear, loss, happiness.

- Recognize the hidden meanings (what did the person mean to say?).

Supportive Strategies (useful in encouraging continued communication and supporting personhood)
- Introduce yourself, and explain why you are there. Reach out to shake hands, and note the response to touch.
- If the person does not want to talk, go away and return later. Do not push or force.
- Sit closely, and face the person at eye level.
- Limit corrections.
- Assume meaningfulness.
- Use multiple ways of communicating (gestures, touch).
- Search for meaning.
- Know the person's past life history as well as daily life experiences and events.
- Recognize feelings, and respond.
- Treat with respect and dignity.
- Show interest through body posture, facial expression, nodding, and eye contact. Assume a pleasant, relaxed attitude.
- Attend to vision and hearing losses.
- Do not try to bring the person to the present or use reality orientation. Go to where the person is, and enjoy the conversation.
- When leaving, thank the person for his or her time and attention as well as information.
- Remember that the quality, not the content or quantity, of the interaction is basic to therapeutic communication.

ADL, Activities of daily living.

---

tant gerontological nursing responses, such as person-centered care, therapeutic communication, and establishing meaningful relationships.

COMMUNICATION IN GROUPS

Group work with the older adults has been used extensively in institutional settings to meet myriad needs in an economical manner. Nurses have led groups of older people for a variety of therapeutic reasons, and expert gerontological nurses such as Irene Burnside, Priscilla Ebersole, and Barbara Haight have extensively discussed advantages of group work for both older people and group leaders and have provided in-depth guidelines for conducting groups. Chapter 5 provides more specific information about conducting reminiscence and life review groups. Some of the advantages of group work (Burnside, 1994) include the following:

1. Group experiences provide older adults with an opportunity to try new roles—those of teacher, expert, storyteller, or even clown.

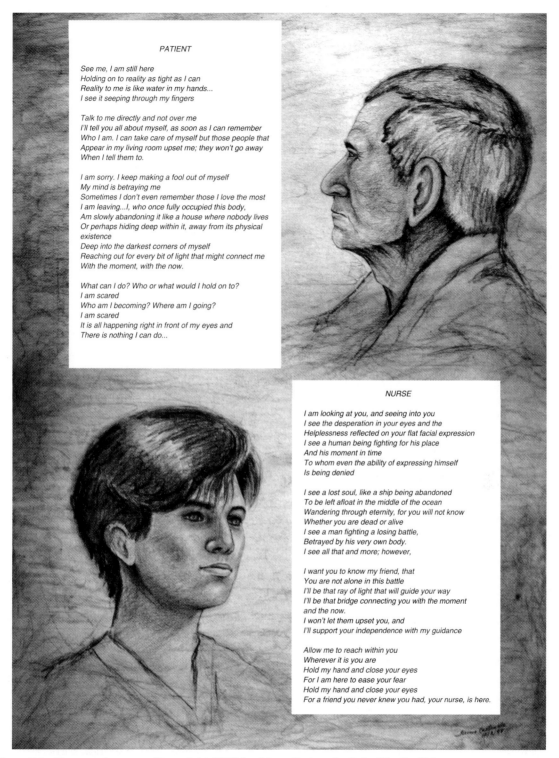

PATIENT

See me, I am still here
Holding on to reality as tight as I can
Reality to me is like water in my hands...
I see it seeping through my fingers

Talk to me directly and not over me
I'll tell you all about myself, as soon as I can remember
Who I am. I can take care of myself but those people that
Appear in my living room upset me; they won't go away
When I tell them to.

I am sorry. I keep making a fool out of myself
My mind is betraying me
Sometimes I don't even remember those I love the most
I am leaving...I, who once fully occupied this body,
Am slowly abandoning it like a house where nobody lives
Or perhaps hiding deep within it, away from its physical
existence
Deep into the darkest corners of myself
Reaching out for every bit of light that might connect me
With the moment, with the now.

What can I do? Who or what would I hold on to?
I am scared
Who am I becoming? Where am I going?
I am scared
It is all happening right in front of my eyes and
There is nothing I can do...

NURSE

I am looking at you, and seeing into you
I see the desperation in your eyes and the
Helplessness reflected on your flat facial expression
I see a human being fighting for his place
And his moment in time
To whom even the ability of expressing himself
Is being denied

I see a lost soul, like a ship being abandoned
To be left afloat in the middle of the ocean
Wandering through eternity, for you will not know
Whether you are dead or alive
I see a man fighting a losing battle,
Betrayed by his very own body.
I see all that and more; however,

I want you to know my friend, that
You are not alone in this battle
I'll be that ray of light that will guide your way
I'll be that bridge connecting you with the moment
and the now.
I won't let them upset you, and
I'll support your independence with my guidance

Allow me to reach within you
Wherever it is you are
Hold my hand and close your eyes
For I am here to ease your fear
Hold my hand and close your eyes
For a friend you never knew you had, your nurse, is here.

Figure 3-1 Nurse and person. (Copyright 1998 by Jaime Castaneda, Lake Worth, FL.)

2. Groups may improve communication skills for lonely, shy, or withdrawn older people as well as those with communication disorders or memory impairment.

3. Groups provide peer support and sharing of common experiences, and they may foster the development of warm friendships that endure long after the group has ended.

4. The group may be of interest to other residents, staff, and relatives and may improve satisfaction and morale. Staff, in particular, may come to see their patients in a different light—not just as persons needing care but as persons.

5. Active listening and interest in what older people have to say may improve self-esteem and help them feel like worthwhile persons whose wisdom is valued.

6. Group work offers the opportunity for leaders to be creative and use many modalities, such as music, art, dance, poetry, exercise, and current events.

7. Groups provide an opportunity for the leader to weekly assess the person's mood, cognitive abilities, and functional level.

Many groups can be managed effectively by staff with clear goals and guidance and training. A basic knowledge of group process and adaptation to older adults, as well as support from a skilled group leader, is important. Volunteers, nursing assistants, and recreation staff can be taught to conduct many types of groups, but groups with a psychotherapy focus require a trained and skilled leader. Group work is personally satisfying to the leader and can increase the health and well-being of older people. Groups can be implemented in many settings, including adult day health, retirement communities, assisted living facilities, nutrition sites, and nursing homes. Some of the possibilities for designing groups to meet special needs are shown in Table 3-1. Groups may be recreation or service oriented, inspirational, informative, or constrained by specific needs or goals. Groups providing interactional support may be formal or informal.

Informal Groups

Informal groups are those that naturally occur and have few restrictions, expectations, or goals. The following are examples of such groups:

- Groups of older adults that spontaneously arise at nutrition sites
- Gatherings of older people in city parks
- Participants in senior citizen activities (these often have formal and informal components)
- Groups that cluster together in long-term care or residential settings
- Any group that occurs sporadically for the purpose of socialization, discussion, or participation in a particular activity

These groupings should be supported in whatever way possible.

Formal Groups

Formal groups are defined by their expectations, dependability, and goals. The intensity of interpersonal exchange varies in accordance with the members' and group's goals. The development and maintenance of peer groups are particularly important when friends are no longer available. The advantage of group affiliations for older adults is in the diffusion of relationship intensity and the constancy over time. A reliable group maintains its function despite the loss or addition of members. This is an important consideration when working with the very old.

Needs Assessment

Groups can be organized to meet any level of human need; some meet multiple needs (Figure 3-2). Using the assessment of social climate and human needs as basic guides, one can begin to determine the type of group most suitable in a given situation.

At least three types of formal groups exist: (1) those that accomplish some identifiable goal, (2) those designed to be psychotherapeutic, and (3) those that facilitate positive communication patterns. The distinction between the second and third types is in the readiness of members. Therapy groups imply some psychological disturbance or conflict and should be led by qualified personnel. Nurses with training in psychotherapy often do an excellent job in such groups. The third type of group does not explore deep psychological needs but, rather, assists individuals in overcoming some communication barriers.

Table 3-1 Choosing a Group According to Need

Needs and Problems	Suggested Group
BIOLOGICAL INTEGRITY	
Poor nutrition	Mealtime groups
Loss of sexual satisfaction or opportunity	Male/female groups
Inadequate rest/excess stress	Relaxation groups
Health education	Health information or health-monitoring groups (e.g., blood pressure)
SAFETY AND SECURITY	
Impaired sensory perception	Sensory awareness training
Immobility	Movement and exercise groups, Tai Chi, yoga
Relocation	Patient councils, environmental planning groups
Communication difficulties	Storytelling, reminiscence
BELONGING	
Isolation	Socialization, activities, reminiscence
Alienation from family	Family groups, cohort groups
Loss of significant others	Grief group
SELF-ESTEEM	
Uselessness	Reminiscing groups
Lack of work	Productive groups, intergenerational groups
Lack of recognition	Discussion groups
Depression	Therapy groups, expressive groups
SELF-ACTUALIZATION	
Spiritual growth	Spirituality or religious groups/wisdom circles
Memory impairment	Support groups for early- to middle-stage memory loss (patients and families), cognitive exercises
Acceptance of cultural myths ("Old dogs can't learn new tricks.")	Discussions, debates, educational groups, creative/expressive groups

Group Goals

Functional goals for groups of older adults include combinations of the following:
- Socialization—interpersonal exchange
- Therapeutic—healing through group
- Entertainment
- Cohort affiliation
- Increased functional levels
- Stimulation/environmental enrichment
- Activation/movement
- Patient and family support and/or education
- Increased autonomy
- Improved communication skills
- Growth and self-actualization

Group Structure and Special Considerations for Groups of Older Adults

Implementing a group follows a thorough assessment of environment, needs, and potential for various group strategies. Major decisions regarding goals will influence the strategy selected. For instance, several older people with diabetes in an acute care setting may need health care teaching regarding diabetes. The nurse sees the major goal as education and restoring order (or control) in each individual's lifestyle. The strategy best suited for that would be motivational or educational. A group of people experiencing early-stage Alzheimer's disease may benefit from a support

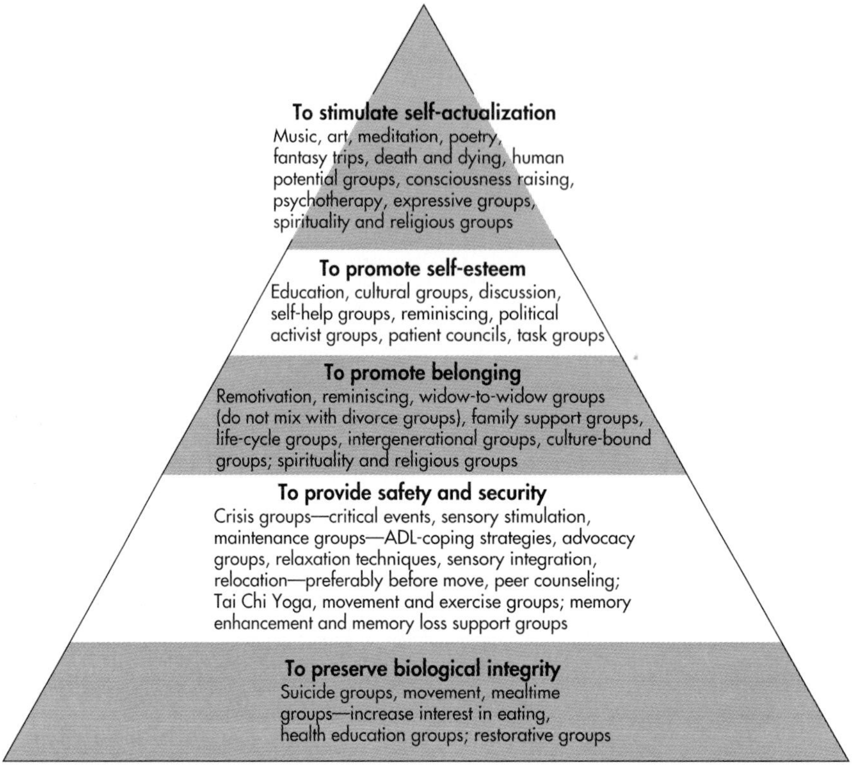

Figure 3-2 Hierarchical needs met in group work with the aged. *ADL*, Activities of daily living.

group to express feelings or a group that teaches memory-enhancing strategies. Successful group work depends on organization, attention to details, agency support, assessment and consideration of the older person's needs and status, and caring, sensitive, and skillful leadership (Burnside, 1994).

Group work with older persons is different from that with younger age groups; and there are some unique aspects that require special skills, training, and an extraordinary commitment on the part of the leader. Although these unique aspects may not apply to all types of groups of older adults, some of the differences include the following:

1. The leader must pay special attention to sensory losses and compensate for vision and hearing loss.

2. Pacing is different, and group leaders must slow down in both physical and psychological actions.

3. Group members often need assistance or transportation in getting to the group, and adequate time must be allowed for assembling the members and assisting them to return to their homes or rooms.

4. Time of day to schedule a group is important. Meeting time should not conflict with bathing and eating schedules, and evening groups may not be a good idea for older people who may be tired by then. For community-based older people, transportation logistics may become complicated in the evening.

5. A warm and friendly climate of acceptance of each member as well as showing appreciation and enjoyment of the group and each member's contribution is important. As a result of ageist attitudes in society, older people's wisdom and contributions are not often valued, making them feel useless or a bother.

6. They may need more stimulation and be less self-motivating. (This is, of course, not true of self-help and senior activist groups such as the Gray Panthers.)

7. Groups generally should include people with similar levels of cognitive ability. Mixing very intact elders with those who have memory and communication impairments requires special skills. Burnside (1994) suggested that in groups of people with varying abilities, alert persons tend to ask, "Will I become like them?" whereas the people with memory and communication impairments may become anxious when they are aware that they cannot perform as well as the other members.

8. Many older people likely to be in need of groups may be depressed or have experienced a number of losses (health, friends, spouse). Discussion of losses and sad feelings can be difficult for group leaders. A leader prone to depression would not be appropriate.

9. Leaders must be prepared for some members to become ill, deteriorate, and die. Plans regarding recognition of missing members will need to be clear. The following example that occurred during a reminiscence group conducted by one of the authors (TT) illustrates: "As I arrived at the nursing home one week for the group, I was told by the nursing home staff that one of our members had died. One of the members had been a priest so we asked him to say a prayer for our deceased group member. He did so beautifully, and the group was grateful. The next week, to our surprise, the supposedly deceased member showed up for the group (she had been in the hospital). We didn't know how to handle the situation, but the other members came to our rescue by saying, 'Father's prayers really worked this time.'" Older people's wisdom and humor can teach us a lot.

10. Leaders are continually confronted with their own aging and attitudes toward it. Group leaders need to plan in advance to incorporate a consistent support person in the group if possible. Co-leaders are ideal. If this is not feasible, someone must be available for planning and recapitulation of group sessions. Students generally should work in pairs and will need supervision. Skills in developing and imple-

menting groups for older adults improve with experience. Burnside (1994) reminds us that "all new group leaders should have guidance from an experienced leader to help them weather the difficult times" (p 43). Box 3-5 presents guidelines for group work with older adults.

LEARNING AND GROWING IN LATER LIFE

In this era of health care restrictions it is imperative that providers and elders understand each other and that necessary information be shared accurately and in a timely fashion. And yet, a 2004 report by the Institute of Medicine (IOM) titled *Health Literacy: a Prescription to End Confusion* revealed that close to one half of adults nationwide have problems understanding and using the health information they receive. Individuals residing in urban settings, those with poor education or low income, minorities, older people, and people for whom English is a second language are more likely to perform at lower levels of literacy (Wilson et al, 2003). Limited literacy skills mean that people have limited ability to read and understand directions on prescriptions, appointment slips, consent documents, insurance forms, and educational materials. People with limited health literacy also face increased hospitalizations and use emergency services more frequently. Nurses should be sensitive to the fact that patients with low literacy skills feel shame and embarrassment and usually do not readily share their reading or understanding difficulties with others. "Limited literacy is, in fact, an occult, silent disability and a secret that most people do not share even with members of their own family" (Dreger, Tremback, 2002).

Reaching some elders with information that is understood and beneficial presents special challenges. Hearing and vision losses, cognitive impairment, and low literacy skills of some elders may create barriers to understanding. Adults aged 60 and over are a heterogeneous group in their characteristics as well as in their literacy skills. However, the National Literacy Survey (Brown et al, 1996) reported that low levels of literacy are a significant problem for a large portion of older adults in the United States. Seventy-one percent of

Box 3-5   Guidelines for Group Work with Older Adults

Before Starting

A. What are the purposes for beginning the group?
B. Are there any known constraints to beginning the group you want to launch?
C. Determine the logistics of the group.
1. How many people will be in the group? Six to eight is the recommended number.
2. What will be the age range? Will you include both men and women? Will they be ambulatory and able to get to the group on their own? If not, consider transportation and room accommodations for wheelchairs.
3. Will the members be alert or cognitively impaired or both?
4. Will it be an open or closed group? (An open group with new members coming in every week complicates leadership and acquiring new friends and confidants, whereas a closed group with the same members each week facilitates cohesion.)
5. How often and where will the group meet, and how long will the meetings be in length?
6. Check the room for temperature, glare, noise, availability, privacy, size, comfortable furniture, and accessibility.
7. Do you have entrée into an agency?
8. How will you gain support of the agency personnel so they will support your group?
9. Are there any costs involved (e.g., food, beverages, supplies), and who will pay for them?
10. How will you inform and invite people to the group (e.g., invitations, posters, flyers, phone calls)?
11. Will you conduct preevaluation and postevaluation of the group to determine outcomes, and if so, what will you use and how will you obtain consent and IRB approval?
12. Do you possess some basic knowledge of group process, or do you need to read more?
13. Do you plan to use a co-leader? If so, how will you share the responsibilities of the group and work together?
14. Are you knowledgeable about the type of group you have selected (e.g., if you have selected a reminiscence group, are you knowledgeable about the techniques)?

15. Is the group modality you have chosen appropriate for the members (e.g., severely cognitively impaired people cannot participate in current events groups)?
16. What talents do you have that you could share with the group as a leader (e.g., music, art)?

During the Group

A. Because the first meeting sets the tone for future meetings, have you made every effort to plan the first meeting to go as smoothly as possible? Also, will you deal with termination during the first meeting?
B. Are you paying attention to the group process?
1. Are you including all people in each meeting by verbally acknowledging them and/or touching them?
2. Are you helping the frail who may ambulate poorly, checking on the batteries in a hearing aid, and/or cleaning eyeglasses?
3. Are you respectful of their schedules (even those in nursing homes who may have to give up television or favorite activities)?
4. Are you attentive to changes in members' behaviors in the group (e.g., withdrawal, appearing to be in pain, sleeping through meetings when previously alert)? What will you do about such behaviors?
5. How will you handle the shy person, the person who monopolizes discussion, the silent member, the late member, and those with physical impairments?

After the Group

A. How will you evaluate the effectiveness of the group?
B. Do you need to write any reports for agency personnel?
C. If you have a co-leader, have you had a debriefing about the group?
D. Have you tabulated the pretest and posttest evaluation data and determined the outcomes of the group?
E. Can you quickly make a list of what you learned during the group to help you in leading future groups or to share with colleagues?
F. Have you written thank-you notes to the group members, agency personnel, and any others who have helped you during the group time?

Adapted from Burnside IM: Group work with older persons, *J Gerontol Nurs* 20(1):43, 1994.
IRB, Institutional review board.

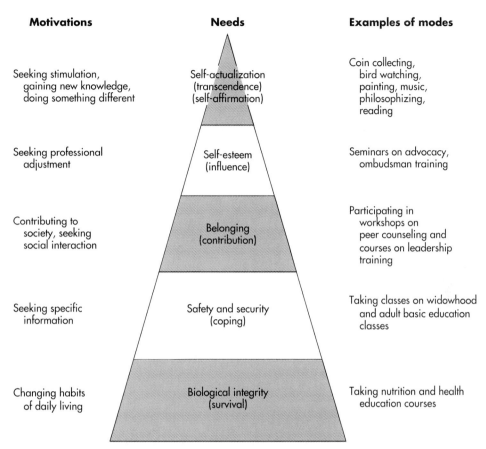

Motivations

Seeking stimulation, gaining new knowledge, doing something different

Seeking professional adjustment

Contributing to society, seeking social interaction

Seeking specific information

Changing habits of daily living

Needs

Self-actualization (transcendence) (self-affirmation)

Self-esteem (influence)

Belonging (contribution)

Safety and security (coping)

Biological integrity (survival)

Examples of modes

Coin collecting, bird watching, painting, music, philosophizing, reading

Seminars on advocacy, ombudsman training

Participating in workshops on peer counseling and courses on leadership training

Taking classes on widowhood and adult basic education classes

Taking nutrition and health education courses

Figure 3-3 Learning and growing in later life. (Developed by Priscilla Ebersole.)

adults 60 and over, or approximately 29 million individuals, demonstrated limited literacy skills. Individuals over 80, those with less education, and those with visual impairments had the lowest skills. Cultural and cohort variations have produced great differences in receptivity to health information. Many elders still have special learning needs based on education deprivation in their early years and consequent anxiety about formalized learning. Box 3-6 summarizes some ways to overcome these problems.

Implications for Gerontological Nursing and Healthy Aging

The nurse's role extends beyond simply giving information. To be useful the nurse must discover the preferred learning mode and setting appropriate to the needs and desires of the elder (Figure 3-3). Also, the nurse should provide the elder with information about media resources that may make knowledge readily available and easier to understand. Increasingly, elders are taking charge of their own learning and scanning the Internet for information about health and lifestyles. Approximately 15% of people 65 and over are online, and these numbers will continue to grow as the baby boomers bring their computers with them into senior citizenship (Clark, 2002). Innovations such as a user-friendly talking computer touch screen are being used with good outcomes to assist low-literacy elders in quality of life studies and health promotion and disease prevention initiatives (Hahn et al, 2004). There are many reliable Internet resources related to health and aging.

Box 3-6   Guiding Older Adult Learners

- Make sure the client is ready to learn before trying to teach. Watch for clues that would indicate that the client is preoccupied or too anxious to comprehend the material.
- Sit facing the client so that he or she can watch your lip movements and facial expressions.
- Speak slowly.
- Keep your tone of voice low; elderly persons can hear low sounds better than high-frequency sounds.
- Present one idea at a time.
- Use extra voice and media amplification
- Emphasize concrete rather than abstract material—make learning practical.
- Encourage the learner to develop various mediators or mnemonic devices (visual images, rhymes, acronyms, self-designed coding schemes).
- Use high contrast on visuals and handout material (e.g., larger-font black print on white paper).
- Pay attention to reading ability; use techniques other than printed material, such as drawings, pictures, and discussion.
- Provide enough time to respond because older adults' reaction times may be longer than those of younger persons.

- Focus on a single topic to help the client concentrate.
- Keep environmental distractions to a minimum.
- Take appropriate breaks and defer teaching if the client becomes distracted or tired or cannot concentrate for other reasons.
- Invite another member of the household to join the discussion.
- Use audio, visual, and tactile cues to enhance learning and help the client remember information.
- Provide regular feedback.
- Use past experience; connect new learning to that already learned.
- Ask for feedback to ensure that the information has been understood.
- Compensate for physical discomfort and sensory decrements.
- Support a positive self-image in the learner.
- Use creative teaching strategies.
- Respond to identified interests of learners.
- Emphasize and integrate emotional and personal values in the acquisition of skills and ideas.

Modified from *Bridging principles of older adult learning: reconnaissance phase final report,* Washington, DC, 1999, SPRY Foundation.

The National Institute of Aging website (http://www.nia.nih.gov/health/) provides excellent resources for learning and teaching health-related topics. The Age Page series is especially helpful and includes a variety of one-page informational sheets for consumers and for health professionals. Nurses are beginning to recognize the necessity of revising the traditional teaching/learning strategies, which often are limited to giving information in the form of brochures and minilectures with return demonstrations. In addition, in designing or referring older adults to instructional materials, attention to literacy skills and cultural variations is important to enhance learning and usefulness.

Numerous opportunities exist for older learners within the established educational institutions or in special programs. Many universities have "senior scholar" or lifelong learning programs designed especially for elders. The Elderhostel program is an example of a program designed for elders to participate in learning combined with travel. Other resources are listed at the end of the chapter. The nurse's role should include providing suggestions of resources available to the elder and encouraging continued learning, self-development, and growth.

APPLICATION OF MASLOW'S HIERARCHY

Skilled, sensitive, and caring individual and group communication strategies with elders are essential

NANDA and Wellness Diagnoses

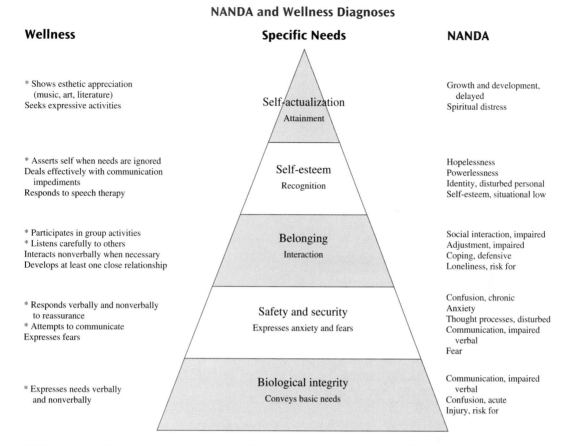

Wellness	Specific Needs	NANDA
* Shows esthetic appreciation (music, art, literature) Seeks expressive activities	**Self-actualization** Attainment	Growth and development, delayed Spiritual distress
* Asserts self when needs are ignored Deals effectively with communication impediments Responds to speech therapy	**Self-esteem** Recognition	Hopelessness Powerlessness Identity, disturbed personal Self-esteem, situational low
* Participates in group activities * Listens carefully to others Interacts nonverbally when necessary Develops at least one close relationship	**Belonging** Interaction	Social interaction, impaired Adjustment, impaired Coping, defensive Loneliness, risk for
* Responds verbally and nonverbally to reassurance * Attempts to communicate Expresses fears	**Safety and security** Expresses anxiety and fears	Confusion, chronic Anxiety Thought processes, disturbed Communication, impaired verbal Fear
* Expresses needs verbally and nonverbally	**Biological integrity** Conveys basic needs	Communication, impaired verbal Confusion, acute Injury, risk for

* Wellness when individual communicates to best of ability through whatever means is available.

These are not all of the possible wellness or NANDA diagnoses that may be identified. The above are frequent examples of nursing diagnoses that should be considered when planning care for the older adult in whatever setting.

to meeting needs at all levels of Maslow's hierarchy. Elders with communication difficulties may have difficulty expressing basic needs for food, water, toileting, sleep, nutrition, and safety and security. Adapting communication to enhance understanding and satisfaction of basic needs not only assists in preserving biological integrity, but also is the basis for the establishment of therapeutic nursing relationships that help patients grow toward self-actualization. Just as all people have the need to communicate and have their basic needs met, they also have the right to experiences that are meaningful and fulfilling. Age, language impairment, or mental status do not change these needs. Creation of care environments that are rich with pleasant experiences—a good cup of coffee, a meal shared with friends, a sunrise, beautiful music, learning something interesting, or sharing experiences from the life one has lived—is as important as getting enough to eat. Our nursing care with older people experiencing cognitive and communication impairments must be more than keeping their bodies alive, safe, and clean, or preventing injury. The unique contribution that nursing brings to care of people is the intimate, personal knowing of the person behind the disease and the creation of relationships and environments of care that support, validate, and celebrate the person as someone of value and worth (Touhy, 2004). Within this framework, gerontological nurses assist in the meeting of needs at all levels. The privilege of nursing older people is sharing the wisdom of those who have lived long lives and can guide us toward life's greatest challenge, achieving self-actualization.

Throughout this chapter we have tried to convey the potential for honest and hopeful communication regardless of the condition of the elder. We must break through the barriers and continue to reach toward the humanity of the individual with the belief that communication is the most vital service we can offer. This is the heart of nursing.

▶ KEY CONCEPTS

- Communication is a basic need regardless of age or communication or cognitive impairment. Respect for the person and knowledge of therapeutic communication techniques are essential skills for gerontological nurses.
- Group work can meet many needs at all levels of Maslow's hierarchy and is satisfying and rewarding for both the older adult and the group leader.
- There are many activities in which older adults can participate to continue learning and growth. Attention to principles of older adult learning, adaptations of teaching methods, literacy level, and cultural variations is important in communicating health-related information.
- Gerontological nursing responses related to communication and learning are focused mainly on using therapeutic communication techniques, providing necessary information, encouraging individuals to express personal interests and preferences, and, when function is impeded, ensuring that basic needs are mutually recognized, discussed, and met to the greatest extent possible.

▶ Activities and Discussion Questions

1. Discuss adaptations to communication for individuals with aphasia or dysarthria.
2. Discuss ways in which you might respond to a person with cognitive impairment who has difficulty expressing thoughts and feelings.
3. Role-play a simulated interaction with an older adult experiencing communication or cognitive impairments such as aphasia, dysarthria, or memory loss.
4. With a partner, plan and discuss an activity that would be appropriate for an individual with cognitive impairment.
5. What would be important considerations in designing a brochure or a lecture on stroke for older adults?
6. Rent the movie *Iris* or *The Notebook,* and discuss effective and ineffective communication strategies with persons experiencing cognitive impairment.

RESOURCES

Books and Publications

Bell V, Troxel D: *A dignified life: the best friends approach to Alzheimer's care, a guide for family caregivers,* Deerfield Beach, FL, 2002, Health Communications.

Feil N, Rubin-Klerk V: *The validation breakthrough: simple techniques for communicating with people with Alzheimer's type dementia,* Baltimore, 2002, Health Professions Press.

Goldsmith M: *Hearing the voice of people with dementia: opportunities and obstacles,* Levittown, Pa, 1996, Jessica Kingsley Publishers.

McGowin D: *Living in the labyrinth,* New York, 1993, Dell Publishing.

Snyder L: *Speaking our minds,* New York, 2000, WH Freeman & Co.

Tan A: *The bonesetter's daughter,* New York, 2002, Ballantine Books.

Organizations

Alzheimer's Association
225 N. Michigan Ave. FL. 17
Chicago, IL 60601
1-800-272-3900
Website: www.alz.org

Alzheimer's Disease Education and Referral Center
P.O. Box 8250
Silver Spring, MD 20907
1-800-438-4380
Website: www.alzheimers.org

American Heart Association, National Center
7272 Greenville Avenue
Dallas, TX 75231
1-800-242-8721
Website: www.americanheart.org

American Stroke Association, National Center
7272 Greenville Avenue
Dallas, TX 75321
Website: www.strokeassociation.org
Also provides information on attending local Stroke
Club meetings.

Aphasia Hope Foundation
2436 West 137th Street
Leawood, KS 66224
Website: www.aphasiahope.org

National Aphasia Association
29 John Street, Suite 1103
New York, NY 10038
Website: www.aphasia.org

On-line stroke support group
www.strokenetwork.org

Adult Education/Teaching and Learning (Web Resources)

AARP's free Directory of Centers for Older Learners. The
state-by-state listing includes the names, addresses,
phone numbers, and sponsors of educational
programs around the United States designed for
older students (www.aarp.org).

American Association for Adult and Continuing Education.
Information and resources on adult education and
lifelong learning (www.aaace.org).

*American Association of Community and Junior
Colleges,* No. 1 Dupont Circle, Suite 410,
Washington, DC 20036, (202) 293-7050
(http://www.aacc.nche.edu).

Elderhostel. Lifelong learning and travel
opportunities for older adults. 50 Federal
Street, Boston, MA 02110, (617) 426-8056
(www.elderhostel.org).

Institutes for Lifetime Learning. A service of the
American Association of Retired Persons (AARP) and
National Retired Teachers Association (NRTA), it
provides classes at institute centers throughout the
United States and a series of radio programs allowing
members of AARP/NRTA to pursue independent
study at their own pace in their own fields of
interest. Contact AARP, (202) 872-4700
(www.aarp.org).

Lifetime Education and Renewal Network (LEARN), a
constituent group of the American Society on Aging
(ASA). Involved in all aspects of education for older
adults and providing information on settings and
programs for lifetime learners. Publishes a newsletter
The Older Learner (www.asaging.org/networks/learn/
about.cfm).

National Institute on Aging, Senior Health. Age Pages,
convenient one-page information sheets on health
and aging (www.nihseniorhealth.gov).

Films and Videos

Best Friends. Discusses the innovative best friends
approach to caring for older people with Alzheimer's
disease and related dementias. Available from Health
Professions Press (www.healthpropress.com).

*Breakfast Club: Enhancing the Communication Ability of
Alzheimer's Patients.* Available from the Alzheimer's
Association (www.alz.org).

Communicating in Alzheimer's Disease. Caregivers
describe their challenges and solutions for
communicating with the person with the disease
(20-minute video). Available from the Alzheimer's
Association (www.alz.org).

Communicating with Oriented Older Adults. Shows how
to listen, empathize, and engage in the give-and-take
of effective conversation. Demonstrates techniques
of getting information, paraphrasing, summarizing,
and clarifying. Available from Mental Health
Outreach Network, Duluth, MN. Also available from
the Alzheimer's Association (www.alz.org).

Communication Strategies for Alzheimer's Patients.
Presents methods of maintaining patient dignity and
self-respect while communicating effectively. Utilizes
actual scenes with patients, family, and staff.
Available from Geriatric Video Productions, P.O. Box
1757, Shavertown, PA 18708-0757, (800) 621-9181
(http://www.geriatricvideo.com).

*Interacting with Alzheimer's Patients: Tips for Family and
Friends: Alzheimer's Disease Do's and Don'ts.* In a
discussion with several caregivers, Alzheimer's
disease expert Peter Rabins identifies the do's and
don'ts of interacting with individuals with
Alzheimer's disease. Available from Video Press,
University of Maryland, School of Medicine,
Baltimore. Also available from the Alzheimer's
Association (www.alz.org).

*Recognizing and Responding to Emotion in Persons with
Dementia.* Discusses emotions in people with
dementia, especially when they can no longer
express their likes and dislikes but can still have
preferences (26 minutes). Available from the
Philadelphia Geriatric Center. Also available from
the Alzheimer's Association (www.alz.org).

What is Aphasia and *Pathways: Moving Beyond Stroke
and Aphasia.* Videos targeted toward stroke survivors
and family members and appropriate for health care
professionals and students. Available from The
Aphasia Hope Foundation at www.aphasiahope.org.

Working with the Confused Elderly. Presents verbal and
nonverbal techniques that increase skills in
understanding communication and behaviors
associated with cognitive impairment. The work
presents some revolutionary methods to deal with
problems such as wandering, paranoia, and
disorientation (21-minute video). Available from Dr.
Joyce Colling, Oregon Health Sciences University,

Nursing School, 3181 SW Sam Jackson Park Road, Portland, OR 97201.

Full-Length Motion Pictures Relevant to Communication with Cognitively Impaired Elders

Iris (2001)
The Notebook (2004)

REFERENCES

Bridging principles of older adult learning: reconnaissance phase final report, Washington, DC, 1999, SPRY Foundation.

Brown H, Prisuta R, Jacobs B, Campbell A: *Literacy of older adults in America: results from the National Adult Literacy Survey, NCES 97-576,* Washington, DC, 1996, U.S. Department of Education, National Center for Education Statistics.

Buckwalter KC, Gerdner LA, Hall GR et al: Shining through: the humor and individuality of persons with Alzheimer's disease, *J Gerontol Nurs* 21(3):11-16, 1995.

Burnside IM: Listen to the aged, *Am J Nurs* 75(10):1800-1803, 1975.

Burnside IM: Group work with older persons, *J Gerontol Nurs* 20(1):43, 1994.

Clark DJ: Older adults living through and with their computers, *Comput Inform Nurs* 20(3):117-124, 2002.

Dreger V, Tremback T: Optimize patient health by treating health literacy and language barriers, *AORN J* 75(2):280-285, 2002.

Dysarthria and Coping with dysarthria. Accessed 7/3/04 from http:www.rcslt.org and www.asha.org.

Hahn EA, Cella D, Dobrez D et al: The talking touch-screen: a new approach to outcomes assessment in low literacy, *Psychooncology* 13(2):86-95, 2004.

Kitwood T: *Dementia reconsidered: the person comes first,* Bristol, Pa, 1999, Open University Press.

Miller L: Effective communication with older people, *Nurs Stand* 17(9), 2002.

Nagley S: Personal communication, Case Western Reserve University, Cleveland, 1988.

Tappen RM, Williams-Burgess C, Edelstein J et al: Communicating with individuals with Alzheimer's disease: examination of recommended strategies, *Arch Psychiatr Nurs* 11(5):249-256, 1997.

Tappen RM, Williams C, Fishman S et al: Persistence of self in advanced Alzheimer's disease, *Image J Nurs Sch* 31(2):121-125, 1999.

Touhy TA: Dementia, personhood, and nursing: learning from a nursing situation, *Nurs Sci Q* 17(1):43-49, 2004.

Wilson FL, Racine E, Tekieli V et al: Literacy, readability and cultural barriers: critical factors to consider when educating older African Americans about anticoagulation therapy, *J Clin Nurs* 12(2):275-282, 2003.

Woods B: The person in dementia care, *Generations* 13(3):35-39, 1999.

Culture and Aging

4

LEARNING OBJECTIVES

Upon completion of this chapter, the reader will be able to:

- Identify factors contributing to personal ethnic and cultural sensitivity.
- Discuss approaches that facilitate an appreciation of diverse cultural and ethnic experiences.
- Explain the prominent health care belief systems.
- Identify nursing care interventions appropriate for ethnic elders.
- Formulate a plan of care incorporating ethnically sensitive interventions.

GLOSSARY

Ethnicity Belonging to or deriving from the cultural, racial, religious, or linguistic traditions of a people or country.

Ethnocentrism The belief in inherent superiority of one's group and culture accompanied by devaluation of other groups or cultures.

Ethnogeriatrics The medical science dealing with disease, disabilities, and care of ethnic elders.

Folk medicine Curing methods originating among the people of a culture and transmitted through the people of that culture.

Interpreter A person who explains the meaning of what is spoken in one language into another language.

Stereotype Belief applied to a group of persons based on actual or assumed knowledge of an individual member of the group.

THE LIVED EXPERIENCE

I feel so out of place here. If my children weren't so busy, I suppose I could live with them, but they seemed so relieved when this retirement home would accept me. I wonder if they knew I was the only Chinese person in this place. A sweet young Chinese student tried to talk with me, but she only spoke Mandarin and that not very well. She had never lived in China. I want so much to talk to someone my age who lived in China.

Shin, a 75-year-old woman

I was interviewing an older black woman. When I got to the part of the interview about race/ethnicity I said, "May I assume you consider yourself African American?" To which she replied, "Well, no dear, you may not, I always considered myself just plain American and never thought of myself in terms of African American."

Kathleen, a 50-year-old white woman of European descent

THE DEMOGRAPHIC IMPERATIVE

The population of the United States is rapidly becoming more diverse. Persons of color, who have long been classified as those from "minority groups," will represent about 50% of the population in the next 50 years. Among those over 65 years of age, the numbers are not as dramatic, but the effect of the growing numbers is being seen in all aspects of gerontological nursing and long-term care. It would not be unusual for nurses working in states with the greatest number of immigrant elders (California, Nevada, Florida, Texas, New Jersey, Illinois) to care for persons from a variety of backgrounds in the same day (Gelfand, 2003).

The nurse of today is expected to be prepared to provide competent care to persons with different life experiences, cultural perspectives, values, and styles of communication. The term *ethnogeriatrics* has entered the language of health care professionals; it is a specialty in which we hope to work sensitively with ethnic elders. The nurse may need to effectively communicate with persons regardless of the languages spoken. In doing so, the nurse may depend on limited verbal exchanges and attend more to facial and body expressions, postures, gestures, and touching. However, how these forms of communication are interpreted is heavily influenced by culture and ethnicity and may be easily misunderstood. To be able to skillfully assess and intervene, nurses must first develop cultural sensitivity through awareness of their own *ethnocentricities*. Nurses must then develop cultural competence through new cultural knowledge about ethnicity, culture, language, and health belief systems. Finally, the nurse must learn new skills to optimize intercultural communication.

INCREASING CULTURAL COMPETENCE AND SENSITIVITY

To optimize the quality of the care provided to older adults of any ethnic group, the nurse moves toward cultural competence, that is, increased awareness, cultural knowledge, and skills. Nurses can learn of their personal biases, prejudices, attitudes, and behaviors toward persons different

from themselves in age, gender, sexual orientation, social class, economic situations, and many other factors. Through increased knowledge, nurses can better assess the strengths and weaknesses of the older adult and know when and how to effectively intervene to support rather than hinder cultural strengths. Cultural competence means having the skills to put cultural knowledge to use in assessment, communication, negotiation, and intervention.

Cultural Awareness

Increased awareness requires openness and self-reflection. If the nurse is white, it is realizing this whiteness often means special privilege and freedoms. Older adults of color may not have had the same advantages or experiences as the nurse (McIntosh, 1989). Cultural awareness means recognizing the presence of the "isms" (racism, social classism, ageism) and how these have the potential to impact not only the pursuit and receipt of health care, but also the quality of life for older adults (Smedley et al, 2002).

If the nurse is younger, awareness means acknowledging that ageism, or negative attitudes toward older persons, is prevalent in society and in health care. *Ageism* is a term coined by Robert Butler, the first Director of the National Institute on Aging, to describe the discrimination that often accompanies old age and is based solely on age. Cole (1997) examined the historic roots of ageism in America. At one time, power in the United States was held almost exclusively by older white males. With the shift to urban industrialism, emphasis on productivity, and shifting philosophies in government, old men lost some of their influence and were replaced by younger men. In contemporary society the concept of aging carries many negative connotations. An old woman may be referred to as a "hag"—a term that once meant a "font of wisdom." An old man is no longer referred to as an elder or older statesman but as an "old fogy" or a "geezer."

Ageism exists among some health care professionals, undoubtedly somewhat influenced by the fact that providers often see older persons who need help or are ill. The influence these negative perceptions have on potential therapeutic outcomes has been largely ignored. The realization that aging is the greatest challenge one will ever face is a reality for the very old. For some, the challenge is exciting; for others, it is a test of the human spirit. As long as old age represents proximity to death, it will be embraced with reluctance.

Before the gerontological nurse provides quality care to ethnic elders it is useful to self-reflect and consider if there are any personal beliefs about persons who look different from the nurse and consider if these beliefs are negative or positive and if they are based on reality or opinion. Box 4-1 outlines approaches to cultural sensitivity and competence as described by Grossman (1994).

Cultural Knowledge

Cultural knowledge is both what the nurse brings to the caring situation and what the nurse learns about older adults, their families, their communities, their behaviors, and their expectations. Essential knowledge includes the elder's way of life (ways of thinking, believing, and acting). This knowledge is obtained formally or informally through the professional experience of nursing and caring. Over time, the nurse builds up a reservoir of information about the beliefs of his or her clients and how they behave.

Some nurses prefer to use what can be called an "encyclopedic" approach to details of a particular culture or ethnic group, such as proper name usage, greeting, eye contact, gender roles, foods, and beliefs about relevant topics, such as pain expression, death practices, or caregiving. This information is available in many well-done compendiums of cross-cultural information (see Resources at the end of this chapter for suggestions). In this chapter we elect to discuss concepts that have more global application to nursing the ethnic elder.

Although cultural knowledge is not only helpful and essential, caution must be used with the application of stereotyping. *Stereotyping* is the application of limited knowledge about one person with specific characteristics applied to other persons with the same characteristics and limits the recognition of the heterogeneity of any group. Relying on knowledge of a positive stereotype can be useful as a starting point in understanding but can also be used to limit understanding of the uniqueness of the individual and

---

| Box 4-1 | Steps to Cultural Sensitivity and Competence |

- Know yourself: examine your own values, attitudes, beliefs, and prejudices and your cultural heritage and identity.
- Confront biases and stereotypes.
- Do not judge: do not measure others' behavior against your beliefs and values.
- Keep an open mind: attempt to look at the world through other cultures' perspectives.
- Respect differences among people: each group has strengths and weaknesses.
- Appreciate inherent worth of diverse cultures, value them equally, and do not consider them inferior to one's own.
- Listen! Develop the ability to hear things that transcend language, and foster understanding of the client and his or her cultural heritage and the resilience that supports family and community that comes from within the culture.
- Be willing to learn: this requires interest in people's beliefs, values, and practices.
- Travel, read, and attend local ethnic and cultural events in the community.
- Develop an awareness and understanding for the complexities of the health care delivery system—its philosophy, problems, biases, and stereotypes—and become keenly aware of the socialization process that brings the care provider into this complex system.
- Be resourceful and creative: there are many ways to accomplish the same thing.
- Adapt your nursing interventions to suit different cultures and individuals.

Data from Grossman D: Enhancing your cultural competence, *Am J Nurs* 94(7):58, 1994; Spector RE: *Cultural diversity in health and illness*, ed 4, East Norwalk, Conn, 1996, Appleton & Lange.

---

impose unrealistic expectations. For example, a common stereotype of older African Americans may be that the church is a source of support. If the nurse simply assumes this to be true it could have a negative outcome, such as fewer referrals for other forms of support (e.g., home-delivered meals). On the other hand, this stereotype can be used to shortcut the assessment. In discussing discharge plans with an African American elder, the nurse may say, "I understand that the church is often a source of support in the African American community. Is this one of the resources you will be able to depend on when you return home?"

First, there is a need to clarify several terms, namely, race, culture, and ethnicity. *Race* is usually defined in terms of underlying skin tones (red, yellow, black, white) and other hereditary traits, such as eye color, facial structure, and hair texture. However, the relative importance of race is diminishing because of widespread mixing of the gene pool so that it is becoming increasingly uncommon for any one person to be genetically homogeneous (Gelfand, 2003).

Culture is the shared and learned beliefs, expectations, and behaviors of a group of people. For example, beliefs about aging may be relatively consistent within one culture group. Cultural knowledge is transmitted from one member to another through the process called *enculturation.* Culture provides directions for individuals as they interact with family and friends within the same group. Culture allows members of the group to predict each other's behavior and respond appropriately (Spector, 2003). *Ethnicity* is a complex phenomenon. It is a social differentiation based on cultural criteria. Most important, it is a shared identity. Although culture and ethnicity frequently are used interchangeably, in reality a distinct difference in meaning exists (Spector, 2003).

Persons from a specific ethnic group may share common geographical origins, migratory status, race, language or dialect, or religion. Traditions, symbols, literature, folklore, food preferences, and dress are often expressions of ethnicity. These persons may or may not share a common race. For example, persons who consider themselves Hispanic (the largest ethnic group in the United States) may be from any race and from any one of a number of countries. However, many Hispanics share the Catholic religion and the Spanish language.

Health beliefs and practices are usually a mixed expression of life experience and cultural knowledge. In most cultures, older adults are likely to treat themselves for familiar or chronic conditions in ways they have found successful in the past, often referred to as folk medicine or folk healing. The basis for much folk medicine is and was making the most of whatever was available. When self-treatment fails, a person will consult with others known to be knowledgeable or experienced with the problem, such as a community or indigenous healer. Only when this too fails do most people seek professional help within the formal health care system of the United States.

The culture of nursing and health care in the United States is one that advocates what is called the Western or biomedical system with its own set of beliefs about the cause of illness and the choice of treatments. In most settings this belief system is considered superior to all others from an ethnocentric perspective. However, many of the world's people have different beliefs, such as those of the personalistic (magicoreligious) system or the naturalistic (holistic) system. Each system is complete with beliefs about disease causation and recommendations for treatment and may have been used for thousands of years. Nurses who are familiar with the range of health beliefs and realize their importance to the followers will be able to provide more sensitive and appropriate care. Without this understanding there is great potential for conflict.

Western or Biomedical System

In the Western or biomedical belief system, disease is believed to be the result of abnormalities in structure and function of body organs and systems, often caused by the invasion of germs or microbes. The objective term *disease* is used by care providers, and *illness* is a subjective term to describe symptoms of discomfort associated with the disease. Assessment and diagnosis are directed at identifying the pathogen or process causing the abnormality, often through laboratory and other procedures. Treatment is based on removing or destroying the invading organism or repairing, modifying, or removing the afflicted body part. Prevention in this belief system is to avoid pathogens, chemicals, activities, and dietary agents known to cause abnormalities.

Personalistic or Magicoreligious System

Those who follow the beliefs of the personalistic or magicoreligious system believe that illness is caused by the actions of the supernatural, such as gods, deities, or non-human beings, such as ghosts, ancestors, or evil spirits. Illness is a punishment for a breach of rules, breaking a taboo, or failure to please the god, ancestor, and so on. Someone may be put under a spell by a disgruntled neighbor so that he or she cannot eat or sleep. A dead relative may be angry that his or her wishes were not followed and send an animal to bite the person, cause a growth, or cause a woman to be infertile. Treatments may consist of or include religious practices, such as praying, meditating, fasting, wearing amulets, burning candles, and establishing family altars. Making sure that social networks with their fellow humans are in good working order is the essence of prevention in this health belief system. It is therefore important to avoid angering family, friends, neighbors, ancestors, and gods. This belief system can be traced back to the ancient Egyptians, thousands of years before the common era, and persists in whole or in parts in many groups. Current practices that would be included in this group include things such as "laying of the hands" and prayer circles. It is not uncommon to hear an older adult pray for a cure or to lament "What did I do to cause this?"

Naturalistic or Holistic Health System

The naturalistic or holistic health belief system is based on the concept of balance and stems from the ancient civilizations of China, India, and Greece (Jackson, 1993). Disturbances in this balance result in disharmony and subsequent illness. Diagnosis requires the determination of the type of imbalance. The appropriate interventions, therefore, are methods that restore balance.

Traditional Chinese medicine is based on this belief, on the balance between yin and yang, darkness and light, hot and cold. Older adults who were raised in one of the countries on the Pacific rim (especially Asia and the Pacific Islands) or in a traditional Native American community frequently rely on these beliefs. The naturalistic system practiced in India and some of its neighboring countries is known as *ayurvedic*.

Another variation is seen in those who follow the hot/cold beliefs, apart from traditional Chinese medicine. Illness is believed to be the result of an excess of heat or cold that has entered the body and caused an imbalance. Hot and cold are generally metaphoric, although at times temperature is an aspect. Various foods, medicines, environmental conditions, emotions, and body conditions, such as menstruation and pregnancy, may possess the characteristics of either hot or cold (Spector, 2003). Diagnosis is concerned with

identifying the type of disease as either hot or cold. Remedies are divided into hot and cold. Treatment then is focused on using the opposite element; if the disease is the result of excess hot, treatment will be with something that has cold properties, and vice versa. The treatments may take the form of herbs, food, dietary restrictions, or medications from Western medicine that have hot and cold properties, such as antibiotics, massage, poultices, and other therapies.

Naturalistic healers are physicians or herbalists who specialize in symptomatic treatment and know which medicines will restore the body's equilibrium. Prevention is directed at protecting oneself from imbalances.

Cultural Skills

Providing the highest quality of care for ethnic elders and enhancing healthy aging require a new or refined set of skills. These skills include listening carefully to the person, especially for his or her perception of the situation, and attending not just to the words but to the nonverbal communication and the meaning behind the stories. Listen to the elder's perception of the situation, desired goals, and ideas for treatment. Cultural skills include the ability to explain your (the nurse's) perceptions clearly and without judgment, acknowledging that there are both similarities and differences between your perceptions and goals and those of the elder. Finally, cross-cultural skills include the ability to develop a plan of action that takes both perspectives into account and negotiate an outcome that is mutually acceptable (Berlin, Fowkes, 1983). Skillful cross-cultural nursing means developing a sense of mutual respect between the nurse and the elder. It is working "with" the client rather than "on" the client.

Use of Interpreters

Working with the client in the cross-cultural nursing situation may also include working with an interpreter. *Interpretation* is the processing of oral language in a manner that preserves the meaning and tone of the original language without adding or deleting anything. The job of the interpreter is to work with two different linguistic codes in a way that will produce equivalent messages (Haffner, 1992). The interpreter tells the elder what the nurse has said and the nurse what the elder has said without adding meaning or opinion.

An interpreter is needed any time the nurse and the elder speak different languages, when the elder has limited English proficiency, or when cultural tradition prevents the elder from speaking directly to the nurse. The more complex the decision making, the more important the interpreter is, such as when determining the elder's wishes regarding life-prolonging measures.

It is ideal to engage persons who are trained in medical interpretation and who are the same gender and social status as the elder. Ideally the interpreter would be a mature individual so that there are not potential problems of age differences. However, often children are called on to act as interpreters. When doing so the nurse must realize that the child or the elder may "edit" comments because of cultural restrictions about the content (i.e., what is or is not appropriate to speak to parent or child about).

When working with an interpreter the nurse first introduces herself or himself to the client and the interpreter and sets down guidelines for the interview. Sentences should be short, employ the active tense, and avoid metaphors because they may be impossible to convert from one language to another. The nurse asks the interpreter to say exactly what is being said, and all conversation is directly to the client.

For more information see Box 4-2 and refer to the detailed guidelines and protocols available from Enslein and colleagues at the University of Iowa (Enslein et al, 2001, 2002).

IMPLICATIONS FOR GERONTOLOGICAL NURSING AND HEALTHY AGING

The contact between elders and gerontological nurses often begins with assessment. During that time, the nurse and the older adult have an opportunity to come to know each other. Listening is the key to the assessment as the nurse tries to understand the situation, problem, and person. A thorough assessment includes a cultural assessment. A comprehensive cultural assessment takes time. Not all situations allow for this, but even if it must be done bit by bit over time, it will be valuable to the nurse in better understanding

---

Box 4-2 | Hints for Working with Interpreters

Before an interview or session with a client, try to meet with the interpreter to explain the purpose of the session.

Encourage the interpreter to meet with the client before the session to identify the educational level and attitudes toward health and health care and to determine the depth and type of information and explanation needed.

Look and speak directly to the client, not the interpreter.

Be patient. Interpreted interviews take more time because long explanatory phrases often are needed.

Use short units of speech. Long, involved sentences or complex discussions create confusion.

Use simple language. Avoid technical terms, professional jargon, slang, abbreviations, abstractions, metaphors, or idiomatic expressions.

Encourage interpretation of the client's own words rather than paraphrased professional jargon to get a better sense of the client's ideas and emotional state.

Encourage the interpreter to avoid inserting his or her own ideas or omitting information.

Listen to the client and watch nonverbal communication (facial expression, voice intonation, body movement) to learn about emotions regarding a specific topic.

Clarify the client's understanding and the accuracy of the interpretation by asking the client to tell you in his or her own words what he or she understands, facilitated by the interpreter.

Modified from Lipson JG, Dibble SL, Minarik PA, editors: *Culture and nursing care: a pocket guide*, San Francisco, 1996, UCSF School of Nursing Press.

---

how to work with and within the culture of the client.

Several tools or instruments can assist the nurse to elicit health care beliefs and at the same time identify to the nurse his or her own perceptions of the beliefs. The explanatory models developed by Kleinman and associates (1978) and Pfeifferling

Box 4-3	Cultural Assessment Related to Client's Health Problem

The clinician may need to identify others who can facilitate the discussion of the client's problem or problems.

1. How would you describe the problem that has brought you here? (What do you call your problem; does it have a name?)
   a. Who in the community and your family helps you with your problem?
2. How long have you had this problem?
   a. When do you think it started?
   b. What do you think started it?
   c. Do you know anyone else with it?
   d. Tell me what happened to them when dealing with this problem.
3. What do you think is wrong with you?
   a. What does your sickness do to you?
   b. How severe is it?
   c. What might other people think is wrong with you?
   d. Tell me about people who do not get this problem.

4. Why do you think this happened to you?
   a. Why has it happened to the involved part?
   b. Why do you get sick and not someone else?
   c. Will it have a long or short course?
   d. What do you fear most about your sickness?
5. What are the chief problems your sickness has caused you?
6. What do you think will help clear up this problem? (What treatment should you receive; what are the most important results you hope to receive?)
   a. If specific tests, medications are listed, ask what they are and do.
7. Apart from me, who else do you think can make you feel better?
   a. Are there therapies that make you feel better that I do not know (may be in another discipline)?

Modified from Kleinman A: *Patient and healers in the context of culture: an exploration of the borderland between anthropology, medicine, and psychiatry,* Berkeley, 1980, University of California Press; Pfeifferling JH: A cultural prescription for mediocentrism. In Eisenberg L, Kleinman A, editors: *The relevance of social science for medicine,* Boston, 1981, Reidel.

(1981) have helped nurses and other health care professionals obtain needed information in a culturally sensitive manner. An adaptation of these models for use in obtaining a meaningful cultural health assessment appears in Box 4-3. Another framework for a meaningful and more detailed cultural assessment was offered by Evans and Cunningham (1996) and is presented in Table 4-1.

Key information in the assessment is the determination of the health beliefs as discussed earlier. Most people (nurses and patients alike) ascribe to more than one belief system combining Western biomedical approaches with those that may be considered more traditional. People choose from among the beliefs or include several of them in their attempt to make sense of health, illness, and treatments. To optimize the healthy aging of the person who depends on the nurse for intervention and caring, the nurse should learn to be sensitive to the possibility that the person may hold one or more of these beliefs. Significant conflict with nurses may result when a patient refuses biomed-

ical treatments because to do so may be viewed as a sign of disrespect for God (as challenging God's will) or when biomedical treatments are not believed to restore balance. Finding out more about the person's beliefs about disease causation and type of treatments believed to be effective will allow the nurse to work between the cultures of medicine and the person to promote better health.

Working between cultures and health beliefs means developing enough rapport with your patient that he or she is willing to tell you of their beliefs, especially during assessment. It means encouraging and incorporating any practices into the plan of care unless they are clearly detrimental. It also may mean working with traditional or alternative healers if the client believes they are important. Encourage family members to prepare specially enjoyed foods and perform significant rituals. Locate priests, monks, rabbis, or ministers, or indigenous healers if the older adult desires. When alternative healing methods are used, respect them as judiciously as those you may be

Table 4-1 Nursing Care for the Ethnic Elder

	Assessment	Interventions
Ethnicity	Number of years living in United States Age at immigration (immigrant vs. refugee) Degree of affiliation with ethnic group or assimilation to U.S. culture	Be sensitive to historical events that influence elders' perception of self and authority of health care providers. Demonstrate respect for elder by using surname and providing care in a manner sensitive to cultural norms. Use interpretor for exchange of health information.
Communication	English as primary or secondary language Level of fluency Barriers to communication, e.g., sensory deficits, lack of privacy, distractions Meaning of nonverbal gestures	Document system for communicating basic needs between patient and staff. Provide patient access to sensory aids (glasses, hearing aids, pocket talkers). Eliminate background noise, and provide optimum lighting. Smile; offer gestures of assistance with basic needs (warm blanket, glass of water).
Health perception	Perception of health problem, causes, prognosis Response to pain, illness, death	Educate patient/family about disease process and medical treatments. Identify and document reasons for behavior. Develop system for identifying and rating pain.
Folk practices	Use of cultural healers, herbal medicines, alternative health practices and beliefs	Obtain order for use of folk remedies as indicated. Educate patient regarding contraindications for folk remedy and discourage use if dangerous.
Health care system	Previous hospitalization experiences Current hospitalization planned or emergency?	Encourage patient to express fears regarding hospitalization and treatments. Keep patient/family informed of patient's progress.
Religion	Spiritual practices and beliefs Level of incorporation of spiritual practices into healing/dying process	Allow privacy and space for religious articles and practices. Arrange for visit from spiritual leader. Refer patients to hospital chaplain. Document beliefs about death and burial.
Food	Beliefs regarding food and healing Use of hot/cold system Specific food preferences	Obtain consultation with dietitian. Incorporate food preferences into menu selection. Ask family to supply familiar foods. Document use of hot/cold practices as they relate to nursing care.
Social support	Current living situation Support of family and/or community	Encourage family participation in care. Encourage visits or phone calls with peers.
Decision making	Primary decision maker for health care How does the patient make decisions? Who is needed for decisions?	Involve family when providing patient with health care information. Arrange for family conference if disparity exists among goals of patient, family, and/or health care team.
Discharge planning	Expectations for care after hospitalization and during future years of aging Financial status that affects discharge planning and long-term health status Ability of patient/family to support discharge needs	Involve family in discharge planning. Obtain consult for social services. Refer patient to community resources for legal advice, transportation, meals, shopping, and emotional support.

From Evans CA, Cunningham BA: Caring for the ethnic elder. Even when language is not a barrier, patients may be reluctant to discuss their beliefs and practices for fear of criticism or ridicule, *Geriatr Nurs* 17(3):105-110, 1996.

implementing. A sense of caring is conveyed in these gestures of personal recognition. Unbiased caring can surmount cultural differences.

Nurses should not attempt to change the client's beliefs. It is difficult if not impossible and usually is counterproductive. However, negotiating options with the client is helpful. The nurse should attempt to preserve helpful beliefs and practices, accommodate beliefs that are neither helpful nor harmful from the point of Western medicine, or help clients to give up beliefs or practices that have been shown to be harmful (Jackson, 1993). The nurse who has little or no knowledge of a belief or practice should study and evaluate it to determine its helpfulness or its potential harm. In this way beliefs and practices can be preserved. Respectfully explaining concern about harmful client practices with the offer of possible alternatives may show the client that the nurse is considering the client's beliefs and practices. The client is less likely to be dissatisfied and not return for future care.

As consumers of health care, ethnic elders are frequently cared for in the home, and nurses must adapt home care strategies to the beliefs and culture of the individual and the family if they hope to be useful. Nursing concerns must focus on their overall health care by assisting them to gain access to needed services. This is done by ascertaining affordability, efficacy, accessibility, and availability of information; client satisfaction; respect for clients' health beliefs; illness perspective; and informal support systems. See Box 4-4 for several guidelines to nursing interventions for ethnic elders.

Ethnic elders can also be found in senior centers, especially those that have introduced culturally appropriate food and activities. The impact of cultural relativism in a senior center was described by Ochoco and Shimamoto as far back as 1987. They found that many of the participants who were ethnically distinct had been passive, dependent, and depressed during the "usual" center activities. Two thirds of the participants were widowed women who had originally emigrated from Japan and were now highly dependent on their children. By introducing ethnic-related activities at a senior center in Hawaii they were able to increase patient self-esteem, independence, and satisfaction. The community health nurse who activated the group

Box 4-4	Guidelines to Nursing Interventions for Ethnic Elders

Respect the cultural preferences in food, music, and religion.

Design teaching to the vocabulary and attitude of the individual.

Listen attentively to complaints because these may be the clues to health problems.

In people of color, the signs of some disorders may be masked by color (pallor, cyanosis, ecchymosis); buccal cavity coloration is significant.

Base physical assessment on norms for the ethnic group.

Adequate light is especially important in skin assessment for turgor, blemishes, and cyanosis; eye lens, nail beds, palms of hands, and soles of feet can be revealing.

Listen for signs of depression, often in the form of hypochondriasis and apathy.

Inquire about losses and the individual's adaptation to them.

Gather information about lifestyle preferences, and incorporate into care plans.

Inquire about health practices the individual finds effective.

Identify spiritual resources important to the elder, and incorporate in care plan; contact minister and church friends.

wished to strengthen the sense of self in group members through a focus on cultural heritage. In addition to health teaching sessions and education about the aging process, the nurse used reminiscence and construction of a collective oral history to stimulate interaction and the sense of accomplishment (see Chapter 5). This model has been adapted in many community and institutional settings. In providing culturally relevant care the uniqueness of the person is honored.

Ethnicity and Long-Term Care

Long-term care refers to the ongoing assistance provided to persons who are physically or mentally fragile and unable to independently perform their own activities of daily living (ADL). Long-term care may occur in family homes, group homes, assisted living and skilled nursing facilities, or hospices. The preference for where this takes place is culturally influenced. In many cultures outside the United States and subcultures in the United States, families are expected to take care of their older members, and thus there may be a reluctance to utilize institutional long-term care.

Historically, the Japanese did not consider nursing home placement for elderly parents, but the modern *nisei* (second generation) and *sansei* (third generation) face the same dilemmas as others when caring for their elderly parents, despite *issei* (first generation) expectations of *oya koko* or "care for parents" (Kitano, 1969). However, as families become more mobile and all members of the family enter the work force, home care is no longer always possible. This disparity in expectations and what is possible can result in considerable conflict between elders and family members, which in turn is experienced by nursing staff at all levels. As the number of ethnic elders increases in institutions, it puts pressure on staff to develop cultural competence, become culturally welcoming, and learn to deal with cultural differences.

The On Lok Project in San Francisco is the ultimate model of the provision of long-term care services to diverse elders. Originally designed to meet the home care needs of Chinese and Italian immigrants, it now has the capacity of providing every level of short- and long-term care to all persons. Services are provided in the language of the elder and in the manner that optimizes each person's cultural heritage (Bodenheimer, 1999; Kornblatt et al, 2002, 2003). Nurses can learn from the work of On Lok and other programs to enhance the care and encourage the health of ethnic elders.

Modifications of existing long-term care services to enhance the well-being of ethnic elders may include the following:
1. Ensuring that the resident has access to professional interpreter services if needed
2. Developing programs that reflect the diversity of the residents and the staff
3. Considering monocultural facilities or units where population demographics warrant
4. Attempting to employ staff that reflects the diversity of the residents

Cultural diversity of physicians and nurses who are choosing to work in fields of aging or long-term care is increasing. These providers of gerontological care are an increasingly heterogeneous cultural group. The countries from which these providers come vary from one part of the United States to another. The positive aspects of this trend are that they (1) may bring respect for the elder, found in other cultures and less in the youth-driven society of the United States, and (2) may have the language skills and understanding to better care for the elders and families of their own cultural background. The concerns are (1) the complexities of cross-cultural communications and decision making when second languages are used and (2) the use of cultural norms not well understood by each other.

The study of the uniqueness and individuality of each elder is one of the most complex and intriguing opportunities of our day. Realistically it is almost impossible to become familiar with the whole range of clinically relevant cultural differences of older adults one may encounter, but to attempt to serve them holistically and sensitively is the most challenging and potentially satisfying opportunity.

Culture, Nursing, and Maslow's Hierarchy of Needs

Promoting healthy aging in the care of ethnic elders frequently provides the gerontological nurse with new challenges and necessitates a slightly different conceptualization of Maslow's hierarchy. Unfortunately, poverty is very common in many households of persons of color, and meeting basic needs, especially food and health care, may be difficult. Older immigrants who have never worked in the United States will not qualify for Medicare and may not qualify for Medicaid. The nurse must be sensitive to this possibility without making assumptions or stereotyping. The nurse can assess the components of biological integrity and, if necessary, facilitate the elder or family obtaining whatever supports (e.g., food stamps, home-delivered meals) that are possible and appropriate.

Although some ethnic elders have been in the United States their entire lives and their move to the United States was not traumatic, there are many others who have experienced horrific events in their home country or during their immigration process and for whom safety and security may have unique meanings. The staff of a Jewish nursing home complained that it was particularly difficult getting some of the residents with dementia to shower. It was some time before they realized that a number of their residents were Holocaust survivors. As the residents' dementia progressed, they were no longer able to distinguish the difference between a shower for hygiene and the fear of "going to the showers" (i.e., to the gas chamber) in the concentration camps of their youths (Weissman, 2003).

A sense of belonging for the ethnic elder may be closely tied to self-esteem. Cultural identity may be one of the major elements of self-concept and a key to self-esteem and increasingly so as a

person becomes more mentally or physically frail. Often ethnic elders are closely tied to family and community and in some cases religious communities. Estrangement from their country of origin may be ameliorated if they live in homogeneous communities and exacerbated if they live in social isolation or away from persons with similar backgrounds. The ethnic community (e.g., barrios, Nihonmachi, Chinatown) serves as a buffer and a means of strengthening cohesiveness for elders and others of various cultural groups. Within the community, members are protected from discrimination and the strange language and customs of the society outside.

Family, religion, community, and history are important reference points for self-worth and iden-

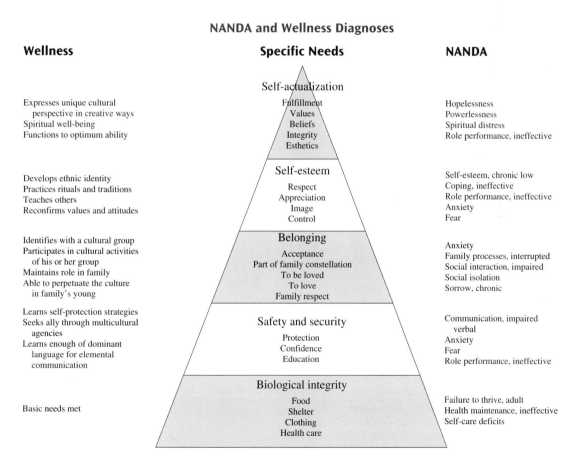

NANDA and Wellness Diagnoses

Wellness	Specific Needs	NANDA
	Self-actualization	
Expresses unique cultural perspective in creative ways	Fulfillment	Hopelessness
Spiritual well-being	Values	Powerlessness
Functions to optimum ability	Beliefs	Spiritual distress
	Integrity	Role performance, ineffective
	Esthetics	
	Self-esteem	
Develops ethnic identity	Respect	Self-esteem, chronic low
Practices rituals and traditions	Appreciation	Coping, ineffective
Teaches others	Image	Role performance, ineffective
Reconfirms values and attitudes	Control	Anxiety
		Fear
Identifies with a cultural group	**Belonging**	
Participates in cultural activities of his or her group	Acceptance	Anxiety
Maintains role in family	Part of family constellation	Family processes, interrupted
Able to perpetuate the culture in family's young	To be loved	Social interaction, impaired
	To love	Social isolation
	Family respect	Sorrow, chronic
Learns self-protection strategies	**Safety and security**	Communication, impaired verbal
Seeks ally through multicultural agencies	Protection	Anxiety
Learns enough of dominant language for elemental communication	Confidence	Fear
	Education	Role performance, ineffective
	Biological integrity	
Basic needs met	Food	Failure to thrive, adult
	Shelter	Health maintenance, ineffective
	Clothing	Self-care deficits
	Health care	

These are not all of the possible wellness or NANDA diagnoses that may be identified. The above are frequent examples of nursing diagnoses that should be considered when planning care for the older adult in whatever setting.

tity for any ethnic group. Familial supports vary among groups, social classes, and subcultures, yet the nuclear or extended family is the chief avenue of transmitting cultural values, beliefs, customs, and practices. The family provides orientation, stability, and often, sanctuary. In a simplistic sense we may say that Asians value familial piety; Hispanics, the extended family (compadres translates to co-parents); African Americans, extended or fictive kin supports; and Native Americans, a system of kinship and line of descent.

Changes are threatening the historical role of the aged and the traditional family. Economic independence and mobility of the younger members of the family are chipping away at the insulation afforded by the community. Intergenerational discontinuities of assimilation create a communication gap between the young and the old. This may cause isolation and estrangement between the oldest and youngest generations. Members of ethnic minorities are extremely vulnerable in old age. They may be devalued because of age and ethnicity. Attitudes and economic inequality contribute to their problems. Nurses can take an active role in facilitating self-actualization by facilitating expression of the uniqueness of the individual, by attending to the elder's spiritual and cultural needs, and by taking the lead at optimizing the abilities of those who seek our care.

▶ **KEY CONCEPTS**

- Population diversity will continue to increase rapidly for many years. This suggests that nurses will be caring for a greater number of ethnic elders than in the past.
- Culture is a complex concept reflecting the interrelationship of many components.
- Culture, social status, and support systems are essential within cultural groups.
- Stereotyping negates the fact that significant heterogeneity exists within cultural groups.
- To increase cultural competence requires cultural awareness, knowledge, and skills.
- Nurses caring for ethnic elders must let go of their ethnocentrism before they can give effective care.
- Many ethnic elders hold health beliefs different from that of the biomedical or Western

system used by most health care professionals in the United States.
- Lack of awareness of the elder's health beliefs has the potential to produce conflict in the nursing situation.
- The more complex the communication or decision-making, the greater the need for skilled interpretor services for persons with limited English proficiency.
- Programs staffed by persons who reflect ethnic elders' background and speak their language are preferred by the elder.

▶ **Activities and Discussion Questions**

1. Discuss your personal beliefs regarding health and illness.
2. Explain the types of questions that would be helpful in assessing an elder's health problem or problems.
3. What strategies would be helpful in planning care for ethnic elders?
4. List the elements that enable the nurse to develop cultural sensitivity and competency.
5. Formulate a nursing care plan utilizing wellness and North American Nursing Diagnosis Association (NANDA) diagnoses.

RESOURCES

Publications

Baker M: Cultural differences in the use of advance directives: a review of the literature, *African Am Res Perspectives* 6(3):35-40, 2002.

Barker J: Recognizing cultural differences: health-care providers and elderly patients, *Gerontol Geriatr Educ* 15(1):9-21, 1994.

Burroughs VJ, Maxey RW, Levy RA: Racial and ethnic differences in response to medicines: towards individualized pharmaceutical treatment, *J Natl Med Assoc* 94(10, suppl):1-26, 2002.

Cortis J: Caring as experienced by minority ethnic patients, *Int Nurs Rev* 47(1):53-62, 2000.

Gibson R, Stoller E: *Worlds of difference: inequalities in the aging experience*, 2002, Thousand Oaks, CA, Pine Forks Publishing.

Kobylarz F, Hernandez G, Hurwitz E: Culturally-sensitive decision making in end-of-life care, *Annals of Long-Term Care* 10(8):40-42, 2002.

Mazanec P, Tyler MK: Cultural considerations in end-of-life care: how ethnicity, age, and spirituality affect decisions when death is imminent, *Am J Nurs* 103(3):50-58, 2003.

McCarty LJ, Enslein JC, Kelley LS et al: Cross-cultural health education: materials on the world wide web, *J Transcult Nurs* 13(1):54-60, 2002.

Tripp-Reimer T, Choi E, Kelley LS et al: Cultural barriers to care: inverting the problem, *Diabetes Spectrum* 14(1):13-22, 2001.

Organizations

National Asian Pacific Center on Aging
Melbourn Tower, Suite 914
1151 Third Avenue
Seattle, WA 98101
(800) 33-NACPA

National Center on Black Aged (NCBA)
1730 M Street NW, Suite 811
Washington, DC 20020

National Hispanic Council on Aging
2713 Ontario Road NW
Washington, DC 20009

National Indian Council on Aging (NICOA)
P.O. Box 2088
Albuquerque, NM 87103

Websites

www.aoa.gov
Then click on "professionals" then "addressing diversity" for another set of statistics and resources and links.

www.aoa.gov/minorityaccess
Stats related to health.

www.aoa.gov/prof/adddiv/cultural/addiv_cult.asp
Achieving Cultural Competence: a Guidebook for Providers of Services to Older Americans and Their Families. Contains text and down-loadable slides.

www.census.gov
See "factfinder" for the most current statistical information available from the U.S. Census Bureau.

www.diversityRx.org
Information, links, down-loadable documents regarding culture and linguistic competence.

www.gasi.org/
Then click on the "diversity" section. Worth a trip—lots of good culture-specific information, such as what to call people.

www.health.qld.gov.au/hssb/cultdiv
The Queensland government (Australia) website with lots of good and helpful information, especially about cross-cultural communication.

www.hhs.gov/ocr
Office of Civil Rights—key information about discrimination and links regarding cultural diversity.

www.lastacts.org
Key word "diversity." End-of-life issues website. See site to obtain excellent document "Last Acts Statement on Diversity and End-Of-Life Care" describing end-of-life issues specific to a number of cultural groups.

www.nccj.org
National Conference for Community and Justice. They advocate for reducing disparities in the name of justice and have an initiative.

www.ncmhd.nih.gov
National Center on Minority Health and Health Disparities, National Institutes of Health (NIH) reporting on the latest research and funding opportunities.

www.omhrc.gov
Office of Minority Health with a wealth of information on persons of any age.

www.stanford.edu
Then search GEC. The Stanford Geriatric Education Center has a series of modules related to various ethnic groups. See their website for a complete listing and ordering information.

www.un.org/esa
The United Nations website—interesting to browse through.

Films

The Angry Heart: the Impact of Racism on Heart Disease Among African Americans. By Jay Fedigan. Available from Fanlight Productions: www.fanlight.com.

The Color of Fear. A film by Lee Mun Wah available from www.stirfryseminars.com. If you search under the title you will also find a number of discussion groups, critiques, and other materials related to the use of this film. Cost: $110 to $460.

Famous Irish Americans. A film by Roger Beebee. Approximately $20 from the filmmaker at rogerbb@english.ufl.edu.

Sources of videos

www.newsreel.org

www.pbs.org/race

www.viewingrace.org
A site of important sources of information about race issues.

REFERENCES

Berlin EA, Fowkes WC: A teaching framework for cross-cultural health care: application in family practice, *West J Med* 139(6):934-938, 1983.

Bodenheimer T: Long term care for frail elderly people—the On Lok model, *N Engl J Med* 341(17):1324-1328, 1999.

Cole T: *The journey of life: cultural history of aging in America*, Cambridge, England, 1997, Cambridge University Press.

Enslein J et al: *Evidence-based protocol: interpreter facilitation for persons with limited English proficiency.* Research Dissemination Core Product, 2001. Available from the University of Iowa Gerontological Nursing Interventions Research Center.

Enslein J, Tripp-Reimer T, Kelley LS et al: Evidence-based protocol: interpreter facilitation for individuals with limited English proficiency, *J Gerontol Nurs* 28(7):5-13, 2002.

Evans CA, Cunningham BA: Caring for the ethnic elder, *Geriat Nurs* 17(3):105, 1996.

Gelfand D: *Aging and ethnicity: knowledge and service*, ed 2, New York, 2003, Springer.

Grossman D: Enhancing your cultural competence, *Am J Nurs* 94(7):58-60, 1994.

Haffner L: Translation is not enough. Interpreting in a medical setting, *West J Med* 157(3):255-259, 1992.

Jackson LE: Understanding, eliciting, and negotiating clients' multicultural health beliefs, *Nurse Pract* 18(4): 30-32, 37-38, 41-43, 1993.

Kitano H: *Japanese Americans*, Englewood Cliffs, NJ, 1969, Prentice-Hall.

Kleinman A, Eisenberg L, Good B: Culture, illness, and care: clinical lessons from anthropologic and cross-cultural research, *Ann Intern Med* 88(2):251-258, 1978.

Kornblatt S, Cheng S, Chan S: Best practices: the On-Lok Model of geriatric interdisciplinary team care. In Howe, JL. *Older people and their caregivers across the spectrum of care*, Binghamton, NY, 2002, Haworth Social Work, pp 15-22.

Kornblatt S, Eng C, Hansen JC: Cultural awareness in health and social services: the experience of On Lok. *Generations* 26(3):46-53, 2003.

McIntosh P: White privilege: unpacking the invisible knapsack. Working paper #189. Wellesley College Center for Research on Women. Available at www.utoronto.ca/acc/events/peggy1.htm.

Ochoco L, Shimamoto Y: Group work with the frail ethnic elderly, *Geriatr Nurs* 8(4):185-187, 1987.

Pfeifferling JH: A cultural prescription for medicentrism. In Eisenberg L, Kleinman A, editors: *The relevance of social science for medicine*, Boston, 1981, Reidel.

Smedley B, Stith, Nelson A, editors: *Unequal treatment: confronting racial and ethnic disparities in health care.* Special report, Institute of Medicine, Washington, DC, 2002, National Academy Press.

Spector RE: *Cultural diversity in health and illness,* ed 6, Upper Saddle River, NJ, 2003, Prentice-Hall Health.

Weisman, G. Personal communication. April 10, 2004.

5

Developing the Life History

LEARNING OBJECTIVES

Upon completion of this chapter, the reader will be able to:

- Understand the significance of the life story of an elder.
- Discuss the modalities of reminiscence and life review.
- Identify several possible legacies and discuss the importance to elders.
- Discuss ways in which nurses can come to know the story of elders to promote individualized care.

GLOSSARY

Ideological A body of ideas characteristic of an individual, group, or culture.

Life review A critical analysis of one's past life with the goal of facilitating integrity.

Reminiscence Sharing of memories.

THE LIVED EXPERIENCE

You know, coming to this group has made me remember things I had forgotten long ago. I told them about working with my father to deliver ice in a horse-drawn wagon, my adventures as a WWII fighter pilot, and all the interesting people I met when I drove a taxi in New York. Why I even met Eleanor Roosevelt and Harry Truman. One day I got out my old uniform and medals and brought them to the day program. I hadn't thought about those things in years, and I think it's helped my memory. I really have had a pretty interesting life.

Sam, age 90

Sam was so quiet when the group first started, he seemed depressed about his memory loss. Now he is the life of the group and has such interesting things to say. It's nice to see him enjoying life again, and I really have learned a lot of history from listening to him. He was quite a guy. You can sure learn a lot about a person listening to their memories. It makes me sad that I don't know more about my own family and their history.

Shelly, a volunteer in the day program, age 21

THE LIFE STORY

The life story as constructed through reminiscing, journaling, psychotherapy, or guided autobiography has held great fascination for gerontologists in the last quarter century. The universal appeal of the life story as a vehicle of culture, a demonstration of caring and generational continuity, and an easily stimulated activity has held allure for many professionals. Stories are a gift in that they image those life events most dear to the storyteller. Stories are an invaluable means of coming to know the beauty, wholeness, and uniqueness of the person (Boykin et al, 1998). Stories are important; as Robert Coles (1989, p 7) states: "The people who come to see us bring us their stories. They hope that they tell them well enough so that we understand the truth of their lives. They hope we understand how to interpret their stories correctly."

The literature is vast, and some especially good sources for further study are cited at the end of this chapter. The work of Haight and Webster (1995, 2002) is among the most comprehensive emanating from the nursing profession. Cole (1992), Birren and Deutchman (1991), and Birren and Cochran (2001) have also been influential in describing the importance of seeking life stories. The International Institute for Reminiscence and Life Review, an interdisciplinary organization bringing together participants to study reminiscence and life review, is another valuable resource for nurses and members of other disciplines involved in research or practice in the field.

Life History

An older person is a living history book, but unlike written history, the story remains flexible and changeable, similar to a kaleidoscope. Each shift, however minor, in the person's self-esteem or interaction brings forth another pattern and colorful image. The most exciting aspect of working with older adults is being a part of the emergence of the life story: the shifting and blending patterns. When we are young, it is important for our emotional health and growth to look forward and plan for the future. As one ages, it becomes more important to look back, talk over experiences, review and make sense of it all, and end with a feeling of satisfaction with the life lived. This is very important work and the major developmental task of older adulthood that Erik Erikson called ego integrity versus self despair. Ego integrity is achieved when the person has accepted both the triumphs and disappointments of life and is at peace and satisfied with the life lived (Erikson, 1963).

A memory is an incredible gift given to the nurse, a sharing of a part of oneself when one may have little else to give. The more personal memories are saved for persons who will patiently wait for their unveiling and who will treasure them. Especially with older adults, listening to stories is a more complete way to know them. Older people bring us complex stories derived from long years of living. Through attentiveness to the stories of those cared for, the gerontological nurse can unfold many wraps of life that influence the present experiences and enhance person-focused care (Boykin et al, 1998). "Storytelling can be thought of as a way of caring: caring for the individual who is telling the story by providing a vehicle for looking over his or her life, and caring for the listener who gains from the wisdom of the storyteller's experiences" (Maloney, 1995, p 108).

Creating a Life History

Becoming whole requires that one integrate all of life's remembered experience into a self-concept that sustains or enhances self-esteem and gives meaning to life as lived. Numerous gerontological nurses have used reminiscence, individually and in groups, as a therapeutic strategy to achieve these goals. Because reminiscence is such a natural function of many elders, it is one of the simplest and most enriching for elder and nurse. Working with older adults in the most mutually satisfying manner requires some knowledge of the individual's life history.

Development of a Life Line
The classic writing of Back and Bourque (1970) suggested that it may be useful to have clients graphically represent life in terms of highs, lows, and plateaus experienced at various ages. Development of a life line in which each decade is marked and important events are placed at appropriate times and places is also useful; noting the feelings and impact of these events may create new understanding. The nurse may then match

the client's life history against the graphical representation to gain a clearer understanding of events, patterns, and the impact of experiences. Development is facilitated by examining the peaks and valleys in one's life and recognizing patterns.

Geographical Memories

Geographical memories of places once lived, sketching or drawing these places, reexperiencing the effect of events attached to places—all are significant to stability of self (Rubinstein, 1996b). The social and physical settings of remembered episodes are potent. Developing a residential life history may have unexpected benefits in revealing surroundings significant to individuality and feelings of attachment and loss. During these activities the awareness of self is continually growing. This may also give a sense of the environmental supports that are particularly meaningful to the elder during translocation experiences.

Collective Histories

The use of a life history and reminiscence for older learners in group and classroom settings is useful in many ways. Often the collective memories are compiled into booklets that convey the experiences of a particular era or place. The reminiscing of elders attending classes in adult education or community college programs may reveal common connections between early life and present interests. With the increased recognition of the value of life history, many organizations such as senior centers and local colleges and universities offer opportunities to participate in life history activities.

Creation of Self Through Journaling

The central activity of humans is creating meaning. Through the personal journal one can, in thoughtful reflection, discover meaning and patterns in daily events. The self becomes a coherent story with successive revisions as old events are reread and perceived in new contexts. The journals of certain elders provide rich descriptions of the interior lives of the authors. May Sarton (1984) and Florida Scott-Maxwell (1968) are two of the most well known. The study of their journals, as well as those of less well-known and less articulate elders, assists nurses in understanding the inner experiences of older people and, perhaps, their own. Encouraging older people to keep a journal (or tape record) can foster continued growth and development and serve as a legacy to others.

Seeking Wisdom

Reflecting on one's life story touches not only the mind but also the imagination and the unconscious depths in a person. The wisdom of old age develops from the ability to elicit new meanings from prior experience. Unlike ordinary knowledge, wisdom leads to an appreciation of reality in its grandest sense. The wisdom of old age involves a crisis of explanation in which the ordinary structures of thought are shaken and the meaning of life is reexamined. It may include the wisdom of questioning assumptions in the search for meaning. This is the rich, self-actualized experience that Maslow identifies as the highest level of human need.

REMINISCING

Reminiscing is an umbrella term that can include any recall of the past. Robert Butler (2002) pointed out that 50 years ago, reminiscing was thought to be a sign of senility or what we now call Alzheimer's disease. Old people who talked about the past and told the same stories again and again were said to be boring and living in the past. From Butler's seminal research (1963), we now know that reminiscence is the most important psychological task of older people. The work of several gerontological nursing leaders, including Irene Burnside, Priscilla Ebersole, and Barbara Haight, has contributed to the body of knowledge about reminiscence and its importance in nursing. Box 5-1 lists several ways that memories and reminiscences can be used effectively for the enrichment of the aging process.

Reminiscing occurs from childhood onward, particularly at life's junctures and transitions. Reminiscing cultivates a sense of security through recounting of comforting memories, belonging through sharing, and self-esteem through confirmation of uniqueness. For the nurse, reminiscing is a therapeutic intervention important in assessment and understanding.

Box 5-1	Suggested Applications of Memories

Life story recording for family (audiotaped or
  videotaped)
Legacy identification
  Products
  Contributions
  Qualities of character
  Talents
Scrapbooks
Photo albums
Establishment of rituals of security and comfort
Work history
Life's turning points—can be mapped out as a
  road map
Fantasy trips—follow the alternate road
Grief resolution
History of homes
Mapping of life geographically
Historical events—cohort identification
Life history of significant persons and why
  significant
Sensory stimulation
Development of memory chains
Inventory of significant items and why
  significant—to whom would he or she like to
  give them?
Dietary history (significant foods of the past
  may stimulate appetite)
Resolution of disappointment
Entertainment

Box 5-2	Reminiscence as a Developmental and Therapeutic Strategy

Maintain continuity.
Extract meaning.
Define and develop personal philosophy.
Identify cycles and themes.
Recapitulate learning and growth.
Enhance self-worth and feeling of
  accomplishment.
Evolve identity.
Provide insight and growth.
Integrate and accept regrets and
  disappointments.
Perceive universality.

Reminiscence can have many goals. It not only provides a pleasurable experience that improves quality of life, but also increases socialization and connectedness with others, provides cognitive stimulation, improves communication, and can be an effective therapy for depressive symptoms (Bohlmeijer et al, 2003; Haight, Burnside, 1993). Reminiscence is important to personal development and is also a very accessible activity with therapeutic implications, as can be seen in Box 5-2. The process of reminiscence can be structured as in a nursing history, or it can occur in a group where each person shares memories and listens to others share memories (Haight, Burnside, 1993). The nurse can learn much about a resident's history, communication style, relationships, coping mechanisms, strengths, fears, affect, and adaptive capacity by listening thoughtfully as the life story is constructed. Box 5-3 provides some suggestions for encouraging reminiscence. The concept of reminiscence also fits well with mechanisms of crisis and grief resolution and is a fitting tool to use to accomplish some of the work in these situations (see Chapters 25 and 26). Group work techniques and the role of the nurse as a group leader are discussed in Chapter 3.

Life Review

Robert Butler (1963) first noted and brought to public attention the review process that normally occurs in the older person as the realization of one's approaching death creates a resurgence of unresolved conflicts. Butler called this process *life review*. Life review occurs quite naturally for many persons during periods of crisis and transition; however, Butler (2002) noted that in old age, putting one's life in order increases in intensity and emphasis. Life review occurs most frequently as an internal review of memories, an intensely private, soul-searching activity. It often occurs sporadically in a long-term trusted relationship.

The goals of life review (Butler, 2002, p 2) include the following:

. . . resolution of past conflicts and issues, atonement for past acts or inaction, and reconciliation with family members or friends . . . The overall benefit of a life review is that it can engender hard-won serenity, a philosophical acceptance of what has occurred in the past, and wisdom. When

Box 5-3   Suggestions for Encouraging Reminiscence

- Listen without correction or criticism. Older adults are presenting their version of their reality; our version belongs to another generation.
- Encourage older adults to cover various ages and stages. Use questions such as "What was it like growing up on that farm?" "What did teenagers do for fun when you were young?" "What was WWII like for you?"
- Be patient with repetition. Sometimes people need to tell the same story often to come to terms with the experience, especially if it was very meaningful to them. If they have a memory loss, it may be the only story they can remember and it is important for them to be a member of the group and contribute. If group members seem bothered by repetition, be sure to acknowledge the person's contribution and then direct conversation to include others.
- Be attuned to signs of depression in conversation (dwelling on sad topics) or changes in physical status or behavior and provide appropriate assessment and intervention.
- Keep in mind that reminiscing is not an orderly process. One memory triggers another in a way that may not seem related; it is not important to keep things in order or verify accuracy.
- Keep the conversation focused on the person reminiscing, but do not hesitate to share some of your own memories that relate to the situation being discussed. Participate as equals, and enjoy each other's contributions.

- Listen actively, maintain eye contact, do not interrupt.
- Respond positively and give feedback by making caring, appropriate comments that encourage the person to continue.
- Use props and triggers such as photographs, memorabilia (e.g., a childhood toy or antique), short stories or poems about the past, favorite foods.
- Use open-ended questions to encourage reminiscing. You can prepare questions ahead of time, or you can ask the group to pick a topic that interests them. One question or topic may be enough for an entire group session. Consider using questions such as the following:

How did your parents meet?
What do you remember most about your mother? father? grandmother? grandfather?
What are some of your favorite memories from childhood?
What was the first house you remember?
What were your favorite foods as a child?
Did you have a pet as a child?
Tell me about your first job.
How did you celebrate birthdays or other holidays?
Tell me about your wedding day.
What was your greatest accomplishment or joy in your life?
What advice did your parents give you? What advice did you give your children? What advice would you give to young people today?

people resolve their life conflicts, they have a lively capacity to live in the present.

Life review should not occur only when we are old or facing death but should be engaged in frequently throughout our lives. This process can assist us to examine where we are in life and change our course or set new goals. Butler commented that one might avoid the overwhelming feelings of despair that may surface when there is no time left to make changes.

Life review can be considered a psychotherapeutic process or technique and involves the review of remote memories (self-revelation), the expression of related feelings (catharsis), the recognition of conflicts (insight), and the relinquishment of viewpoints that are self-inhibiting (decathexis). The process of life review is very directive and structured and occurs on a one-to-one basis. Gerontological nurses participate with older adults in both reminiscence and life review, and it is important to acquire the skills to be effective in achieving the purposes of both.

Life review therapy (Butler, Lewis, 1983), guided autobiography (Birren, Deutchman, 1991), and structured life review (Haight, Webster, 1995) are psychotherapeutic techniques based on the concept of life review. An important setting for life review therapy is in hospice and palliative care. The Hospice Foundation of America published

A Guide for Recalling and Telling Your Life Story that nurses and families may find helpful (http://www.hospicefoundation.org). When working with the elderly in a life review process, it is important to have a clear understanding of goals:

1. Is the person reviewing the life course preparatory to letting go? If so, the main goal will be acceptance of what has been.
2. Is the individual facing a major crisis in self-esteem or need? The goal will be to identify past coping strategies and, from those, gather strategies that will be currently effective. Evaluating times when one was effective will sustain confidence in future effectiveness.
3. Is the individual bound in a morass of regret? The goal will be to reenergize the person for present and future functioning by developing alternative views of past failures.
4. Is the individual suffering the effects of institutionalization? The goal will be to stimulate clear memories of what one has been and has accomplished to reaffirm uniqueness and individuality.
5. Has the person held long-standing grievances against significant others? The goal will be to explore the complexity of those relationships and provide opportunities for interpersonal resolution with the individuals involved.

These and many other exploratory statements will facilitate the life review. Do not ask if you are not prepared to listen carefully and without judgment or advice. It is usually helpful to begin with descriptions of events, since those are less threatening than sharing fears, failures, and feelings. During any interview it is important to comment on increasing evidence of anxiety and tension and ask if the interviewee wishes to continue, to sit quietly, or to be left alone. When life review occurs during group reminiscing, it can produce anxiety or agitation in the individual. In that situation we would verbally validate the discomfort and move the focus to another group member by saying, "I can see that this was a very difficult experience for you. When the group is over, I would like to spend a few minutes alone with you." Sometimes memories are painful and may produce tears or lead to anxiety, guilt, or depression. The nurse must be skilled in providing support and appropriate interventions and referrals if indicated. Box 5-4 provides guidelines for life review therapy.

Reminiscing and Storytelling with Individuals Experiencing Cognitive Impairment

Cognitive impairment does not necessarily preclude older adults from participating in reminiscence or storytelling groups. Opportunities for telling the life story, enjoying memories, and achieving ego integrity and self-actualization should not be denied to individuals based on their cognitive status. Modifications must be made based on the cognitive abilities of the person, and although individual life review from a psychotherapeutic approach is not an appropriate modality, individuals with mild to moderate memory impairment can enjoy and benefit from group work focused on reminiscence and storytelling.

When the nurse is working with a group of cognitively impaired older adults, the emphasis in reminiscence groups is on sharing memories, however they may be expressed, rather than specific recall of events. There should be no pressure to answer questions such as "Where were you born?" or "What was your first job?" Rather, discussions may center on jobs people had and places they have lived. Additional props, such as music, pictures, and familiar objects (e.g., an American flag, an old coffee grinder), can prompt many recollections and sharing. The leader of a group with participants who have memory problems needs to be more active. Many resources are available to guide these groups, including books such as *I Remember When* (Thorsheim, Roberts, 2000), that offer numerous ways to adapt the reminiscing process for those with cognitive impairment. Other helpful resources are listed at the end of the chapter.

Bastings (2003) has described a storytelling modality designed for individuals with cognitive impairment called *Time Slips*. Group members, looking at a picture, are encouraged to create a story about the picture. The pictures can be fantastical and funny, such as from greeting cards, or more nostalgic, such as Norman Rockwell paintings. All contributions are encouraged and welcomed, there are no right or wrong answers, and everything that the individuals say is included in the story and written down by the scribe. Stories are read back to the participants during the session, using their names to identify their contributions. At the beginning of each session, the story from the last session is read to the participants. Care is

Box 5-4	Guidelines for Life Review Therapy

1. Share with older adults the characteristics and normalcy of the life review process.
2. Provide opportunities for older adults to recapitulate events in their lives (e.g., "What has most influenced the course of your life?" "Who has most influenced the course of your life?").
3. Assist older adults to view their life experiences in a broader or different context (e.g., "As you explain your regrets, can you think of other factors that contributed to those events?" "How would you have changed your life then?" "What factors influenced your course of action?" "What would you do differently now, and what difference might it have made?")
4. Facilitate connections among past hopes, present events, and future expectations.
5. Be aware that the process may be carried out sporadically over several months. It can be a painful examination of the past and is sometimes avoided. Be open and encourage sharing, but do not force it.
6. As difficult events are remembered, focus on affirming and acknowledging the strengths of the person. Coping strategies that got them

through can be brought forward to deal with current difficulties.
7. Conflicts or regrets may emerge, and the process may assist the individual to come to terms with these feelings or events. This may involve reconciling with an estranged friend or family member, or it may mean forgiving oneself or another and letting go of the negative feelings associated with the memory. This may give new meaning to life and assist in preparation for death by decreasing anger, fear, and anxiety.
8. Life review can be thought of as a time of "sorting," a time of doing a "balance sheet" and ending up with the feeling that despite some rocky times, people did the best they could. The outcome of life review is to achieve resolution, celebrate a life well lived, provide hope, and encourage personal growth and integrity.
9. Goals of life review include integrity, resolution of conflicts, serenity and peace, and preparation for death.
10. Life review therapy requires a skilled listener with knowledge and experience in psychotherapeutic techniques.

taken to compliment each member for his or her contribution to the wonderful story. The stories created are full of humor and creativity and often include discussions of memories and reminiscing. John Killick (1999, p 49), writer in residence at a nursing home in Scotland, stated: "Having their words written down is empowering for people with dementia. It affirms their dignity and gives an assurance that their words still have value . . . One woman said, 'Anything you can tell people about how things are for me is important. It's a rum do, this growing ancient . . . The brilliance of my brain has slipped away when I wasn't looking.'"

One of the authors (TT) has used the storytelling modality extensively with mild to moderately impaired older people with great success as part of a research study on the effect of therapeutic activities for persons with memory loss. Potential outcomes include increased verbalization and communication, socialization, alleviation of depression, and enhanced quality of life. Qualita-

tive responses from group participants and families indicate their enjoyment with the process. At the end of the 16-week group, the stories are bound into a book and given to the participants with a picture of the group with each member's name listed. Many of the participants and their families have commented on the pride they feel at their "book" and have even shared them with grandchildren and great-grandchildren. In Basting's work (Bastings, 2003), some of the stories were presented as a play. Although further research is indicated in relation to the outcomes of this intervention, it seems to have potential as a beneficial and cost-effective therapeutic intervention in many settings.

LEGACIES

A legacy is one's tangible and intangible assets that are transferred to another and that may survive the bequeather's mortality. Both giver and receiver are part of the concept of legacy; a recipient, individually or collectively, is essential (Frolik, 1996; Kivnick, 1996). Doers leave their products and live through them. Powerful figures are remembered in fame and infamy. The quiet, unobtrusive person survives in the memory of intimates and in family anecdotes. The intangible, nonmaterial legacy of our elders is embodied in the courage, wisdom, and insights that they show. The search for immortality seems to be the basic motivation for leaving a legacy. Characteristics of older adults significant to legacy development are seen in Box 5-5.

Throughout life, shared experiences provide satisfaction, but in the last years the identification of a legacy allows one to gain a clearer perspective on how one's existence has had enduring meaning. Older people must be encouraged to identify that which they would like to leave and whom they wish the recipients to be. This process has interpersonal significance and prepares one to leave the world with a sense of having truly lived. It can provide a transcendent feeling of continuation and ties with survivors. If transfers of significant items are made before death, the individual has the joy of seeing another appreciate treasured objects (Tobin, 1996). However, many families are reluctant to discuss the transfer of cherished belongings, because it brings one into direct awareness of the death of the elder. Many older people would welcome the opportunity to talk about this with their families, and the nurse should encourage both in this effort.

Childless individuals are becoming more prevalent with each passing generation, and they must find a way to outlive the self through a legacy. Many choose a "social" legacy (Rubinstein, 1996a). Florence Nightingale would be one such person. The legacy of her thinking and accomplishments has influenced and will influence nurses for generations to come (Macrae, 1995).

Legacies are diverse and may range from memories that will live on in the minds of others to bequeathed fortunes. The list is as diverse as individual contributions to humanity. Legacies are both generative and integrative. The activity involved in legacy identification reinforces integrity and life satisfaction. Certain questions, such as the following, may stimulate thoughts and discussions of legacies:

Box 5-5	**Special Characteristics of Older Adults**

- Desire to leave a legacy provides a sense of continuity.
- "Elder" function is a natural propensity of the old to share with the young accumulated knowledge and experience.
- Attachment to familiar objects gives a sense of continuity; aids the memory; and provides comfort, security, and satisfaction.
- Change in the sense of time is experienced as a sense of immediacy, of here and now, of living in the moment.
- Older adults have a personal sense of the entire life cycle.
- Creativity, curiosity, and surprise may promote active and productive lives in the absence of disease and social problems.
- Feeling of consummation or fulfillment in life that brings "serenity" and "wisdom."

- Have you thought of writing your autobiography?
- What would you like to leave the younger generation?
- What contributions have you made in your life that particularly please you?

Legacies Expressed Through Others

There are many ways that one's legacy is expressed through the development of others: in a teaching/learning situation or through mentorships, patronage, shared talents, and organ donations. Some examples may illustrate this type of legacy:

- An aged man cried as he talked of his grandson's great talent as a violinist. They shared their love for the violin, and the grandfather believed that he had genetically and personally contributed to his grandson's development as a musician.
- An older woman worried about preserving the environment for future generations, so she took young children on nature walks to stimulate their interest in birds, plants, and animals. She also donated land for a natural park.

Some creative works and research studies are evolving legacies, left to successive generations

NANDA and Wellness Diagnoses

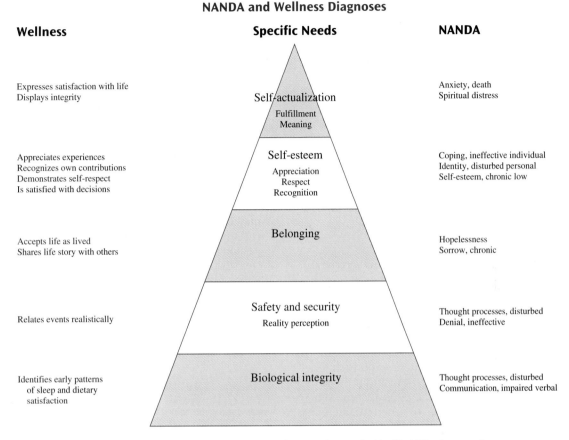

Wellness	Specific Needs	NANDA
Expresses satisfaction with life Displays integrity	Self-actualization Fulfillment Meaning	Anxiety, death Spiritual distress
Appreciates experiences Recognizes own contributions Demonstrates self-respect Is satisfied with decisions	Self-esteem Appreciation Respect Recognition	Coping, ineffective individual Identity, disturbed personal Self-esteem, chronic low
Accepts life as lived Shares life story with others	Belonging	Hopelessness Sorrow, chronic
Relates events realistically	Safety and security Reality perception	Thought processes, disturbed Denial, ineffective
Identifies early patterns of sleep and dietary satisfaction	Biological integrity	Thought processes, disturbed Communication, impaired verbal

These are not all of the possible wellness or NANDA diagnoses that may be identified. The above are frequent examples of nursing diagnoses that should be considered when planning care for the older adult in whatever setting.

for continued modification and growth (Philip, 1995). In other words, one's legacy may be a product of his or her own thought, brought to fruition through someone else who may become an intermediary in the further development of the product or thought. A professor emeritus spoke of visiting his son in a distant state and hearing him expound ideas that had been partially developed by his father, the professor, before him. Thus people and generations are tied in sequential development. People who amass a fortune and allocate certain funds for the endowment of artists, scientific projects, and intellectual exploration are counting on others to complete their legacy.

Developing a Legacy

The following are suggestions for assisting elders in identifying and developing their legacy:
1. Find out the older person's lifelong interests.
2. Establish a method of recording.
3. Identify recipients—either generally or specifically.
4. Record the person's legacy.
5. Distribute as planned.
6. Provide for systematic feedback of results to the person.

It is gratifying to the elderly if a legacy can be converted into some tangible form, ensuring that it will not be readily dismissed or forgotten. The following vehicles often serve that function:

- Published summation of life work
- Photograph albums, scrapbooks
- Written memoirs
- Taped memoirs (video or audio)
- Artistic representations
- Memory gardens
- Mementos
- Genealogies
- Recorded pilgrimages

See Chapter 26 for additional discussion of legacies.

IMPLICATIONS FOR GERONTOLOGICAL NURSING AND HEALTHY AGING

The greatest privilege a nurse has is to accompany an aged individual in the final journey of life (Cole, 1992). As each person confronts individual mortality, there is a need to integrate events and to then transcend the self. The human experience, the person's contributions, and the poignant anecdotes within the life story bind generations together, validate the uniqueness of each brief journey in this level of awareness, and provide the assurance that one will not be forgotten. When the nurse takes the time to listen to an older person share memories and life stories, it communicates respect and valuing of the individual and his or her life as something very important to be treasured. What more can one ask at the end of life than to know that who one is and what one has accomplished are meaningful personally and to others? This characterizes the final tasks of life—ego integrity and self-actualization.

▶ KEY CONCEPTS

- In a rapidly changing society the shared life histories of elders provide a sense of continuity among the generations.
- The life history of an individual is a story to be developed and treasured. This is particularly important toward the end of life.
- Personal integration of life events through reminiscing facilitates acceptance of life as lived.
- Wisdom is achieved through integration, revision, and reconsideration of experiences and knowledge.

- Life review is the spontaneous recollection of guilt and disappointments and can be a growth experience when nonjudgmental, supportive persons are available.
- Establishing a legacy allows the individual to develop a sense of immortality and is a significant late-life task.

▶ Activities and Discussion Questions

1. Listen to the life story of one of your older relatives, and discuss the significance to you and to the elder.
2. Discuss your earliest memories and how they may or may not have shaped your life.
3. Discuss with your peer group the concept of wisdom and how it is shown.
4. Discuss the elements of life review that are different from ordinary remembering.
5. How would you encourage someone to record his or her life story?
6. Discuss your ideas about legacy, and define a legacy that you would like to leave to others.

RESOURCES

Publications

Akeret R: *Photolanguage: how photos reveal the fascinating stories of our lives and relationships,* New York, 2000, WW Norton & Co.

Albom M: *Tuesdays with Morrie,* New York, 1997, Doubleday.

Bastings A, Killick J: *The arts and dementia care: a resource guide.* Available from the National Center for Creative Aging, 138 Oxford Street, Brooklyn, NY 11217, (718-398-3870). Website: http://www.creativeaging.org.

Gibson F: *Using reminiscence in health and social care,* Baltimore, 2004, Health Professions Press.

Murphy C: *It started with a sea shell: life story work and people with dementia,* Stirling, UK, 1994, Dementia Services Centre, University of Stirling.

Rainer T: *Your life as a story: discovering the "new autobiography" and writing memoir as literature,* New York, 1997, Penguin Putnam.

Organizations

International Society for Reminiscence and Life Review

Center for Continuing Education/Extension

University of Wisconsin-Superior
P.O. Box 2000
Superior, WI 54880-4500
(800) 370-9882
website: http://www.reminiscenceandlifereview.org

National Center for Creative Aging
138 S. Oxford Street
Brooklyn, NY 11217
(718) 398-3870
website: http://www.creativeaging.org

National Time Slips Project
Center on Age & Community
P.O. Box 413
Milwaukee, WI 53211
(414) 229-2740
website: http://www.timeslips.org

Films

Emil and Fifi: the Story of My Grandfather. An image of aging videotaped by a grandson of Emil Synek, a Czech playwright, journalist, and statesman, and Emil's constant companion, Fifi, a poodle (50 minutes). Filmakers Library (http://www.filmakers.com).

Giants of Time. Celebrates elders whose lives have already spanned two centuries and who are approaching their third (57 minutes). Filmakers Library (http://www.filmakers.com).

Life Review. Video illustrating the therapeutic process of life review and the use of living history. Available from Connecticut Association of Therapeutic Recreation Directors, Inc. (www.catrd.com/resources/videos).

May Sarton: Writing in the Upward Years. A 30-minute documentary focuses on the role of aging in the creative process and, in particular, how it has affected Sarton's life and writing. Available from Terra Nova Films (http://www.terranova.org).

Reminiscence Through Music. Video illustrating the therapeutic effects of music, group interaction, and practical musical interventions for residents of long-term care facilities. Available from Connecticut Association of Therapeutic Recreation Directors, Inc. (www.catrd.com/resources/videos).

Reminiscing: Reaching Back, Moving Forward. Video featuring how reminiscence can be used as a therapeutic tool. Available from Connecticut Association of Therapeutic Recreation Directors, Inc. (www.catrd.com/resources/videos).

In Times Past: Radio Days. An entertaining history of the golden days of radio bringing back many wonderful memories. Available from Terra Nova Films (http://www.terranova.org).

Games and Kits

The Baby Boomer Memory Bank (http://www.boomerbaby.com) and *The Fifties Web Site* (http://www.fiftiesweb.com). Fun websites for nostalgia of the boomer generation.

Bi-Folkal Reminiscing Kits. Theme-based kits with slide show, narration, music, and activities chosen to bring back memories. Remembering is the first word of every kit title (e.g., Remembering County Fairs, Remembering African American Lives, Remembering Summertime.) A newsletter and other products for use in reminiscence groups are also available. Bi-Folkal Productions, Inc., 809 Williamson Street, Madison, WI 53703, (800) 568-5357, or e-mail bifolks@bifolkal.org. Website: http://www.bifolkal.org. Check with your local library to see if they have these kits.

Reminiscing: the Game for People Over 30. This game is available from TDC Games (Item 1110), 1456 Norwood Drive, Itaska, IL 60143, (800) 292-7676.

Tell Me a Story. A simple reminiscence tool for visitors as well as family and professional caregivers of people with Alzheimer's disease. Available from Elder Books, Forest Knolls, Calif.

REFERENCES

Back KW, Bourque LB: Life graphs: aging and cohort effects, *J Gerontol* 25(3):249-255, 1970.

Bastings A: Reading the story behind the story: context and content in stories by people with dementia, *Generations* 27:25-29, 2003.

Birren JE, Cochran KN: *Telling the stories of life through guided autobiography groups,* Baltimore, 2001, Johns Hopkins University Press.

Birren JE, Deutchman DE: *Guiding autobiography groups for older adults: exploring the fabric of life,* Baltimore, 1991, Johns Hopkins University Press.

Bohlmeijer E, Smit F, Cuijpers P: Effects of reminiscence and life review on late-life depression: a meta-analysis, *Int J Geriatr Psychiatry* 18(12):1088-1094, 2003.

Boykin A, Parker M, Touhy T: Discovering the beauty of older adults—opening doors, *J Clin Psychol* 4(3):205-210, 1998.

Butler R: Age, death, and life review. Available at http://www.hospicefoundation.org, 2002. Accessed 6/24/04.

Butler R, Lewis M: *Aging and mental health: positive psychosocial approaches,* ed 3, St Louis, 1983, Mosby.

Butler RN: The life review: an interpretation of reminiscence in the aged, *Psychiatry* 26:65-76, 1963.

Cole TR: *The journey of life: a cultural history of aging in America,* Cambridge, UK, 1992, Cambridge University Press.

Coles R: *The call of stories,* Boston, 1989, Houghton Mifflin Co.

Erikson EH: *Childhood and society,* ed 2, New York, 1963, WW Norton & Co.

Frolik LA: Legacies of possessions: passing property at death, *Generations* 20(3):9, 1996.

Haight B, Webster J: *The art and science of reminiscing: theory, research, methods and applications,* Washington, DC, 1995, Taylor & Francis.

Haight BK, Burnside IM: Reminiscence and life review: explaining the differences, *Arch Psychiatr Nurs* 7(2):91-98, 1993.

Haight B, Webster J: *Critical advances in reminiscence work: from theory to application,* New York, 2002, Springer.

Killick J: 'What are we like here?' Eliciting experiences of people with dementia, *Generations* 13(3):46-49, 1999.

Kivnick HQ: Remembering and being remembered: the reciprocity of psychosocial legacy, *Generations* 20(3):49, 1996.

Macrae J: Nightingale's spiritual philosophy and its significance for modern nursing, *Image J Nurs Sch* 27(1):8-10, 1995.

Maloney MF: A Heideggerian hermeneutical analysis of older women's stories of being strong, *Image J Nurs Sch* 27(2):104-109, 1995.

Philip CE: Lifelines, *J Aging Stud* 9(4):265, 1995.

Rubinstein RL: Childlessness, legacy and generativity, *Generations* 20(3):58-61, 1996a.

Rubinstein RL: *Feelings for the past: reminiscences about former residences.* Paper presented at the meeting of the Gerontological Society of America, Washington, DC, Nov 19, 1996b.

Sarton M: *At seventy: a journal,* New York, 1984, WW Norton & Co.

Scott-Maxwell F: *The measure of my days,* New York, 1968, Knopf.

Thorsheim H, Roberts B: *I remember when: activity ideas to help people reminisce,* Forest Knolls, Calif, 2000, Elder Books.

Tobin S: Cherished possessions: the meaning of things, *Generations* 20(3):46, 1996.

Communication Through Documentation

6

LEARNING OBJECTIVES

Upon completion of this chapter, the reader will be able to:

- Describe the reasons for accurate and thorough documentation in gerontological nursing.
- Identify potential problems in documentation.
- Identify ways in which errors in documentation and communication can potentially harm patients.
- Describe the major assessment methods used in acute, long-term care and home care.
- Identify some of the responsibilities of the nurse in protecting the privacy of patients.
- Identify ways to reduce the possibility of medication errors through the use of documentation.

GLOSSARY

HIPAA Health Insurance Portability and Accountability Act of 1996, which legislated the handling of confidential patient information.

JCAHO The Joint Commission on the Accreditation of Healthcare Organizations, which sets voluntary standards for the quality of patient care in the United States.

Medicaid An insurance plan for children, persons over the age of 65, and selected others with low incomes. This plan is supported jointly by the federal government and each state, with wide variation in eligibility and benefits from state to state.

Medicare Government-sponsored insurance plan for legal residents in the United States who are over 65 years old or who have been totally and permanently disabled for at least 2 years. Does not include payment for services that are considered "custodial."

Taxonomy As used in this chapter, the orderly classification of diagnoses based on categorical relationships.

THE LIVED EXPERIENCE

I was so happy to be able to make a big difference in Mrs. Jones's life. She was 97 and had grown slowly confused over the years. She was also very hard of hearing. Between the two things, we really could not communicate very effectively with her, we could just show her we cared. Eventually she became acutely ill, and a decision needed to be made about CPR. When we tried to find out what her wishes were we could not immediately find any record of them and she had no living relatives or friends, just an attorney. I searched and searched and finally found it. We were able to provide her the comfort she wanted because of a nurse's careful documentation years before.

Kathleen, RN

DOCUMENTATION

Nursing documentation is an age-old practice of making a permanent record of the conditions of our patients, our actions, and the patients' responses to our actions or those of others. There is probably not a nurse alive who does not know the mantra "if you didn't document it—you didn't do it!"

Careful and accurate documentation is important for a number of reasons. Clinical documentation chronicles, supports, and communicates the condition of the patient or resident at all times. Good documentation will help the nurse identify, monitor, and evaluate treatment or intervention. The recorded assessment provides the data needed for the careful development of the individualized plan of care and the evaluation of patient outcomes. Documentation also provides the communication needed to ensure that the persons will get the ongoing care that is needed; in other words, good documentation leads to continuity of care. The nurse who provides care to a patient for whom the previous nurse did not document well will see the potential errors that can be made and the added burden to both the patient and the nurse. Documentation is the major means for the nurse to demonstrate the high level of care he or she provides. In certified long-term care nursing facilities and home health agencies, documentation also serves as a basis for the calculation of the amount of reimbursement or payment for the nursing care provided.

Documentation begins whenever a client enters the health care system, sometimes even before the client is seen. It cannot be effectively done in a haphazard or careless manner. Done correctly, ongoing documentation not only provides the basis for care, but also forms the basis of the information needed when a patient moves from one setting to another or returns home. Documentation in gerontological nursing is even more important because of the complexity of the problems that many elders have and the great risk they are under at having less than ideal outcomes from our interventions and medical treatments.

Documentation also includes the recording of the wishes of our patients. These wishes include who they want involved in their care, who they want to have access to their records, and their wishes related to everything from organ donation to the use of CPR (cardiopulmonary resuscitation) and the handling of their bodies after death. Patients often discuss these things with nurses during quiet moments or during times of stress. By recording these conversations in the medical or clinical record we are able to share this important information with other members of the health care team and better ensure that the patient's wishes are respected.

Documentation is essential not only to ensure the highest quality of care but also to ensure appropriate reimbursement for the care that is provided by the nurse. This chapter reviews nursing documentation in the acute care, long-term care, and home health settings.

Documentation in the Acute Care Setting

Documentation in the acute care setting has undergone a significant shift in recent years. Computers can be found at the bedside, in nurses' pockets, and in strategic locations around the unit. Nurses are given passwords that may be more important than their name tags. The use of standardized tools has become the norm (see Chapter 14), as has the use of checklist and flow sheets for everything from vital signs to discharge planning. Care maps are used to predict and document the care provided with "narratives" or hand-written notes used only when the patient does not follow the anticipated trajectory.

In order to reduce the errors associated with the administration and documentation of medications the use of bar codes has been mandated by the U.S. Food and Drug Administration (FDA). The bar code on the medication is scanned and matched to the bar code on the patient's wristband. Adoption of this method has resulted in a reduction of medication-related errors by 86.2% (Hampton, 2004).

However, in some settings, some "lower tech" approaches are still used. There documentation, after the detailed baseline assessment, is done in the form of problem-oriented notes made in the clinical record. The patient is assessed (usually with a checklist); nursing diagnoses may be identified using the diagnoses of the North American Nursing Diagnosis Association (NANDA); and care plans of interventions using the Nursing

Interventions Classification (NIC) are created or selected from preprinted forms. NANDA diagnoses and NIC/Nursing Outcomes Classification (NOC) are the taxonomies most often used by nurses to categorize their findings, interventions, and outcomes; they allow standardization of language and ease of communication among nurses.

When the nurse needs to document a particular event in the course of the patient stay, a SOAP note may be used, again for the standardization of the presentation of information. SOAP is the acronym for *subjective*, *objective*, *assessment*, and *plan*. If SOAPE is used, the E represents *education*. The subjective section of the note, also called the chief complaint, represents the patient's own words related to how he or she is doing or feeling. The objective portion includes the data that the nurse can measure, see, feel, touch, or smell related to the chief complaint. The assessment is the result of the nurse's analysis of the situation considering both the subjective and objective data. The assessment may be written out in NANDA language. The plan is those nursing interventions that have been done or will be done associated with the chief complaint, and NIC language may be used. The education section, if included, is the patient teaching that has been done or is needed, again related to the chief complaint (Box 6-1). This system is very useful for the succinct communication of information related to a specific problem. If the patient has multiple problems, as do many older adults, this form of documentation can be complicated and lengthy.

Documentation in Long-Term Care

When persons enter long-term care facilities they are often functionally impaired because of physical problems, cognitive limitations, the onset or exacerbation of an acute problem, or other related factors. Long-term care occurs in an assortment of locations, including home, assisted living (board and care homes), rehabilitation hospitals, nursing facilities, and "swing beds" in rural hospitals (beds that serve as either acute or long-term care, depending on the patient's needs). Although licensed nurses are not involved in all long-term settings, when they are involved, documentation is required. The documentation is used not only to record what the nurse has done, but also to evaluate the effectiveness of nursing actions

Box 6-1	Example of a SOAP Note

S: "I have to go to the toilet too much and it burns . . . started last week and getting worse." Denies history of urinary tract infections.

O: 72-year-old white female. Temp 99, pulse 94, blood pressure 140/86, respirations 18. Urine is dark yellow with strong foul odor, skin slightly damp, face flushed, abdomen tender.

A: Altered elimination, elevated temp, mild distress, possible infection.

P: Call nurse practitioner with report, ask patient to drink extra water every hour, check vital signs every 4 hours until this is resolved.
N. Nurse, RN

and communicate information from one shift to another. Documentation in long-term care nursing facilities encompasses the recording of day-to-day events, such as vital signs, but also includes regularly scheduled comprehensive assessments. Documentation is the definitive basis for the calculation of payment for services that are covered under Medicare, Medicaid, and a number of insurance companies.

Documentation in long-term care nursing facilities includes standardized tools (see below), narrative progress notes, flow sheets, and checklists. Good documentation is an expectation of both trained and licensed staff who provide professional care for others; however, in most cases the nurse is ultimately responsible for both the quality of the care provided and the completeness and accuracy of the documentation of the care.

Resident Assessment Instrument

In 1986 the Institute of Medicine (IOM) completed a study indicating that elders in long-term care facilities were receiving an unacceptably low quality of care (although there was considerable variation). As a result of this study, nursing home reform was legislated as part of the Omnibus Budget Reconciliation Act (OBRA) of 1987. OBRA recognized the challenging work of caring for sicker and sicker persons discharged from acute care settings to long-term care settings and, along with this, the need for comprehensive assessment and complex decision making regarding the care required, care planning, implementation, and evaluation. In an attempt to improve the quality of care provided and help long-term care residents achieve the highest level of functioning and highest quality of life possible, OBRA began requiring that all facilities complete the Resident Assessment Instrument (RAI) on all residents receiving Medicare and Medicaid (CMS, 2002).

Nurses are often responsible for the coordination of the completion of a standardized assessment shortly after admission, at preset intervals (see current requirements at www.cms.gov), and at any time the resident's condition changes dramatically. At all times the RN is responsible for verifying completion of the assessment with his/her signature. The RAI is used to gather definitive information on the resident's functioning through the completion of the portion known as the Minimum Data Set (MDS). The data are summarized in the resident assessment protocols (RAPs), which are structured, problem-oriented frameworks for the organization and direction of the nurse. An identified actual or potential social, medical, or psychological problem that appears in the RAP is known as a trigger. The trigger directs the nurse to conduct a more detailed assessment surrounding it, following utilization guidelines (UGs). Individualized care planning is the result of the trigger, with the actual or potential problem addressed by the optimal means possible. When the MDS is completed jointly by all members of the interdisciplinary team a more holistic plan results.

In many settings the data of the RAI are entered into software packages for ease of analysis and communication of patient needs. Some facilities submit their aggregate data into a national database used to better understand the needs of residents in long-term care facilities and to help inform health policy.

The RAI process is dynamic and solution oriented. As MDS reassessments are done, the nurse and other members of the care team are able to both document and track the progress toward the resolution of the triggered problems and make changes to the plan of care as necessary. The type and level of documentation required in the RAI facilitate reliable and measurable communication and, when used properly, improved outcomes for residents. The picture of the resident is as clear as possible. For persons who will benefit from active rehabilitation the outcomes include discharge to a lower level of care, such as returning home. For persons whose condition is one of progressive decline, the RAI process can lead to increased comfort and appropriate care. Elements of the MDS can be found in the Condensed Minimum Data Set in Table 6-1 and Figure 6-1.

Documentation and Reimbursement

In an attempt to control the increasing costs associated with long-term care, the Balanced Budget Act of 1997 set the reimbursement rate for long-term care in a skilled nursing facility (SNF) on a prospective payment system (PPS). In SNFs, the daily rate is calculated based on the results of the MDS through the use of resource utilization groups (RUGs). This means that the payment is determined by which RUG the resident falls in and includes the relative weight of the amount of staff time that is expected to be needed for the specific person with specific problems, strengths, and weaknesses. Like the DRGs (diagnostic-related groups) used in the acute care setting, the payment is preset and not based on the actual costs. Facilities whose nurses provide efficient care have the potential to benefit financially, whereas those who are inefficient will incur more costs than payment to be received.

Documentation in Home Care

Persons are often cared for in the home setting. Care in this setting is provided informally by family and friends (see Chapter 23) and formally by nurses both in a private arrangement where payment is considered "out of pocket" and by nurses employed by home health agencies, which are certified and reimbursed by Medicare, Medicaid, or other insurance companies.

Family caregivers will often develop documentation systems of their own, relating to appointments, medication schedules, and health care provider instruction. This system may be available to each caregiver who enters the home to increase the continuity of care, including the private duty nurse. The nurse may assist the family in developing effective systems.

For care in the home that is provided by nurses and staff from certified home health agencies, Medicare and Medicaid have very strict criteria for

Table 6-1 Minimum Data Set (MDS) Version 2.0 (Condensed) for Nursing Home Resident Assessment and Care Screening

Identification Information	Name, gender, birthday, Social Security and Medicare numbers, provider number, reasons for assessment
Background Information	Assessment reference date, date of entry, marital status, payment sources, responsible person, advance directives
Demographic Information	Date of entry, situation prior to admission, occupation, education, language, mental health history and conditions related to MR/DD status
Customary Routine	Usual cycle of daily events, eating patterns, functional ability in activities of daily living, social involvement
Cognitive Patterns	Consciousness, memory, recall ability, decision-making skills, delirium, disordered thinking, changes in cognitive status
Communication/Hearing Patterns	Hearing, communication devices/techniques, modes of expression, speech clarity, ability to understand, changes in communication or hearing
Vision Patterns	Vision, specific limitations/difficulties, visual appliances
Mood and Behavior Patterns	Indicators of depression, anxiety, sad mood, mood persistence, mood changes, behavioral symptoms, changes in behavioral symptoms
Psychosocial Well-Being	Sense of initiative/involvement, unsettled relationships, past roles
Physical Functioning and Structural Problems	Activities of daily living (ADL) self-performance: bed mobility, transfer, walking/locomotion, dressing, eating, toileting, personal hygiene, bathing, range of motion, modes of transfers, modes of locomotion, functional and rehabilitation potential, changes in ADL function
Continence in Last 14 Days	Self-control categories, bowel continence, bladder continence, bowel elimination pattern, appliances and programs, changes in urinary continence
Disease Diagnoses	Diseases, infections, other diagnoses
Health Conditions	Problem conditions, pain symptoms, pain site, accidents, stability of conditions
Oral/Nutritional Status	Oral problems, height and weight, weight changes, nutritional problems, nutritional approaches, parenteral or enteral intake
Oral/Dental Status	Oral status and disease prevention, tooth decay, disintegration; buccal cavity exam; dentures, bridges, missing teeth
Skin Condition	Ulcers, type of ulcers, history of unresolved ulcers, other skin problems or lesions, skin treatments, foot problems and care
Activity Pursuit Patterns	Time awake, time involved in activities, preferred activity settings, general activity preferences, prefers change in daily routines
Medications	Number of medications, new medications, injections, days received the following medications (antipsychotic, antianxiety, antidepressant, hypnotic, diuretic)
Special Treatments and Procedures	Treatments, procedures, and programs; intervention programs for mood, behavior, cognitive loss, nursing rehabilitation/restorative care, devices and restraints, hospital stays, emergency room visits, physician visits, physician orders, abnormal lab values
Discharge Potential and Overall Status	Discharge potential, overall change in care needs
Resident Participation in Assessment	Resident, family members, significant other

documentation. Like the requirements for standardized documentation in the long-term care setting above, home care was also affected by the Balanced Budget Act of 1997. The Outcomes and *Assessment Information Set* (OASIS) was implemented to provide the format for the comprehensive assessment, which forms the basis for measuring patient outcomes for the purposes of outcome-based quality improvement (OBQI) (CMS, 2004). The data collected, focused on outcomes, can be used for care planning. As with all other documentation systems, it is used both to improve the quality of the communication about the individual and to serve as a guide for reimbursement for care provided. Often OASIS is completed in the person's home, recorded directly on portable or hand-held computers, and later transferred to a central operating system. Home health agencies are required to electronically transmit OASIS data to a standard state system provided by the federal Centers for Medicare and Medicaid (CMS). OASIS data began to be used as the basis for the determination of payment in 2000.

It is important to note that nurses will need to supplement the data collected in OASIS to fully assess the health status and care needs of patients. For example, vital signs are not part of the data set.

PROTECTION OF PATIENT PRIVACY

Documentation relating to clients, patients, or residents, whether it is written on paper or entered into a computer, contains highly personal and private information. For many years the confi-

PROCEDURES FOR COMPLETING THE RESIDENT ASSESSMENT PROTOCOLS (RAPs)

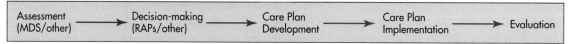

Assessment (MDS/other) → Decision-making (RAPs/other) → Care Plan Development → Care Plan Implementation → Evaluation

The Resident Assessment Protocols (RAPs) are used to assess conditions identified by the Minimum Data Set (MDS) triggering mechanism. The goal of the RAPs is to guide the interdisciplinary team through a structured comprehensive assessment of a resident's functional status. Functional status differs from medical or clinical status in that the whole of a person's life is reviewed with the intent of assisting that person to function at his or her highest practicable level of well-being. Going through the RAI process will help staff set resident-specific objectives in order to meet the physical, mental, and psychosocial needs of residents.

What are the Resident Assessment Protocols (RAPs)?

The MDS alone does not provide a comprehensive assessment. Rather, the MDS is used for preliminary screening to identify potential resident problems, strengths, and preferences. The RAPs are problem-oriented frameworks for additional assessment based on problem identification items (triggered conditions). They form a critical link to decisions about care planning. The RAP Guidelines provide guidance on how to synthesize assessment information within a comprehensive assessment. The triggers target conditions for additional assessment and review, as warranted by MDS item responses; the RAP Guidelines help facility staff evaluate "triggered" conditions.

There are 18 RAPs in Version 2.0 of the RAI. The RAPs in the RAI cover the majority of areas that are addressed in a typical nursing home resident's care plan. The RAPs were created by clinical experts in each of the RAP areas.

The care delivery system in a facility is complex yet critical to successful resident care outcomes. It is guided by both professional standards of practice and regulatory requirements. The basis of care delivery is the process of assessment and care planning. Documentation of this process (to ensure continuity of care) is also necessary.

The RAI (MDS and RAPs) is an integral part of this process. It ensures that facility staff collect minimum, standardized assessment data for each resident at regular intervals. The main intent is to drive the development of an individualized plan of care based on the identified needs, strengths, and preferences of the resident.

Figure 6-1   Resident assessment protocols. (Modified from *Minimum Data Set [MDS] Version 2.0 for Nursing Home Resident Assessment and Care Screening*, Form 1728HH, Des Moines, 1995, Briggs Corp.)

RESIDENT ASSESSMENT PROTOCOL TRIGGER LEGEND FOR REVISED RAPS (FOR MDS VERSION 2.0)

Resident _____   Numeric Identifier _____

Key:
- ● = One item required to trigger
- ② = Two items required to trigger
- ★ = One of these three items (Psychotropic Drug Use), plus at least one other item required to trigger
- ●★ = Psychotropic Drug Use triggered only when at least one of the three items (O4a, O4b, O4c) identified by ★ apply
- (a) = When both ADL triggers present, maintenance takes precedence

Proceed to RAP Review once triggered

MDS 2.0 ITEM AND DESCRIPTION		CODE	1 Delirium	2 Cognitive Loss/Dementia	3 Visual Function	4 Communication	5A ADL-Rehabilitation Trigger A (a)	5B ADL-Maintenance Trigger B (a)	6 Urinary Incontinence and Indwelling Catheter	7 Psychosocial Well-Being	8 Mood State	9 Behavioral Symptoms	10A Activities Trigger A (Revise)	10B Activities Trigger B (Review)	11 Falls	12 Nutritional Status	13 Feeding Tubes	14 Dehydration/Fluid Maintenance	15 Dental Care	16 Pressure Ulcers	17 Psychotropic Drug Use	18 Physical Restraints	ITEM
B2a	Short term memory	1		●																			B2a
B2b	Long term memory	1		●																			B2b
B4	Decision making	1,2		●																			B4
B4	Decision making	3		●		●																	B4
B5a-B5f	Indicators of delirium	2	●																		●★		B5a-B5f
B6	Change in cognitive status	2	●																		●★		B6
C1	Hearing	1,2,3				●																	C1
C4	Understood by others	1,2,3				●																	C4
C6	Understand others	1,2,3		●		●																	C6
C7	Change in communication	2																			●★		C7
D1	Vision	1,2,3			●																		D1
D2a	Side vision problem	√			●																		D2a
E1a-E1p	Indicators of depression, anxiety, sad mood	1,2									●												E1a-E1p
E1n	Repetitive movement	1,2																			●★		E1n
E1o	Withdrawal from activities	1,2								●													E1o
E2	Mood persistence	1,2									●												E2
E3	Change in mood	2	●																		●★		E3
E4aA	Wandering	1,2,3										●	●										E4aA
E4bA-E4dA	Behavioral symptoms	1,2,3										●											E4bA-E4dA
E5	Change in behavioral symptoms	1										●											E5
E5	Change in behavioral symptoms	2	●																		●★		E5
F1d	Establishes own goals	√								●													F1d
F2a-F2d	Unsettled relationships	√								●													F2a-F2d
F3a	Strong id, past roles	√								●													F3a
F3b	Lost roles	√								●													F3b
F3c	Daily routine different	√								●													F3c
G1aA	Bed mobility	1					●																G1aA
G1aA	Bed mobility	2,3,4					●													●			G1aA
G1aA	Bed mobility	8																		●			G1aA
G1bA-G1jA	ADL self-performance	1,2,3,4					●																G1bA-G1jA
G2a	Bathing	1,2,3,4					●																G2a
G3b	Balance while sitting	1,2,3																			●★		G3b
G6a	Bedfast	√																		●			G6a
G8a,b	Resident, staff believe capable	√					●																G8a,b
H1a	Bowel incontinence	1,2,3,4																		●			H1a
H1b	Bladder incontinence	2,3,4							●														H1b
H2b	Constipation	√																			●★		H2b
H2d	Fecal impaction	√																			●★		H2d
H3c,d,e	Catheter use	√							●														H3c,d,e
H3g	Use of pads/briefs	√							●														H3g
I1i	Hypotension	√																			●★		I1i
I1j	Peripheral vascular disease	√																		●			I1j
I1ee	Depression	√																			●★		I1ee
I1jj	Cataracts	√			●																		I1jj
I1ll	Glaucoma	√			●																		I1ll
I2j	UTI	√													●								I2j

Form 1729HH BRIGGS, Des Moines, IA 50306 (800) 247-2343 PRINTED IN U.S.A.

MDS 2.0 RAP TRIGGER LEGEND
MDS 2.0 10/18/94N

Figure 6-1 *Continued.*

SECTION V. RESIDENT ASSESSMENT PROTOCOL SUMMARY Numeric Identifier________________

Resident's Name:	Medical Record No.:

1. Check if RAP is triggered.
2. For each triggered RAP, use the RAP guidelines to identify areas needing further assessment. Document relevant assessment information regarding the resident's status.
   - Describe:
     –Nature of the condition (may include presence or lack of objective data and subjective complaints).
     –Complications and risk factors that affect your decision to proceed to care planning.
     –Factors that must be considered in developing individualized care plan interventions.
     –Need for referrals/further evaluation by appropriate health professionals.
   - Documentation should support your decision-making regarding whether to proceed with a care plan for a triggered RAP and the type(s) of care plan interventions that are appropriate for a particular resident.
   - Documentation may appear anywhere in the clinical record (e.g., progress notes, consults, flow sheets, etc.).
3. Indicate under the *Location of RAP Assessment Documentation* column where information related to the RAP assessment can be found.
4. For each triggered RAP, indicate whether a new care plan, care plan revision, or continuation of current care plan is necessary to address the problem(s) identified in your assessment. The Care Planning Decision column must be completed within 7 days of completing the RAI (MDS and RAPs).

A. RAP Problem Area	(a) Check if Triggered	Location and Date of RAP Assessment Documentation	(b) Care Planning Decision—check if addressed in care plan
1. DELIRIUM	☐		☐
2. COGNITIVE LOSS	☐		☐
3. VISUAL FUNCTION	☐		☐
4. COMMUNICATION	☐		☐
5. ADL FUNCTIONAL/ REHABILITATION POTENTIAL	☐		☐
6. URINARY INCONTINENCE AND INDWELLING CATHETER	☐		☐
7. PSYCHOSOCIAL WELL-BEING	☐		☐
8. MOOD STATE	☐		☐
9. BEHAVIORAL SYMPTOMS	☐		☐
10. ACTIVITIES	☐		☐
11. FALLS	☐		☐
12. NUTRITIONAL STATUS	☐		☐
13. FEEDING TUBES	☐		☐
14. DEHYDRATION/FLUID MAINTENANCE	☐		☐
15. ORAL/DENTAL CARE	☐		☐
16. PRESSURE ULCERS	☐		☐
17. PSYCHOTROPIC DRUG USE	☐		☐
18. PHYSICAL RESTRAINTS	☐		☐

B. ____ 2. ☐☐ – ☐☐ – ☐☐☐☐
1. Signature of RN Coordinator for RAP Assessment Process   Month Day Year

____ 4. ☐☐ – ☐☐ – ☐☐☐☐
3. Signature of Person Completing Care Planning Decision   Month Day Year

TRIGGER LEGEND

1 - Delirium
2 - Cognitive Loss/Dementia
3 - Visual Function
4 - Communication
5A - ADL-Rehabilitation
5B - ADL-Maintenance
6 - Urinary Incontinence and Indwelling Catheter
7 - Psychosocial Well-Being
8 - Mood State
9 - Behavioral Symptoms
10A - Activities (Revise)
10B - Activities (Review)
11 - Falls
12 - Nutritional Status
13 - Feeding Tubes
14 - Dehydration/Fluid Maintenance
15 - Dental Care
16 - Pressure Ulcers
17 - Psychotropic Drug Use
18 - Physical Restraints

Figure 6-1 *Continued.*

dentiality of health and medical information was protected through professional codes, standards, and ethics and enacted through facilities' policies and procedures. The expectation has been that the nurse and other health care providers only access information that relates to a specific individual that they are providing care to and that knowledge is shared only with those other professionals who have a "need to know" the information. Nursing students are taught to avoid talking about patients in hallways, elevators, and lunch rooms or with persons outside their clinical groups, such as friends and family members. The nurse who notes that a neighbor has been admitted to the unit is expected to not review the chart unless the nurse is assigned to provide the care.

Unfortunately, we have not been as respectful of people's privacy as we should be. This, coupled with the increasing use of electronic documentation, has significantly increased the risk of breaches of confidentiality. In 1996 the Health Insurance Portability and Accountability Act (HIPAA) was passed legislating the expectations of health care personnel in relation to health and medical records and implemented nationwide on April 14, 2003. The Department of Health and Human Services has been charged with enforcing these new rules.

The privacy regulations put in place through HIPAA that relate especially to nurses include the following (USDHHS, 2003):

Access to medical records. Patients and those directly involved in their care have access to records; however, no one else does. The patient may specifically designate anyone of their choosing to have access as well, but this is up to the adult patient or guardian and no one else.

Notice of privacy practices. Patients must be provided a notice of how their information will be both used and protected. For elders with vision problems the nurse may need to read the notices to them and ensure their understanding. For persons with limited English proficiency, the information must be translated or given by an interpreter.

Limits on use of personal medical information. The information obtained about a person in the context of a health care setting can only be used for purposes relating to health care, and only the minimum amount of information necessary should be shared, if any.

Confidential communication. Patients may request that reasonable steps be taken to ensure that their communications are done in such a way as to provide confidentiality, such as closing the patient's/resident's door prior to having health-related conversations or staff avoiding discussing patient/residents' needs or condition in a location where it could be overheard, for example, hallways, some nurses' stations.

REDUCING ERRORS IN DOCUMENTATION

The number of medical and nursing errors has increased dramatically over the last several years. Although most do not result in any lasting harm to the patient, some of these have caused increases in both morbidity and mortality. Problems with documentation and communication have been one of the factors contributing to the rise in the rate of errors and the subsequent rise in patient deaths, with medication errors those most frequently seen. Of the more than 300 medication errors with serious effects reported to the FDA in 2003, 19% of these were related to problems with communication (Hampton, 2004).

The Joint Commission on Accreditation of Healthcare Organizations (JCAHO) established a special safety goal in 2004 to reduce the errors associated with ambiguous documentation, specifically the use of abbreviations. The use of several of the most common abbreviations can result in nurses and others misinterpreting a letter or symbol, and because of this, administering a wrong medication or dose or giving it at the wrong time or with the wrong frequency (JCAHO, 2004).

Five abbreviations long used in documentation are on the "do not use/do" list; these are U (as in units); IU (as in international units); QD and QOD (daily and every other day); the use of a trailing zero, such as 1.0, and failure to use a leading zero, such as 0.1; and the use of the abbreviations for morphine and magnesium, MS, MSO_4, or $MgSO_4$ (Beyea, 2004). In the first case, the U could easily be misread as an O. It has also been mistaken for a zero, a four, and a cc (cubic centimeters). This is most dangerous in its use with insulin. The nurse may read "gave 10U regular insulin" as "gave 100 regular insulin." The word *units* should be written out ("gave 10 units of regular insulin") to be absolutely clear. Similarly, IU can be misread as IV or 10; it should be written out as "international units." QD and QOD can be mistaken for each other; if periods are used, a Q.D. (daily) can be mistaken for QID (four times per day) with serious consequences. The dosages with trailing zeros are fraught with potential for errors; it would be very easy to mistake 4.0 mg for 40 mg—with disastrous effects; .0 should never be used after whole numbers. Some medications are used in small doses, less than one. Thyroid medications, such as levothyroxine (Synthroid), and the heart medication digoxin are two of these commonly used with older adults. Leading zeros should always be used to record their doses; for example, a dose of digoxin should be recorded as 0.25 mg rather than .25 mg, which could be mistaken for 25 mg, with this being a fatal dose. Finally, the use of abbreviations should not be used for any medication or other notation with more than one representation or use. MS and MSO_4 both stand for morphine sulfate, although sometimes nurses also mistakenly use the abbreviation "MS" for "mental status" even further confusing the communication among staff members. MSO_4 and $MgSO_4$ are so similar they are easily misinterpreted; therefore it is reasonable to expect the nurse to write these out in their full names of morphine sulfate and magnesium sulfate in order to ensure clear documentation and patient safety.

JCAHO has a goal of 100% compliance of all organizations that they accredit to no longer use any of the above abbreviations and to identify three others at a minimum that they have stopped using. Additional abbreviations to avoid are µg mistaken for mg, resulting in a 1000-fold drug overdose; mcg or even micrograms should be used instead. H.S. may stand for either half strength or at bedtime; use instead "half-strength" or "at bedtime." T.I.W. is mistaken for three times per day or twice weekly (instead of three times per week). Neither S.Q. nor S.C. (both used for subcutaneous) should be used to avoid confusion with S.L. (sublingual). The abbreviation D/C is understood to mean either discharge or discontinue. Discharge can be from a wound or from a facility, confounding communication. A more complete listing of common medication-related documen-

tation errors can be found at the website for the Institute for Safe Medication Practice (www.ismp.org).

Communication through documentation has become critical to ensure patients' rights, adequate care, and the economic survival of providers. It is the responsibility of the nurse to make sure that communication and documentation are of the highest quality so as to provide error-free appropriate care and continuity and to maximize both patient outcomes and reimbursement.

KEY CONCEPTS

- Excellence in documentation sets the stage for excellence in patient care.
- Standardized instruments for patient evaluation are integral to consistent determination of patient acuity and appropriate reimbursement.
- Documenting patient status and needs accurately is a key responsibility of the licensed nurse.
- Nurses have a responsibility to protect patient confidentiality at all times, both in spoken information and in the clinical record.
- A decreased reliance on the use of abbreviations in the health care setting will decrease the risk for error and consequently, the risk for patient injury or death.

Activities and Discussion Questions

1. Discuss the origins and purpose of the development of standardized documentation systems.
2. Discuss problems you have experienced with incomplete data or poor documentation in a health facility.
3. Discuss the potential uses of the RAI/MDS and OASIS.
4. Discuss ways in which patient confidentiality is breached and what the nurse can do about this.
5. Explain the reasons why documentation is critical to patient care.
6. Discuss the documentation errors that have been observed in the clinical setting, and describe their possible effects.

RESOURCES

Publication

MDS 2.0; *The Long Term Care Facility Resident Assessment Instrument (RAI) User's Manual.* Obtain copies from Briggs Health Care Products, Customer Service Department, (800) 247-2343.

Websites

Center for Medicare and Medicaid Services
www.cms.gov

Institute for Safe Medication Practice
www.ismp.org

JCAHO
www.jcaho.org

NANDA
www.nanda.org

NIC/NOC
www.nursing.uiowa.edu/centers/ncce/noc

REFERENCES

Beyea SC: Best practices for abbreviation use, *AORN J* 79(3):641-642, 2004.

Center for Medicare and Medicaid Services (CMS): *CMS's RAI version 2.0 manual,* Washington, DC, 2002, U.S. Government Printing Office. Available at www.cms.hhs.gov.

Center for Medicare and Medicaid Services (CMS): *OASIS: an overview,* 2003. Available at www.cms.hhs.gov.

Hampton T: Bar codes mandated for hospital meds, *JAMA* 291(4):1685-1686, 2004.

Joint Commission on Accreditation of Healthcare Organizations (JCAHO): *2004 National patient safety goals: FAQ,* 2004. Available at www.jcaho.org.

United States Department of Health and Human Services (USDHHS): *Fact sheet: protecting the privacy of patients' health information,* 2003. Available at www.hhs.gov.news/facts/privacy.html.

7

Physical Changes of Aging

LEARNING OBJECTIVES

Upon completion of this chapter, the reader will be able to:

- Identify normal age changes.
- Begin to differentiate normal changes with aging from those that are potentially pathological.
- Make a plan of care for the older adult that reflects prevention and maintenance associated with some of the changes with age.

▶ **GLOSSARY**

Creatinine clearance (CrCl) A calculated measurement reflective of the level of kidney functioning.

Ectropion Eversion or turning outward of the margin of the eyelid.

Edentulous Toothless.

Entropion Inversion or turning inward of the margin of the eyelid.

Glomerular filtration rate (GFR) The rate at which the kidneys are able to filter the blood in the glomeruli.

Kyphosis C-shaped curvature of the cervical vertebrae.

Osteoporosis Significant reduction in the density, or the strength, of the bones.

Presbycusis Progressive, bilaterally symmetrical perceptive hearing loss occurring with age, usually of high-frequency sounds.

Presbyopia Diminished accommodation of the lens of the eye occurring normally with age, usually resulting in farsightedness.

Xerostomia Excessive drying of the mouth.

▶ **THE LIVED EXPERIENCE**

Strange how these things creep up on you. I really was surprised and upset when I first realized it was not the headlights on my car that were dim but only my aging night vision. Then I remembered other bits of awareness that forced me to recognize that I, that 16-year-old inside me, was experiencing normal changes that go along with getting old.

Sally, age 60

*L*ater life is a time of challenge and opportunities. Among the challenges are those related to physical changes. Some changes are considered a normal part of aging, whereas others relate to the development of pathological conditions that, although they are not part of the normal aging process, become increasingly common over time.

Aging does not begin in late life. It is a process that begins at birth, with building of the organism until the late teens or early twenties and then a slow decline in the functional capacity of the organ systems. Physiological aging is universal, progressive, decremental, intrinsic, and unavoidable (Goldman, 1979). Most of the time, changes with aging, such as wrinkling, graying of hair, hearing loss, or decreased close vision, are not noticeable until the forties or fifties. The factors that affect when the signs of aging become noticeable include genetics, wear and tear (often associated with athletic activity), injury or abuse of the body earlier in life, and stress or environmental factors, such as exposure to smoke or other pollutants.

Aging is not a disease, nor is it a condition that is correctable by medical or surgical intervention. It is a series of complex changes that occurs in all living organisms. Most of these changes are intrinsic; others are a result of extrinsic influences specific to one's way of life. Just why the changes occur has been an interest of gerontologists for decades.

In this chapter we will examine each body system and discuss the common physical changes with normal aging. We will also discuss some of the common pathological conditions seen in older adults in the United States so that the nurse can begin to differentiate normal aging from possible pathological conditions. We begin with a review of the major theories that have been developed to attempt to explain the process of physical aging.

BIOLOGICAL THEORIES OF AGING

A theory is an explanation of a phenomenon that makes sense to us. Theories remain reasonable explanations until someone finds them to be incorrect. Most theories cannot be proved or disproved, but they are useful as a point of reference. Like many other phenomena, there are a number of theories about the mechanics and causes of physical aging. Scientists persist in piecing together the puzzle of aging. Each theory in its own right provides a clue to the aging process. However, many unanswered questions remain. New and exciting data concerning biological theories of aging have emerged recently through the application of more sophisticated methods of unlocking the secrets of the cell. We are beginning to confirm some of the previous suppositions and to develop a more thorough understanding of the genetic, molecular, and biochemical basis of the cellular changes of aging. The biological explanations about physical aging fall into two categories, stochastic and nonstochastic theories.

Stochastic theories suggest that aging events occur randomly and accumulate with time. Three of the most common stochastic theories are the theories of error, free radical, and wear and tear. Error theory proposes that aging is the result of the accumulation of errors in deoxyribonucleic acid (DNA) or ribonucleic acid (RNA) synthesis. The accumulation of errors over time eventually leads to failure of cellular activity and the changes we associate with aging. Free radical theory postulates that as fats, proteins, and carbohydrates oxidize, they create what are called *free radicals,* which attach to other molecules and damage them. The damage is random, and as it accumulates aging occurs and ultimately death of the damaged organism (i.e., person). Aging is also often described as "worn out" (Jett, 2003). In the wear-and-tear theory, aging is caused by the accumulation of repeated and random injury and overuse of cells, tissues, organs, or systems.

Nonstochastic theories suggest that aging is genetically programmed for the specific life span of an organism and includes senescence, or aging of the entire organism (Hayflick, 1983). This category includes programmed, immunological, and neuroendocrine theories. The programmed theory explains aging as a result of an inner "biological clock" for each cell. In other words, each cell is "born" with a limited number of replications. When they are done, the cell dies. When enough cells die, the organism does as well. From an immunological (theoretical) perspective, over time there is an alteration of B and T cells that leads to the loss of cellular regulation. The altered cells are recognized as foreign bodies, and antibodies are produced to fight them, as seen in autoimmune diseases. Finally, the neuroendocrine theory proposes that over time, the efficiency of the control mechanism of the organs is altered or lost (especially in the pituitary and hypothalamus), resulting in aging and death.

It is important for the nurse to understand that the exact cause of aging is unknown, that there is considerable variation in the aging process, and that what is normal in an older adult may be abnormal in an adult of a younger age with the same condition. Also, the approach to the care of the younger adult and older adult with the same condition may be considerably different. Individual variations are enormous at every age and in

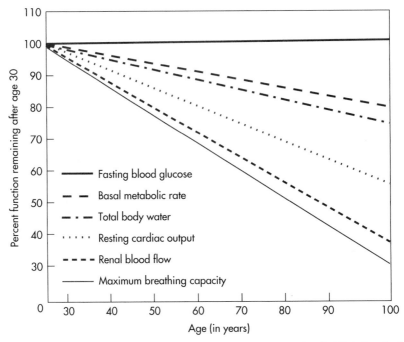

Figure 7-1 Changes in biological function with age. (Modified from Shock NW. In Carlston LA, editor: *Nutrition in old age: tenth symposium of the Swedish Nutrition Federation*, Uppsala, Sweden, 1972, Almquistand Wilksell.)

every part of the body. Figure 7-1 and Table 7-1 provide a summary of selected biologic, anatomical and physiological changes with aging of healthy adults.

INTEGUMENT

The skin is looked on as having esthetic and cosmetic appeal. Artists have portrayed its delicate, flawless qualities, and poets have extolled its virtues through descriptive phrases. Today, art, poetry, and conversation still include similar depictions. Changes in the skin are part of the normal aging process. Changes occur as a result of genetic (intrinsic) factors and environmental (extrinsic) factors, such as the sun and harsh weather. Whether these changes are genetic or environmental, all older persons will have some degree of dryness, thinning of the skin, decreased elasticity, and prominence of small blood vessels.

Changes thought to be part of the initial process of aging are products of extrinsic causes, such as cigarette smoking, which causes coarse wrinkles, and the sun, which is responsible for photodamage, including rough, leathery texture, itching, and mottled pigmentation of the skin. Skin tears, purpura, and xerosis are common.

The rate at which the skin ages is in part genetic but also is proportional to the degree of exposure to environmental elements, such as wind and the irradiation of the sun. The face and hands are the most constantly exposed areas of the body; thus aging is considerably faster in these areas than in those that are rarely exposed. Visible changes of the skin—quality of color, firmness, elasticity, and texture—affirm that one is aging. Skin coloration varies with blood flow. Paleness is apparent with diminished blood flow; conversely, flushing occurs when blood flow increases. Decreased hemoglobin in capillary blood flow that has lost most of its oxygen produces cyanosis. Circulatory

Table 7-1 Summary of Selected Anatomical and Physiological Changes with Aging in Healthy Adults

System Affected	Change Noted	Age Span (yr)
Height	Average loss 2 inches	40-80
Weight		
Men	Peaks in mid-fifties, then declines	
Women	Peaks in mid-sixties, then declines	
Total body water		
Men	Declines from 60% to 54%	20-80
Women	Declines from 54% to 46%	20-80
Muscle mass	30% decrease	30-70
Taste buds	70% decrease	30-70
Cardiac reserve	Decrease from 4.6 to 3.3 times resting cardiac output	25-70
Maximum heart rate	155-195 beats/min	25-70
Lung vital capacity	17% decrease	30-70
Renal perfusion	Reduced by 50%	30-80
Cerebral blood flow	Reduced by 20%	30-70
Bone mineral content	Reduced by 25%-30% in women; 10%-15% in men	40-80
Brain weight	Reduced by 10%	20-80
Amount of light reaching retina	Diminished by 70%	20-65
Plasma glucocorticoid levels	No change	30-70

Modified from Kenney PA: *Physiology of aging: a synopsis*, Chicago, 1982, Year Book Medical Publishers; Shock NW et al: *Normal human aging: the Baltimore study of aging*. NIH pub no 84-2450, Washington, DC, 1984, U.S. Government Printing Office; Timiras P: *Physiological basis of aging and geriatrics*, New York, 2002, CRC Press; Beers MH, Berkow R, editors: *The Merck manual of geriatrics*, ed 3, Whitehouse Station, NJ, 2000, Merck Research Laboratories.

disorders affect skin coloration; skin loses its color, and blood vessels become more fragile. There are many changes that occur in normal, healthy, aging skin. Some of these changes are inconsequential, and others have important meaning for the health and healing of the individual and the response by the nurse.

The integument does more than keep the skeleton from falling apart. As the largest, most visible organ of the body, its various layers mold and model the individual to give much of his or her personal identity; glands and hair provide recognizable characteristics and sexual identity. The skin is important both in health and in illness. It provides clues to hereditary, racial, dietary, physical, and emotional conditions.

Epidermis

The skin is composed of the epidermis, dermis, and subcutaneous layers. The aged epidermis pro-

duces varying cell shapes and sizes. The loss of conelike projections, called *rete ridges,* changes the previously textured skin to thinner, fragile, shiny, and flatter tissue. The skin serves as an impermeable barrier, preventing the loss of fluids and intrusion of substances from the environment. Melanocytes are in the basal layer of the epidermis. Melanin gives the skin its color. Areas of the skin exposed to the sun have two to three times the melanocytes as unexposed skin. Hormonal activity causes changes in skin pigmentation. Melanin is affected by the melanocyte-stimulating hormone (MSH), which is similar to adrenocorticotropic hormone (ACTH). Moles, nevi, and freckles are all products of melanin distribution. Melanocytes increase in size but decrease in number over time; it is the degree of this activity that creates the uneven pigmentation. In highly pigmented persons there may be an increase in pigmentation seen in darkened creases and elbows. In lighter-pigmented persons pigment spots may appear. Sometimes these spots take the form of increased number of freckles (nevi) and, at other times, the development of lentigo (age or liver spots) and seborrheic keratosis, especially in sun-exposed areas, such as the back of the hands and face. The loss of melanocytes increases the elder's risk for problems with sun exposure, such as skin cancers, and the nurse should reinforce the use of sun block with persons of all ages. Not only is the epidermis thinner, but also cell renewal time increases by up to one third after 50 years of age, requiring 30 or more days for new epithelial replacement. The implications for healing are clear: wounds that take a few days to heal in a younger person may take weeks to heal in an older person.

Added to this is an altered inflammatory response. T-cell function declines, and there may be a reactivation of latent conditions such as herpes zoster (shingles), herpes simplex, or mycobacterium. Delayed healing should be expected. In a younger adult, if the skin is injured with a cut or a scrape, the surrounding area becomes erythematous almost immediately. This inflammatory response is the first step in the natural healing process. In an older adult, this inflammatory first step toward healing may take 48 to 72 hours. A laceration that becomes inflamed several days after the event may be misinterpreted by the nurse as having become "infected," when in reality, the healing process has just started. Evidence of true skin infection in older adults is no different than in younger adults, namely, increasing redness and purulent drainage.

Dermis

The dermis, lying beneath the epidermis, is a supportive layer of connective tissue composed of a matrix of yellow elastic fibers that provide stretch and recoil, white fibrous collagen fibers that provide tensile strength, and an absorbent gel between the two types of fibers. In addition, the dermis also supports hair follicles, sweat and sebaceous glands, nerve fibers, muscle cells, and blood vessels, which provide nourishment to the epidermis. With age, the dermis elasticity and suppleness are lost as a result of cross-link changes of the elastin and collagen components. Dermal cells also are replaced more slowly, and tactile sensory receptors do not transmit sensations as rapidly.

Loss of elasticity accentuates jowls and elongated ears and contributes to the formation of a "double" chin. Sun exposure accelerates skin tissue changes by hastening collagen fiber alterations. Breasts that were full and firm begin to sag and become pendulous as the glandular envelope of fat atrophies and the skin elasticity weakens. Nipples may also invert because of the shrinkage and fibrotic changes.

Subcutaneous Layer

The subcutaneous, inner layer is composed of fat and the base of the eccrine, apocrine, and sebaceous glands and is instrumental for both protection and thermal regulation. With age, some areas of subcutaneous tissue atrophy, especially in the hands, face, and lower legs. As the natural insulation of the subcutaneous layer diminishes, persons are more sensitive to cold environmental temperatures. Other areas of subcutaneous fat (e.g., around the thighs of women and the waist, which is more prominent in women than in men) hypertrophy.

Gland activity is influenced by the hormonal and nervous systems; thus as the hormonal and nervous stimulation decreases, glandular activity diminishes significantly. *Eccrine glands,* or sweat glands, are located all over the body and respond to thermostimulation and neurostimulation. The usual body response to heat is to produce moisture or sweat from these glands and thus cool the skin by evaporation. When this ability is lost, individuals are at significant risk for overheating. When caring for frail older adults, gerontological nurses can assist their patients in avoiding extremes of temperature.

Apocrine glands are associated with hair follicles and are located in the axillary, genital, and perianal areas and in the external ear canal. These glands are larger than the eccrine glands, depend on hormones, and are responsive to emotions. They become active at puberty, but this activity diminishes slightly with advanced age.

Sebaceous glands secrete sebum and depend on hormonal stimulation. Sebum protects the skin by preventing the evaporation of water from the keratin, or horny, layer of the epidermis; it possesses bactericidal properties and contains a precursor of vitamin D. When the skin is exposed to sunlight, vitamin D is produced and absorbed into the skin. With a decrease in androgen levels and in the blood supply to sebaceous glands, sebum production decreases with age, resulting in increased risk for infection and interruptions in the integument.

Hair and Nails

Hair, as part of the integument, has a biological, psychological, and cosmetic value for both men and women. Hair is composed of tightly fused horny cells that arise from the dermal layer of the skin and obtain coloration from melanocytes. The hormones testosterone and estrogen influence hair distribution in both men and women.

Men and women in all racial groups have less hair as they grow older. Race, gender, gender-linked genes, and hormones determine the maximum amount of body and scalp hair that one has and the changes that will occur with it throughout life. Hair on the head thins. Scalp hair loss is prominent in men, beginning in their twenties for some. For others, hair patterns increase until the forties and then begin to recede. Women have less pronounced scalp hair loss. For some, the hair color of their youth persists, but for most, there is a gradual loss of pigmentation (melanin) and it becomes dryer and coarser. Older women develop chin and facial hair because of decreased estrogen in relation to testosterone. Leg, axillary, and pubic hair tends to diminish with age in post-menopausal women and in some instances disappears. The absence of leg hair is sometimes misinterpreted as a sign of peripheral vascular disease in the older adult, when it is a normal part of aging.

The various races have distinctive hair characteristics, which should be kept in mind when caring for or assessing the aged. Almost all Asians have sparse facial and body hair that is dark, straight, and silky. Blacks have slightly more head and body hair than Asians; however, the hair texture varies widely. It is always fragile, and it ranges from straight to spiraled, and thick. Whites have the most head and body hair, with an intermediate texture and form ranging from straight to curly, fine to coarse, and thick to thin.

The nail becomes harder and thicker, more brittle, dull, and opaque. It changes shape, becoming at times flat or concave instead of convex. Vertical ridges appear because of decreasing water,

calcium, and lipid content. The blood supply, as well as the rate of nail growth, decreases. The half moon (lunule) of the fingernail may entirely disappear, and the color of the nails may vary from yellow to gray. The development of a fungal infection of the nails, or onychomycosis, is not the result of aging but is quite common. The fungus invades the space between the layers of the nails, leaving a thick and unsightly appearance. The slowness of the growth and reduced circulation in the older nail make treatment very difficult.

MUSCULOSKELETAL

As seen with the skin, changes in the musculoskeletal system are influenced by many factors, such as age, gender, race, and environment, with signs becoming obvious in the forties. By the time a person is in the sixties or seventies, his or her height is $1\frac{1}{2}$ to 2 inches less than that found on the driver's license (Lamb, 1996). The trunk shortens as a result of gravity and of dehydration of the vertebral disks. If the person also has osteoporosis of the vertebral column, a loss of 2 to 3 inches is not uncommon. With the shortened appearance, the bones of the arms and the legs may appear disproportionate in size.

A mild reduction of bone strength, or reduced bone mineral density, is a normal part of aging, often seen in the slightly stooped posture, or kyphosis. Kyphosis, curvature of the cervical vertebrae because of decreased bone mineral density, is aggravated by atrophic processes of cartilage and muscle. As a result, the person may have a stooped, forward-bent posture, with the hips and knees somewhat flexed and the arms bent at the elbows, raising the level of the arms. If the kyphosis is more advanced, to maintain eye contact it is necessary for the person to tilt his or her head backward in order to maintain eye contact, which makes it appear that the person is jutting forward.

For many women and a few men, the bone loss accelerates to the point of pathology, called osteoporosis. Osteoporosis is four times more prevalent in women than men. In women, the bone loss is associated with the normal loss of estrogen after menopause. In men it is more likely the result of long-term steroid use.

Skeletal and abdominal muscles decrease in size and number of fibers, and the lean tissue is replaced with adipose tissue. This change is most noticeable in men in the area of the waist and in women between the umbilicus and the symphysis pubis. Disuse of the muscles accelerates the loss of strength. The nurse can encourage older adults to exercise, especially weight-bearing exercises, to help maintain healthy bones and muscles and flexibility.

Finally, the musculoskeletal changes that have the most effect on function are related to the ligaments, tendons, and joints; over time these become dry, hardened, more rigid, and less flexible. In joints that had been subjected to trauma earlier in life (injuries or repetitive movement) these changes can be seen earlier and more severely. As joint space is reduced, arthritis is diagnosed. Statistically, arthritis is the number one cause of disability in persons over the age of 65 (Ham et al, 2002).

CARDIOVASCULAR

Cardiac

The normal changes in the healthy heart are known as presbycardia. The maximum coronary artery blood flow is decreased with the resultant decreased stroke volume and cardiac output. Cardiac irritability and contractile recovery are delayed. The left ventricle wall thickens as much as 50% by 80 years of age, and the left atrium also increases in size slightly—an adaptation that enhances ventricular filling (Taffet, Lakatta, 2003). Because of these changes, a fourth heart sound may be audible but is not considered pathological in older adults. However, the size of the heart remains relatively unchanged in healthy adults.

For the person who has lived a healthy lifestyle earlier in life, these changes do not affect function under normal, nonstressful conditions. Diminished cardiac output only becomes significant when the older adult is environmentally, physically, or psychologically stressed. Sudden demands for more oxygen and energy may be particularly troublesome. It takes longer for the heart to accelerate to meet the demands placed on it and to return to its baseline rate. The tachycardia usually seen in younger persons in association with anxiety, pain, hemorrhage, or infection is not as evident in the aged as in the young. Box 7-1 lists

Box 7-1	General Risk Factors That Can Stress the Heart or Aggravate Existing Conditions

Stressors
Continued high intake of dietary animal fat, salt, and calories
Obesity and excessive weight
Long-term cigarette smoking
Lack of regular exercise
Internalization of emotions
Air pollution

Extra Demand or Aggravating Events
Existing chronic conditions
Infection
Anemia
Pneumonia
Cardiac dysrhythmias
Surgery
Fever
Diarrhea
Hypoglycemia
Malnutrition
Avitaminosis
Circulatory overload
Drug-induced condition
Renal disease
Prostatic obstruction

possible stressors and conditions that produce extra cardiac demand. The nurse promoting healthy aging needs to be aware of noncardiac signs of stress and can encourage regular steady exercise and skills in stress management.

However, gerontological nurses are much more likely to care for persons with heart disease than persons with healthy hearts. Cardiovascular disease is the number one cause of death for all elders, of every ethnic and racial group in the United States. The nurse frequently works with persons who have coronary artery disease, dyslipidemia, heart failure, and hypertension. Myocardial infarctions are commonly manifested by "silent" symptoms or without the classic symptoms seen in younger adults. Valvular conditions in the aged are considered residual effects of earlier rheumatic infections and arteriosclerosis.

Aortic and mitral valves are the most often affected and result in slight to moderate regurgitation of blood. The majority of elders have mild systolic ejection murmur, especially of aortic origin, heard as a swooshing sound somewhere between auscultation of S_1 and S_2 (Taffet, Lakatta, 2003). Arrhythmias may be primary or secondary, but the majority of rate irregularities in the aged are attributed to myocardial damage either by interference with the coronary circulation or by valvular insufficiency and concomitant interference of the neurological mechanisms essential to heart action. These conditions are so common that it is easy to imagine that they represent normal aging, but they do not.

Peripheral Vascular

Like the skin, blood vessels, particularly the arteries, become less elastic and more brittle. Elastic fibers fray, split, straighten, and fragment. Calcium that leaves the bone is deposited in the vessels. When combined with the reduction of smooth muscle noted above, the lumen size of the blood vessels is chemically and anatomically decreased and causes a reduction in blood supply to various organs and an increase in peripheral resistance. Change in flow to the coronary arteries and the brain is minimal, but perfusion of the liver and kidneys shows significant change.

In healthy aging, the body is able to compensate for these changes. However, for many older adults the changes lead to an increase in blood pressure. In older adults this increase is rarely in the diastolic interval and is usually restricted to what is called *isolated systolic hypertension (ISH)*. In part because of the frequency of this finding, ISH was thought to be acceptable and was not treated. The most recent clinical advisory statement for the management of high blood pressure published by the National Institutes of Health, as recommended by the *JNC 7 Report,* indicates that all blood pressure readings above 120/90 are cause for concern and readings above 140/90 are no longer acceptable, regardless of the age of the individual (JNC 7, 2003).

Untreated elevations in blood pressure combined with decreased elasticity of arteries and arterioles damage the heart, liver, and kidneys. Dilation and elongation of the aorta occur as a result of collagen and elastin changes and calcium deposition from degenerating elastin. Increased resistance to peripheral blood flow occurs at a rate of about 1% per year, with a moderate decrease in circulation to the coronary arteries. Weakness of vessel walls and varicosities can lead to abnormal swelling of the lower extremities when the vessel walls and varicosities are subjected to increased pressure. Some atherosclerosis is normal with aging, but it can be exacerbated to a pathological state by a diet high in saturated fat (Beare, Myers, 1998).

RESPIRATORY

The normal aging changes in the respiratory system are related to both structure and function. The changes occur gradually and are unnoticed in everyday conditions. However, like the heart, when an older adult is confronted with unusual or stressful circumstances and the demand for oxygen surpasses the available supply, a significant respiratory deficit may occur.

The prominent effects of age-related changes on the respiratory systems are reduced efficiency in ventilation and gas exchange. Starting in the fifties, respiratory muscles begin to weaken, chest wall compliance begins to decrease, and there is a loss of elastic recoil. The elastin and collagen changes caused by cross linkage and deterioration result in a decrease of outward movement and inward pull, with the end result being slightly smaller total lung capacity, increased residual capacity and residual volume, and early airway closure.

Skeletal defects, such as kyphosis and scoliosis, also contribute to restricting chest expansion by further reducing the size of the chest cavity area in which the lungs can expand. The outcomes of these changes are increased dead space, decreased vital capacity, and decreased expiratory flow.

Ossification of the costal cartilage and the downward slant of the ribs further limit chest expansion. Intercostal and accessory muscles and the diaphragm become "floppier" as a consequence of muscle weakness. The potential for greater lung expansion exists but cannot be realized because of structural limitations that develop in the thoracic walls. Total lung capacity is not significantly altered but, rather, is redistributed. The residual capacity increase that occurs with the diminished inspiratory and expiratory thoracic muscle strength results in hyperinflation of the lung apices and underinflation of the lung bases (see Appendix 7-A).

These combined changes affect the blood oxygen (Po_2) level but not the blood carbon dioxide (Pco_2). The blood oxygen level remains relatively constant at about 80 mm Hg from the age of 65 to 90 (Enright, 2003), compared with 90 to 95 mm Hg in the younger adult (Timaris, 1994). There is a decline in the transmural gradient that holds airways open. Airway collapse limits the ability of the lungs to empty and decreases the exhalation of Pco_2. This places a greater demand on cardiac function to increase cardiac output to compensate for less oxygen delivery to body tissues. Diminished elastic recoil of the lungs makes gaseous exchange across alveolar membranes more difficult. Chemoreceptor function is altered or blunted at the peripheral and central chemoreceptor sites in the central nervous system, with reduced ability to respond to hypoxia or hypercapnia.

The changes that occur in the anatomical structures of the chest and the altered muscle strength do not lend themselves to the forcefulness needed to expel material that accumulates or causes an obstruction in the airway. In addition, the respiratory cilia are less effective. Therefore the less effective cough response or cough reflex is a problem for elders, placing them at high risk of potentially life-threatening infections. However, if other clearing mechanisms are intact, the cough reflex is not essential for respiratory clearance. With impairments such as dysphagia or decreased esophageal motility, an intact cough reflex is a necessity. The lack of basilar inflation, an ineffective cough response, and a less efficient immune system pose potential problems for the aged who are sedentary, bedridden, or limited in activity.

RENAL

Renal blood flow decreases by about 10% per decade (Wiggins, 2003). Blood flow through the kidney decreases from 1200 ml/min in young adults to 600 ml/min by the age of 80 as a result of the vascular and fixed anatomical and structural changes. The kidneys lose as many as 50% of the millions of nephrons with little change in the body's ability to regulate the chemical composition of body fluids and the ability to maintain adequate fluid homeostasis day to day (Horowitz, 2000). The age-related decrease in size and function occurs primarily in the kidney cortex, begins in the thirties, and becomes significant by the seventies. Contour remains relatively smooth, and the decline in size parallels the general decrease in size and weight of other body organs.

By the seventies, 30% of the glomeruli are lost and there is evidence of age-related glomerular sclerosis. The cause of sclerosis of the glomeruli is unclear, but it is thought that a high-protein diet or glomerular ischemia may be responsible (Rowe, 1995).

Changes in the arterioglomerular units affect the cortical area (hyalinization and collapse of the glomerular tufts), with the preglomerular arterioles becoming obliterated, reducing the blood flow. The medullary area of the kidney shows sclerosis and loss of the glomeruli and shrinking between the afferent and efferent arterioles; however, the arteriolae rectae verae preserve blood flow to the medullary area. Age does not decrease the number of arterioles in this area.

In general, these changes pose little threat to day-to-day well-being. However, renal reserve is lost and the ability to respond to either a salt or water load or deficit is compromised. We observe for the changes in the glomerular filtration rate (GFR) and creatinine clearance. The GFR depends on the number of glomeruli and steadily declines; this is perhaps the change that is most important relating to nursing intervention. Approximately one third of elders do not show a decline in GFR, suggesting that factors other than age-related change may be responsible for altered renal function (Lindeman, 2000).

Whereas plasma creatinine is constant throughout life, urine creatinine shows a decline even in healthy aging because of the reduced lean muscle mass. The creatinine clearance, a measurement of GFR, is decreased to 100 ml/min by the age of 80. The urine creatinine clearance is an important indicator for appropriate drug therapy in the aged, reflecting the ability to handle medications through the kidneys. Persons with a reduced creatinine clearance usually need a reduction in the dosages of their medications to avoid potential toxicity and caution must be used in the administration of fluids. Unfortunately, this number must be calculated and is not a part of standard laboratory reports. The Cockcroft-Gault equation is used to determine a male's creatinine clearance (CrCl). The calculation for females uses the same formula, but the answer is multiplied by 0.85 or 85%.

$$CrCl = \frac{140 - Age\,(Weight\,in\,kg)}{72 \times Serum\,creatinine}$$

Finally, lower renin levels are associated with a parallel reduction of the same proportions in aldosterone. This decreases the kidneys' ability to conserve sodium and delay the response of the acid/base loading. A reduced ability to concentrate urine and conserve water resulting from medullary loss makes the collecting ducts less responsive to antidiuretic hormone (ADH).

The importance of the age-related kidney changes is that elders are more susceptible to fluid and electrolyte imbalance and renal damage from medications and contrast media of diagnostic tests. Under normal circumstances, kidney function is sufficient to meet the regulation and excretion demands of the body. However, with the stress of disease, surgery, or fever, the kidneys have reduced capacity to respond.

ENDOCRINE

Hormones are responsible for and control reproduction, growth and development, maintenance of homeostasis, and energy production. Two principles must be kept in mind when considering hormonal control and effects: (1) a particular hormone may have an effect on many body systems and functions, and (2) one body function may require the coordinated action of many hormones. Most glands atrophy and decrease their rate of secretion. However, there is no uniform direction of change.

Insulin secretion from the beta cells and glucose metabolism change little throughout life. The age-related change is in the decreased sensitivity of receptor sites to insulin and is thought to be caused by a change in the molecular makeup of naturally produced insulin. In addition, higher levels of circulating proinsulin are found in older adults than in younger adults. When the pancreas is stressed with sudden concentrations of glucose,

blood levels are higher and prolonged (see Appendix 7a). These temporary levels of increased blood glucose make the diagnosis of diabetes or glucose intolerance difficult.

Thyroid function remains adequate with age, as do the secretions of thyroid-stimulating hormone (TSH) and the serum concentration of thyroxine (T_4). However, a significant decline in triiodothyronine (T_3) occurs with age, which is thought to reflect reduced conversion of T_4 to T_3 in extrathyroidal locations. Collective signs, such as a slowed basal metabolic rate, thinning of the hair, and dry skin, are characteristic of hypothyroidism in the young but are normal manifestations in the aged who have no history of thyroid deficiencies, making the recognition of thyroid disturbances also difficult.

Slightly reduced cortisol, an important glucocorticoid of the adrenal cortex, does not seem to have an adverse effect on the aging body. Likewise, the effect of decreased ACTH production has not been elucidated. Epinephrine, norepinephrine, and dopamine produced by the adrenal medulla decrease with age, but again the significance is unclear.

The pituitary gland, with its diverse functions and central role in the complex hormone feedback system, decreases in volume. The significance of this change is unclear in light of the maintenance of adequate hormonal secretions.

Adrenogenic, estrogenic, and gonadotropic hormones undergo secretory and stimulatory changes resulting in decreases. Diminished hormone levels lead to atrophy of the ovaries, uterus, and vaginal tissue in aged women. For men, the refractory period between erections lengthens and ejaculatory volume decreases. Interest in and need for sexual activity continue; however, sexual capacity may diminish.

GASTROINTESTINAL

Digestion begins in the mouth and depends on adequate mastication and saliva, which contains ptyalin. Normally, saliva production is unchanged with age, but many systemic disorders or their treatments result in decreases leading to impaired digestion and dry mouths, or xerostomia. It is also still common to care for elders who are edentulous, with or without dentures, which can interfere with mastication. It is important that the nurse ensure the fit and cleanliness of the dentures or their replacement if lost, to maximize wellness.

In the esophagus, the number of muscle movements increases but does not yield effective propulsion of its contents and actually results in decreased peristalsis. The decreased esophageal peristalsis is a result of diminished muscle strength and motility. The sluggish emptying of the esophagus, or presbyesophagus, also forces the lower end to dilate and sustain greater stress, which increases the risk of hiatal hernias and causes digestive discomfort. Complaints of indigestion and reflux are common.

The reduction of hydrochloric acid (HCl) in the stomach occurs at about age 60, with a decline of pepsin starting in the forties and continuing in a sharp decline to the sixties. The pepsin level then levels out and remains at a constant low. Increased stomach pH interferes with the protective alkaline viscous mucus, resulting in increased susceptibility to gastric irritation, bleeding, and ulceration. Loss of smooth muscle in the stomach delays emptying time and also exposes the epithelial lining to extended contact with gastric contents. This can increase or delay the absorption time of nutrients and medications affected by the stomach pH.

The glandular secretions of the digestive system from the liver, gallbladder, and pancreas are altered with age. The liver continues to function throughout life even with a decrease in volume and weight (mass) and a concomitant decrease in liver blood flow of 30% to 40% by the late nineties (Hall, 2003), with implications for impaired drug metabolism and associated with an increased half-life of fat-soluble medications. Liver regeneration, although slow, is not greatly impaired, and liver function tests remain unaltered with age.

The gallbladder, which stores the bile manufactured by the liver, does not seem to change, but those 70 years of age and older account for one third of gallbladder surgeries (Tompkins, 1995; Welch, 1995). It is thought that this may be caused by the increased lipogenic composition of bile from biliary cholesterol or by an age-related decline in pancreatic secretions and enzyme output, which decreases the tolerance for fatty foods. A decrease in bile salt synthesis is also thought to increase the incidence of cholelithiasis and cholecystitis.

Smooth muscle, Peyer's patches, and lymphatic follicles of the small intestine decrease with age. Changes in motility, epithelial membranes, vascular perfusion, and gastrointestinal membrane transport may affect absorption of lipids, amino acids, glucose, calcium, and iron. Calcium use is affected by lack of adequate gastric acid and slow active transport in the body. The tendency toward vitamin and mineral deficiency is caused partly by the faulty absorption of vitamins B_1 and B_{12}, calcium, and iron and by inadequate dietary intake.

It is difficult to determine changes in the large intestine even though there is structural atrophy of the layers and glands and a decrease in mucous secretions. The internal sphincter of the large intestine loses some of its muscle tone, which can create problems in bowel evacuation. Weakness of the intestinal walls may also lead to outpouching of small segments of the colon (diverticula), which may or may not be symptomatic. The external sphincter, which retains much of its original tone, cannot by itself control the bowels. Slower transmission of neural impulses lessens the awareness of sensations of a forthcoming bowel evacuation. The outcome of this may be either fecal incontinence or constipation.

NEUROLOGICAL

Contrary to popular beliefs the older nervous system, including the brain, is remarkably resilient. The changes do not cause loss of function, only delayed function. It is not a normal part of aging to lose cognitive function or become depressed, although both of these are very commonly observed. Both indicate pathological conditions.

Central Nervous System

Nurses are sometimes alarmed when they review the computed tomography (CT) scan of an elder's brain, with the diagnosis "brain atrophy." However, this is a normal finding and has no clinical meaning. On autopsy increased deposits of the pigment lipofuscin and the amyloid protein, senile plaque, and an occasional neurofibrillary tangle are also found. Each of these changes has been found in the brains of persons both with and without dementing illnesses, such as Alzheimer's disease (Joynt, 2000).

Changes are also seen in the amount of dopaminergic and cholinergic neurotransmitters. Choline acetylase, dopamine, serotonin, and catecholamines decrease. The enzyme monoamine oxidase (MAO) increases. These changes may make the older adult more at risk for serotonin-related depression; however, the exact ramifications of these changes are not yet known.

Nerve cell loss is minimal in the brainstem but more profound in the hippocampus. By the eighties, the cerebral ventricles have enlarged three to four times. The brain has the ability to compensate for areas of injury or destruction, with compensation more effective in the higher centers. The spinal cord is less able to do so.

Intellectual performance of the elder without brain dysfunction remains constant; however, the performance of tasks may take longer, which is an indication that central processing is slowed. Slight forgetfulness may be normal, such as missing birthdates or one's car keys. More significant memory loss, such as the directions to favorite places, indicates a pathological condition and requires a full evaluation.

Peripheral Nervous System

The most important effect of the normal changes in the aging peripheral nervous system is the increased risk for injury. Vibratory sense in the lower extremities may be nonexistent. Somesthetics, or tactile sensitivity, decreases with the loss of a large number of nerve endings in the skin. This is most notable in the fingertips, palms of the hands, and lower extremities. This decreased sensitivity is translated into delayed reactions to things such as hot surfaces, significantly increasing the risk for burns and the extent of burns should they occur. The presence of a functioning smoke detector is particularly important for healthy aging.

Kinesthetic sense, or proprioception (one's position in space), is altered because of changes in both the peripheral and central nervous systems. If one is less aware of body position and has less tactile awareness (sensitivity) the risk for falling is dramatically increased. The person may be walking on a flat surface when an uneven surface is suddenly encountered, such as an uneven side-walk. It takes just a little longer to realize the surface is uneven and a little longer to realize that one has tripped (changed position in space). Where a younger person would be able to immediately right herself or himself and prevent a fall, this slight delay often results in a fall in an older adult. Conditions such as arthritis, stroke, some cardiac disorders, or damage to the structures of the inner ear may affect peripheral and central mechanisms of mobility. Further discussion of sensory alterations appears in Chapter 9.

Eye and Vision

Changes in vision and eyes are both functional and structural and combine changes in the nervous system with changes in the skin and in associated organs.

Structurally, eyelids droop (senile ptosis) as a result of the loss of elasticity and skin atrophy and can interfere with vision if the lids sag far enough. A decrease in the orbicular muscle strength of the eyes may result in ectropion or entropion. Ectropion may cause the lower lid to roll outward, exposing the palpebral conjunctiva. This may result in nonclosure of the lids and leads to corneal dryness at sleep and excessive tearing while awake. Spasms of the orbicular muscle may cause the eyelashes, particularly of the lower lid, to turn inward (entropion), with scratching and irritation to the cornea, and may require a surgical repair.

Visually, a gray-white to silver ring or partial ring, known as *arcus senilis,* may be observed 1 to 2 mm inside the limbus or outer edge of the iris; it is composed of deposits of calcium and cholesterol salts. It does not appear to have any clinical significance and is considered a normal part of aging.

The conjunctiva, the thin membrane over the sclera, contains goblet cells that provide mucin, essential for eye lubrication and movement. In normal aging the number of goblet cells decreases, resulting in a deficiency of lubrication for the eye and potential for irritation and what is known as dry eye syndrome. A flatter, less smooth, and thicker cornea is noticeable by its loss of sparkling transparency.

Functionally, visual acuity, accommodation, and light and color sensitivity are affected by the aging process. The decreased ability of the eyes to accommodate to close and detailed work (presbyopia) begins in the thirties and continues throughout the rest of one's life. Suspensory ligaments, ciliary muscles, and parasympathetic nerves contribute to the decreased accommodation that occurs. Nearly everyone between ages 40 and 45 requires glasses for close vision acuity. For those who are myopic (nearsighted), their distance vision improves. Peripheral vision (visual fields) also deteriorates with less clarity at the edges of vision.

In addition, the pupils have more limited or slowed dilation and constriction. Changes in dilation and constriction cause problems when the person moves from one level of lighting to another. Because of the slow ability of the pupils to accommodate to changes in light, glare is a major problem. Glare is a problem created not only by sunlight outdoors, but also by the reflection of light on any shiny object, especially light striking polished or linoleum floors (Meisami et al, 2003).

The pupils become smaller with a need for more light for visual clarity. Older people require three times as much light to see things as they did when they were in their twenties. It is more effective to place high-intensity light on the object or surface that is involved than to increase the intensity of the light in the entire area or room. For example, it would be more effective to focus a light directly on the newspaper a person was reading than to try to increase the light in the whole room.

Lens opacity or cataracts begin to develop in the forties. The origins are not fully understood, although ultraviolet rays of the sun contribute to the problem, with cross linkage of collagen creating a more rigid and thickened lens structure. Linked in part to this opacity, color clarity diminishes by 25% in the fifties and by 59% in the seventies. Color is less accurate with blues, violets, and greens of the spectrum; light colors such as reds, oranges, and yellows are more easily seen.

Intraocular changes occur as well, although they are not usually assessed by the nurse. The vitreous humor, which gives the eye globe its shape and support, loses some of its water and fibrous skeletal support with age. Opacities other than cataracts are described by persons as lines, webs, spots, or clusters of dots moving rapidly across the visual field with each movement of the eye. These opacities, known as *floaters,* are bits of coalesced vitreous that have broken off from the peripheral or central part of the retina. Mostly they are harmless but annoying until they dissipate or one gets used to them. If, however, the person says that he or she sees a shower of these and a flash of light, this requires immediate medical attention, since it might indicate an acute retinal problem.

On inspection, the retina has less distinct margins and is duller in appearance than in younger adults. The fovea of the macula may not reflect as brightly. Drusen (yellow-white) spots may appear during the ophthalmoscopical examination. As long as these changes are not accompanied by distortion of objects or a decrease in vision they are not clinically significant. If the person has had hypertension for a long time, arteriovenous (AV) nicking may be visible or distortions of the ocular veins as they pass over the arteries. Resorption of the intraocular fluid becomes less efficient with age and may lead to eventual breakdown in the absorption process. This creates the potential for the pathological condition known as *glaucoma.*

Ear and Hearing

The most notable changes in the older ear are its appearance (especially in men) and the normal age-related hearing loss known as *presbycusis.* The auricle, or pinna, loses flexibility and becomes longer and wider as a result of diminished elasticity. The lobule sags, elongates, and develops wrinkles. Together these changes make the ear appear larger. The periphery of the auricle develops coarse, wiry, stiff hair in men. The tragus also becomes larger in men.

The auditory canal narrows, causing inward collapsing. Stiffer and coarser hair lines the ear canal. Cerumen glands atrophy, causing thicker and dryer cerumen, which is more difficult to remove and is a substantial cause for hearing impairment. The gerontological nurse should be sensitive to this and be skilled at assisting with ear hygiene to maximize hearing.

On otoscopical examination the tympanic membrane appears dull, retracted, and gray. Structurally, the ossicle joints between the malleus and the stapes develop calcification, causing joint fixation or reduced vibration of these bones and reducing transmitted sound.

Auditory changes occur subtly. Normal decrements in hearing acuity, speech intelligibility, level of auditory threshold, and discrimination of pitch, especially in the speech frequencies, are referred to as *presbycusis,* the "hearing loss of aging." Presbycusis is the type of loss, not the cause of the loss, and can be classified according to the structural source of impairment. Further discussion of vision and hearing is addressed in Chapter 9. In sensory hearing loss there is a decrease in vestibular sensitivity as a result of degeneration of the organ of Corti in the cochlea and otic nerve loss and subsequent impaired transmission of sound waves to the brain. Neural hearing loss is the result of the loss of cochlear neurons that occurs in late life (even with the preservation of the organ of Corti) and is considered to be related to genetic factors. Familial tendencies in middle life associated with electrophysiological function of the organ of Corti are the basis of metabolic hearing loss. Altered motion of the cochlear ducts occurs in middle age and is considered cochlear conductive hearing loss. The role of basilar membrane stiffening as a possible cause of this type of hearing loss is not proved. All these types of loss are presbycusis. Many elders have a combination of causes for their hearing deficit.

Constant or recurring high-pitched tinnitus (clicking, buzzing, roaring, ringing, or other sounds in the ear) is usually caused by impairment of the otic nerve accompanying the aging process,

NANDA and Wellness Diagnoses

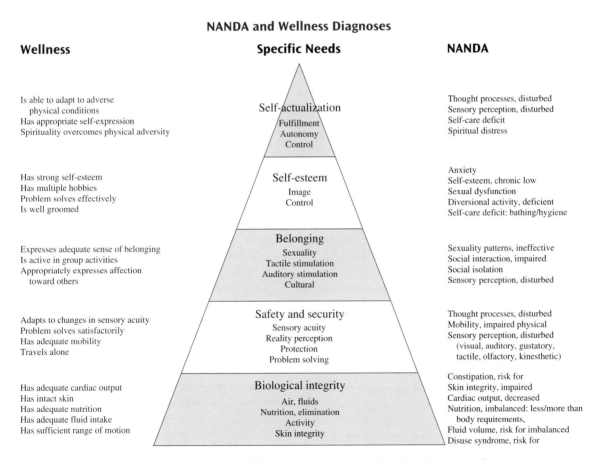

Wellness

Is able to adapt to adverse
  physical conditions
Has appropriate self-expression
Spirituality overcomes physical adversity

Has strong self-esteem
Has multiple hobbies
Problem solves effectively
Is well groomed

Expresses adequate sense of belonging
Is active in group activities
Appropriately expresses affection
  toward others

Adapts to changes in sensory acuity
Problem solves satisfactorily
Has adequate mobility
Travels alone

Has adequate cardiac output
Has intact skin
Has adequate nutrition
Has adequate fluid intake
Has sufficient range of motion

Specific Needs

Self-actualization
Fulfillment
Autonomy
Control

Self-esteem
Image
Control

Belonging
Sexuality
Tactile stimulation
Auditory stimulation
Cultural

Safety and security
Sensory acuity
Reality perception
Protection
Problem solving

Biological integrity
Air, fluids
Nutrition, elimination
Activity
Skin integrity

NANDA

Thought processes, disturbed
Sensory perception, disturbed
Self-care deficit
Spiritual distress

Anxiety
Self-esteem, chronic low
Sexual dysfunction
Diversional activity, deficient
Self-care deficit: bathing/hygiene

Sexuality patterns, ineffective
Social interaction, impaired
Social isolation
Sensory perception, disturbed

Thought processes, disturbed
Mobility, impaired physical
Sensory perception, disturbed
  (visual, auditory, gustatory,
  tactile, olfactory, kinesthetic)

Constipation, risk for
Skin integrity, impaired
Cardiac output, decreased
Nutrition, imbalanced: less/more than
  body requirements,
Fluid volume, risk for imbalanced
Disuse syndrome, risk for

These are not all of the possible wellness or NANDA diagnoses that may be identified. The above are frequent examples of nursing diagnoses that should be considered when planning care for the older adult in whatever setting.

although it may be caused by medications, infection, cerumen accumulation, or a blow to the head. Tinnitus may be unilateral or bilateral and becomes most acute at night or in quiet surroundings. It is a nuisance that is difficult to combat or treat. The most helpful strategy is to use masking techniques that introduce another, competing sound. White noise (soft static between FM radio stations) on low volume can be soothing, but it can also be irritating. The nurse who understands these changes can actively develop other interventions to promote healthy aging.

KEY CONCEPTS

- There are many physical changes with aging; however, a number of these are relatively insignificant in the absence of disease or unusual stress.
- Physiological aging is universal, progressive, decremental, intrinsic, and unavoidable.
- There are enormous individual variations in the rate of aging of body systems and functions.
- Many of the normal changes with aging may be misinterpreted as pathological, and some pathological conditions may be mistaken as normal changes of aging.
- Careful assessment of individual aging changes, lifestyle, and desires is fundamental to good nursing care of the old.

Activities and Discussion Questions

1. Identify at least two normal changes with aging and two abnormal physical/physiological changes that are commonly seen in older adults, for each body system.
2. Discuss the age changes you would find most difficult to accept.
3. Obtain the creatinine level and prescribed medication from the chart of several aged persons. Calculate the urine creatinine levels to identify the GFR and to determine if there is a danger of drug toxicity from the medication or medications being taken.
4. Develop a nursing care plan using wellness and North American Nursing Diagnosis Association (NANDA) diagnoses.

REFERENCES

Beare P, Myers J: *Adult health nursing,* ed 3, St Louis, 1998, Mosby.

Enright PL: Aging of the respiratory system. In Hazzard WR et al, editors: *Principles of geriatric medicine and gerontology,* ed 5, New York, 2003, McGraw-Hill.

Goldman R: Decline in organic function with age. In Rossman I, editor: *Clinical geriatrics,* ed 2, Philadelphia, 1979, Lippincott.

Hall KE: Effect of aging on gastrointestinal function. In Hazzard WR et al, editors: *Principles of geriatric medicine and gerontology,* ed 5, New York, 2003, McGraw-Hill.

Ham RJ, Sloane PD, Warshaw GA: *Primary care geriatrics,* ed 4, St Louis, 2002, Mosby.

Hayflick L: Theories of aging. In Cape R, Coe R, Rossman I, editors: *Fundamentals of geriatric medicine,* New York, 1983, Raven Press.

Horowitz M: Aging and the gastrointestinal tract. In Beers MH, Berkow R, editors: *The Merck manual of geriatrics,* ed 2, Whitehouse Station, NJ, 2000, Merck Research Laboratories.

Jett KF: The meaning of aging and the celebration of years among rural African-American women, *Geriatr Nurs* 24(5):290-293, 2003.

Joint National Committee on Detection, Evaluation, and Treatment of High Blood Pressure: JNC 7 Report. Available at www.nhlbi.nih.gov. Accessed 7/2/04.

Joynt JR: Aging and the nervous system. In Beers MH, Berkow R, editors: *The Merck manual of geriatrics,* ed 3, Whitehouse Station, NJ, 2000, Merck Research Laboratories.

Lamb KV: Musculoskeletal function. In Lueckenotte AG: *Gerontologic nursing,* St Louis, 1996, Mosby.

Lindemann RD: Aging and the kidney. In Beers MH, Berkow R, editors: *The Merck manual of geriatrics,* ed 3, Whitehouse Station, NJ, 2000, Merck Research Laboratories.

Meisami E, Brown CM, Emerle HF: Sensory systems: normal aging, disorders, and treatments of vision and hearing in humans. In Timiras PS, editor: *Physiological basis of aging and geriatrics,* ed 3, New York City, 2002, CRC Press.

Rowe JW: Aging process: renal changes and disorders. In Abrams WB, Beers MH, Berkow R, editors: *The Merck manual of geriatrics,* ed 2, Whitehouse Station, NJ, 1995, Merck Research Laboratories.

Taffet GE, Lakatta EG: Aging of the cardiovascular system. In Hazzard WR et al, editors: *Principles of geriatric medicine and gerontology,* ed 5, New York, 2003, McGraw-Hill.

Timiris PS: *Physiological basis of aging and geriatrics,* ed 3, New York, 2002, CRC Press.

Tompkins RG: Surgery: preoperative evaluation and interoperative and postoperative care: surgery of the gastrointestinal tract. In Abrams WB, Beers MH, Berkow R, editors: *The Merck manual of geriatrics,* ed 2, Whitehouse Station, NJ, 1995, Merck Research Laboratories.

Welch CE: Surgery: preoperative evaluation and intra-operative and postoperative care: surgery of the gas-trointestinal tract. In Abrams WB, Beers MH, Berkow R, editors: *The Merck manual of geriatrics,* ed 2, Whitehouse Station, NJ, 1995, Merck Research Laboratories.

Wiggins J: Changes in renal function. In Hazzard WR et al, editors: *Principles of geriatric medicine and gerontology,* ed 5, New York, 2003, McGraw-Hill.

Appendix 7-A Physiological Changes and Functional Effects with Age: Implications and Interventions

System	Physiological Changes	Functional Effect	Nursing Implications*	Possible Interventions*
Integument	Skin loses elasticity: wrinkles, folds, sagging, dryness	Easy tearing; itching Incisions, cuts, bruises heal more slowly than in younger adults	Introduction of organisms leading to infections Bath or shower water temperature should be between 95° and 105° F	Nurse should keep own nails short; handle patient's skin with care; limit bathing to every other day; bathe perineal area daily; lubricate skin with lotion at least once daily
	Spotty pigmentation in sun-exposed areas; face paler (even without presence of anemia)			Apply sunscreen before going outside; wear a hat and sunglasses
	Atrophy of epidermal arterioles		Prone to pressure ulcers; slow wound healing	Inspect skin when bathing; check pressure areas at least every 2h if patient is bedridden; if sitting in chair, as soon as medically possible; if ambulating, at least every few days; maintain immaculate aseptic technique
	Atrophy of oil, moisture, and sweat glands	Dryness Prone to hyperthermia	Potentially life threatening	Hydrate; wear light, cool clothing; stay in cool area; apply ice to back of neck or head to keep cool
	Decreased subcutaneous fat; fat deposition mainly through trunk, less on extremities	Altered thermoregulation (hypothermia)	Potentially life threatening	Maintain warm environment; use warm blankets; warm intravenous (IV) fluids postoperatively if necessary or if very chilled; in cold weather provide warm environment and maintain humidity at 60%; adequate warm clothing

	Hair thins on scalp, axillae, and pubic areas; decreases on upper and lower extremities; decreased facial hair in men; women may develop chin and upper lip hair		Intentional or unintentional scratching	
	Nail growth slows	Nails prone to snagging, chipping, ragged edges, tearing		Keep nails clipped short and filed; offer periodic basic manicure; buff nails or apply nail polish
Respiratory	Nose elongates	Decreased cough reflex	Congestion	Place in upright position when eating, drinking, or having respiratory problems; limit exposure to airborne viruses, bacteria, pollutants; adequate ventilation; yearly flu immunization
	Stiffer pharynx and larynx	Decreased removal of mucus, dust, irritants	Voice pitch higher	Establish exercise program (walking or stationary bike riding, etc.); pace activity; provide adequate rest periods
	Decreased cilia	Decreased vital capacity	Potential for upper respiratory tract infections	Deep-breathing exercises; ascertain that patient has Pneumovac immunization (1 time after age 65); auscultate lungs; smoking cessation program
	Increased anteroposterior chest diameter	Decreased chest expansion reduces recoil		
	Rigidity of chest wall	Decreased endurance		
	Fewer alveoli	Hyperinflation of apices; underinflation of bases		
	Airway resistance			
Cardiovascular	Thickening of walls of blood vessels	Lower cardiac output	Fatigue, shortness of breath	Pace activities; monitor blood pressure; establish aerobic exercise program; smoking cessation program
	Narrowing of vessel lumen	Increased pulmonary vascular tension; increased systolic pressure; decreased peripheral circulation	Dependent edema	Check for swelling and pitting edema; wear support hose; elevate feet periodically during day
	Loss of vessel elasticity	Left ventricle hypertrophy (only in fiber size)	Decreased cardiac output	
	Lower cardiac output		Dysrhythmias	
	Decreased number of heart muscle fibers		Murmurs	
			Dizziness from too-rapid change of position	

Continued.

Data from Saxon SV, Etten MJ: *Physical change and aging*, ed 3, New York, 1994, Tiresias Press; Abrams WB et al: *The Merck manual of geriatrics*, ed 2, Whitehouse Station, NJ, 1995, Merck Research Laboratories; Copstead LEC: *Perspectives on pathophysiology*, Philadelphia, 1995, Saunders; Stanley M, Beare PG: *Gerontological nursing*, Philadelphia, 1995, Davis; Ebersole P, Hess P: *Toward healthy aging: human needs and nursing response*, ed 5, St Louis, 1998, Mosby.
*Provides examples of some implications and interventions.

Appendix 7-A Physiological Changes and Functional Effects with Age: Implications and Interventions—cont'd

System	Physiological Changes	Functional Effect	Nursing Implications*	Possible Interventions*
Cardiovascular, cont'd	Decreased elasticity and calcification of heart valves Decreased baroreceptor sensitivity	Decrease in rate, rhythm, and tone (heart rate normal at rest)		Auscultate heart and lungs; if on medications ascertain that they are taken (given) correctly; teach client about taking medications Overall teaching for heart-healthy diet: decrease intake of fat, sodium, sugar; control weight Instruct on proper way to get up after lying in bed, sitting for extended periods of time; how to bend over and get up
	Decreased efficiency of venous valves	Poor venous return	Venous pooling, stasis dermatitis; stasis ulcers; varicosities; dependent edema	Inspect for color and swelling, beginnings of stasis dermatitis or ulcers; palpate for temperature; wear support hose; no crossing of legs at knees
Gastrointestinal	Periodontal disease; loss of teeth	Change in jaw/mouth contour; poor mastication	Changes in food intake; fetid breath; edentulousness	Appropriate oral hygiene regimen: brushing teeth 2-3 times daily, use of dental floss; minimum of yearly teeth cleaning and checkup (every 6mo is best) If dentures: clean daily; remove at night; keep in good repair
	Decrease in saliva production	Dry mouth	Breakdown of tissue integrity of oral mucosa	Chew gum to create moist environment; use artificial saliva; drink adequate fluids (minimum 1500ml/day); monitor/instruct on chewing food slowly and thoroughly

System	Physiological Change	Problem	Nursing Intervention
	Decrease in secretion of digestive juices Pancreas less active—decrease in production of insulin Decreased smooth muscle Decreased esophageal peristalsis Decreased small intestinal peristalsis	Food intolerances; difficulty with digestion Improper eating patterns; dependency on antacids	Assess for food intolerance; avoid offending foods
Musculoskeletal	Decreased muscle mass Skeletal changes	Muscle strength diminishes	Unable to do tasks done when younger; danger of injury	Muscle-strengthening exercises (weight training)
	Decalcification of bones	Brittle bones	Fractures; osteoporosis; thoracic-vertebral hump	Adequate calcium intake; flexibility exercises and weight-bearing exercises (walking)
	Degenerative joint changes	Stiffer joints; restricted movement; aches and pains with movement; femoral joint angle causes legs to turn outward	Limited mobility; arthritis; potential for gait changes, falls	Gentle exercise (water aerobics); use of acceptable analgesics as necessary (topical, systemic); application of heat, cold
	Dehydration of intervertebral disks	Decreased height	Shorter stature; flexed posture	
Neurological	Nerve cell degeneration and atrophy (25%-40%)	Some degree of recent memory loss (age associated—benign)	Forgetfulness; requires longer time for response	Approach learning projects slowly
	Decrease in neurotransmitters Decrease in rate of nerve cell conduction impulses	Learning occurs as usual but more slowly	Potential for dementing processes Client becomes frustrated Longer reaction time to questions and response to danger	Use memory aids (adhesive notes, calendars, word association, etc.) Assess mental status using clock drawing and Mini-Mental Status Examination as appropriate Assess environment for safety Use reminiscence as appropriate
Sensory (Refer to Appendix 9-A.)	Eyes: pupils decrease in size; less light enters eyes; lens yellows	Presbyopia: decreased accommodation to near/far; difficulty adjusting to light and dark	Difficulty reading small print, seeing objects in distance, dealing with fine detail of objects	Adjust lighting to decrease glare Increase light intensity—direct light directly over area where client is working
		Color distortion Glare Cataracts	Poor accommodation to rapid light changes in environment	Use bright and contrasting colors; stay away from dark end of spectrum

Continued.

Appendix 7-A   Physiological Changes and Functional Effects with Age: Implications and Interventions—cont'd

System	Physiological Changes	Functional Effect	Nursing Implications*	Possible Interventions*
Sensory, cont'd		Decreased tear production	Difficulty seeing colors at dark end of spectrum (greens, blues, violets, browns)	Provide magnifying glass or magnifying sheet for reading labels or small print; print information in larger type
			Squinting or pain from bright light or sunshine	Slowly change light intensity from bright to dim and vice versa
			Decreased ability to see	
	Ears: thickening of tympanic membrane; sclerosis of inner ear; ear wax buildup	Presbycusis: loss of high-frequency sounds; decreased mobility of ossicles; impaired hearing	Dry, scratchy eye Difficulty hearing instructions during teaching	Decrease environmental sounds and distractions Speak clearly and face-to-face with patient
	Taste: may have fewer taste buds on tongue, mouth Smell: often diminished Touch: decreased skin receptors Proprioception: decreased awareness of body position in space	Correlation between taste and smell		
Genitourinary	Gradual loss of nephrons (30%-50%)	Decreased absorption of tubules; decreased glomerular filtration rate (GFR)	Increased potential for inadequate excretion of drug metabolites	Monitor renal function carefully
	Decrease in renal blood flow	More time needed for filtration; urine may be more dilute		
	Decreased bladder capacity Women: may develop lax sphincter	Need to urinate frequently; incontinence; decreased bladder tone		Remove barriers to getting to toilet Answer call lights or bell as quickly as possible and provide assistance to toilet as needed

System	Age-related change	Potential	Interventions
	Men: enlargement of prostate	Benign prostatic hypertrophy; potential for urinary retention	Increased potential for urinary treat infections	Assess pattern of voiding with continence log if incontinence is occurring; look at circumstance that might be responsible; establish a toileting plan Use continence pads or pants as needed, but make sure they are checked and changed when wet Provide commode if toilet is too far away As a last resort, catheterize
Reproductive	Women: decreased estrogen production; ovaries degenerate; vagina atrophies; uterus and breasts atrophy	Lose ability to procreate; vaginal dryness; uncomfortable intercourse; menopause	Increased potential for sexual difficulties	Discuss types of hormone replacement therapy, from natural products to medical prescriptions Explore various vaginal lubricants for dryness Explain normal age changes that occur to both men and women
	Men: sperm count diminishes; testes smaller; less firm erections take longer to occur	Erectile dysfunction concerns	Increased potential for sexual difficulties	Discuss importance of using condoms if individuals are single (never married, widowed, divorced) or live an alternative lifestyle Dispel myths of loss of sexual drive Discuss impotence and need for professional consultation
Endocrine	Alteration in hormone regulation	Decrease in ability to respond to stress	Impaired physiological and psychological responses	Modulate environment to reduce physical, psychological, and social stressors
Thyroid	Decreased thyroid hormone	Temperature intolerance; decreased target organ sensitivity	Feels too cold or too hot; possible depression or nervousness; weight gain or loss	Periodic thyroid-stimulating hormone (TSH) check
Thymus	Involution of thymus gland	Decreased cell-mediated immunity	More susceptible to infection	Good hand washing; ensure that flu and Pneumovac inoculations are updated; limit exposure to obvious pathogens; maintain aseptic technique in dressing changes and any invasive procedures
Cortisols/glucocorticoids	Increased antiinflammatory hormone	Slower ability to respond to inflammatory process	Decreased speed of tissue repair; slower ability to respond to inflammatory process	
Pancreas	Increased fibrosis; decreased secretions and enzymes	Effect on glucose metabolism	Potential for diabetes mellitus	Periodic blood glucose test

Psychological, Cognitive, and Social Aspects of Aging

8

LEARNING OBJECTIVES

Upon completion of this chapter, the reader will be able to:

- Explain the major cognitive, psychological, and sociological theories of aging.
- Understand several normal cognitive changes of aging.
- Recognize that culture and cohort affect psychological and social adaptation.
- Identify several social roles that elder members of a society usually fulfill.
- Discuss several "buffers" that make transitions to new roles somewhat easier.
- Compare some of the differences you would expect between the retirement adjustment of women and men.
- Explain the major issues in adaptation to a major role change, such as retirement or widowhood.

GLOSSARY

Cognition The mental process characterized by knowing, thinking, learning, and judging.

Cross-sectional A study design that includes several groups, assessing these subjects at different points in a process. An example of this would be cohort studies that involve several cohorts and survey their experience around a given event.

Depersonalization As used in this chapter, not a severe psychiatric disturbance but, rather, the loss of identity and sense of self that occurs when a person is treated as an object.

Longitudinal research A study design that studies a group of subjects over time, assessing their experiences

at predetermined stages. The Harvard Nurses' Study is an example of this in that a large group of nurses have been assessed every few years for more than 20 years.

Psychometrics The development, administration, and interpretation of psychological and intelligence tests.

Psychosocial Pertaining to a combination of psychological and social factors.

Regeneration Rebuilding of impaired or injured tissues.

Synaptogenesis To form a connection between neurons.

THE LIVED EXPERIENCE

IF I HAD MY LIFE TO LIVE OVER

I'd dare to make more mistakes next time, I'd relax, I would limber up. I would be sillier than I've been this trip. I would take fewer things seriously. I would take more chances. I would climb more mountains and swim more rivers. I would eat more ice cream and less beans. I would perhaps have more actual troubles, but I'd have fewer imaginary ones.

You see, I'm one of those people who live sensibly and sanely hour after hour, day after day. Oh, I've had my moments, and if I had to do it over again, I'd have more of them. In fact, I'd try to have nothing else. Just moments, one after another, instead of living so many years ahead of each day. I've been one of those persons who never goes anywhere without a thermostat, a hot water bottle, a raincoat and a parachute. If I had it to do again, I would travel lighter than I have.

If I had my life to live over, I would start barefoot earlier in the spring and stay that way later in the fall. I would go to more dances. I would ride more merry-go-rounds. I would pick more daisies.

Source: Stair N: If I had my life to live over. In Martz S, editor: If I had my life to live over
I would pick more daisies, Watsonville, Calif, 1992, Papier Mache Press, p 1.

*T*here are normal psychological, cognitive, biological, and social changes in the process of aging. The biological changes are fully explained in Chapter 7. This chapter is meant to provide the reader with information on the psychosocial aspects of aging. The student can then identify normal cognitive, psychological, and sociological changes and begin to detect those that go beyond the normal changes and need attention. All the psychosocial aspects of aging are less measurable than the biological changes, and there is much to be learned about the aging process. Each individual has unique life experiences and because of this must be seen holistically, through the lens of his or her time, place, and personal history.

LIFE SPAN DEVELOPMENT THEORY

Human development goes on throughout life and is a lifelong process of adaptation. Life span development refers to an individual's progress through time and an expected pattern of change: biological, sociological, and psychological. A summary of the key principles of the life span developmental approach provided by Papalia et al (2002) is based on the work of Paul Baltes and colleagues (Baltes, 1987; Baltes et al, 1998). Principles include the following:

- Development is lifelong. Each part of the life span is influenced by the past and will affect the future. Each period of the life span has unique characteristics and value; none is more important than any other.
- Development depends on history and context. Each person develops within a certain set of circumstances or conditions defined by time and place. Humans are influenced by historical, social, and cultural context.

- Development is multidimensional and multidirectional and involves a balance of growth and decline. Whereas children usually grow consistently in size and abilities, in adulthood, the balance gradually shifts. Some abilities, such as vocabulary, continue to increase, whereas others, such as speed of information retrieval, may decrease. New abilities, such as wisdom and expertise, may emerge as one ages.
- Development is pliable or plastic. Function and performance can improve throughout the life span with training and practice. However, there are limits on how much a person can improve at any age.

The course of behavior throughout the life span appears to have three major forces: hereditary, cultural, and individual choice (Birren, Cunningham, 1985). The close relationship among biological, social, and psychological development that exists through childhood and adolescence varies more in adulthood because of the greater variations in life experiences and demands as one matures.

People age in a number of ways. Aging can be viewed in terms of chronological age, biological age, psychological age, and social age. These ages may or may not be the same. *Chronological age* is measured by the number of years lived. *Biological age* is predicted by the person's physical condition and how well vital organ systems are functioning. *Psychological age* is expressed through a person's ability and control of memory, learning capacity, skills, emotions, and judgment. Maturity and capacity will direct the manner in which one is able to adapt psychologically over time to the requirements of the physical and social environment. *Social age* may be quite different from chronological age and is measured by age-graded behaviors that conform to an expected status and role within a particular culture or society. A person may be chronologically aged 80 but biologically aged 60 because he or she has remained fit with a healthy lifestyle. Or, a person with a chronic illness may be biologically aged 70 but psychologically is much younger because he or she has remained active and involved in life.

Buhler (1964) was one of the first humanistic psychologists who saw the uniqueness and potential in each phase of the life span. Lehman (1953) and Kuhlen (1968) added to the picture of the varied nature of adult development, and Jung (1971) considered the importance of different personality types as they develop. The idea is that individuals will develop in particular ways because of their heredity or social environment. Factors often ignored are cultural and gender differences. These are discussed throughout the text when there are important differences.

PSYCHOSOCIAL THEORIES OF AGING

The three major psychosocial theories of aging—disengagement, activity, and continuity—are important because they influence the expected behaviors of the older adult. It is important to remember that much of the early research on theories of aging (i.e., biological, psychosocial, cognitive, social) was conducted with elders who were ill or impaired. We are just beginning to study aging in healthy older adults, and this is changing the nature of what we know about growing old. As future generations of elders move through this period of life development, many of the ideas we have about this period of life are being redefined.

Disengagement Theory

The disengagement theory states that "aging is an inevitable, mutual withdrawal or disengagement, resulting in decreased interaction between the aging person and others in the social system he belongs to" (Cumming, Henry, 1961, p 2). This means that withdrawal from one's society and community is natural and acceptable for the older adult and his or her society. The measures of disengagement are based on age, work, and decreased interest or investment in societal concerns. The theory is seen as universal and applicable to older

people in all cultures, although there are expected variations in timing and style.

Activity Theory

The activity theory is based on the belief that remaining as active as possible in the pursuits of middle age is the ideal in later life. Because of improved general health and wealth, this is more possible than it was 40 years ago when Maddox (1963) proposed this theory. The activity theory may make sense when individuals live in a stable society, have access to positive influences and significant others, and have opportunities to participate meaningfully in the broader society if they continue to desire to do so. Attempts at clarifying activity theory as a general concept of satisfactory aging have not been supported.

Continuity Theory

The continuity theory, proposed by Havighurst and co-workers (1968), explains that life satisfaction with engagement or disengagement depends on personality traits. Three ideas about personality (Neugarten et al, 1968) are important to understanding continuity theory:
1. In normal aging, personality traits remain quite stable as men and women age.
2. Personality influences role activity and one's level of interest in particular roles.
3. Personality influences life satisfaction regardless of role activity.

In all three of the psychosocial theories of aging, the importance of opportunity, ethnicity, gender, and social status is largely ignored. None of the three theories can be clearly supported with data. In addition, they have little to do with personal meaning and motivation.

PSYCHOLOGICAL ASPECTS OF AGING

The psychology of aging is the study of changes in behavior that characteristically occur after young adulthood. Healthy psychological aging involves coping in ways that ensure one's psychological integrity. The self-view must be maintained and appreciated.

Retaining dignity and self-respect in the face of the losses accompanying aging is a poorly understood psychological component of successful aging (Lenker, Polivka, 1996). Some individuals maintain a strong sense of self regardless of devastating changes. These are the psychologically "hardy" persons (Bowsher, Keep, 1995). The hardy ones are capable of enduring physical and emotional stressors because they maintain a sense of control and challenge. Each event is seen as an open door on new experience and one that allows for choice (Kobasa, 1979; Ebersole, 1996).

Self-Efficacy

Some older persons are *hardy* individuals who believe that their personal actions and decisions are effective (perceived self-efficacy [Bandura, 1977]). These individuals are able to manage well even in circumstances that overwhelm others. They are able to do so partially because they have developed strong social networks and adequate financial resources (McAvay et al, 1996). Hardiness involves control, competence, and challenge. Some also add a fourth characteristic—compassion. Indeed, it seems that those who manage best against all odds are those whose central concerns go beyond self to include others. This presupposes some underlying altruism and a sense of humor. Nurses can further self-efficacy by respecting elders' decisions, commenting on areas of competence, and asking about challenges. By listening thoughtfully, one hears the compassion and sense of humor that are often present.

Personality Styles and Phases

One's personality under ordinary conditions is assumed to remain quite stable across the adult life span. Personality traits such as interiority (tending toward introversion), extroversion (sociability), stability, creativity, sensitivity, and openness to experience do not seem to change when studied over time and during different life stages. Two of the most important of these for older adults are interiority and stability.

Interiority
The last half of life is often a time of inner discovery, quite different from the biological and social issues that demand a great deal of outward attention during the first half of life (Jung, 1971). The last half of life, ideally, is less intensely demanding and allows more time for inner growth, self-awareness, and reflective activity. The

development of the psyche and the inner person is accompanied by a search for personal meaning and the spiritual self. However, many older persons may not be released from the demands of daily living and have little time for such indulgences. Others do not value psychological exploration and remain action oriented. Spirituality is an important aspect of development in later life and the means by which one becomes whole and develops the integrity described by Erikson. Wholeness may be achieved by doing, as well as reflecting. Seeing a valued activity toward completion may be a very enlightening experience.

Stability
Stability of personality over time is in itself a personality characteristic. Some persons act in very predictable ways throughout their life. These individuals will accept the demands of aging just as they do every other event in their lives. Age does not in itself appear to affect personality traits in healthy, community residents. Some serious disease states, especially pathological brain conditions, and institutional living may bring about major personality changes.

Psychological Tasks of Aging

Theories are the organizing framework from which tasks quite naturally will arise. Box 8-1 summarizes some of the concepts, dynamics, issues, and tasks that have been formulated by various life span theorists over the years to explain human development. These, like the biological theories of aging, all have some elements of truth but must be seen only as the particular theories that various groups ascribe to. Psychosocial theories of human development are much less clear than biological theories because there are many variables—culture, cohort, and gender being the most significant. The most recognized theories are those of Jung and Erikson. Jung has not established tasks but, as explained previously, sees a natural shift in concerns in the aging process. Erikson has provided the most useful framework for human development considerations.

Establishing Integrity
Erikson (1963) saw the last stage of life as a vantage point from which one could look back with integrity or despair on one's life. Erikson believed in a predetermined order of development

Box 8-1 **Summary of Theories of Human Development**

I. Life stages model
    A Jungian (popular)
        1. Anchored in psychoanalytical theory
            a. Mid-life shift—second stage of development
                (1) Anima—female; emergence of in men
                (2) Animus—male; emergence of in women
        2. Issues
            a. Masculinity-femininity
            b. Creativity-destructiveness
            c. Attachment-loss
    B. Eriksonian—psychosexual stages
        1. Organized in sequences of life structures and transitions (6- to 10-year average)
            a. Stability-disruption (1- to 3-year average)
            b. Equilibrium-imbalance
            c. Denial, rebirth (Kübler-Ross)
            d. Socially and personally motivated with genetic and chronological influence
    C. Levinsonian—mentors (7 to 10 years older) to guide
        1. 35- to 45-year shift
            a. Guided by a dream
            b. Mid-life crises
            c. End of dream
            d. Death of youth

II. Adaptational model (Valliant)
    A. Basic premises
        1. Gradual shifting of self and understanding
        2. Incremental-decremental shifts
        3. Tradeoffs
        4. Holding on and letting go—critical
    B. Examples
        1. Sensory decrease/quality of perception increase
        2. Excitement decrease/experience increase
        3. Physical decrease/wisdom increase
    C. Quantity versus quality
        1. What are you willing to let go of or diminish?
        2. What is not worth pursuing?
        3. What are your best assets?
        4. What is possible?
            a. Undiscovered self
            b. New births of self
         5. Stay with growing edge of self
         6. Bargaining is the essence

III. Life structure and transitions (Lowenthal) (based on organizational life cycles)
    A. Family life cycles
    B. Transitions
        1. College
        2. Marriage
        3. Retirement
    C. Premises
        1. Significant others may not be in the same sequence
        2. Evidence from clinical world
        3. Accelerated life structure transitions
            a. Toffler—*Future Shock*
        4. Choice—intolerance of change or creative change

IV. Dialectical/ecological/systems (Riegel)
    A. Premises
        1. Based on social psychology
        2. No life span approach
        3. Intersection of events produces change by breaking equilibrium
            a. Triggering event
            b. Turning point
            c. Timing of events (Rossi)
        4. Discover self by reaction
        5. Perspective on development by looking backward
        6. Metaphorical conceptualizations
        7. Restoration of balance
        8. Essence in energy exchanges with impact
    B. Examples
        1. World events, trends, culture, milieu
            a. Geography
            b. Ideational
            c. Situational
            d. Micro and macro systems
            e. Health evolution

V. Fielding model—Roger Gould—psychoanalytical consultation
    A. Premises
        1. Become finest self
            a. Give up safety
            b. Creativity reaches beyond myth of safety
            c. Self-actualizing
                (1) Maslow
                (2) Bueler
            d. Past life, future self
            e. Autonomy/control/taking charge
            f. Pilgrimage of the self
                (1) Teleological
                (2) Future oriented
                (3) Proactive
                (4) Goal oriented
                (5) Shaping one's own world
    B. Agenda for mature adulthood
        1. Individualization
        2. Recreation
        3. Undo the boring—trigger a transition, renewal
        4. Endings and beginnings—the essence of development

that proceeded by critical steps, all dependent on timing and sequence. However, he also theorized that individuals return again and again to the stages that have been poorly resolved. It is assumed that certain inner biological and outer sociological conditions are required to achieve integrity in late life. Thus some elders will be struggling with much earlier developmental needs. In later years Erikson and his wife, Joan, reconsidered his seminal work from the perspective of their own aging (they were both octogenarians at the time). They reframed their presentation of the theoretical framework as achieving balance at each stage of life. Thus ego integrity is tinged with some regrets, wisdom is balanced with frivolity, and letting go is balanced with hanging on. The Eriksons define wisdom as "detached concern with life itself, in the face of death itself. It maintains and learns to convey the integrity of experience, in spite of the decline of bodily and mental functions" (Erikson et al, 1986, p 38).

Peck (1968) identified discrete tasks of old age that must be addressed to establish integrity:

- *Ego differentiation versus work role preoccupation.* The individual can no longer be defined by his or her work.
- *Body transcendence versus body preoccupation.* The body is cared for but does not consume the interest and attention of the individual.
- *Ego transcendence versus ego preoccupation.* The self becomes less central, and one feels a part of the mass of humanity, their struggles, and their destiny.

It is clear that to achieve integrity by Peck's model, one must develop the ability to redefine self, to let go of occupational identity, to rise above body discomforts, and to establish meanings that go beyond the scope of self-centeredness. Although these are admirable and idealistic goals, they place a considerable burden on the older person. Not everyone may have the courage or energy to laugh in the face of adversity or surmount all of the assaults of old age. The wisdom of old age involves a crisis of understanding in which the ordinary structures are shaken and the meaning of life is reexamined. It may include the wisdom of questioning assumptions in the search for meaning in the last stage of life.

Cynthia Kelly (1990) identified the three *R's* that define the tasks of aging as (1) accepting reality, (2) fulfilling responsibility, and (3) exercising rights. Realities have to do with accepting one's capacities in the health, social, and financial realms; responsibilities include planning for one's survivors and for making the best choices regarding the remainder of life; and rights include exercising the right to move at one's own pace, the right to privacy, the right to respect, the right to refuse what one does not desire, and the right to participate in plans and decisions related to one's own life. Developmental tasks, as defined by several theorists, are included in Figure 8-1.

Maintaining Caring and Continuity

For many, caring remains focused on children and grandchildren. Reflecting on the successes of children confirms older persons' own success as parents. The aspect of caring, so predominant during the generative stages in the adult years, is the quality that provides the greatest sense of continuity. As individuals nurture their young and watch their descendants nurture their young, they experience a connectedness with the repetitious cycles of life and at times an opportunity to redo their youth. Continuity and vicarious fulfillment are experienced as one sees qualities in grandchildren that were identified in the self or in the parents or grandparents of self. As many as six generations may be viewed in continuous progression. Others find caring and connectedness through ideas, creative works, mentoring, and contributing to progress in their fields of expertise. Grandparenting is discussed in Chapter 23.

COGNITION AND AGING

Cognition is both a biological and a psychological factor that must be considered in caring for the older adult. The abnormal biological aspects of brain function are dealt with in Chapter 21; normal functions are addressed in this chapter and in Chapter 7.

In general, cognitive performance in testing is poorer for the very old than for those 60 to 80 years old (Poon et al, 1992). Most tests were designed by adults to test children or young adults and do not include cultural or ethnic differences. Therefore these tests may have little relevance for daily function. Ecological validity and context are important in testing normal cognitive capacities. That is, psychometric tests of intelligence must

Intrinsic

Continue to develop curiosity
Transcend ego

Achieve inner peace and self-
    acceptance
Separate identity from work role
Cultivate anima (feminine) and animus
    (masculine)

Accept one's share of responsibility
    for the past
Accept death of spouse
Identify a legacy and a plan of
    dispersal

Learn to tolerate losses and
    depressive episodes
Accept help when needed

Monitor body function
Adapt to physical limitations
Transcend body

Extrinsic

Share wisdom
Teach others to live and die
    uniquely

Develop latent abilities that may
    be dormant
Develop flexible social roles

Serve as a historian for younger
    persons
Maintain significant relationships
Relate to age peers
Develop new, less intense
    relationships, particularly with
    younger persons
Plan for death (i.e., living wills,
    home care, services, burial methods)

Budget income and energy to meet
    important needs
Find a suitable living situation
    allowing maximal independence

Seek adequate health maintenance
    services

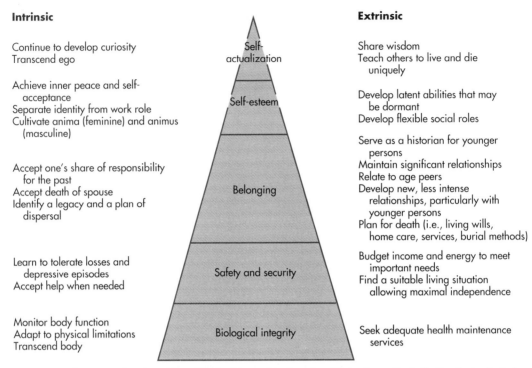

Pyramid levels (top to bottom): Self-actualization; Self-esteem; Belonging; Safety and security; Biological integrity

Figure 8-1 Developmental tasks of late life in hierarchical order. (Data from Peck R: *Psychological develop-ments in the second half of life.* In Neugarten B, editor: *Middle age and aging,* Chicago, 1968, University of Chicago Press; Havinghurst R: *Developmental tasks and education,* New York, 1972, McKay.)

have relevance to the daily lives of older adults if they are to be useful. However, cognitive development of the older adult is often measured against the norms of young or middle-age people, which may not be appropriate to the distinctive characteristics of the older adults. Intelligence in old age is dynamic, and certain abilities change and even improve with age (Figure 8-2).

More and more theorists are now speculating about the possibility of the unique cognitive powers of old age, as did Plato. Reflective regression (intense reliving and reviewing of old memories) and life review seem to be a form of cognitive development characteristic of late life. Individuals focus more on memories and meanings.

The determination of intellectual capacity and performance has been the focus of a major portion of gerontological research. In general, cognitive functions may remain stable or decline with increasing age (Beers, Berkow, 2000). The cogni-

tive functions that remain stable include attention span, language skills, communication skills, comprehension and discourse, and visual perception. The cognitive skills that decline are verbal fluency, logical analysis, selective attention, object naming, and complex visuospatial skills (Beers, Berkow, 2000). In general, intellectual abilities appear to plateau in the fifties and sixties and begin to decline in the seventies.

Late adulthood is no longer seen as a period of growth cessation and arrested cognitive development; rather it is seen as a life stage programmed for plasticity and the development of unique capacities. Education, pulmonary health, general health, and activity levels all influence cognitive activity in later life. Other reasons have been advanced for the variations of intellectual performance of the older adult being tested (Box 8-2). Crowley (1996) says that if brain function becomes impaired in old age, it is a result of disease, not aging.

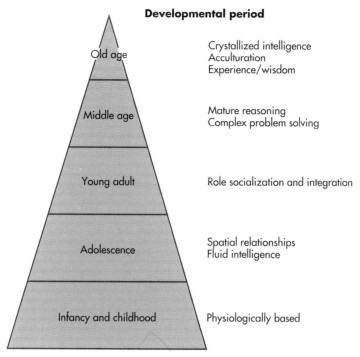

Developmental period

Old age — Crystallized intelligence / Acculturation / Experience/wisdom

Middle age — Mature reasoning / Complex problem solving

Young adult — Role socialization and integration

Adolescence — Spatial relationships / Fluid intelligence

Infancy and childhood — Physiologically based

Figure 8-2   Life span cognitive developmental strengths. (Developed by Priscilla Ebersole.)

The Aging Brain

It has been generally believed that cognitive function declines in old age because of a decreased number of neurons, decreased brain size, and diminished brain weight. Although these losses are features of aging, they are not consistent with deteriorating mental function (Sugarman, 2002), nor do they interfere with everyday routines. Neuron loss occurs mainly in the brain and spinal cord and is most pronounced in the cerebral cortex. The neuronal dendrites atrophy with aging, resulting in impairment of the synapses and changes in the transmission of the chemical neurotransmitters dopamine, serotonin, and acetylcholine. This causes a slowing of many neural processes. However, overall cognitive abilities remain intact. We now understand that continued development requires appropriate levels of challenge and stimulation throughout life. There is untapped potential for patterning and learning through stimulating brain cells to expand function. This is shown most remarkably in the retraining of speech and other functions following a stroke. When working with the older adult to improve cognitive functions, there must be regular input and "exercise" of the brain around ideas that are significant and interesting to the older person. The phrase "use it or lose it" applies to cognitive function as well as physical.

Memory Retrieval

Memory is defined as the ability to retain or store information and retrieve it when needed. Memory is a complex set of processes and storage systems. Three components characterize memory: immediate recall; short-term memory (which may range from minutes to days); and remote or long-term memory (Gallo et al, 2003). Biological, functional, environmental, and psychosocial influences affect memory development throughout adulthood. Recall of newly encountered information seems to decrease with age, and memory declines are noted for complex tasks and strate-

Box 8-2	Complexities of Accurately Assessing Intellect in Old Age

- The old are most frequently compared with college students, whose chief occupation is proving their intellectual capacity.
- Young adults are in the habit of being tested and have developed test wisdom, a skill never developed by the elderly or one that has grown rusty with disuse.
- Test material may not be relevant to the world of older adults, especially those of different cultures.
- The ability to concentrate is inversely related to anxiety.
- Intellectual function declines differentially. The old are assumed deficient in encoding during learning, storing information for retention, and/or speed of retrieving stored information.
- Adrenal or stress hormones may be responsible for some of the gradual changes in the brain during aging.
- Older persons always perform more slowly than younger people in tasks involving neuromuscular learning because of slower reaction time and an increase in cautious behavior.
- Older people often perform poorly on test items because they are less likely to guess and more likely not to answer any items that seem ambiguous to them.
- Cautiousness has often been described as the reason why older adults do not perform as well as younger people in memory tasks. Other personality traits, such as greater activity levels, less impulsiveness, and greater emotional stability, also seem to influence how well older people perform on memory tests.
- Older people may have difficulty focusing attention and ignoring irrelevant stimuli.
- Subject attrition in longitudinal studies of older adults shows evidence of the survival of the intellectually superior.
- There is no evidence of general slowing of central nervous system activity in old age as had been commonly presumed and reported by researchers.
- Intellectual performance relying on verbal functions shows little or no decline with age, but speeded tests using nonverbal psychomotor functions show a great decline.
- Social cognition and social context are related in terms of elder function. The elderly who maintain the best cognitive function are also those with a high social interactional level.

gies. Even though some older adults show decrements in processing information, reaction time, perception, and attentional tasks, the majority of functioning remains intact and sufficient. Familiarity, previous learning, and life experience compensate for the minor loss of efficiency in the basic neurological processes. In unfamiliar, stressful, or demanding situations, these changes may be more marked.

Age-associated decline in memory is a major focus of research in aging and dementia. Normal older adults may complain of memory problems, but their symptoms do not meet the criteria for dementia. The term *age-associated memory impairment* (AAMI) has been used to describe memory loss that is considered normal in light of the person's age and educational level. *Mild cognitive impairment* (MCI) (Gallo et al, 2003; Petersen, 2004) is used to describe memory impairment beyond that which is felt to constitute normal aging, but other aspects of cognitive functioning remain intact. Some research indicates that people with MCI may go on to develop Alzheimer's or a related dementing illness. Others may have medical or psychiatric difficulties (depression, anxiety) that influence memory abilities. Clearly, the knowledge about memory and changes related to aging is still developing. Nurses should encourage older adults with memory complaints to have a comprehensive evaluation to rule out reversible and irreversible causes and receive appropriate treatment.

Scientists are finding that nerve cell regeneration does occur in the hippocampus of the brain, where memory formation occurs (National Institutes of Health, 2002). They have found that stress decreases the capacity for generation of new nerve cells, and present research focuses on the factors linking stress and nerve cell regeneration. Still other research on the "plasticity" of the brain is based on physical changes that occur in the brain that result from new memories and the addition of new neurons. This is good evidence for us to continue to learn and grow and experience the world around us even into very old age.

Cognitive stimulation and memory training utilizing techniques such as mnemonics (strategies to enhance coding, storage, and recall), internal and external aids, cognitive games (e.g., Scrabble, chess, crossword puzzles), and spaced retrieval techniques (Camp, 1989) may be helpful for cognitively intact elders as well as those with cognitive impairment. There are currently many games and aids on the market that may be useful to enhance memory and stimulate cognitive function. All older adults should remain active and engaged in stimulating activities for the mind as well as for the body. Ruth Tappen and colleagues at Florida Atlantic University are studying the effect of several therapeutic interventions, including cognitive games and memory training techniques, on the function of mild to moderately impaired older adults.

Elders seem to learn best when new information or expectations can be related to familiar concepts and prior knowledge. Mood is extremely important in terms of what individuals (old and young) will recall. In other words, when we attempt to measure recall of events that may have occurred in a crisis situation or an anxiety state, recall will be impaired. This is significant for health care workers who give information to elders when the elders are ill or upset. They are very likely not to remember it.

SOCIOLOGICAL AGING

Sociological aging is composed of the performance of expected social roles appropriate to one's chronological age, culture, and capacity. Terms that are associated with sociological aging are *age norms, social time clocks, age grading,* and *social time.* All of these are descriptive of the place individuals should occupy in a society at any given time in their lives. The great diversity of individuals in the United States has made social aging complex and social norms virtually nonexistent. Social scientists are now focusing more attention on the interaction of age, origins, historical period, and cohort in attempts to study the social aspects of aging from a life course perspective.

Life Course

The life course is composed of elements that make up the overall structure and timing of events in one's life from cradle to grave. It must be examined and taken into account to understand an older individual. This is the basis for longitudinal studies. Life structure is composed of roles (occupational, social, family), relationships (intimate, personal, professional), and inner structure (goals, values, motives, memories). The progress of all these aspects of life can be considered a life course. Helping elders record and understand the story of their lives, as explained in Chapter 5, clarifies the life course and structure.

Life Transitions

The transitions throughout the life course include major shifts in social expectations and responsibilities as a result of age, role, occupation, family, and economics. Figure 8-3 outlines the distribution of these transitions.

Age Norms

Norms are socially shared expectations of the "shoulds" and "oughts" of behavior. As mentioned earlier, norms are difficult to identify in a multicultural society. The large population of extremely old persons lacks predictable transitions, and thus after age 80 norms are virtually nonexistent.

Status and Role Changes

Status and role are the concepts around which norms, relationships, conformity and deviance, and stability and change are organized. The role of the older person in our society remains highly variable. The major issues to be considered are the number and significance of an elder's roles as personally defined and valued.

Social Support

Social support is derived from the assurance of love, esteem, and belonging to a network of individuals with common goals and mutual concerns. Social support has traditionally come from intimates, family, friends, and neighbors.

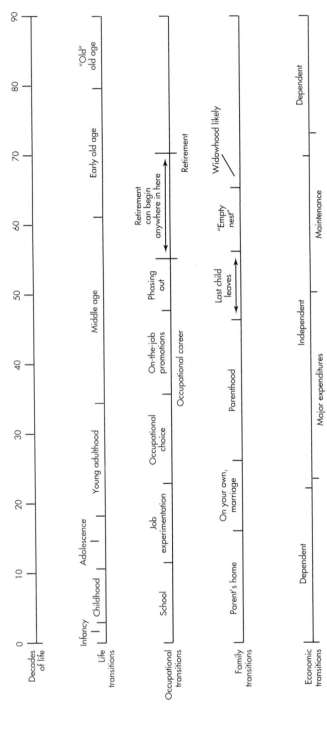

Figure 8-3   Life transitions. (From Cunningham W, Brookbank J: *Gerontology: the psychology, biology, and sociology of aging*, New York, 1988, Harper & Row.)

Nurses often become important providers of social support for older adults, particularly those in nursing homes. In a study investigating hope, spirituality, and connectedness with others among institutionalized older adults, 35% of the participants named nurses as confidants and significant providers of social support in their lives (Touhy, 2001). In the age of electronic communication and travel ease, many elders receive a great deal of social support through less intense but frequent involvement with others, such as through e-mail, on-line chat groups, and Elderhostel travel groups.

Reciprocity

Many of our elders grew up feeling self-sufficient and highly independent. Yet in this nuclear age we are all aware that we must depend on others and be depended on if we are to survive individually and culturally. The concept of reciprocity in relationships and society is basic to survival. In old age, as people become physically and functionally dependent in various ways, their contribution often involves sharing their history and wisdom and demonstrating their survival capacities to younger persons. Elders become our teachers of life. Many also think of reciprocity in terms of payback time: elders spent much of their lives assisting the younger generations, and then it becomes time for the younger ones to assist the elders.

ROLES OF ELDERS

Numerous minor role changes occur in the aging process, but the transitions expected by most elders are related to the work role and the role of spouse or partner. From a life course perspective, the transitions and adaptations required produce both stability and change in individual preferences, capacities, expectations, and behavior. Age-related transitions are socially created, shared, and recognized. A transition is socially recognized and entails a reorientation of perceptions and expectations of and by the individual. Cohort and gender differences exist in all of life's major transitions.

Concepts Related to Role Transitions

To the degree that an event is perceived as expected and occurring at the right time, a role transition may be comfortable and even welcomed. Those persons who must retire "too early" or are widowed "too soon" will have more difficulty adapting than those who are of an age when these events are expected. The speed and intensity of a major change may make the difference between a transitional crisis or a gradual and comfortable adaptation. Role changes that produce crises are usually abrupt losses of familiar functions at a time when meaningful substitute functions are not available. Anticipatory planning, awareness of potential problems, positive or negative attitudes, and a sense of control (by far, the most important) make role transitions easier.

During the transition from familiar roles to new ones, an individual needs the freedom to try various possibilities in an accepting atmosphere that encourages success, tolerates failure, and recognizes that progress is not accomplished by slow, even steps. In real life, progress follows a more wayward, uneven course. One is easily distracted and often falls back to the familiar. A nurse is most helpful in providing an accepting milieu that encourages independence and exploration, as well as the awareness that transitions all create some anxiety. Useful nursing interventions will assist the older adult in maintaining self-esteem and developing new and satisfying roles.

The most common roles of older people are retiree, parent, grandparent, great-grandparent, spouse, homemaker, widow, kin, friend, citizen, volunteer, church member, club member, acquaintance, patient, and service recipient. In cases of role accumulation, such as that of grandparent, some previous development will be applicable, with modification, to the new role. Likewise, the shifts in parent-child relationships are gradual and do not require complete role deletion or role reversal. Those transitions that make use of past skills and adaptations may be least stressful. Cohort and gender differences are inherent in all of life's major transitions.

Role Reversal

Developmental transitions in relationships have received insufficient attention. An interesting area of investigation would be that of the elder's experience of moving from caregiver to care recipient. Most attention has been given to the experience of the caregiver and little to that of elders and their adjustment to the need to be a care recipient. When a strong and independent elder retires because of failing health, the reaction to dependency and role reversal with the spouse may sap the patience and energies of both. Long-standing relationship dynamics may reverse in the illness of old age.

Sometimes a passive, dependent spouse may be unable to make the transition without considerable help. (See Chapter 23 for additional discussion of caregiving.) Assuming an unfamiliar role is difficult for both parties. The nurse should discuss with the couple particular activities that the couple can maintain that are symbolic of their previous roles. For example, perhaps the man always wrote the checks or the woman always determined the need for household supplies. The man may have organized outings and the woman decided on holiday activities. These routines can be sustained with some creative methods devised by nurses. The nurse should be alert to situations in which health care personnel may be able to provide the supports and resources that make it possible for an individual to sustain important habitual activities and assume new responsibilities without being totally overwhelmed.

When a spouse is ill and the mate needs to take over functions for both, it is essential that someone be available to give reinforcement, encouragement, and relief. An adult day care program, routine visits from a community health nurse, or periodic assistance from a home health aide or a housekeeper may make it possible for the couple to continue to live together. One important consideration is counseling the couple to maintain as much independent function as possible for both persons.

Gender Considerations in Role Transitions

Although women are thought to have greater continuity in their late lives, the roles of old women are generally judged less attractive than those of old men (Barer, 1993). Women are considered "old" earlier than men and are more often eco-

nomically and vocationally disadvantaged when single, divorced, or widowed. However, throughout their lives women are confronted with more frequent and visible physical and social transitions and thus may become more adept at adapting to new roles. They have also generally developed a larger network of friends that is not necessarily work related, whereas men are more likely to have closest relationships with those with whom they have worked. These trends have changed somewhat and are expected to continue changing with the emergence of the baby boomers on the aging scene. With few exceptions, all elders must adapt to two major changes that occur with aging: changes in the work role and in the role of spouse or partner.

Retirement

Retirement is no longer just a few years of rest from the rigors of work before death. It is a developmental stage that may occupy 30 years of one's life and involve many stages. The transitions are blurring because numerous pursuits and opportunities may occur after one has "retired." Tafford (2002) is addressing this relatively new segment of adult life. She examines the unprecedented aging in the life cycle and contends that people know as little about it as they did about adolescence at the turn of the century (Age Beat on Line, 2002). The numerous patterns and styles of retiring have produced more varied experiences in retirement. More and more older people are working longer or changing careers after formal retirement. Some do so because of economic need whereas others have a desire to remain involved and productive.

Older adults who did not expect retirement at the time when they left the work force may suffer detrimental effects and be in need of counseling or assistance. They may experience job separation as a crisis and a traumatic role transition triggered by an unplanned job termination resulting from illness or company *downsizing*, a euphemistic term for cutting out jobs.

Others, given the opportunity to work past retirement age, must weigh the benefits. Part-time work during retirement is viewed by the working public of all ages as a desirable option. Employers seek older workers because they are more reliable and dependable. Seniors over the age of 65 can now earn any amount without endangering Social Secu-

Box 8-3	Issues in Retirement Potential

1. Financial need versus resources
2. Employability
3. Rewards derived from employment
   - Wages sufficient for needs and morale
   - Satisfaction level, possibility for resolution of job frustrations
   - Meaning of job, contact with friends, source of prestige
4. Psychosocial characteristics—attitudes toward retirement
   - Attitudes of significant others (advising? directing?)
   - Strength of work ethic
   - Effect of retirement on prestige
5. Personality factors
   - Time orientation (past, present, future)
   - Active versus passive in planning
   - Rationalism versus fatalism as life stance
   - Type-A versus type-B personality (hard driving versus easy going)
   - Inner directed versus other directed (enjoyment of self or need for high level of external motivation)
6. Level of information about retirement
   - Planning programs on job, adult education, or community programs
   - Awareness of friends and family who have retired and how influenced by them
7. Pressures to retire
   - Compulsory, age discriminatory
   - Unemployment (how long?)
   - Job retrogression (being moved down the ladder)
   - Skill obsolescence (opportunities for developing other skills?)
   - Peer pressure, organized or informal
   - Employer pressure (reduced incentives to continue work, increased incentives to retire)
   - Family pressure (spouse's working status)
   - Health discomfort or disability interfering with job performance and dependability

rity benefits. Obviously, health status and financial status affect decisions and abilities to continue work or engage in new work opportunities.

Labor Force Participation

Just as Social Security was initially seen as a mechanism for resolving unemployment, early retirement is a means of regulating the labor supply. Employers encourage early retirement of older, more expensive workers by offering attractive incentives. Early retirement packages may be so attractive that individuals retire earlier than they had planned or expected and without sufficient preparatory time.

Clearly, the goals of government and industry are in conflict related to the older work force. Government cannot afford a large body of nonworking individuals, and industry cannot afford to keep these individuals in top salaried positions. With recent events that have seriously threatened pension security and portability, more workers are remaining in the work force. "The long term trend toward ever-earlier retirement has halted" (Ekerdt, Dennis, 2002, p 1). The work scene continually changes and becomes more complex as government policies, technology, and world economics continually destroy jobs and create new ones. The balance between downsizing and creating new jobs is variable across regions and industries.

Retirement Intentions

Decisions to retire are often based on attitude toward work, chronological age, health, and self-perceptions of ability to adjust to retirement (Taylor, Shore, 1995). Retirement intentions are variable and include four types of "retirement": to retire from work, to change jobs, to partially retire, or to work for self (Ekerdt et al, 1996). It is important to know just what an individual means when discussing retirement. Issues to consider are summarized in Box 8-3.

Working couples must plan together for retirement. Decisions will depend on their career goals, shared future interests, and the quality of their interpersonal relationship.

The following are some questions one must weigh when deciding to retire or continue working:
- What do I want to do?
- Who needs me, and what are my best opportunities?
- What am I best able to do?

- What is the meaning of my life?
- What should my life accomplish or contribute?
- Am I financially independent for the rest of my life if I live 30 more years?
- Am I in good physical condition, and do I enjoy spending time with my spouse?
- Can I afford to completely retire from paid work?

Individuals who are retiring in poor health, minority persons, and those in lower socioeconomic levels may experience greater concerns in retirement and may need specialized counseling. As noted by Stanford and Usita (2002), retirement security depends on the "three-legged stool" of Social Security, pensions, and savings and investments. Older people with disabilities, those who have lacked access to education or held low-paying jobs with no benefits, and those not eligible for Social Security, are at economic risk during retirement years. Minority older persons, women, immigrants, and gay and lesbian couples often face greater challenges related to adequate income and benefits in retirement. The traditional idea of retirement as a time of increased leisure, new interests, and relaxation and enjoyment may not be possible for many older people. "Future retirement policies will need to consider the rapidly changing demographics of the aging population and the special barriers faced by older people of color, women, immigrants, and gays and lesbians" (Stanford, Usita, 2002, p. 47).

Many older persons preparing for retirement are also caring for older adult parents. Increasingly, large corporations are developing employee assistance programs that provide support and resources in coping with the needs of these elders. Legislation now supports the right to unpaid leave from jobs for parental or spousal care; however, many persons cannot afford this.

Women are often called on to retire earlier than anticipated because of family needs. A recent study from Cornell University, reported by Family Caregiver Alliance, National Center on Caregiving (2002), found that late mid-life women are five times more likely to retire early to care for an ill or disabled husband than those who are not caregivers. The study also found that male caregivers who are caring for their wives retire earlier than those who are caring for a person other than a spouse. Most men have always worked outside the home, but it has been only within the last 30 years that this has been the expectation of women. Therefore large cohort differences exist.

Traditionally, the variability of women's work histories, interrupted careers, the residuals of sexist pension policies, Social Security inequities, and low-paying jobs created hazards for adequacy of income in retirement. The scene is gradually changing in many respects, but the gender bias remains. Basing retirement calculations on gender and projected survival statistics is now illegal, although until the early 1980s, women were allotted less pension income based purely on their expected longevity in comparison with men. Although this is no longer true, women who retired 20 or 25 years ago remain penalized because of gender.

Older women are very likely to have several years of no earnings calculated in the averages that determine the amount of their Social Security benefits. Some women find that they will receive more if Social Security is calculated on their husband's earnings; this may be true even though these women are widowed or divorced. The Social Security Administration must be contacted regarding these issues because many variables may be used. The complexity of the issues includes a difference between retirement patterns of single and married women and men. Single and married women differ in the degree of dependency on their own benefits and work history. Pension coverage and health are useful predictors of retirement for men but not as much for women. For single women, recent income is an important factor in the decision to retire. For women and men, the most significant factors in adaptation to retirement are health, income, and social involvement.

Retirement Planning for Domestic Partners

Those couples who have lived together for years and have jointly acquired assets may experience undue discrimination in retirement and death benefit planning. Barriers to equal treatment in retirement include job discrimination, unequal treatment under Social Security, pension plans, and 401(k) plans. Domestic partners are not eligible for Social Security survivor benefits, and unmarried partners cannot claim pension plan rights after the death of the pension plan participant. These policies clearly put domestic partners at a disadvantage in retirement planning.

Nurse's Role in Retirement Preparation

Questions a nurse may introduce to clients considering retirement include the following:

- What are the chief work-related satisfactions, and what might compensate for the loss of those?
- Are friendship networks tied to the job?
- How do spouse and family enter into the decision-making process?
- Is there an opportunity to test partial work status or nonworking status before actual retirement?
- Has sufficient information been available regarding retirement planning?
- Is the work situation more stressful than it is satisfying?
- How much of self is defined by job status?
- Is competitive activity an important source of satisfaction?

Successful retirement adjustment depends on socialization needs, energy levels, health, variety of interests, amount of self-esteem derived from work, presence of intimate relationships, and general adaptability. Nurses counseling older adults can use the following guidelines:

1. Talk to clients over 50 years of age about any retirement plans they may have.
2. Make clients aware that the transition to retirement is experienced as a crisis with manifestations of grief in many people.
3. Work with couples whenever retirement may be a possible stressor in their relationship.
4. Institute nursing research regarding the effects of retirement.

The inequities inherent in various work roles result in major differences in retirement compensation and comfort. To our dismay, the service industries that employ caregiving professionals are among the least likely to provide health care and adequate retirement for their employees (Hirshorn et al, 1996). The increasing number of nurses working in long-term care at various levels and at numerous sites must band together and give retirement planning a high priority for themselves. The American Nurses Association and other nursing organizations must expand their efforts beyond the hospital nurse. We as members must institute action. Nurses need to think of and plan for their own retirement needs. Just as we often say, "Physician, heal thyself," we would admonish, "Nurse, take care of thyself."

Satisfaction in Retirement

The most powerful factors in retirement satisfaction are health status, sufficient income, and the option to continue working. Adequate income is often tied to the ability to continue some type of remunerative activity. Health conditions are the least subject to control by the retiree and apparently the most critical to perceived quality of life (Dorfman, 2002). In the best of situations, retirement offers couples, both of whom have been working, an opportunity for more relaxed interactions and pursuit of mutual interests that may have been neglected while fulfilling obligations. With more time and resources, retirees have the opportunity to develop special relationships with their grandchildren. Phases of retirement can be found in Box 8-4.

Volunteer Role

Retirement is often thought of as a time to develop secondary interests and challenges. Many older people volunteer and contribute to filling gaps in services that might otherwise be unmet. Some of the formal volunteer programs for older adults include the National Network on Aging (Nursing Home Ombudsman Program, National Nutrition Program), ACTION (Foster Grandparents [FGP], Retired Senior Volunteer Program [RSVP], Volunteers in Service to America [VISTA], Senior Companion, Peace Corps, Legal Service Corporation, SCORE (Small Business Administration), Depart-

---

Box 8-4	Phases of Retirement

Remote: Future anticipation with little real planning

Near: Preparation and fantasizing regarding retirement

Honeymoon: Euphoria and testing of the fantasies

Disenchantment: Letdown, boredom, sometimes depression

Reorientation: Developing a realistic and satisfactory lifestyle

Stability: Personal investment in meaningful activities

Termination: Loss of role resulting from illness or return to work

ment of Veterans Affairs, and National Volunteer School Program (teacher aides). Many of these volunteers are paid or given other inducements to supplement low incomes. Numerous other volunteer opportunities are available in local communities including community agencies, hospitals, and other health care facilities. Some of the many ways volunteers may be involved are seen in Box 8-5.

Volunteer Training

Training programs, supervision, and ongoing support are critical to the success of volunteer programs. The following considerations guide the development of successful volunteer programs:

Box 8-5   Volunteer Community Services

Perform in a choral group in nursing homes.
Sew for institutionalized children.
Help deprived persons obtain entitlements.
Provide widow-to-widow help.
Perform American Cancer Society clerical work.
Assist at nutrition programs.
Make dolls for hospitalized children.
Assist children in school remedial reading programs.
Organize food co-op, sell to elders at discount prices.
Raise money with bazaars, white elephant sales for nutrition programs.
Serve as musicians for senior dances.
Teach language classes in senior centers.
Become "fix it" men.
Prepare kits for Red Cross Blood Mobile.
Telephone the homebound.
Present puppet shows to schoolchildren, bringing history alive.
Serve coffee and act as language interpreters at gerontological centers.
Help residents settle into new living arrangements, nursing or retirement homes.
Assist with shopping, walking around.
Teach remedial math to schoolchildren.
Present slide shows as museum volunteers in churches and senior centers.
Assist in child care shelters.
Work with developmentally disabled—teach swimming, cooking, and activities of daily living.
Alert isolated elderly to services and Supplemental Security Income (SSI).

- Administrative support of volunteers
- Clearly determined goals for the program
- A specific orientation program with printed support materials to give volunteers
- Buddy systems to orient and reinforce the volunteer role and expectations
- Periodic evaluations and modifications as needs are indicated by volunteer participants
- Determination of specific awards and rewards to sustain interest and involvement

Individuals should be encouraged to begin minimal participation in volunteer programs before discontinuing the work role. This can serve as a bridge of continuity. There are certain identifiable steps in the full development of a role as a volunteer. These can be seen in Box 8-6. Group involvement and group meetings will solidify and strengthen the identification with the volunteer role. Some, such as the Foster Grandparents program, are particularly fulfilling.

Our present elders are perhaps the only ones who have, in large numbers, the health, vitality, education, affluence, and opportunity to make retirement the most creatively productive and gratifying stage of life. Retirement can be the time when the individual is free to pursue a lifelong avid interest. For the fortunate individuals, retirement years can indeed be the best years of their lives and the most gratifying.

Box 8-6   Steps in Development of Volunteer Role

1. Volunteer role uses skills from previous work or community experience. A gain in status, prestige, and community sanction is experienced.
2. Volunteer role improves interest in self and others. Dependence is reduced, and interdependence is created.
3. Feedback is gained from recipients of services. Self-view is improved, and resourcefulness is recognized.
4. Social and psychological stimulation is found in volunteer settings. Personal growth and development occur as skills are refined.
5. Community rewards and recognition are awarded. New roles of social significance are internalized.

Widows and Widowers

Losing a partner, when a close and satisfying relationship has lasted a long time, is the most difficult adjustment one can face, aside from the loss of a child. The loss of a spouse is a stage in the life course that can be anticipated but seldom is. Nearly 50% of all women and 12% of all men age 65 and older are widowed (DeVries, 2001). The death of a life partner is essentially losing one's self and one's core. The mourning is as much for self as for the individual who has died. Part of oneself has died with the partner, and even with satisfactory grief resolution, that self will never return. Even those widows and widowers who reorganize their lives and invest in family, friends, and activities often find that many years later they still miss their "other half" profoundly. With the loss of the intimate partner several changes occur simultaneously that involve social status, economics, and self-image. Individuals who have been self-confident and competent seem to fare best. The transitional phase of grief, if handled appropriately, leads to the confirmation of a new identity, the end of one stage of life, and the beginning of another. Seldom in life is there such an abrupt and distinct breach that creates intense pain but offers the opportunity for the emergence of a new identity.

Patterns of adjustment can be seen in Box 8-7. Knowing the stages of the transition to a new role as a widow or widower may be useful, although each individual is unique in this respect. Individuals respond to losses in ways that reflect the nature and meaning of the relationships as well as the unique characteristics of the bereaved (DeVries, 2001). Gender differences are found in the literature on widowhood. Bereaved husbands may be more socially and emotionally vulnerable. Many studies have found that widowers adapt more slowly than widows to the loss of a spouse and often remarry quickly. Common bereavement reactions of widowers are listed in Box 8-8 and should be discussed with male clients. When the long-frozen winter is over, the woman or man emerges, shedding the intense grief and ready to cultivate strength and independence to the fullest. The self, previously "halving" identity with another, tries to emerge from the cocoon. This is not always done successfully, but those who do emerge gain a new identity.

Box 8-7   Patterns of Adjustment to Widowhood

Stage One: Reactionary (first few weeks)
Early responses of disbelief, anger, indecision, detachment, and inability to communicate in a logical, sustained manner are common. Searching for the mate, visions, hallucinations, and depersonalization may be experienced.
INTERVENTION: Support, validate, be available, listen to talk about mate, reduce expectations.

Stage Two: Withdrawal (first few months)
Depression, apathy, physiological vulnerability occur; movement and cognition are slowed; insomnia, unpredictable waves of grief, sighing, and anorexia occur.
INTERVENTION: Protect against suicide, and involve in support groups.

Stage Three: Recuperation (second 6 months)
Periods of depression are interspersed with characteristic capability. Feelings of personal control begin to return.

INTERVENTION: Support accustomed lifestyle patterns that sustain and assist person in exploring possibilities.

Stage Four: Exploration (second year)
Individual begins new ventures, testing suitability of new roles; anniversaries, holidays, birthdays, and date of death may be especially difficult.
INTERVENTION: Prepare individual for unexpected reactions during these times. Encourage and support new trial roles.

Stage Five: Integration (fifth year)
Individual will feel fully integrated into new and satisfying roles if grief has been resolved in a healthy manner.
INTERVENTION: Assist individual in recognizing and sharing own pattern of growth through the trauma of loss.

Box 8-8	Common Widower Bereavement Reactions

The search for the lost mate
The neglect of self
The inability to share grief
The loss of social contacts
The struggle to view women as other than wife
The erosion of self-confidence and sexuality
The protracted grief period

Nurse's Role with Widows and Widowers

Nurses working with the bereaved will need to review Lindemann's classical grief studies to understand the initial somatic responses of the bereaved (Lindemann, 1944). Feelings of the bereaved one are not orderly or progressive; they are conflicted, ambivalent, suicidal, full of rage, and often suspicious. Widows and widowers may exhibit personality disorganization that would be considered mentally aberrant or frankly psychotic under other circumstances. Some people handle grief with less apparent decompensation. Grief reactions must be accepted as personally valid and useful evidences of healing. DeVries (2001) discusses the ongoing bonds and connections (dreaming of the deceased, ongoing daily communication, "checking in") with the deceased that persist long after death and counsels professionals to reexamine the idea that there is a timetable for "resolution" of grief. Rather, according to DeVries, "Grief reflects the intimacy of relationships that need not end with the physical absence of individuals" (p 79).

With adequate support, reintegration can be expected in 2 to 4 years. People with few familial or social supports may need professional help to get through the early months of grief in a way that will facilitate recovery. Supporting the grieving person requires an extension of self to reconnect the severed person with a world of warmth and caring. No one nurse or one family member can accomplish this task alone. Hundreds of small, caring gestures build strength and confidence in the grieving person's ability and willingness to survive. Additional information about dying, death, and grief can be found in Chapter 26.

Divorce and the Elderly

In the past, divorce was considered a stigmatizing event, although today it is so common that a person is inclined to forget the ostracizing effects of divorce from 60 years ago. There are large generational and individual differences in expectations from marriage, but older couples are becoming less likely to stay in an unsatisfactory marriage (Lanza, 1996). Health care professionals need to avoid assumptions and be alert to the possibility of marriage dissatisfaction in old age. Nurses need to ask, "How would you describe your marriage?"

At age 65 and beyond, 11.5% of women and 9.2% of men are divorced (U.S. Bureau of the Census, 2001). People who divorce in late life have been largely neglected in research and support services. The number of people who seek divorce after that age is unknown, but divorce, as well as marriage and remarriage, must often be considered within the context of economics. In the last few years, the number of divorced elders has increased much more rapidly than the increase in the elderly population. This statistic may largely be a cohort effect. As divorces increase in couples of all ages, many more enter the ranks of the aged. At present 50% of all first marriages and 60% of remarriages end in divorce (U.S. Divorce Statistics, 2002). Long-term relationships are varied and complex, with many factors forming the glue that holds them together. Lanza (1996) studied the divorces of older women and found them attributed to their husbands' infidelity, retirement, or simply growing apart. Wives often tended to blame themselves, believing that they were in some way deficient and that otherwise the divorce would not have occurred. Lanza concluded that marital breakdown is more devastating in old age because it is often unanticipated and may occur concurrent with other significant losses.

Health care workers must be concerned with supporting a client's decision to seek a divorce and with assisting him or her in seeking counseling in the transition. A nurse should alert the client that a divorce will bring on a grieving process similar to the death of a spouse and that a severe disruption in coping capacity may occur until adjustment to one's new life is made. The grief may be more difficult to cope with because no socially sanctioned patterns have been established, as is the case with widowhood. In addition, tax and fiscal policies favor married couples, and many a divorced elderly lady is at a serious economic disadvantage in retirement.

ALONENESS, ISOLATION, AND LONELINESS

The sociology of aging examines the integration of individuals into society, and when a great number of these individuals are alone, lonely, and isolated, the responsive society must address their special needs.

Living Alone

The United States has a large number of elders living alone. This reflects the affluence of our times, the likelihood of widowhood for women, the involvement of families willing to assist elders in maintaining an independent lifestyle, and the cultural value of individual independence that is highly treasured in parts of our society. Cultures vary significantly in this respect.

Living alone does not equate with loneliness. The size and quality of the social network and the life patterns of the elder are far more significant than whether the elder has a partner. Those elders who are alone but have supportive friendships may treasure their independence and times of solitude.

Men living alone or with someone other than their spouse are thought to be at a disadvantage in terms of survival, whereas the living situation seems to make less difference to women. Both genders are affected by income, race, physical activity, and employment, but these variables are not necessarily related to being alone. To be alone is to be solitary, apart from others, and undisturbed. Many people have a strong need to be alone.

Isolation

Isolation is a response to conditions that inhibit the ability or opportunity to interact with others or is a result of the desire not to interact. At times, self-imposed isolation by individuals enhances creativity, individuality, and integrity, but when isolation is externally imposed by life situations, it is rarely satisfying.

The classical study by Berkman and Syme (1979) showed that socially isolated individuals were more prone to certain diseases, such as ischemic heart disease, cancer, and cerebrovascular and circulatory disorders. They concluded that circumstances that create social isolation may have pervasive health consequences and that the lack of social involvement may influence host resistance and disease vulnerability. Other researchers have since replicated these findings. Isolation increases vulnerability to disease, suicide, and death; yet there are many who are isolated from the mainstream by age, race, culture, frailty, poverty, geography, appearance, sexual orientation, or stereotypical thinking.

Social isolation has many causes and numerous defining characteristics: absence of supportive significant others; lack of purpose or challenges; aloneness imposed by others; or withdrawal because of hearing deficits, feelings of rejection, limited mobility, or visual impairment. Social isolation and emotional isolation are not necessarily equivalent. Older adults are particularly susceptible to social isolation because of environmental strictures, loss of familiar friends, and inability to perform certain activities. In addition, they may voluntarily disengage from some activities and become more intensely involved in those that are more valued. This is characteristic of healthy adaptation, but enforced isolation is likely to have detrimental effects. Emotional isolation involves unfilled needs for affiliation and often results from the loss of significant others.

Assessing elders for vulnerability to undesired social isolation and devising proactive measures to prevent or delay debilitating emotional isolation are nursing functions. Assessing vulnerability involves determination of the following: sensory status and decrements that interfere with communication and participation; absence of interactional opportunities; degree and intensity of losses experienced; and alterations to the sense of self. Interventions in general will involve compensating for sensory deficits, increasing opportunities for interaction with others, working through grief processes, and restoring self-esteem.

Care of the social isolate must be planned based on the source of the isolation, the level, the pattern, and the degree of vulnerability. Isolation concep-

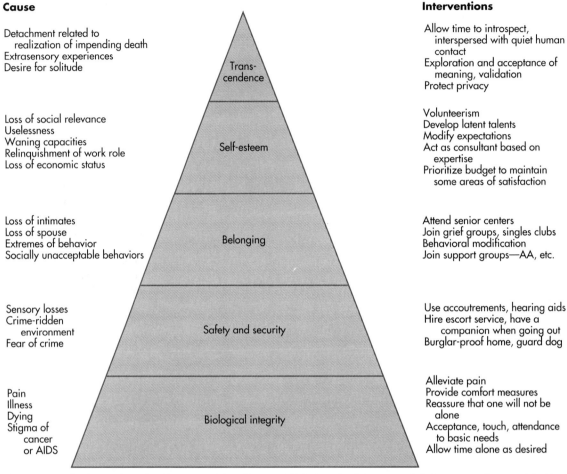

Cause

Detachment related to
    realization of impending death
Extrasensory experiences
Desire for solitude

Loss of social relevance
Uselessness
Waning capacities
Relinquishment of work role
Loss of economic status

Loss of intimates
Loss of spouse
Extremes of behavior
Socially unacceptable behaviors

Sensory losses
Crime-ridden
    environment
Fear of crime

Pain
Illness
Dying
Stigma of
    cancer
    or AIDS

Interventions

Allow time to introspect,
    interspersed with quiet human
    contact
Exploration and acceptance of
    meaning, validation
Protect privacy

Volunteerism
Develop latent talents
Modify expectations
Act as consultant based on
    expertise
Prioritize budget to maintain
    some areas of satisfaction

Attend senior centers
Join grief groups, singles clubs
Behavioral modification
Join support groups—AA, etc.

Use accoutrements, hearing aids
Hire escort service, have a
    companion when going out
Burglar-proof home, guard dog

Alleviate pain
Provide comfort measures
Reassure that one will not be
    alone
Acceptance, touch, attendance
    to basic needs
Allow time alone as desired

Pyramid levels (top to bottom): Trans-cendence, Self-esteem, Belonging, Safety and security, Biological integrity

Figure 8-4 The hierarchy of isolation and loneliness. *AIDS,* Acquired immunodeficiency syndrome; *AA,* Alcoholics Anonymous. (Idea from Ravish T: Prevent social isolation before it begins, *J Gerontol Nurs* 11[10]:10-13, 1985.)

tualized in levels of a hierarchy and life patterns provides a more accurate assessment of issues and possible interventions (Figure 8-4 and Box 8-9).

Loneliness

Loneliness seems to increase in direct proportion with perceptions of physical incapacity for both men and women. Lonely persons visit the physician oftener, take more medications, and have lower energy levels and multiple psychosomatic illnesses.

Tornstam (1990) studied loneliness among Swedish people and identified four distinct variables of loneliness: intensity and quantity (how often and how painful), inner loneliness (personality introversion), and positive loneliness (isolation sought). Early developmental experiences and present situations remain important factors in the loneliness experienced by older adults. The important contribution of Tornstam's study is his attempt to show loneliness as a complex and multidimensional effect. It is not a categorical condition of the aged.

For nurses, this indicates the need to assess and discuss loneliness in depth rather than simply identify it as a possible factor in the existence of clients. Loneliness is a passive, possessive, and

Box 8-9	Patterns of Isolation

Type 1: Lifelong extrovert isolated by condition or situation
- Ameliorate the situation to the greatest extent possible.
- Seek to bring in contact with individuals and groups through the Internet, distance learning.
- Help to identify like individuals who may enjoy frequent telephone contact.
- Establish pen pal network.

Type 2: Retiree whose contacts were mostly through work and who is now bereft of socialization opportunities
- Seek ready-made groups with some shared interests, often similar to work skills and expertise.
- Interest person in volunteer activities that will use particular skills.
- Provide opportunities to express particular skills in arenas where others will appreciate abilities.

Type 3: Active extrovert who withdraws in late life because of events causing shame (e.g., divorce, alcoholism, poverty)
- Assist with grief resolution, suggest counseling, seek support, self-help group.
- Help find resources addressing specific alienating condition.

Type 4: Lifelong isolate
- Assist in finding resources to augment areas of interest, hobbies.
- Initiate dyadic interactions if individual is willing.

painful emotion, whereas aloneness, solitude, and isolation may be actively sought, enhancing, and creative. Nurses need to assess whether clients are lonely or like to be alone. Nursing care plans for the alone and those for the lonely will be distinctly different. To make an adequate assessment, one must understand loneliness as different from being alone:
- Loneliness is an affective state of longing, emptiness, and feeling bereft.
- Lonely people may be physically alone or surrounded by others.
- Self-growth comes from one's ability to recognize and cope with loneliness.

- Loneliness accompanies self-alienation and self-rejection.
- Loneliness is evidence of the capacity for love. The degree of attachment is directly correlated with the felt loss when detachment occurs.

The Gerontological Orphan

The gerontological orphan is an older adult with no close friends or family members surviving or available to provide supports (Boyack, 1983). He or she has had significant others and lost them to death, distance, or fractured relationships. The gerontological orphan has not desired to be alone. In the event that such individuals are the last surviving member of their clan, nurses may encourage them to talk about those they have lost. Some have serious "survivor's guilt" that they need to express, particularly if the individual is the eldest and last survivor of a large sibling group. They can be assured that this is an aspect of grief that is often experienced. The survivor may say, "I was always the sickly one. I never expected to live so long. Why me and not them?" The sensitive nurse will resist platitudes and will respond, "Tell me about them."

For some gerontological orphans it may be a relief to be among others in a congregate or institutional setting, whereas others may find it depressing and react much better to friendly visits from younger people. Nurses are urged to make a loneliness assessment with their clients and discuss with them ways in which they could establish contact with others.

Assessing Loneliness

Luggen and Rini (1995) found it useful to assess the social network of community elders to predict those at risk of isolation. Almost half of the sample were found (based on the Luggen Social Network Scale) to be at great risk of isolation and detrimental loneliness. The greatest risk factor was childlessness. The following questions can be asked to assess loneliness:
- Does the patient initiate contact?
- Is the patient anxious, withdrawn, apathetic, or hostile?
- Does the patient cling to others or attempt to detain them?
- Is the patient unable to articulate his or her own needs?

- Is the patient eager for visitors and distressed when they leave?
- Does the patient exhibit contempt for his or her condition or self?
- Has there been a major disruption in the number of contacts with the patient?
- How often does the patient feel lonely and under what circumstances?
- Does the patient provoke to gain attention?

Interventions
- Ask about loneliness.
- Spend time with the patient in silence or in conversation.
- Assist the patient in keeping contact with people important to the patient.
- Let the patient know when you will be available.
- Explore the nature of the loneliness with the patient, as well the phenomenon of loneliness.
- Guide the person in reviewing life experiences related to loneliness to gain insight (for the patient) and data (for you).
- See or call the client frequently for brief periods.

Combating Loneliness with Pets

Pets often enhance an older person's quality of life, increasing happiness, decreasing loneliness, and improving physical functioning and emotional health (Suthers-McCabe, 2001). In 1859 Florence Nightingale (reprint, 1992) wrote that pets were excellent companions for persons confined with long-term illnesses. Studies of the value of animals for older people began to appear in 1980.

Pets provide comfort; intimacy; unquestioning, uncritical, and unconditional affection; and the opportunity to nurture and care for another being (Suthers-McCabe, 2001). Touching and fondling a pet may provide a substitute for human touch. In addition, a dog may provide a sense of protection and safety. Individuals recovering from a major loss or those who are institutionalized seem to experience beneficial effects from a pet. The positive effects of animal-assisted therapy in residential facilities have been documented in the literature and include reduced anxiety and behavioral problems and increased socialization and participation (Suthers-McCabe, 2001). See

Resources for more information on animal-assisted therapy.

A consideration in the selection of a pet may be potential longevity, because the loss of a pet can produce deep grief. Older people who lose a pet often grieve intensely but may not find others responding to their grief. Older people entering institutional care often have to give up a beloved pet. Staff may not appreciate the effect of grief responses on adjustment. Recognizing the significance, nurses may inquire about pets and the attachment and validate the grief. At these times it is important to make every effort to assist the elder in finding a support system. These individuals may need some sort of funeral or memorial for their pet. It may be useful to consider establishing grief groups for individuals whose pets have died. The American Veterinary Medical Association (AVMA) lists resources, including pet-loss hotlines, on their website (http://www.avma.org/care4pets/losshotl.htm). We sometimes become so preoccupied with "serious" issues that we do not fully understand the meaning of the loss of a pet in the life of a lonely elder.

GOVERNMENTAL POLICIES AND THE AGING EXPERIENCE

More than any other factor, the biopsychosocial aspects of aging have been influenced by governmental policies related to aging. Research dollars influence the rate and substance of new knowledge; Social Security and retirement policies influence income adequacy in later life; and health care policies have a major impact on the last years of life. Today, funding for social services is often tied to stringent governmental requirements. Although we hear about shifting the funding responsibility from federal agencies to state agencies, we have yet to see the full effects of this action. One of the paradoxes that hinders delivery of services to older adults in the United States is that America is both a capitalistic and a socialistic society, with health care moving rapidly into a highly competitive marketing mode. Therefore life-sustaining services are now designed for profit, although we simultaneously federally subsidize them. Box 8-10 lists the political events that have had a major impact on the psychosocial

Box 8-10   Political Events Influencing Aging

1935   Social Security Act signed by Franklin D. Roosevelt.

1937   National Institute of Health established first of the special institutes to study diseases common to older people.

1948   Hospital Construction and Facilities Act (Hill-Burton) provided funds for construction of long-term care facilities.

1950   First National Conference on Aging held in Washington, D.C.

1951   Federal Committee on Aging and Geriatrics created to coordinate federal programs for the aging.

1952   First Federal-State Conference on Aging held in Washington, D.C.

1956   Special Staff on Aging established within U.S. Department of Health, Education, and Welfare (HEW). Federal Council on Aging replaced Intradepartmental Working Group on Aging.

1959   Senate subcommittee authorized to consider problems of the aged and aging. Federal Council on Aging reconstituted at cabinet level.

1960   First appropriation passed for Section 202, Housing Act of 1959, authorizing direct loans for housing for the elderly.

1961   First White House Conference on Aging held in Washington, D.C. Senate Special Committee on Aging established as advocate for older Americans. First Annual Conference of State Executives held in Washington, D.C.

1962   Federal Council on Aging became President's Council on Aging.

1963   John F. Kennedy sent Congress the first presidential message on elderly citizens; designated May as Senior Citizens Month. Special Staff on Aging became Office of Aging in HEW's new Welfare Administration.

1965   President Johnson signed Older Americans Act, creating Administration on Aging (AOA). Amendments to the Social Security Act established Medicare program. Foster Grandparent Program initiated by Office of Economic Opportunity and Administration on Aging.

1967   Age Discrimination in Employment Act brightened job outlook for Americans 40 to 65 years old.

1970   Older Americans White House Forums held across the nation to identify problems and issues for upcoming White House Conference on Aging.

1971   Second White House Conference on Aging held in Washington, D.C. Cabinet-level Domestic Council Committee on Aging created. ACTION—the federal volunteer agency—established and given responsibility for senior volunteer programs previously administered by AOA.

1972   New act passed establishing Nutrition Program for the Elderly to be administered by AOA.

1973   Amendments to Older Americans Act called for state agencies on aging to establish area agencies on aging to plan for comprehensive, coordinated service delivery systems for older people at the local level.

Establishment of a National Clearinghouse on Aging and a Federal Council on the Aging with members appointed by the president. Amendments included a separate Older Americans Community Employment Act with responsibility for administering given to Department of Labor.

Federal Aid Highway Act of 1973 provided funds for a demonstration program of public transportation in rural areas with an emphasis on the needs of the elderly and handicapped.

1974   Research on Aging Act established National Institute on Aging within National Institute of Health; Robert N. Butler appointed director.

Amendments to Urban Mass Transportation Act of 1964 made funds available to nonprofit private organizations and corporations for transportation vehicles and equipment for the elderly and handicapped. National Mass Transportation Act mandated reduced fares for the elderly and handicapped on all public transportation systems assisted by the act.

1975   House of Representatives Special Committee on Aging established. Amendments to the Older Americans Act established four new priority areas under Title IV:

Continued.

Box 8-10	Political Events Influencing Aging—*cont'd*

	a. Transportation	1984	Sexual discrimination in pension benefit payments outlawed by U.S. Supreme Court.
	b. Home Services		
	c. Legal Services	1988	Medicare Catastrophic Coverage Act.
	d. Residential Repair and Renovation	1989	Medicare Catastrophic Coverage Act repealed.
1976	Title V of the Older Americans Act received an appropriation for the first time since inception of the act in 1965. Five million dollars was appropriated "to pay part of the cost of acquisition, alteration, or renovation of community facilities that will serve as multipurpose Senior Centers."	1991	Fourth White House Conference on Aging stalled. AOA funds cut drastically.
		1992	Proposals from multiple sources for rescue of health care system.
		1995	Fourth White House Conference on Aging. Focused on preservation of Medicare, Medicaid, Social Security, and the Older Americans Act (OAA).
1977	Title V re-funded at rate of $20 million annually.	1996	Majority of elders moved through Medicare changes to managed care systems.
1981	Third White House Conference on Aging held in Washington, D.C. Mandatory retirement laws revised.	1998	Congress considers privatizing Social Security.
1982	T. Franklin Williams appointed director of National Institute of Aging.	2000	Numerous methods of reducing drug costs are proposed.
1983	Diagnostic-related groups (DRGs) instituted by the Health Care Financing Administration to control costs of Medicare.	2004	Prescription drug plans instituted.
		2005	Medicare payment for preventive benefits expanded.

experience of the aged in the past 70 years. Nurses need some basic understanding of these major changes in the way the government has dealt with the older adult population.

IMPLICATIONS FOR GERONTOLOGICAL NURSING AND HEALTHY AGING

Knowledge about the process of life span development and the various ways people experience growing older assists gerontological nurses in understanding the meaning of healthy aging for each individual. Future generations of older adults will redefine what we now consider "norms" for aging. Role transitions and losses often characterize the aging experience. For some older adults, these can be devastating and will require support from nurses and other health professionals. Nurses can provide anticipatory guidance to assist older people in preparing for these transitions. It is important to build on the strengths of older adults' life experiences and coping skills and

to provide appropriate counseling and support to assist older people to continue to grow and develop in meaningful ways. What constitutes healthy aging will be different for each person based on individual life experiences. Our goal as gerontological nurses is to create opportunities for each older adult to thrive, not merely survive, in late life.

APPLICATION OF MASLOW'S HIERARCHY

Throughout this chapter we have presented the various psychosocial theories and aspects of aging that may result in both inner satisfaction and distress. Nurses can provide the opening for elders to discuss the process of aging and its psychological and social effects. In our highly biomedicalized approach to aging, it is imperative that we seek to know individuals beyond the problem that brings them to the attention of the health care team. Ask elders, "How has aging affected your inner life and

NANDA and Wellness Diagnoses

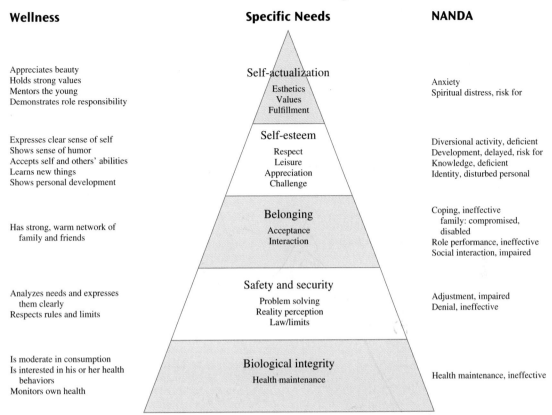

Wellness

Appreciates beauty
Holds strong values
Mentors the young
Demonstrates role responsibility

Expresses clear sense of self
Shows sense of humor
Accepts self and others' abilities
Learns new things
Shows personal development

Has strong, warm network of
   family and friends

Analyzes needs and expresses
   them clearly
Respects rules and limits

Is moderate in consumption
Is interested in his or her health
   behaviors
Monitors own health

Specific Needs

Self-actualization
Esthetics
Values
Fulfillment

Self-esteem
Respect
Leisure
Appreciation
Challenge

Belonging
Acceptance
Interaction

Safety and security
Problem solving
Reality perception
Law/limits

Biological integrity
Health maintenance

NANDA

Anxiety
Spiritual distress, risk for

Diversional activity, deficient
Development, delayed, risk for
Knowledge, deficient
Identity, disturbed personal

Coping, ineffective
   family: compromised,
   disabled
Role performance, ineffective
Social interaction, impaired

Adjustment, impaired
Denial, ineffective

Health maintenance, ineffective

These are not all of the possible wellness or NANDA diagnoses that may be identified. The above are frequent examples of nursing diagnoses that should be considered when planning care for the older adult in whatever setting.

outlook?" "What gives your life meaning and purpose?" Listen and learn. We are all aging, and those we serve are our best teachers.

KEY CONCEPTS

- Normal aging involves a gradual process of biopsychosocial change over the course of time.
- Life span development theorists tend to study the total life course of cohort groups to determine the influence of major historical events on their development.
- The impact of gender, culture, and cohort must always be considered when discussing the validity of biopsychosocial theories.

- It is becoming more generally accepted that personality characteristics, as well as biological characteristics, are to some degree inherent in the individual and that they remain relatively stable throughout life.
- Role transitions may be more difficult than in the past because there are fewer constant and relevant models in a rapidly changing society.
- Loneliness in old age is prevalent because of loss of longtime friends, companions, and family members.
- The totality of the aging experience is greatly influenced by the place, time, and general health of individuals as they reach the age of retirement.
- Governmental policies greatly impact the aging experience.

▶ **Activities and Discussion Questions**

1. Discuss some of the problems of adequately testing the cognitive function of elders.
2. Identify and discuss the major flaws in the sociological theories of aging.
3. Select one role that you might assume as an older person, and discuss pros and cons of this role.
4. What are some of the factors elders should consider when contemplating retirement?
5. Is retirement essentially different for older women than for older men and, if so, in what ways?
6. Discuss the variables that must constantly be considered when assessing the psychosocial aspects of the aging experience. Identify and discuss those that seem most significant.

RESOURCES

Organizations

Animal Assisted Therapy Foundation
P.O. Box 698
Troup, TX 75789
website: http://www.therapet.com

American Association of Retired Persons (AARP)
601 E Street NW
Washington, DC 20049
e-mail: member@aarp.org
website: http://www.aarp.org
AARP has numerous publications regarding consumer, economic, health, legal, and work issues. Most are available in English and Spanish.

Delta Society: The Human-Animal Health Connection
875 124th Avenue NE, Suite 101
Bellevue, WA 98005
website: http://www.deltasociety.org

Social Security Administration
(800) 772-1213
website: www.ssa.gov
Phone books list local offices under the Government section.

REFERENCES

Age Beat on Line: *The Newsletter of the Journalists Exchange on Aging* 2(15), July 2002. Available at paul@asaaging.org.

Baltes PB: Theoretical propositions on life-span developmental theory: on the dynamics between growth and decline, *Dev Psychol* 23(5):611-626, 1987.

Baltes PB, Lindenberger U, Staudinger U: Life-span theory in developmental psychology. In Lerner R, editor: *Handbook of child psychology*, vol 1. *Theoretical models of human development*, New York, 1998, Wiley.

Bandura A: Self-efficacy: toward a unifying theory of behavioral change, *Psychol Rev* 84(2):191-215, 1977.

Barer BM: Men and women aging differently, *Int J Aging Hum Dev* 38(1):29-40, 1993.

Beers MH, Berkow R: *Merck manual of geriatrics*, ed 3, Whitehouse Station, NJ, 2000, Merck Research Laboratories.

Berkman LF, Syme SL: Social networks, host resistance, and mortality: a nine-year follow-up study of Alameda County residents, *Am J Epidemiol* 109(2):186-204, 1979.

Birren J, Cunningham W: Research on the psychology of aging: principles, concepts, and theory. In Birren J, Schaie K, editors: *Handbook of the psychology of aging*, ed 2, New York, 1985, Van Nostrand Reinhold.

Bowsher JE, Keep D: Toward an understanding of three control constructs: personal control, self-efficacy, and hardiness, *Issues Ment Health Nurs* 16(1):33-50, 1995.

Boyack V: The geriatric orphan: Research and practice perspectives. Paper presented at the annual convention of the Western Gerontological Society, Albuquerque, NM, March 18, 1983.

Buhler C: The human course of life in its goal aspects, *J Hum Psychol* 4:1, 1964.

Camp CJ: Facilitation of new learning in Alzheimer's disease. In Gilmore G et al, editors: *Memory and aging: theory, research and practice*, New York, 1989, Springer.

Crowley SL: Aging brain's staying power, *AARP Bull* 37(4):1, 1996.

Cumming E, Henry W: *Growing old*, New York, 1961, Basic Books.

Cunningham W, Brookbank J: *Gerontology: the psychology, biology and sociology of aging*, New York, 1988, Harper & Row.

DeVries B: Grief: intimacy's reflection, *Generations* 25(2):75-79, 2001.

Dorfman LT: Health conditions and perceived quality of life in retirement, *Health Soc Work* 20(3):192, 2002.

Ebersole PR: May your goals never be fully accomplished, *Geriatr Nurs* 17(5):258-259, 1996.

Ekerdt DJ, Dennis H: Introduction to retirement: New chapters in American life, *Generations* 26(11), 2002.

Erikson EH: *Childhood and society*, ed 2, New York, 1963, WW Norton & Co.

Erikson EH, Erikson JM, Kivnick HQ: *Vital involvement in old age: the experience of old age in our time*, New York, 1986, WW Norton & Co.

Family Caregiver Alliance, National Center on Caregiving: *Caregiving Policy Digest* 11(11):3, 2002.

Gallo JJ, Fulmer T, Paveza G: *Handbook of geriatric assessment,* ed 3, Boston, 2003, Jones and Bartlett.

Havighurst RL, Neugarten BL, Tobin SS: Disengagement and patterns of aging. In Neugarten BL, editor: *Middle age and aging,* Chicago, 1968, University of Chicago Press.

Hirshorn BA, Tetrick LE, Sinclair RR: Understanding the provision of postretirement health care and pension benefits: which firm characteristics are most explanatory, *Gerontologist* 36(5):637, 1996.

Jung C: The stages of life. In Campbell J, editor: *The portable Jung,* New York, 1971, Viking Press (translated by RFC Hull).

Kelly C: Perspectives of gerontic nurse pioneers. In Ebersole P, Hess P, editors: *Toward healthy aging: human needs and nursing response,* ed 3, St Louis, 1990, Mosby.

Kobasa SC: Stressful life events, personality, and health: an inquiry into hardiness, *J Pers Soc Psychol* 37(1):1-11, 1979.

Kuhlen R: Developmental changes in motivation during the adult years. In Neugarten B, editor: *Middle age and aging,* Chicago, 1968, University of Chicago Press.

Lanza ML: Divorce experienced as an older woman, *Geriatr Nurs* 17(4):166-170, 1996.

Lehman H: *Age and achievement,* Princeton, NJ, 1953, Princeton University Press.

Lenker LT, Polivka L: Project rationale and history, *J Aging Identity* 1(1):3-6, 1996.

Lindemann E: Symptomatology and management of acute grief, *Am J Psychiatr* 101(2):141-148, 1944.

Luggen AS, Rini AG: Assessment of social networks and isolation in community based elderly men and women, *Geriatr Nurs* 16(4):179-181, 1995.

Maddox G: Activity and morale: a longitudinal study of selected older adult subjects, *Soc Forces* 42:195, 1963.

McAvay GJ, Seeman TE, Rodin J: A longitudinal study of change in domain-specific self-efficacy among older adults, *J Gerontol* 51B(5):243-253, 1996.

National Institutes of Health: Memory loss, 2002. Available at www.ninds.nlm.nih.gov/medlineplus/ency/article/003257.htm.

Neugarten B, Havighurst R, Tobin S: Personality and patterns of aging. In Neugarten B, editor: *Middle age and aging,* Chicago, 1968, University of Chicago Press.

Nightingale F: *Notes on nursing,* Philadelphia, 1992, Lippincott (originally published in 1859).

Papalia D, Sterns H, Feldman R, Camp C: *Adult development and aging,* Boston, 2002, McGraw-Hill.

Peck R: Psychological developments in the second half of life. In Neugarten B, editor: *Middle age and aging,* Chicago, 1968, University of Chicago Press.

Petersen R: MCI as a useful clinical concept, *Geriatric Times* 5(1), 2004. Available at http://www.geriatrictimes.com/g040215.html.

Poon LW et al: Biomarkers of aging, *Generations* 16(4):11-14, 1992.

Stanford P, Usita P: Retirement: Who is at risk? *Generations* 26(11):45-48, 2002.

Sugarman RA: Structure and function of the nervous system. In McCance KL, Huether SE, editors: *Pathophysiology: the biologic basis for disease in adults and children,* ed 4, St Louis, 2002, Mosby.

Suthers-McCabe H: Take one pet and call me in the morning, *Generations* 25(2), 2001.

Tafford A: *The bonus decades,* New York, 2002, Basic Books.

Tappen R, Touhy T, Sparks D, et al: The effectiveness of a pilot program of therapeutic activities in early stage memory loss. Unpublished data.

Taylor, MA, Shore RM: Predictors of planned retirement age: An application of Beehr's model, *Psychol Aging* 10(1):76, 1995.

Tornstam L: Dimensions of loneliness, *Aging* 2(3):259, 1990.

Touhy TA: Nurturing hope and spirituality in the nursing home, *Holist Nurs Pract* 15(4):45-56, 2001.

U.S. Bureau of the Census: *Statistical abstract of the United States 2002,* ed 122, Washington, DC, 2001, U.S. Government Printing Office.

U.S. Divorce Statistics: DivorceMagazine.com, December 2002. Available at www.divorcemag.com/statistics/statsUS.shtml.

Sensory Changes of Aging

> ## LEARNING OBJECTIVES

Upon completion of this chapter, the reader will be able to:

- Identify sensory changes accompanying aging that alter the perceived world of the aged.
- Discuss vision and hearing impairments and diseases that may occur in older adults.
- Describe nursing assessment and interventions that can be implemented to help elders with decreased vision and hearing problems.

> ## GLOSSARY

Agnosia Loss of comprehension of auditory, visual, or other sensations, although the sensory sphere is intact.

Paresthesia Sensation of numbness, prickling, tingling or heightened sensitivity.

Presbycusis Normal decrement in hearing acuity, speech intelligibility, auditory threshold, and pitch discrimination that occurs with aging.

Presbyopia Decreased ability of the lens of the eyes to accommodate for close and detailed work as one advances in age.

Sensory deprivation A condition in which there is insufficient stimuli to sensory apparatus to allow integrative perceptions to develop.

Sensory overload Bombardment of the sensory apparatus by environmental stimuli that reaches levels that are physically and psychologically overwhelming.

> ## THE LIVED EXPERIENCE

I DON'T HEAR AS WELL AS I USED TO

I don't hear as well as I used to
People have to shout and repeat things.
Frankly, a lot of what they have to say
Isn't worth repeating.
And the world's too noisy anyway.
The important thing is, I can hear,
Not with my ears, but with my heart,
What I really want to:
The children, when they were little,
Saying, "I love you Mama."
Dan, when we lost our savings,

Saying, "Hold me, Anne."
Stephen in front of all those people,
Saying, "My mother should be receiving this honor
Instead of me."
My father-in-law, dying, laying his hand on my hair,
"You're a good gel, Annie, carry on."
It's no fun going deaf,
But there are worse things,
And I do have a lot of good memories
To listen to.

From Maclay E: Green winter: celebrations of old age, New York, 1977,
Copyright ©1977 Elise Maclay.

APPRECIATION OF SENSORY CHANGES AND EXPERIENCES

All senses gradually lose their acuity with old age. The normal changes result from the accumulated atrophy of sensory receptors in the eye, ear, nose, buccal cavity, and peripheral afferent nerves, substantially reducing the vividness of environmental impressions. Events no longer alert the nervous system with such clarity as in youth. Habituation to certain sensations may also diminish their impact. The normal gradual diminution of the senses during the aging process is usually well accommodated by experience. When the experience remains within the boundaries of constancy and familiarity, normal sensory loss is not detrimental to function. It may in fact be desirable. An older person, because of lowered energy and concentration, may be more vulnerable to sensory overload than to sensory deprivation. We are all subject to alterations in our sensory experience, and with increasing age it is likely that these circumstances will occur more frequently and perhaps be more devastating.

The issues of concern to nurses include the following: devising methods to keep the organismic senses functional enough to negotiate the environment effectively by keeping the environment within reach; supplementing sensory loss with additional pleasures to the remaining senses; and providing touch, color, and variety. The sensory environment is to be revered and cultivated. Therein lie many problems. Growing older may subject one to decreased appreciation of the environment through drugs, machines, treatments, paresthesias, presbyopia, presbycusis, and agnosia. Life may be more cautiously sampled. Stored experiences often come to the rescue, and older people remember things they can no longer perceive.

When describing the capacities and changes in the various sensory apparatuses, we must understand that they all work in consensus. Situations are experienced through sight, sound, smell, and touch simultaneously (Sacks, 1989). The senses are tightly interwoven in forming the perceptual base of our world. Possibly the "sixth sense" (intuition, or the power of perception that goes beyond that of the five senses) is really the consensus of all the senses in an acutely aware individual. In some cases a disorder of one of the senses may stimulate the others in a compensatory manner.

Age-related declines are variable and cannot be generalized to all sensory systems or to all older individuals. Personal hardiness and an environment that conveys order and meaning contribute in ways yet unidentified to good perceptual processing and high-level functioning. It is not uncommon that elders are thought to be cognitively impaired when in fact attention to enhanced sensory function through an adapted environment and appropriate assistive devices reveals much higher functional levels. General perceptual organization and efficiency are modified by health status, frailty of aging, illness, medications, fatigue, and stress and anxiety.

Those who care for older adults are concerned about manipulating stimuli and enhancing sensory stimuli to induce an optimal functional level of perceptual adequacy. When the senses are grossly underloaded or overloaded, perception and reactions are distorted. The world becomes an alien, confusing place. Fear and anxiety increase, or one withdraws into a fabricated world that provides security. Altered sensory experience will affect one's view of self and one's ability to relate to others. Isolation and loneliness may be the result. Emotional responses to altered sensory input include boredom, diminished concentration, incoherent thoughts, anxiety, fear, depression, and even hallucinations. Clear and sometimes repetitive data about the environment must be given when perceptions are impaired. Manipulating the environment to reduce demands and enhance sensory function should decrease these symptoms, although studies show that signs may persist for several days. Adequate input is essential to continued cognitive development. This chapter discusses sensory deprivation and sensory overload as well as vision and hearing changes affecting sensory functioning. Changes in taste and smell also affect older adults and will be discussed in Chapter 10.

Sensory Deprivation

There are at least three types of sensory deprivation: (1) reduced sensory capacities, (2) elimination of patterns and meaning from input, and (3) restrictive, monotonous environments. Certain

Box 9-1	Effects of Sensory Deprivation

- Sensory deprivation tends to amplify existing personality traits.
- Perceptual disorganization occurs in visual/motor coordination, color perception, apparent movement, tactile accuracy, ability to perceive size and shape, and spatial and time judgment.
- Sensory deprivation alters mechanisms of attention, consciousness, and reality testing (similar to brain anoxia).
- Marked changes of behavior occur, such as inability to think and solve problems, affectual disturbance, perceptual distortions, hallucinations and delusions, vivid imagination, poor task performance, increased anxiety and aggression, somatic complaints, temporal and spatial disorientation, emotional lability, and confusion of sleep and waking states.
- Monotony produces a disruption of the capacity to learn and the ability to think.
- In the absence of varied stimulation, brain function becomes less.
- Illness often increases perceptual confusion, particularly in older adults.

effects thought to be "confusion" or "old age" may arise from sensory deprivation. Any situation lacking varied environmental stimuli deprives the senses of adequate material for perceptual integrity. Box 9-1 summarizes some effects of sensory deprivation.

Common contributors to sensory deprivation, particularly in the frail older adult, such as poor vision, decreased energy, poor hearing, extended periods in a supine position, debilitating illness and chronic disorders, few pleasant sounds, and limited meaningful contact with others, often result in disorientation. Late afternoon may aggravate the deprivation if daylight is diminished and there is inadequate indoor lighting. Open the drapes and the window; the sights, sounds, and smells of outdoors and life can be enjoyable and reassuring. Turn on lights; raise the head of the bed, or assist the person to a chair bolstered comfortably with pillows; bring a flower to the room; sit down; speak; touch; and listen to the client's feelings and perceptions. Discuss the isolated person's interests; radio, television, computers,

books, puzzles, and handicrafts may all amuse the solitary person. It is essential to plan with the elderly, not for them. When these efforts fail, it is because of inadequate assessment. If the individual is concerned about more fundamental issues, such as maintaining biological integrity, attention to surroundings and the environment will not be a priority. Life, at all ages, is meant to be savored, not endured.

When the ambience is one of monotony, even a small stimulus may trigger a strong response. Knowing this makes it easier to understand the overreactions displayed when a routine is interrupted. People are more sensitive to change of any sort when there are so few changes and they feel deprived of control. There is a good response to gradual environmental enrichment. Rapid increases and overstimulation may produce anxiety, fear, and confusion. Meanings and patterns that throughout life have formed the basis of precepts, and on a preconscious level have sorted data in ways meaningful to the individual, may be shattered in crises, unnatural events, and catastrophes. The senses are no longer reliable.

Sensory Overload

Sensory overload can occur from unexpected, abrupt environmental change such as those brought on by accident or hospitalization. These are situations of sensory overload precipitated by actual or perceived environmental demands. Sensory overload is a contributing factor to the development of delirium in older adults who are hospitalized. An individual with marginal adaptation and cognitive decrements is particularly vulnerable. Sensory overload is a very individual matter, often related to cognitive capacity. It can be recognized by certain symptoms—thoughts may race, and attention may scatter in many directions. People find it difficult to sit still. Aberrant thoughts or actions may occur. Evidence of anxiety is present. The amount of stimuli necessary for healthy function varies with each individual; the relevance and familiarity of stimuli may be more important than the amount. Biorhythms are another important consideration. Individuals may be more subject to environmental overload at one time than at another. Sensations are generally most acute in the late afternoon.

Sensory overload cannot always be avoided, but when one is extremely stressed and bombarded with adaptive demands, time must be arranged for peacefulness and frequent rest periods. It is often helpful to sit quietly with the person, saying very little, or engage him or her in a nondemanding repetitive activity that will help focus attention on something that provides security and reduces stress. Walking can be beneficial. Careful assessment of behavior is important to determine both internal and external precipitants for changes.

VISION AND VISUAL IMPAIRMENT IN THE AGED

Visual acuity and accommodation normally decrease with age. These changes begin making themselves felt in the mid-forties for many people and are mainly an inconvenience rather than a problem. Major aging of the eye (presbyopia) occurs between 45 and 55 years of age; still, 80% of the aged have fair to adequate vision past 90 years of age. Much can be done to improve vision for the majority of elders.

Several ophthalmological changes that occur with aging are not serious but may cause discomfort or alarm in the elder experiencing them. Headache accompanied by eye muscle pain can be caused by the tendency with aging for a gradual decrease in the tone of the medial rectus muscle, which turns the eye inward while focusing on close objects. This then creates exophoria (slight turning outward of the eye) and may result in headache when one is doing close work for an extended period. Headaches associated with this condition can be remedied by taking more rest breaks while doing close work, doing close work early in the day, and engaging in eye muscle exercises three times daily for 5 minutes each session. Symptomatic relief is usually achieved in 4 to 6 weeks.

A decrease in pupil size, which hinders light from reaching the retina, is a major factor in visual changes of aging. Small objects cannot be seen at a distance. Adaptation to darkness is also deficient in old age, with depletion of certain retinal functions. Night vision decreases, which may become a source of great insecurity and potential danger to those older persons who must drive at night. Many limit themselves to daytime driving. Many

safety factors are obviously attached to visual adequacy, although people with limitations often adapt remarkably well. Reduced translucency of the cornea, lens, and vitreous humor results in a decrease of up to two thirds of ambient light reaching the retina in a 60-year-old person as compared with a 20-year-old person (Ham et al, 2002). Chapter 7 provides an in-depth discussion of vision and eye changes in aging.

Presbyopia

The problem with accommodation, or the ability to focus on objects at various distances, is noticeable by the mid-forties. This is when most people become aware of the need to hold objects farther away to properly focus their gaze. This change is presbyopia. For most individuals the reading lens must be increased in strength every 2 or 3 years between the ages of 45 and 65. Presbyopia tends to occur earlier in persons with farsightedness (hyperopia) than in those with nearsightedness (myopia). As lens opacity increases, some refractive power increases at the same time that accommodation, or lens resilience, decreases. The result is a temporary shift toward myopia and improved close vision. Thus some individuals at 60 or 70 years of age develop "second sight" in which they can again read without glasses (Kupfer, 1995a). Superimposed on these natural changes of aging can be a number of diseases affecting vision.

Diseases Affecting Vision

For elders with visual impairments, the consequences for functional ability, safety, and quality of life can be profound. The major diseases affecting vision are glaucoma, cataracts, macular degeneration, and diabetic retinopathy. With appropriate eye care, these diseases are readily diagnosed, but many older people, particularly minorities, do not receive necessary care. It is estimated that 40% of blindness and visual impairment is treatable or preventable. The problem of undiagnosed visual disorders is increasing, and the number of blind and visually impaired elders is expected to double in the next three decades (Rowe et al, 2004). For the first time, vision objectives have been included in *Healthy People 2010* and are focused on the early detection of cataracts, glaucoma, and diabetic eye disease (Miller, 2004).

The Lighthouse National Survey on Vision Loss reported that more than one fourth of elders over the age of 75 are classified as visually impaired, and half report that a vision problem interferes with their daily lives (accessed 7/5/04 from www.lighthouse.org/research_nationalsurvey.html). Impaired vision is a serious concern among nursing home residents, with estimates of impairment ranging from 21% to 52%. Women completely lose vision more frequently than men, and in both genders it is common to have better vision in one eye than in the other. The following section will discuss the major causes of vision impairment in older adults.

Glaucoma

The most common cause of blindness in Americans over age 65 is primary open-angle glaucoma, a chronic, progressive, degenerative disease involving increased intraocular pressure (IOP), usually bilaterally, that can lead to permanent damage of the optic nerve. The disease affects about 2.2 million Americans age 40 and over, half of whom are not aware they have the disease. Open-angle glaucoma accounts for about 80% of cases and is asymptomatic until very late in the disease, when there is a noticeable loss in visual fields (Kupfer, 1995a, 1995b). Glaucoma has been described as the "silent thief" because it will steal vision with no forewarning. However, if detected early, glaucoma can usually be controlled and serious vision loss prevented (Higginbotham et al, 2004).

Age is the single most important predictor of glaucoma, and older women are affected twice as frequently as older men. Glaucoma is six to eight times more common in African Americans than in Caucasians. African Americans develop glaucoma at younger ages and with more frequency than whites. Glaucoma accounts for 19% of all blindness among African Americans, compared with 6% of Caucasians (Higginbotham et al, 2004). Asians, particularly the Chinese, and those with Spanish heritage are also prone to develop glaucoma. Many drugs with anticholinergic properties or those that cause pupillary dilation will exacerbate glaucoma in older adults.

The etiology of glaucoma is variable and often unknown; however, when the natural fluids of the eye are blocked by ciliary muscle rigidity and the buildup of pressure, damage to the optic nerve

occurs. A family history of glaucoma, diabetes, and past eye injuries have been noted as risk factors for the development of glaucoma. Among African Americans, other factors that may contribute to the high incidence of the disease include earlier onset of the disease compared with other races, later detection of the disease, and economic and social barriers to treatment. An acute attack of closed-angle glaucoma is characterized by a rapid rise in intraocular pressure accompanied by redness and pain in and around the eye, severe headache, nausea and vomiting, and blurring of vision.

Eye drops that relieve the pressure can control glaucoma. These medications lower eye pressure, either by decreasing the amount of aqueous fluid produced within the eye or by improving the flow through the drainage angle. Usually medication can control glaucoma, but laser surgery treatments (trabeculoplasty) may be recommended for some types of glaucoma. Surgery is usually recommended only if necessary to prevent further damage to the optic nerve. In a recent study (McGwin et al, 2004) it was found that statins and other cholesterol-lowering medications may be associated with a reduced risk of glaucoma, particularly among those with cardiovascular and lipid diseases. Further research is warranted.

Glaucoma screening is an important way to identify this silent condition. A dilated eye examination and tonometry are necessary to diagnose glaucoma. These procedures can be performed by a primary care provider, an optometrist, or a nurse practitioner, who will then refer the person to an ophthalmologist if glaucoma is suspected. A simple hand-held noncontact method of tonometry that can be used to identify 90% of patients with IOPs greater than 22 mm Hg has been used since 1972 (Ralston et al, 1992). Ordinarily, a tonometry reading of 10 to 20 is considered acceptable, although there are many complicating factors. Persons with pressure measurements above 21 mm Hg are "ocular hypertensives" and may not yet need treatment but will need visual field testing at 6-month intervals (Kupfer, 1995b). Many elders may have undiagnosed glaucoma that has not been screened for or evaluated. It is recommended that adults 65 and over be evaluated annually and those with medication-controlled glaucoma be examined at least every 6 months (Kupfer, 1995a). Individuals of African descent or those with a family history of glaucoma should begin having eye examinations more frequently and at an earlier age.

Cataracts

Cataracts are a prevalent disorder among the older adults caused by oxidative damage to lens protein and fatty deposits (lipofuscin) in the ocular lens. After age 75, as many as 70% of Americans have cataracts that are significant enough to impair their vision (accessed 7/10/04 from http://www.mayoclinic.com).

When lens opacity reduces visual acuity to 20/30 or less in central vision, it is considered a cataract. Cataracts are categorized according to their location within the lens. They are virtually universal in the very old but may be only minimally visible, particularly in individuals with pale irises. Cataracts are recognized by the clouding of the ordinarily clear ocular lens. The most common causes of cataracts are hereditary and advancing age. They may occur more frequently and at earlier ages in individuals who have been exposed to excessive sunlight, have poor dietary habits, or have diabetes.

The cardinal sign of cataracts is the spraying of light and blurriness around the edges of objects. Other common symptoms include blurring, seeing double moons, decreased perception of light and color, and sensitivity to glare. The hallmark of cataracts is painless, progressive loss of vision (Kupfer, 1995b). Cataract surgery is considered whenever the visual disturbance becomes an impediment in the individual's daily life and is the most common surgery performed in the United States (Ham et al, 2002). Most often, cataract surgery involves removing the entire lens capsule and replacing it with a plastic intraocular lens (IOL). These are often slipped into place without the need for suturing. When necessary, cataract surgery has the potential to improve not only sight but also quality of life. Unfortunately, glaucoma and cataracts often occur simultaneously, which complicates the management of each. Individuals who have had cataract surgery are less likely to be candidates for surgical treatment of glaucoma.

Diabetic Retinopathy

Some visual disabilities are acquired through the deleterious effects of elevated blood glucose levels because of diabetes, which creates microaneurysms in retinal capillaries, the source of diabetic retinopathy. Because of vascular and cellular changes accompanying diabetes, there is often rapid worsening of other visual pathological conditions as well. Diabetic retinopathy accounts for 7% of the blindness in the United States, and the incidence curves upward abruptly with increasing age (Kupfer, 1995b). Constant, strict control of blood glucose, cholesterol, and blood pressure and laser photocoagulation treatments can halt progression of the disease (Hamm et al, 2002). Early detection of the disease can prevent substantial vision loss. Annual dilated fundascopic examination of the eye is recommended beginning 5 years after diagnosis of type 1 diabetes and at the time of diagnosis of type 2 diabetes.

Macular Degeneration

Age-related macular degeneration (AMD) is the most common cause of legal blindness (Snellen reading of 20/200) and the most common visual impairment of individuals over age 50. The prevalence of AMD increases drastically with age, with more than 15% of Caucasian women over the age of 80 having the disease. With the projected increases in the number of older adults over the next 20 years, AMD has been called a growing epidemic (Bressler, 2004). AMD is a degenerative eye disease that affects the macula, the central part of the retina at the back of the eye responsible for clear central vision. The disease causes the progressive loss of central vision, leaving only peripheral vision intact. It usually starts in one eye, but there is a high risk (greater than 40%) that the disease will affect the other eye within 5 years (Bressler et al, 2003).

AMD results from systemic changes in circulation, accumulation of cellular waste products, tissue atrophy, and growth of abnormal blood vessels in the choroid layer beneath the retina. Although etiology is unknown, risk factors are thought to include genetic predisposition, smoking, and excessive sunlight exposure. AMD is more common in women, people with blue eyes, and Caucasians. There are two forms of macular degeneration, the "dry" form and the "wet" form. Dry AMD accounts for the majority of cases, rarely causes severe visual impairment, but can lead to the more aggressive wet AMD. With wet AMD, the severe loss of central vision can be rapid and many people will be legally blind within 2 years of diagnosis. Peripheral vision usually remains normal, but the person will have difficulty seeing at a distance or doing detailed work, such as sewing or reading. Faces may begin to blur, and it becomes harder to distinguish colors. An early sign may be distortion that causes edges or lines to appear wavy. In the advanced forms, the person may begin to see dark or empty spaces that block the center of vision. Patients in the early stage of the disease may attribute the vision problems to normal aging or to cataracts. Early diagnosis is key, and individuals over the age of 50 should have an eye examination at least every 2 years. The Age-Related Eye Disease Study (AREDS) found that a combination of antioxidants plus zinc can reduce the risk of developing AMD (Sackett, Bressler, 2001). Treatment of wet AMD includes photodynamic therapy (PDT) and laser photocoagulation (LPC).

Implications for Gerontological Nursing and Healthy Aging

Visual impairment can have profound consequences for function and quality of life. Gerontological nurses are responsible for preventive teaching regarding health of the eye, as well as identification of risk factors and symptoms of existing impairment and environmental adaptations to enhance vision. Teaching older adults about risk factors for the development of eye diseases as well as modifiable health behaviors to prevent eye diseases is important. All older adults should have annual dilated eye examinations, but routine assessment by the nurse includes checking distant vision using a Snellen chart, assessing visual fields, and evaluating near vision and reading ability. An excellent source for health information and teaching aids is the National Eye Institute website (www.nie.nih.gov). The website also provides vision simulators where images can be viewed as they might appear to a person with glaucoma, diabetic retinopathy, and AMD.

Because visual impairment affects most daily activities, such as driving, reading, maneuvering safely, dressing, cooking, and social activities, assessing the effect of vision changes on functional abilities, safety, and quality of life is most important. Decreased vision has also been found

to be a significant risk factor for falls. Certain signs and behaviors of visual problems that should alert the nurse to action are noted in Box 9-2.

General principles in caring for the elder with visual impairment include the following: use warm incandescent lighting, control glare by using shades and blinds, suggest yellow or amber lenses to decrease glare, suggest sunglasses that block all ultraviolet light, select colors with good contrast and intensity, and recommend reading materials that have large, dark, evenly spaced printing (Stuen, 1996). The intensity of illumination needs to be three times greater to produce the same visual capacity for older adults as for younger people. Intensity must be tempered by appropriate diffusion to avoid glare. Sharply contrasting colors assist people with visual impairment. It is much easier to locate a bright towel than a white towel hanging on a beige wall. Box 9-3 offers ideas

---

Box 9-2   Signs and Behaviors That May Indicate Vision Problems

Individual May Report:
Pain in eyes
Difficulty seeing in darkened area
Double vision/distorted vision
Migraine headaches coupled with blurred vision
Flashes of light
Halos surrounding lights
Difficulty driving at night
Falls or injuries

Health Care Staff May Notice:
Getting lost
Bumping into objects
Straining to read or no reading
Stumbling/falling
Spilling food on clothing
Social withdrawal
Less eye contact
Placid facial expression
TV viewing at close range
Decreased sense of balance
Mismatched clothes

Modified from McNeely E, Griffin-Shirley N, Hubbard A: Teaching caregivers to recognize diminished vision among nursing home residents, *Geriatr Nurs* 13(6):332-335, 1992.

for communicating and caring for the elder with severe visual impairment or blindness.

Gerontological nurses must be familiar with the resources and vision aids available when attempting to help the visually impaired elder achieve the visual activities that are important to his or her quality of life. The following section discusses low-vision assistive devices and programs.

Low-Vision Assistive Devices

Technological advances in the last decade have produced some low-vision assistive devices that may be used successfully to improve the quality of life for the visually impaired elder. People with severe visual impairment may qualify for disability and financial and social services assistance through government and private programs including vision rehabilitation programs. An array of low-vision devices are now available, including insulin delivery and glucose-monitoring equipment, talking watches, large-print books, magnifiers, and computers with low-vision devices (Goldzweig et al, 2004).

Eyeglasses, once heavy and bulky, are now cosmetically appealing. Many also incorporate prismatic lenses that expand the visual field. Sunglasses are designed to filter out ultraviolet rays that may be harmful to sensitive retinas. Some eyeglasses adjust to the light source and become darker in the sun. Magnifiers have been redesigned for ease of changing batteries and bulbs, positioning, and grasping. Telescopic lens eyeglasses are smaller, are easier to focus, and have a greater range. It is now possible to electronically magnify video- and computer-generated text. Some software converts text into artificial voice

---

Box 9-3	**Suggestions for Communicating with and Caring for Visually Impaired Elders**

Remember, there are many degrees of blindness; allow as much independence as possible.

- Assess your position in relation to the individual. One eye or ear may be better than the other.
- When in the presence of a blind person, speak promptly and clearly identify yourself and others with you. State when you are leaving to make sure the person is aware of your departure.
- Make sure you have the individual's attention before you start talking.
- Speak descriptively of your surroundings to familiarize the blind person, and state the position of the people who are in the room.
- Speak normally but not from a distance; do not raise or lower your voice, and continue to use gestures if that is natural to your communication. Do not alter your vocabulary; words such as *see* and *blind* are part of normal speech. When others are present, address the blind person by prefacing remarks with his or her name or a light touch on the arm.
- Try to minimize the number of distractions.
- Use the analogy of a clock face to help locate objects. Describe positions of food on the plate in relation to clock positions (e.g., 3 o'clock, 6 o'clock).
- Check to see that the best possible lighting is available.

- Try to keep the individual between you and the window; you will appear as a dark shadow.
- Whenever possible, choose bright clothing with bold contrasts.
- Do not change the room arrangement or arrangement of personal items without explanation.
- Speak before handing a blind person an object.
- Keep color and texture in mind when buying clothes.
- When walking with a blind person, offer your arm. Pause before stairs or curbs; mention them. In seating, place the person's hand on the back of the chair. Let him or her know the position in relation to objects.
- Blind people like to know the beauty that surrounds them. Describe flowers, scenery, colors, and textures. People who have been blind since birth cannot conceive of color, but it adds to their appreciation to hear full descriptions. Old people most frequently have been sighted and can enjoy memories of beauty stimulated by descriptive conversation.
- Use some means to identify residents who are known to be visually impaired.
- *Be careful about labeling a resident as confused.* He or she may be making mistakes as a result of poor vision.

output. Gerontological nurses must be familiar with the resources and vision aids available when attempting to help the visually impaired elder achieve the visual activities that are important to his or her quality of life. Because individual needs are unique, it is recommended that before investing in any of these vision aids, the client be advised to consult with a low-vision center or low-vision specialist. For further information contact the organizations for the blind listed in the Resources at the end of this chapter.

Orientation Strategies for the Blind

Methods to assist those individuals with total lack of sight are not generally included in nursing curricula. Methods in common use include the following: (1) the clock method, in which the individual is simply told where the food or item is as if it were on a clock face; (2) the sighted guide, in which a companion guides the visually impaired and enables safe mobility; (3) the cane sweep, which encounters obstacles; (4) sound signals (e.g., at street crossings); (5) varied-textured surfaces; and (6) guide dogs.

Sighted Guides

Ask the blind person if he or she would like a "sighted guide." A strong element of dependency and trust is necessary in this method, and many people would rather manage on their own. Initially, as a person is adjusting to blindness, it can be helpful. If assistance is accepted, offer your elbow or arm. Instruct the person to grasp your arm just above the elbow. If necessary, physically assist the person by guiding his or her hand to your arm or elbow.

Go a half step ahead and slightly to the side of the blind person. The shoulder of the person should be directly behind your shoulder. If the person is frail, place his or her hand on your forearm. With this modified grasp, the person will be positioned laterally to your body. Relax and walk at a comfortable pace. Tell the person when approaching doorways, uneven surfaces, or a narrow space.

Cane Sweep

White canes, or "long canes," are used by about 109,000 persons in the United States. The person sweeps the space in front of him/her with the cane just prior to forward movement and in doing so both alerts others of his/her presence and alerts the blind person of obstacles in the space ahead (accessed 7/10/04 from http://www.afb.org).

Sound Signals

In some U.S. cities and most European and Japanese cities, intermittent sound signals alert the person with limited vision when it is safe and unsafe to cross the street—a simple solution, surprisingly not common in the United States.

Guide Dogs

There are 14 guide dog schools in the United States, and about 10,000 persons use guide dogs to assist them in mobility. Trained guide dogs are matched to individuals' needs and personalities, and those elders who have guide dogs have had several during the course of their adult years (accessed 7/10/04 from http://www. guided dogs.com). Each dog becomes a companion, as well as a guide. It is important for the nurse to teach others to avoid petting or otherwise interacting with the dog while it is "working" to allow the dog to maintain focus.

HEARING AND HEARING IMPAIRMENT IN THE AGED

Hearing loss is the third most common chronic condition in older adults, after hypertension and arthritis. It is estimated that 30% of persons over age 65 living in the community have a hearing problem. The prevalence increases with age, and approximately 65% of 85 year olds report some hearing problem. Hearing impairment is under-diagnosed and undertreated in older people. For example, only 25% of people with hearing loss receive hearing aids and less than 10% of internists offer hearing tests to their patients over the age of 65. Assessment of hearing loss and hearing aids have not been covered under Medicare or other health plans, contributing to the problem of unremediated age-related hearing problems (Ham et al, 2002).

Hearing loss contributes to decreased function, increased social isolation, depression, decreased quality of life, falls, and loss of self-esteem (Crews, Campbell, 2004). Older people are often initially unaware of hearing loss because of the gradual manner in which it usually develops. They may believe others are mumbling and may become irritated at individuals around them who they perceive as not speaking up. Impaired hearing increases isolation and suspicion that sometimes progresses to what appears to be paranoia. Because older people with a hearing loss may not understand or respond appropriately to conversation, they may be inappropriately diagnosed with dementia. It is essential that appropriate assessment and testing be done to determine the nature of the loss, how much it interferes with communication, whether it is treatable, and whether a hearing aid will be useful or attainable. Recent advances in hearing aid technology make it possible to find appropriate hearing aids for some who have not found them satisfactory in the past. *Healthy People 2010* identifies several goals in relation to hearing, including reduction of adult hearing loss and increased access to hearing rehabilitation services and adaptive devices.

Forms of Hearing Loss

The two major forms of hearing loss are conductive and sensorineural. Sensorineural hearing loss (presbycusis) is related to aging and is the most common cause of hearing loss in the United States. Sensorineural hearing loss is treated with hearing aids. Conductive hearing loss usually involves abnormalities of the external and middle ear, such as otosclerosis, perforated eardrum, fluid in the middle ear, or cerumen accumulation.

Presbycusis

Presbycusis primarily affects individuals over age 50, but it is not a universal change, and although age related, it may really be more reflective of environmental conditions and lifestyle. The influence of genetics, noise exposure, cardiovascular status, central processing capacity, certain medications, smoking, diet, personality, and stress have all been implicated to varying degrees in the etiology of hearing impairment. Presbycusis is a bilateral and symmetrical sensorineural hearing loss that also affects the ability to understand speech. Men seem to experience more severe presbycusis than women of the same age. Changes in the middle

and inner ear make many elders intolerant of loud noises and incapable of distinguishing among some of the sibilant consonants, such as *z, s, sh, f, p, k, t,* and *g*. People often raise their voice when speaking to a hearing impaired person. When this happens, more consonants drop out of speech, making hearing even more difficult. Without consonants, the high-frequency–pitched language becomes disjointed and misunderstood. Consider the simple sentence "How are you today?" To the individual with presbycusis it might sound like "hOw arE yOU tOdAy?"

Older persons with presbycusis have difficulty filtering out background noise and often complain of difficulty understanding women and children, as well as conversations in large groups or when there is background noise. The condition progressively worsens with age. The environment is teeming with distracting sounds and noise, such as traffic, television, appliances, crowds, and noisy restaurants and shopping malls. Institutions in which elders may be patients are also noisy with many distracting sounds that make communication difficult for sensory and cognitively impaired elders: intercoms, clattering equipment, meal and medication carts, intercoms or pagers, and "canned music." Use of rapid speech when conversing with an elder with a hearing impairment will make sounds garbled and unintelligible, and even through the problem is related to presbycusis, it is one that can be easily remedied. The common but treatable problem of cerumen in the ear canal, particularly seen with hearing aid use, intensifies hearing difficulties for the person with presbycusis.

Cerumen Impaction

Cerumen impaction is the most common and easily corrected of all interferences in the hearing of the aged. Cerumen interferes with the conduction of sound through air in the ear drum. The reduction in the number of cerumen-producing glands and activity of the glands results in a tendency toward cerumen impaction in the aged. Long-standing impactions become hard, dry, and dark brown. Many elderly persons admit to using foreign objects to clean their ears. Some have perforated the tympanic membrane in the process, resulting in severe hearing loss in the injured ear. Individuals at particular risk of impaction are African Americans and older men with large

Box 9-4   Protocol for Cerumen Removal

- Assess for ear pain, traumas, abnormalities, drainage, surgeries, or perforations. These or any other unusual findings should be referred to an otolaryngologist.
- When aural examination reveals cerumen impaction with no other abnormalities, the nurse may irrigate for cerumen removal using the following techniques:
  1. Carefully clip and remove hairs in ear canal.
  2. Instill a softening agent, such as slightly warm mineral oil, 0.5 to 1 ml twice daily or ear drops such as Cerumenex, Debrox, or Murine ear drops for several days until wax becomes softened. Allergic reactions to Cerumenex have been noted if used for longer than 24 hours.
  3. Protect clothing and linens from drainage of oil or wax by placing small cotton ball in each external ear canal.
  4. When irrigating the ear, use hand-held bulb syringe, 2- to 4-ounce plastic syringe, or otological syringe (20- to 50-ml syringe equipped with an angiocath or Jelso catheter rather than a needle) with emesis basin under ear to catch drainage; tip head to side being drained.
  5. Use solution of 3 ounces 3% hydrogen peroxide in quart of water warmed to 98° to 100° F; if client is sensitive to hydrogen peroxide, use sterile normal saline.
  6. Place towels around neck; empty emesis basin frequently, observing for residue from ear; keep client dry and comfortable; do not inject air into client's ear or use high pressure when injecting fluid.
  7. If the cerumen is not successfully washed out, begin the process again of instilling a softening agent for several days.

Modified from Meador JA: Cerumen impaction in the elderly, *J Gerontol Nurs* 21(12):43-45, 1995.

amounts of ear canal hair that tends to become entangled with the cerumen, which prevents dislodgment.

Others who may develop excessive cerumen are those who habitually wear hearing aids, those with benign growths that narrow the external ear canal, and those who have a predilection to cerumen accumulation. This can be removed and must be before accurate audiometry can be done. Irrigation is contraindicated if the tympanic membrane has been perforated, because it may induce an infection. Cautions are also necessary for those with especially sticky cerumen, which can damage the mechanism of a hearing aid and involve costly repairs. The factory cost for placing a wax guard is approximately $100; however, adhesive covers and wire baskets are available for less than $10. A protocol for cerumen removal is described in Box 9-4.

Prelingual Deafness

Prelingual deafness in older adults is rarely addressed because it is assumed that individuals deaf since childhood have learned to communicate early in life through the use of sign language. Until 50 years ago, it was common for deaf children to be placed in a state school for the deaf to develop within a culture of their own; therefore many elders with prelingual deafness will have had an entirely different childhood than those with hearing. The prelingual deaf often learn audible speech and/or sign language and lip reading very well. However, their reading and writing skills may be impaired even though their intelligence is normal. Communication can also be compromised for those dependent on visual cues when vision changes occur. For these individuals, signing is their first language and English their second. Subtleties of verbal communication may be lost to them, although they often compensate and become extremely alert to nonverbal cues and feelings. At times a certified interpreter, well enmeshed in the world of the deaf, will be needed.

Tinnitus

Tinnitus (ringing, buzzing, hissing, whistling, or swishing sounds arising in the ear) is a condition that affects many older persons. In addition to being very irritating, it can interfere with hearing. It is estimated that nearly 50 million adults in the

United States are affected, 12 million severely enough to seek medical help (accessed 7/9/04 from http:www.ata.org). The incidence of tinnitus peaks between ages 65 and 74 and then seems to decrease in men.

Tinnitus can be caused by loud noises, excessive cerumen or auditory canal obstruction, disorders of the cervical vertebrae or the temporomandibular joint, allergies, an underactive thyroid, cardiovascular disease, tumors, conductive hearing loss, anxiety, depression, degeneration of bones in the middle ear, infections, or trauma to the head or ear. In addition, more than 200 prescription and nonprescription drugs list tinnitus as a potential side effect, aspirin being the most common (accessed 7/10/04 from http://www.ata.org). Tinnitus has a significant impact on daily life even in those with normal or very mildly impaired hearing. It is exacerbated by noise and increases in severity over time in many elders.

Tinnitus may be described as pulsatile (matching the beating of the heart) or nonpulsatile, and as unilateral, asymmetrical, or symmetrical. Tinnitus may be subjective (audible only to the person) or objective (audible to the examiner). The mechanisms of tinnitus are unknown but have been thought to be like cross talk on telephone wires, phantom limb pain, or transmission of vascular sounds, such as bruits, and are sometimes hallucinatory.

A Tinnitus Handicap Questionnaire developed by Newman et al (1995) measures physical, emotional, and social consequences of tinnitus. It also can be used to assess the changes the individual experiences with treatment. Some persons with tinnitus never find the cause; for others the problem may arbitrarily disappear. Therapeutic modes of treating tinnitus include transtympanal electrostimulation, iontophoresis, biofeedback, tinnitus masking with alternative sound production, dental treatment, cochlear implants, and hearing aids. Interestingly, the benefits of a hearing aid prove helpful to some, but for others hearing aids increase the problem. Some have found hypnosis, acupuncture, chiropractic, naturopathic, allergy, and drug treatment effective. See Chapter 7 for additional discussion of tinnitus.

Nursing actions include discussions with the client regarding times when the noises are most irritating; having the person keep a diary may identify patterns. There is some evidence that caffeine, alcohol, cigarettes, stress, and fatigue may exacerbate the problem. Assess medications for possible contribution to the problem. Discuss lifestyle changes and alternative methods that some have found effective. Also, refer clients to the American Tinnitus Association for research updates, education, and support groups. See Resources at end of chapter.

Assessment of Those with Impaired Hearing

Assessment of a hearing disability may be done in a superficial manner by almost any observant health care professional. However, the responsibility for the initial identification of hearing problems usually falls on the nurses, and therefore rapid, reliable, effective screening methods must be available to them. Screening should include the use of the Hearing Handicap Inventory for the Elderly–Screening (HHIE-S), visual inspection of the ear, pure-tone screening, and the client's history. The Hartford Institute for Geriatric Nursing's *Try This* Series provides guidelines for hearing screening (http://www.hartfordign.org), and the HHIE-S is available from http://www.msu.edu/~asc/hhi/. Because many elders are very sensitive about admitting losses, they may be reluctant to share such information. It can best be obtained by first establishing rapport with the elderly person and then proceeding to open interviewing with a comment such as "Many people have difficulty hearing in certain situations. Have you experienced any difficulty? Describe these situations for me." If friends and relatives have insisted that the older person needs a hearing evaluation, he or she may be doubly resistant. A self-administered screening for hearing impairment is presented in Box 9-5.

Otoscopical examination allows visualization of the ear canal and tympanic membrane for possible discovery of cerumen impaction or a perforated eardrum. Weber's test, placement of a vibrating tuning fork on the forehead of the individual, will determine the presence of unilateral conductive hearing loss. This is a screening test and does not measure bilateral hearing loss. The Rinne test screens for difficulty in air and bone conduction. The audioscope (similar to the ear

Box 9-5	Do I Have A Hearing Problem?

Do I have a problem hearing on the telephone?

Do I have trouble hearing when there is noise in the background?

Is it hard to me to follow a conversation when two or more people talk at once?

Do I have to strain to understand a conversation?

Do many people I talk to seem to mumble (or not speak clearly)?

Do I misunderstand what others are saying and respond inappropriately?

Do I have trouble understanding the speech of women and children?

Do people complain that I turn the TV volume up too high?

Do I hear a ringing, roaring, or hissing sound a lot?

Do some sounds seem too loud?

Source: National Institute on Deafness and Other Communication Disorders. Retrieved 7/10/04 from http://www.nidcd.gov/health/hearing/older.asp.

thermometer) is used to determine the frequency range of hearing. Human speech is usually heard below the 2000- to 3000-Hz range. Those who have used the audioscope find it a highly valid screening instrument. It is a simple, fast, and accurate method of screening for hearing loss. Audiometry is still needed for more precise information. Details for these techniques can be found in nursing health assessment textbooks.

Every older adult should have a complete and thorough audiometric examination if there is any doubt about adequate hearing capacity. Early detection of hearing loss often depends on a nurse's observational assessment. Box 9-6 provides assessment and interventions that can help the nurse make a significant difference in an elder's ability to hear. Before concluding that any of these signs are evidence of a cognitive impairment, consider the possibility of a hearing problem. When there is any doubt, referral should be made to an otologist or otolaryngologist to identify possible medical conditions and then to an audiologist or a speech-hearing clinic for an audiological

evaluation before contacting a hearing aid representative.

Nurses are reminded that the best judgment of adequate hearing capacity will come from the older individual's own evaluation. Older persons are often unaware of mild to moderate hearing loss because of the gradual manner in which it usually develops. Wearing hearing aids is problematic in the minds of many, whether because of cost or inconvenience, and unless hearing loss significantly impairs one's quality of life, it may be ignored.

Interventions for Those with Impaired Hearing

Physical examination, interview, self-assessment, relative or friend assessment, and audiometric findings are all necessary to arrive at a meaningful recommendation for the hearing-impaired older person. Counseling includes specific information regarding the problem, encouragement that sensorineural loss can often be partially counteracted by a hearing aid, assistance in the adjustment phase of wearing a hearing aid, and working with family members to improve their communication techniques.

Hearing Aids

A hearing aid is a personal amplifying system that includes a microphone, an amplifier, and a loudspeaker. The appearance and effectiveness of hearing aids have greatly improved in recent years. Hearing aid miniaturization may present difficulties for the aged with visual deficits, loss of finger sensation, or arthritic hands. A recent advance has been the introduction of a remote control device that contains an on/off switch and volume device. There are approximately 50 different manufacturers of hearing aids, and thus the informed consumer has a broad selection from which to choose. A hearing aid generally improves hearing by about 50%, and it is important that hearing impaired elders understand that the goal is to improve communication and quality of life, not to restore normal hearing (Karev, Bartz, 2001).

Although hearing aids have improved considerably, only 20% of older adults with hearing impairment purchase and consistently wear them (Fozard, Gordon-Salant, 2001). Many factors may

Box 9-6 **Assessment and Interventions for Hearing-Impaired Elders**

Assessment

History

In the past 3 months, have you had discharge from your ears?

In the past 3 months, have you experienced dizziness (not related to sudden changes in position)?

In the past 3 months, have you had pain in your ears?

In the past 3 months, have you noticed a sudden or rapid change in your hearing?

Have you ever experienced tinnitus, vertigo, or sudden or gradual hearing loss?

In which situations do you have difficulty hearing?

In the past, have you experienced ear infections, surgery, treatment, or hearing aid use?

Is there a family history of hearing loss?

What drugs have you used or are you now using (note particularly toxic levels of streptomycin, neomycin, or aspirin)?

Observations by family and/or caregiver

Does the person often seem inattentive to others?

Does the person respond with inappropriate anger or irritation when spoken to?

Does the person believe people are talking about him or her?

Does he or she lack a movement response to sounds in the environment?

Does the person have difficulty following clear directions?

Is he or she withdrawn and alone much of the time?

Does the person frequently ask to have something repeated?

Does he or she tend to turn one ear toward a speaker?

Does the person have a monotonous or unusual voice quality?

Is speech unusually loud or soft?

Interventions

General

Never assume hearing loss is from age until other causes are ruled out (infection, cerumen buildup).

Inappropriate responses, inattentiveness, apathy may be symptoms of a hearing loss.

Face the individual, and stand or sit on the same level.

Gain the individual's attention before beginning to speak.

You may need to sit or stand closer to decrease interpersonal space. Assess the individual's comfort with this, and make sure individuals know you are there before touching them or when coming from behind.

If hearing aid is used, make sure it is on, is clean, and has batteries.

Speakers need to keep hands away from their mouth and project their voice by controlled diaphragmatic breathing.

Avoid conversations in which the speaker's face is in glare or darkness.

Enunciate carefully, and speak in a normal cadence.

Careful articulation and moderate speed of speech are helpful.

Avoid eating, chewing, or smoking while speaking.

Facial and hand expressions used liberally facilitate understanding.

Pause between sentences or phrases to confirm understanding.

Restate with different words when you are not understood.

Some languages and some cultural levels of verbal expressiveness facilitate understanding more than others (romance languages and stoic, stolid individuals are more difficult to understand).

When changing topics, preface the change by stating the topic.

Provide visual cues to locate noise direction, since there appears to be an age-related deficit to picking up directional cues.

In most cases there is a better ear.

Reduce background noise.

If paranoia has developed, the individual may not respond well to touch. A handshake is a benign gesture and will signal acceptance or rejection of your efforts to communicate.

The hospitalized or institutionalized hearing impaired

Note on the intercom button and the patient's chart whether the patient is deaf.

Note the most effective way to communicate with the patient.

Never restrict movement in the arms of deaf patients who use sign language as the primary means of communication.

Use charts, pictures, or models to explain medications and procedures.

Do not shout.

Talk TO a hard of hearing person, not ABOUT him or her.

In group situations, speak one at a time.

Use assistive devices such as pocket talkers (audio-amplified units).

Adequate lighting is essential.

If the patient has a hearing aid, encourage its use and make sure it is fitted properly and in good working order.

Determine a means of readily identifying the hearing impaired.

Obtain a certified sign language interpreter for obtaining consent for any procedure. It is essential that the patient understand possible risks and outcomes.

Be PATIENT.

influence an individual's ability and willingness to wear a hearing aid. If the person has been taught to use an aid gradually and correctly and yet does not do so, the nurse should attempt to discover the reasons: the appearance of having an infirmity, the difficulty manipulating a small object, poor vision, inadequate training and support, lack of energy, uncomfortable fit, forgetfulness, and cost. In this era of highly sophisticated, personalized, and computerized hearing aids, most individuals can obtain some hearing enhancement. Hearing aids have changed dramatically in recent years, both in effectiveness and appearance, but many individuals, having tried one a number of years ago, have decided against using them.

The law requires that audiological testing be preceded by an examination by a physician to rule out ear, nose, and throat (ENT) disorders. Many ENT specialists have an audiologist and audiological testing available in the office. Audiologists may favor certain models, and it is wise for a client to shop around for fit and sound regardless of what the physician and audiologist recommend. The investment in a good hearing aid is considerable, and a good fit is crucial. Hearing aids range in price from about $500 to several thousand dollars a piece.

Numerous hearing aids and assistive devices to improve hearing exist. The behind-the-ear aid looks like a shrimp and fits around behind the ear; it is less commonly used now than the small in-the-ear aid, which fits in the concha of the ear. The analog hearing aids are designed to be worn at all times; other devices are designed to solve specific problems. Some products are designed to overcome the effects of noise and distance. These transform sound waves to a different energy spectrum, such as infrared or electromagnetic waves that are then transmitted from the microphone to the receiver and delivered as a clear signal directly in the person's ear. Digitally programmed hearing aids that have more than 1 million different settings from which to select are becoming available. These are matched to the individual's hearing loss.

In the past 5 years a miniaturized computer with a memory chip has been integrated into a hearing aid that eliminates many major hearing aid problems, such as adjustment levels, background noise, and whistling. These aids automatically electronically separate incoming sound without the need to adjust the volume. While these can offer great benefit, they may be prohibitively expensive for many. Because of the rapidly developing technology, it behooves the hearing-impaired individual to be thoroughly evaluated in an audiological center that is not marketing specific hearing aids. Many hospitals and health centers have such services and may have dozens of models an individual can try until the most suitable one is found.

In most states, the purchase of a hearing aid comes with a 30-day trial during which time the purchase price is fully refundable. For programmable devices, the purchaser must be seen a number of times during the month until an optimal adjustment is found. If problems occur during that time, the person should return to the audiologist for assistance. Recent federal regulations have influenced hearing aid manufacturers toward more careful marketing and fitting procedures. It is important to advise clients that charges for hearing aids or routine hearing loss examinations are not paid for by Medicare or private insurance. Suggestions for using and caring for a hearing aid are given in Box 9-7. Considering the high cost of hearing aids and the consequences of not being able to hear, it is important for nurses, particularly those working in hospitals and long-term care facilities, to be knowledgeable about the care and maintenance of aids.

Assistive Listening and Adaptive Devices

Assistive listening devices (also called personal listening systems) should be considered as an adjunct to hearing aids or in place of hearing aids for people with hearing impairment. These devices are available commercially and can be used to better understand speech in large rooms such as theaters and auditoriums, use the telephone, and listen to television. Text messaging devices for telephones and closed caption television, now required on all televisions with screens 13 inches or larger, are other examples. Alerting devices, such as vibrating alarm clocks that shake the bed or activate a flashing light and sound lamps that respond with lights to sounds such as doorbells, telephones, babies crying, or other noises, are also available. Assistive devices, such as pocket talkers (audio-amplified units), are helpful in health care situations where accurate communication and privacy are essential. Some very innovative people have developed ideas and products to enrich the

Box 9-7	The Use and Care of Hearing Aids

Hearing Aid Use

Initially, wear aid 15 to 20 minutes daily.

Gradually increase time until 10 to 12 hours.

Hearing aid will initially make client uneasy.

Insert aid with canal portion pointing into ear; press and twist until snug.

Turn aid slowly to one-third or one-half volume.

A whistling sound indicates incorrect ear mold insertion.

Adjust volume to a level comfortable for talking at a distance of 1 yard.

Do not wear aid under heat lamps or hair dryer or in very wet, cold weather.

Do not wear aid while bathing or perspiring heavily.

Concentrate on conversation; request repeat if necessary.

Sit close to speaker in noisy situations.

Continue to be observant of nonverbal cues.

Be patient with self, and realize the process of adaptation is difficult but ultimately will be rewarding.

Care of the Hearing Aid

Insert battery when hearing aid is turned off.

Store hearing aid in a marked container in a safe place when not in use. Remove batteries.

Remove or disconnect battery when not in use.

Batteries last 1 week with daily wearing of 10 to 12 hours.

Clean cerumen from tip weekly with pipe cleaner.

Common problems include switch turned off, clogged ear mold, dislodged battery, twisted tubing between ear mold and aid.

Ear molds need replacement every 2 or 3 years.

Check ear molds for rough spots that will irritate ear.

Avoid exposing aid to excessive heat or cold.

Clean batteries occasionally to remove corrosion; use a sharpened pencil eraser and gently scrape.

---

lives of the hearing impaired. Music especially for the profoundly hearing impaired that is focused only in the low-frequency cycles (which are most easily heard) has been recorded. Assistive listening and adaptive devices can be purchased from hearing aid dealers, telephone companies, electronic and appliance shops, or catalogs. In some states, there is a monthly surcharge on all users' phone bills, which pays for free phones with adjustable volume controls for all persons with documented hearing losses. Resources for hearing assistance are found at the end of the chapter.

A program called Hearing Dogs for the Deaf has gained recognition. Seventeen locations in the United States train hearing dogs. In some locations the Society for the Prevention of Cruelty to Animals (SPCA) trains shelter dogs; some dogs are especially bred and raised to be hearing dogs; and in some locations the individual's own dog is trained appropriately. Hearing dogs serve to warn the hearing impaired of impending danger, audible signals, phones ringing, fire and smoke alarms, emergencies, and intruders. Although there are other, electronic means of dealing with many of these problems, the hearing impaired consistently comment on the alleviation of the sense of isolation that so often accompanies hearing impairment. With a hearing dog companion, elders may experience renewed courage, confidence, and freedom.

Any facility that receives financial aid from Medicare is required by the Americans with Disabilities Act to provide equal access to public accommodations. Such facilities are required to have sign language interpreters, telecommunication devices (TDDs), flashing alarm systems, and telecaptioning devices on televisions for the deaf. Unfortunately, these are seldom seen.

Cochlear Implants

Cochlear implants are increasingly used for older adults who are profoundly deaf as a result of sensorineural hearing loss. Considerable refinement has been achieved, and implants have shown the most success for those elders who have not been deaf for long and have a strong desire to hear. Unlike hearing aids that amplify sound, the cochlear implant converts sound waves into electrical impulses and transmits them to the inner ear. A cochlear implant is surgically implanted in the mastoid bone behind the ear and electrically stimulates the primary hearing organ, the cochlea, setting the cilia in motion and transmitting impulses along the auditory nerve to the brain's hearing center. For people whose hearing loss is so severe that amplification is of little or no benefit, the cochlear implant is a safe and effective method of auditory rehabilitation. Most insurance plans cover the cochlear implant procedure (Ham et al, 2002). The implant carries some risk because the surgery destroys any residual hearing that remains. Therefore cochlear implant users can never revert back to using a hearing aid. Individuals with cochlear implants need to be advised not to undergo magnetic resonance imaging (MRI) because the implanted devices are not compatible with MRI (Miller, 2004).

Implications for Gerontological Nursing and Healthy Aging

When vision and hearing are diminished, the elder has lost major sensory input, which has a direct effect on his or her everyday life. Decreases in these senses can potentiate isolation, depression, withdrawal, and loss of self-esteem; raise personal safety issues; and affect health. Inadequate communication with deaf or hearing impaired patients can also lead to misdiagnosis and medication errors. In interviews with hearing impaired patients about their communication concerns during medical visits and procedures, interviewees described not understanding therapeutic regimens, not understanding medication doses and side effects, and not knowing what to expect during physical examinations and procedures. Some suggestions to improve communication included using lights as signals for required actions such as holding one's breath during a mammogram and finding alternatives to lengthy phone message menus, such as e-mail or fax. Health care staff should be able to use telecommunication devices and receive training in communication with the hearing impaired (Iezzoni et al, 2004).

To promote healthy aging and quality of life, gerontological nurses in all settings must be knowledgeable about the impact of hearing and vision changes on the functional abilities and quality of life of older adults, vision and hearing assessment, prevention and treatment of diseases affecting vision and hearing, effective communication techniques, and ways to assist the individual in adapting to and compensating for these losses.

Age-related vision and hearing sensory changes, along with outcomes and health prevention, promotion, and maintenance, appear in Appendix 9-A.

APPLICATION OF MASLOW'S HIERARCHY

Hearing and vision impairments can contribute to challenges at all levels of the hierarchy from meeting biological integrity needs, such as activity, and safety and security needs to the higher-level needs, such as a sense of belonging, feeling of self-esteem, and self-actualization. The consequences of these impairments severely affect quality of life and predispose the individual to isolation, depression, falls, lack of adequate health care, fear, discomfort, and embarrassment. Despite age or impairments experienced, continued growth and development toward self-actualization, the task of aging, require interactions and environments in which the older adult is assured that basic needs are met and meaningful interactions and stimulating and satisfying experiences continue to be a part of life.

KEY CONCEPTS

- The nurse is in a key position to initiate the assessment of the person suspected of having a sensory impairment.
- Environmental sensory deprivation or sensory overload may have seriously disorienting consequences for the elderly.
- Environments and environmental changes have major effects on sensory input available to elders.
- Visual impairment is only one third as common as hearing loss; total vision loss is rare and is due to pathological processes rather than aging per se.
- Those with hearing impairment may find it difficult to adjust to hearing aids.
- Elders with visual impairment usually greatly appreciate it when nurses announce their pres-

NANDA and Wellness Diagnoses

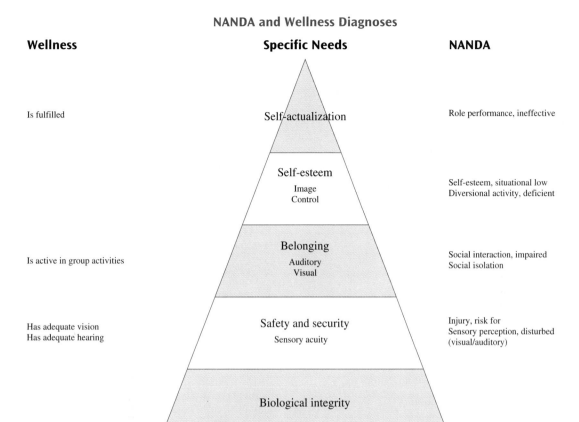

Wellness

Is fulfilled

Is active in group activities

Has adequate vision
Has adequate hearing

Specific Needs

Self-actualization

Self-esteem
Image
Control

Belonging
Auditory
Visual

Safety and security
Sensory acuity

Biological integrity

NANDA

Role performance, ineffective

Self-esteem, situational low
Diversional activity, deficient

Social interaction, impaired
Social isolation

Injury, risk for
Sensory perception, disturbed
(visual/auditory)

These are not all of the possible wellness or NANDA diagnoses that may be identified. The above are frequent examples of nursing diagnoses that should be considered when planning care for the older adult in whatever setting.

ence and provide vivid, detailed descriptions of the surroundings.

- Nurses need to be knowledgeable about the effect of hearing and vision impairments on health, functional ability, and quality of life so that appropriate communication, environmental adaptations, screening, and health promotion and prevention strategies are implemented.
- Presbycusis or age-related hearing loss results in a decreased ability to understand speech.
- To optimize communication with a person with a hearing impairment, the nurse can reduce unnecessary environmental noise.

Activities and Discussion Questions

1. Which of the various sensory/perceptual changes would you find the most difficult to cope with? Why?
2. Try a simulation exercise in which students wear glasses smeared with petroleum jelly (Vaseline) or wear ear plugs as they attempt to take notes, listen, converse with each other, or participate in other daily activities.
3. What measures would you suggest to a person with changes in his or her visual perception?
4. Discuss the stigma of hearing loss and hearing aids.

5. Discuss why individuals do not wear their hearing aids. What suggestions would be helpful in adapting to the wearing of a hearing aid?
6. Use wellness and North American Nursing Diagnosis Association (NANDA) diagnoses to develop a nursing care plan or plans for an aged individual with sensory changes.

RESOURCES

Visual Impairment

American Foundation for the Blind
11 Penn Plaza, Suite 300
New York, NY 10001
(800) 232-5463
e-mail: afbinfo@afb.net
website: http://www.afb.org

The Glaucoma Foundation
116 John Street, Suite 1605
New York, NY 10038
(212) 651-1888
e-mail: info@glaucomafoundation.org
website: http://www.glaucomafoundation.org

Glaucoma Research Foundation
490 Post Street, Suite 1427
San Francisco, CA 94102
(800) 826-6693
e-mail: info@glaucoma.org
website: http://www.glaucoma.org

Health information for older adults in large print
    and "talking" function that reads text aloud
www.NIHSenior.gov

Lions Clubs International
300 West 22nd Street
Oakbrook, IL 60523-8842
(630) 571-5466
website: http://www.lionsclubs.org

National Association for Visually Handicapped
22 West 21st Street
New York, NY 10010
(212) 889-3141
website: http://www.navh.org

National Eye Institute
31 Center Drive, MSC 2510, Building 31, Room
    6A32
Bethesda, MD 20892-2510
(301) 496-5248
website: http://www.nei.nih.gov

See for Yourself: Vision and Older Adults Program
website: http://www.nei.nih.gov/nehep/
    seeforyourself.asp

Vision Simulator (to experience visual impairments)
website: http://visionsimulator.com

Hearing Impairment

American Tinnitus Association
PO Box 5
Portland, OR 97207-0005
(800) 634-8978
website: http://www.ata.org

International Hearing Dog, Inc.
5901 E. 89th Avenue
Henderson, CO 80640
(303) 287-3277
website: http:/www.ihdi.org

National Institute on Deafness and Other
    Communication Disorders
National Institutes of Health
31 Center Drive, MSC 2320
Bethesda, MD 20892-2320
e-mail: nidcdinfo@nidcd.nih.gov
website: http://www.nidcd.nih.gov

Self-Help for Hard of Hearing People
7910 Woodmont Avenue, Suite 1200
Bethesda, MD 20814
(301) 657-2248 voice; (301) 657-2249 TTY
website: http://www.shhh.org

Assistive and Adaptive Equipment

Independent Living Aids, Inc.
PO Box 9022
Hicksville NY 11802-9022
(800) 537-2118
e-mail: can-do@independentliving.com
website: http://www.independentliving.com

REFERENCES

American Foundation for the Blind. www.afb.org

Bressler NM, Bressler SB, Congdon NG et al: Age-related macular degeneration is the leading cause of blindness, *JAMA* 291(15):1900-1901, 2004.

Bressler NM et al: Potential public health impact of Age-Related Eye Disease Study results: AREDS report no. 11, *Arch Ophthalmol* 121(11):1621-1624, 2003.

Crews JE, Campbell VA: Vision impairment and hearing loss among community-dwelling older Americans: implications for health and functioning, *Am J Public Health* 94(5):823-829, 2004.

Fozard J, Gordon-Salant S: In Birren JE, Schaie KW, editors: *The psychology of aging*, San Diego, 2001, Academic Press.

Goldzweig CL, Rowe S, Wenger NS et al: Preventing and managing visual disability in primary care: clinical applications, *JAMA* 291(12):1497-1502, 2004.

Ham R, Sloane P, Warshaw G: *Primary care geriatrics*, ed 4, St Louis, 2002, Mosby.

Healthy People 2010: understanding and improving health, Washington, DC, 2001, U.S. Department of Health and Human Services.

Higginbotham EJ, Gordon MO, Beisner JA et al: The Ocular Hypertension Treatment Study: topical medication delays or prevents primary open-angle glaucoma in African American individuals, *Arch Ophthalmol* 122(6):813-820, 2004.

Iezzoni LI, O'Day BL, Killeen M et al: Communicating about health care: observations from persons who are deaf or hard of hearing, *Ann Intern Med* 140(5):356-362, 2004.

Karev M, Bartz S: Hearing aids. In Mezey MD, editor: *The encyclopedia of elder care*, New York, 2001, Springer.

Kupfer C: Measuring quality of life in low vision patients, *Aging Vision News* 7(2):5, 1995a.

Kupfer C: Ophthalmologic disorders. In Abrams WB, Beers MH, Berkow R, editors: *The Merck manual of geriatrics*, ed 2, Whitehouse Station, NJ, 1995b, Merck Research Laboratories.

Maclay E: *Green winter: celebrations of old age*, New York, 1977.

McGwin G Jr, McNeal S, Owsley C et al: Statins and other cholesterol-lowering medications and the presence of glaucoma, *Arch Ophthalmol* 122(6):822-826, 2004.

Miller C: *Nursing for wellness in older adults*, ed 4, Philadelphia, 2004, Lippincott Williams & Wilkins.

Newman CW, Wharton JA, Jacobsen GP: Retest stability of the tinnitus handicap questionnaire, *Ann Otol Rhinol Largyngol* 104(9, pt 1):718-723, 1995.

Ralston ME, Choplin NT, Hollenbach KA et al: Glaucoma screening in primary care: the role of noncontact tonometry, *J Fam Pract* 34(1):73-77, 1992.

Rowe S, MacLean CH, Shekelle PG: Preventing visual loss from chronic eye disease in primary care: scientific review, *JAMA* 291(12):1487-1495, 2004.

Sackett K, Bressler S: Age-related eye disease study results. 2001. Accessed 7/5/04 from www.nei.nih.gov.

Sacks O: *Seeing voices: a journey into the world of the deaf*, Berkeley, 1989, University of California Press.

Stuen C: Vision care and rehabilitation, *Focus Geriar Care Rehabil* 10(1):157, 1996.

Appendix 9-A

Age-Related Vision and Hearing Changes; Outcomes; and Prevention, Health Promotion, and Maintenance Approaches

Age-Related Changes	Outcomes	Health Prevention, Promotion, and Maintenance
VISION		
Lid elasticity diminishes	Pouches under the eyes	
Loss of orbital fat		
Decreased tears	Excessive dryness of eyes	Use isotonic eye drops as needed
Arcus senilis become visible		
Sclera yellows and becomes less elastic		
Yellowing and increased opacity of cornea	Lack of corneal luster	
Increased sclerosis and rigidity of iris		
Decrease in convergence ability	Presbyopia	Have eyes examined at least once per year
Decline in light accommodation response	Lessened acuity	Use magnifying glass and high-intensity light to read
Diminished pupillary size	Decline in depth perception	Increase light to prevent falls
Atrophy of ciliary muscle	Diminished recovery from glare	Clip-on sunglasses, visors, sun hat, nonglare coating on prescription glasses/sunglasses
Night vision diminishes	Night blindness	Do not drive at night
		Keep night-light in bathroom and hallway
		Paint first and last step of staircase and edge of each step in-between with a bright color or a reflective color
Yellowing of lens	Diminished color perception (blues, greens)	
Lens opacity	Cataracts	Surgical removal of lens (lens implants)
Increased intraocular pressure	Rainbows around lights	Have a yearly eye examination, including tonometer testing
	Altered peripheral vision	

Shrinkage of gelatinous substance in the vitreous
Vitreous floaters appear
Ability to gaze upward decreases
Thinning and sclerosis of retinal blood vessels
Atrophy of photoreceptor cells
Degeneration of neurons in visual cortex

HEARING

Thinner, drier skin of external ear	Impaired hearing	Check ears for wax or infection
Longer and thicker hair in external ear canal (of men)	Difficulty hearing high-frequency sounds (presbycusis)	Formal hearing test
Narrowing of auditory opening		
Increased cerumen		
Thickened and less resilient tympanic membrane		
Decreased flexibility of basilar membrane	Gradual loss of sound	Consultation for proper hearing and speaking tone
Ossicular calcification	Reduced speech discrimination	
Diminished neuron, endolymph, hair cells, and blood supply to inner ear and auditory nerve		
Degeneration of spiral ganglion and arterial blood vessels		

10

Nutrition and Aging

Upon completion of this chapter, the reader will be able to:

- Discuss nutritional requirements for older adults.
- Identify factors affecting the nutrition of older adults.
- Discuss interventions that can aid or provide better nutrition for older adults.
- Discuss involuntary weight loss and malnutrition in older adults, identifying appropriate assessment and interventions to prevent and treat these conditions.
- Identify strategies to assist in ensuring adequate nutrition for older adults experiencing hospitalization, institutionalization, and physical and cognitive impairments.
- Discuss interventions that promote healthy bowel function for older people.

Chemosenses The senses of taste and smell.
Dysphagia Sensation of impaired passage of food from the mouth to the esophagus and stomach; difficulty swallowing.
Gastroesophageal reflux disease (GERD) Backward flow of stomach contents into the esophagus.

Presbyesophagus Age-related change in the esophagus affecting motility.
Soul food Food possessing emotional significance and providing personal satisfaction; often has some cultural or traditional origins.
Xerostomia Dry mouth.

"The end of my soul's dominion will surely arrive on the day that I find myself lined up in a hallway in a row of wheelchairs waiting to be loaded into an elevator, then transported to a dining room and positioned into a row of waiting mouths. I may overhear one staff member say to another, 'I've got to cut this one's meat, then I'll feed that one.' At this juncture, I will have become an object rather than a subject. I will have become that one who must be acted upon, rather than as a person engaged in her own life. I will have become someone's task. I will have become my needs.

If I do reach the point when I can no longer feed myself, I hope that the hands holding my fork belong to someone who has a feeling for who I am. I hope my helper will remember what she learns about me and that her awareness of me will grow from one encounter to another. Why should this make a difference? Yet, I am certain that my experience of needing to be fed will be altered if it occurs in the context of my being known."
From Lustbader W: Thoughts on the meaning of frailty, Generations 13(4):21-22, 1999.

*W*ell-being is influenced by the triad of aging, nutrition, and health. Proper nutrition means that all of the essential nutrients (carbohydrates, fat, protein, vitamins, minerals, water) are adequately supplied and used to maintain optimal health and well-being. Proper nutrition provides the energy and building blocks necessary to maintain body structure and function. The variances in nutritional requirements throughout the life span are not well established for older adults, and this should continue to be an area of emphasis in gerontological research (Wakimoto, Block, 2001). *Healthy People 2010* has several goals related to nutrition in older adults, including counseling and education related to diet and nutrition, dental care, healthy weight, blood cholesterol levels, and food security (presence of adequate food) (accessed 7/18/04 from http://www.healthypeople.gov).

Although some age-related changes in the gastrointestinal system do occur, these changes are rarely the primary factors in inadequate nutrition. Fulfillment of an older person's nutritional needs is more often affected by numerous other factors, including lifelong eating habits, socialization, income, transportation, housing, food knowledge, health, and dentition. Older adults face complex issues affecting their nutritional status. Changes in living situations, such as a move to a senior housing site, loss of a spouse, functional impairments, inadequate income, and changes in health are some of the many issues that may have a negative effect on nutrition.

Adequate nutrition is critical to preserving the health of older people and an integral part of health, happiness, independence, quality of life, and physical and mental functioning; yet nutritional deficiencies and malnutrition occur frequently in older adults and are an area of major concern. National attention and health policy discussions have focused on the issue of malnutrition in older adults, and the research of gerontological nurses, such as Jeannie Kayser-Jones, has contributed to our understanding of the significance of this problem, particularly among those residing in nursing homes.

This chapter discusses dietary needs of older adults, age-related changes affecting nutrition, risk factors contributing to inadequate nutrition, bowel function in aging, the effect of diseases and functional impairments on nutrition, malnu-

trition, and special considerations for older adults with cognitive and physical disabilities.

DIETARY NEEDS OF OLDER ADULTS

Although older adults require the same nutrients as younger people, some changes occur as a result of the aging process. These changes relate particularly to calorie, protein, fat, fiber, dietary supplements, and water intake.

Caloric and Protein Needs

Energy requirements and energy intake gradually decrease from middle to advanced age as a result of lower basal metabolic rate and decreased physical activity. Lowered basal metabolic rate is associated with the decrease in metabolically active skeletal muscle mass, declining from 45% of body weight in young adults to about 27% by age 70 (Ham et al, 2002). Older adults need approximately 1600 calories per day, but that number may vary depending on physical activity, current weight, and concomitant illnesses. Although caloric needs decrease, it is important to ensure that the quality of calories, or the nutritional density, of foods consumed remains high, while intake of foods containing little or no nutrients is decreased. With estimates that up to 20% of community-dwelling ambulatory older adults are malnourished, decreased caloric intake without attention to the quality of calories consumed is a significant concern. In the old-old (over age 85), there is a tendency to lose weight and adipose tissue mass, placing the individual at significant risk of developing malnutrition when illnesses occur (Morley, 2002). The incidence of malnutrition in hospitalized elders and those in nursing homes is extremely high and the subject of national attention. Special considerations for frail elders will be discussed later in the chapter.

Adequate protein intake and protein reserves remain important, with recommendations of a minimum daily protein intake of 1 g/kg of body weight with 10% to 20% of daily calories obtained from protein. Protein-rich foods, such as fish, meats, and dried beans and peas, are important to include in a daily diet. Adequate protein intake helps prevent muscle loss, and adequate protein intake, in concert with calcium and vitamin D supplementation, may be protective for bone health (Dawson-Hughes, Harris, 2002). Protein needs increase with acute illnesses, surgical procedures, and the presence of pressure ulcers or other wounds.

Fats

Intake of fat should be 20% to 25% of daily caloric intake with fat calories coming from foods low in saturated fat. Lowering intake of fat in the diet is an important lifestyle change associated with controlling cholesterol. A direct relationship exists between lower low-density lipoprotein (LDL) cholesterol levels and reduced risk for major coronary events. The 2004 practice guidelines on cholesterol management recommend even more intensive treatment of hyperlipidemia, including lower treatment goals for LDL and the initiation of cholesterol-lowering therapy at lower LDL levels than in the past (Grundy et al, 2004). A copy of the guidelines can be obtained at http://www.nhibi.nih.gov/guidelines/cholesterol/index.htm.

Fiber

Fiber (roughage) is important for health of the digestive system, decreased coronary artery disease risk, and proper bowel function. Dietary fiber comes from many sources, including whole fruits and vegetables, whole grains, cereals, beans, nuts, and legumes. A total of 20 to 35 g of fiber is recommended each day for optimal health, but the average American diet contains approximately half that amount. Older adults should be counseled to eat high-fiber food (pears, dried beans and peas, corn, dates, 100% bran cereals, potatoes with skins) daily. Commercially available fiber supplements, such as Metamucil, Citrucel, and FiberCon, can be used if dietary intake is inadequate. Adequate fluid intake is essential when taking supplements; recommendations are to drink 8 to 12 oz of water when fiber supplements are taken (Ham et al, 2002).

Dietary Supplements

Older adults may not absorb vitamins and minerals required for healthy aging because of changes in metabolism or restricted food choices related to medical conditions. Half of all older adults have a vitamin and mineral intake less than the recommended dietary allowance, and 10% to 30% of older adults have abnormally low serum levels of vitamins and minerals. Vitamin D and vitamin B_{12} deficiencies are also common in older adults, particularly the more frail and those living in nursing homes (Johnson et al, 2002; Meyyazhagan, Palmer, 2002). Dietary supplements of calcium, vitamin D, and vitamin B_{12} are recommended for older adults in addition to healthy food choices. Total daily calcium intake should be 1500 mg, the equivalent of three servings of calcium-rich foods, such as milk, hard cheese, yogurt, greens, sardines, canned salmon with bones, dried peas and beans, and tofu. Calcium supplements, such as calcium citrate and calcium carbonate, are available to make up dietary deficiencies. Daily vitamin D intake should be 600 to 800 international units. Vitamin D is required for calcium absorption. Sunlight provides vitamin D as well, but many older people have limited exposure. Milk and fortified cereals are sources of vitamin D. Both calcium and vitamin D are essential to bone health and prevention and treatment of osteoporosis.

Vitamin B_{12} can be a problem nutrient for older people related to a decrease in the amount of stomach acid that releases the vitamin from animal proteins. Deficiency may also be caused by atrophic gastritis, *Helicobacter pylori* infection, vegetarian diets, or gastric or ileal surgery. Prolonged use of antacids or proton-pump inhibitors may also decrease absorption and increase deficiencies of vitamin B_{12} (van Asselt et al, 1998; Ham et al, 2002). Fortified breakfast cereals can help because they contain vitamin B_{12} in a form that the body can absorb. A total of 2.4 mcg is recommended each day. Taking a multivitamin for seniors will ensure an adequate intake of both vitamin B_{12} and vitamin D.

Folate intake, as well as vitamins B_{12} and B_6, are related to homocysteine levels. High blood homocysteine (>10 to 15 µmol/L) is associated with a twofold to fortyfold increased risk of coronary artery disease, stroke, and peripheral vascular disease (McDowell, Lang, 2000). Although folate supplementation to prevent or treat vascular disease needs further research, older adults should try to consume 400 to 1000 mcg/day, primarily from fruits and vegetables, in addition to the recommended vitamin B_{12} supplementation (Ham et al, 2002).

Whereas some vitamins, particularly those with antioxidant properties (C, E, and the carotenoids), may have protective effects against certain diseases, such as macular degeneration, further research is needed. Supplementation should remain within accepted guidelines since higher than recommended doses can be dangerous (Meydani et al, 1998; Russell, 2000). Megavitamin therapy (the ingestion of large amounts of a specific vitamin or many different vitamins) is nonessential and dangerous. Risks exist in megavitamin therapy: bone meal, a source of calcium, may contain lead and thus cause lead poisoning; high doses of zinc cause zinc toxicity; and kelp, with its high iodine content, can cause goiter in those with preexisting thyroid enlargement. High intake of niacin is discouraged because of a high incidence of cardiac dysrhythmias and gastrointestinal problems. The money spent on unneeded vitamins by older adults could buy more economical foods that benefit the individual's health. Older people should be advised to consult their health care provider before starting any dietary supplements, and dietary supplements should be included in any review of medications.

Water

Water is needed to regulate body temperature, carry out chemical reactions in the body, remove body waste, and prevent constipation. The proportion of total body water decreases in aging and may be further compromised by poor fluid intake secondary to age-related factors, such as diminished thirst sensation, as well as the practice of limiting fluids to prevent frequent toileting. Whereas approximately 80% of a child's weight is water, the total body water of an older adult is approximately 43.4% for women and 50.8% for men. This predisposes older adults to dehydration, and the condition is commonly associated with malnutrition, particularly in frail older adults (Bennett, 2000). A daily total of 1500 to 2000 ml (six to eight 8-oz glasses of fluid) of noncaffeinated fluids, preferably plain water, is recommended to maintain adequate hydration. Alcohol and caffeine-containing beverages should be limited, with the recommendation that women consume no more than one drink per day and men no more than two. Dehydration is discussed in more detail in Chapter 11.

FOOD GUIDE PYRAMID

The current guide for proper nutrition across the life span is the Food Guide Pyramid. As a result of research on the unique nutritional needs of older adults, a modified food pyramid for older adults has been developed by the U.S. Department of Agriculture's Human Nutrition Research Center on Aging (Figure 10-1). Key differences in the modified food pyramid include the following: the addition of at least eight 8-oz glasses of fluid each day; an emphasis on fiber intake; and a flag at the top of the pyramid indicating a recommendation for the dietary supplements calcium, vitamin D, and vitamin B_{12}. The pyramid is also narrower than the traditional pyramid because older individuals may be less active and require less food to maintain the same weight. The pyramid emphasizes nutrient-dense foods, such as darker-colored vegetables and fruits that have higher levels of vitamins. The minimum number of servings recommended on the modified pyramid, including some fat, will total about 1600 calories, the amount recommended for older adults. The Food and Nutrition Information Center provides information on ethnic and cultural adaptations of food pyramid guides (http://www.nal.usda.gov).

Dietary reference intakes (DRIs) and dietary guidelines (DGs) have been developed for the Older Americans Act (OAA) nutrition programs, Title III and Title VI. The programs provide congregate and home-delivered meals to about 3 million older adults each year (National Policy and Resource Center on Health and Aging, 2002). These programs and all federal programs must comply with DGs and DRIs, which are revised every 5 years. The DRIs include specific modifications for adults aged 51 to 70 and those 70 years and over. DRIs are formulated for healthy older adults and will need adjustment for older people with medical conditions and nutrient deficiencies and for those who are malnourished or very frail.

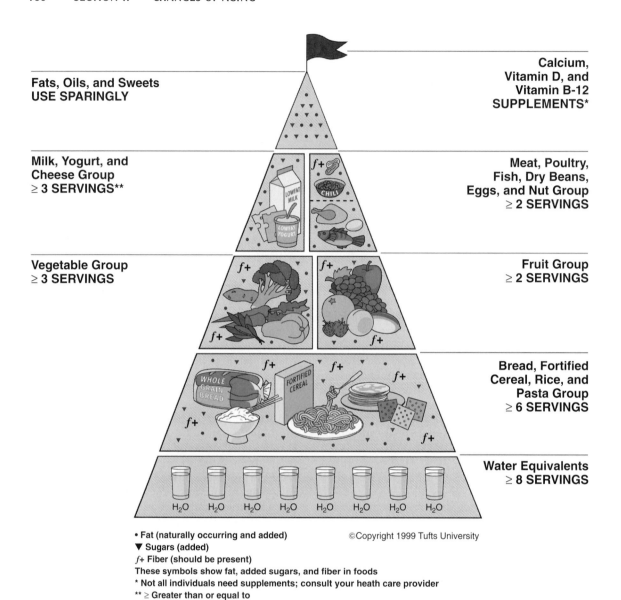

Figure 10-1 Modified Food Guide Pyramid for mature (70+) adults. (Copyright © 1999 Tufts University, Medford, Mass.)

FACTORS AFFECTING FULFILLMENT OF NUTRITIONAL NEEDS

Age-Related Changes Affecting Digestion and Appetite

Some age-related changes in the senses of taste and smell (chemosenses) and the digestive tract do occur as an individual ages and may affect nutrition. For most older people, these changes do not seriously interfere with eating, digestion, and enjoyment of food. However, combined with other factors affecting fulfillment of nutritional needs, they may contribute to inadequate nutrition and decreased eating pleasure.

Taste

The sense of taste has many components and primarily depends on receptor cells in the taste buds. Taste buds are scattered on the surface of the tongue, cheek, soft palate, the upper tip of the esophagus, and other parts of the mouth and throat. Components in food stimulate taste buds during chewing and swallowing, and tongue movements enhance flavor sensation. Fine, subtle taste to discriminate between flavors is an olfactory function, whereas crude taste (e.g., sweet and sour) depends on the taste buds. Individuals have varied levels of taste sensitivity that seem predetermined by genetics and constitution, as well as age variations. A small decline in the number of taste cells occurs with aging, beginning around age 60.

Age-related changes do not affect all taste sensations equally, and with age, the ability to detect sweet taste seems to remain intact whereas the ability to detect sour, salty, and bitter tastes declines. Many denture wearers say they lose some of their satisfaction in food, possibly because dentures cover the palate and because texture is a very important element in food enjoyment. Difficulty in flavor appreciation comes from individual variables, such as smoking, olfactory sensitivity, attitude toward food and eating, and the presence of moistening secretions. There are also aberrations in flavor sensation caused by certain medications and medical conditions. The addition of flavor enhancers (bouillon cubes) and concentrated flavors (jellies or sauces) can amplify both taste and smell. Fresh herbs and spices also give an extra boost to flavor and may increase enjoyment and interest in eating. The bland diets often found in hospitals and institutions contribute to decreased appetite. Refer to Appendix 7-A for age-related changes in taste.

Smell

The sense of smell declines in aging and has a significant influence on food enjoyment, perhaps more significant than declines in taste ability. The ability to detect and identify odors begins to decline at about age 30 and continues into later years. Decrease in the sense of smell may be related to many factors, including the following: nasal sinus disease, repeated injury to olfactory receptors through viral infections, age-related changes in the central nervous system functioning, cigarette smoking, medications, periodontal disease and other dentition problems, and systemic diseases such as dementia and diabetes.

Smell occurs when nerve receptors in the nose send messages to the brain. The interaction of the oral and nasal senses blends together to give us the impression of a certain food or increases the sensory perceptions we receive. Smells also create emotional responses (positive or negative) to food because emotions and smell sensations overlap in the brain. Think how the smell of freshly baked chocolate chip cookies makes you feel compared with the smell of burned popcorn. Many older people, particularly those in institutions, no longer cook and never have the experience of smelling food cooking, an important appetite stimulant. Many long-term care institutions have adapted kitchens and dining rooms so that the residents can smell the food cooking and even participate in the preparation of food as a way of increasing interest and enjoyment in food.

Digestive System

Age-related changes in the oral cavity, esophagus, stomach, liver, pancreas, gallbladder, and small and large intestines may contribute to nutritional status in concert with other factors. However, normal age-related changes do not significantly affect function, and the digestive system remains adequate throughout life. Presbyesophagus, a decrease in the intensity of propulsive waves, may be an age-related change in the esophagus. Some of these changes may be more attributable to pathological conditions rather than to age alone. The functional impact of presbyesophagus seems to be minimal, but combined with other conditions, may contribute to dysphagia. Aging may also be associated with slowed gastric emptying in the stomach and a decrease in the ability of the fundus of the stomach to accommodate large volumes of food. This results in food passing more rapidly from the fundus to the antrum of the stomach, which causes increased antral stretch, a major signal for fullness. This may explain the feeling of early satiation (feeling full with less food) that many older individuals may experience (Morley, 1997). The presence of respiratory and cardiovascular diseases may also contribute to early satiation. Declines in gastric secretions and pepsin, essential for digestion, seem to be minimal and should not contribute to digestive problems. However, conditions such as *Helicobacter pylori* and atrophic gastritis, as well as certain medications, may cause diminished secretions that interfere with the digestive process (Jensen et al, 2001; Miller, 2004).

Structural changes in the small intestine related to aging include atrophy of muscle fibers and mucosal surfaces, reduction in the number of lymphatic follicles, and shortening and widening of the villi. These changes do not significantly affect motility, permeability, or transit time but may have an effect on absorption of some nutrients, such as calcium and vitamin D (Miller, 2004). Changes in the large intestine related to age include reduced secretion of mucus and diminished elasticity and rectal muscle tone. Although not affecting motility or absorption, these changes do contribute to the common problem of constipation discussed later in the chapter.

The liver becomes smaller as one ages, and blood flow decreases to about one third of younger individuals. Although not affecting digestive function, the decreased blood flow can have an impact on drug metabolism. Enzyme production of the pancreas remains intact in aging; however, diminished insulin secretion may be a contributing factor to increased glucose intolerance and adult-onset diabetes mellitus. Morley (2002) suggested that the higher levels of cholecystokinin secreted by the gallbladder may suppress the appetite in older adults. The mechanisms contributing to regulation of appetite are discussed in the following section.

Regulation of Appetite

Appetite is influenced by factors such as physical activity, functional limitations, smell, taste, mood, socialization, and comfort. However, there is also a physiological basis to appetite regulation that differs in older adults compared with younger adults. Although the effect of these changes still needs further research, neurotransmitter regulators of appetite have been implicated in impaired appetite and decreased intake associated with aging. Appetite is regulated by a combination of a peripheral satiation system and a central feeding drive. Gastrointestinal hormones, such as cholecystokinin, also regulate satiety to varying degrees. Cholecystokinin levels increase with age and contribute to decreased appetite, muscle wasting, and inhibition of albumin synthesis. Disease states also increase cytokine as a result of its release by diseased tissues. Increase in cholecystokinin levels also occurs in malnourished individuals, which may further decrease appetite. There is also some suggestion that alterations in the endogenous opioid feeding and drinking drive may decline in aging, further contributing to decreased appetite (Morley, 2003). Several appetite-stimulating (orexigenic) medications are currently available for the treatment of anorexia, undernutrition, and malnutrition in older adults. Further evaluation of the usefulness and side effects of these medications in older people is indicated. Additional discussion of the importance of considering the myriad of factors involved in appetite and nutrition when choosing appropriate interventions is included later in this chapter.

Lifelong Eating Habits

The nutritional state of a person reflects the individual's dietary history and present food practices. Individuals establish their diets and eating patterns for various reasons. Food patterns are described in Box 10-1. Lifelong eating habits are also developed out of tradition, ethnicity, and religion, all of which collectively can be called *culture*. Krebs-Smith et al (1995) found that food habits established since childhood influenced the intake of older adults. Anorexia nervosa can recur in older women who experienced this in younger years and is called anorexia tardive. Weight loss may be more common in older persons who have

Box 10-1   Food Patterns

Physician prescribed/suggested. Treatment for or prevention of disease (e.g., reduction of sodium, fat, sugar, weight).

Change in food use. Factors beyond individual's control (e.g., alteration in taste, isolation, income), all of which are linked to a decrease in food intake.

Self-prescribed diets. Implemented by the individual, not the physician. Similar to prescribed diet, but individual puts self on, for example, high-fiber or low-fat diet because of family history of disease (e.g., heart disease, diabetes mellitus, cancer).*

Overall reduction of food intake. Through a conscientious effort to maintain healthy body weight and decrease health problems.*

Maintenance of lifelong food use. Continuous conscious diet pattern has been incorporated into healthy dietary practices long before old age.*

*Self-determined.

practiced dietary restraint throughout their life. Malnutrition may be seen in older people attempting to lower their cholesterol to prevent heart disease, a condition known as *cholesterol phobia* (Morley, 2003). Strict low-cholesterol or other rigid therapeutic diet regimens are not recommended for frail older adults in long-term care facilities and may contribute to malnutrition and other poor outcomes (Morley, 2003).

Eating habits do not always coincide with fulfillment of nutritional needs. Rigidity of food habits may increase with age as familiar food patterns are sought. Ethnicity determines if traditional foods are preserved, whereas religion affects the choice of foods possible. Throughout life, then, preferences for particular foods bring deep satisfaction and possess emotional significance. Such foods are called *soul food* or *comfort food*. Preferences for soul food influence food choices and affect nutrient intake. Foods prepared or served in a special way provide "soul" and are not unique to any one group but, rather, are found all over the world. Rice with every meal and homemade chicken soup given to the individual when ill are examples of what people consider their soul food.

Culturally and religiously appropriate diets should be available in any institution or congregate dining program.

Lifelong habits of dieting or eating fad foods also echo through the later years. There are a number of suggestions that particular foods or supplements may partially or completely cure various ailments or make one look younger and feel more vital and extend life. Whereas some of these suggestions may be important, older adults should be counseled to base decisions on valid research and consultation with their primary care provider before adjusting the diet. Skipping meals is another practice that one finds with older adults and may be due to decreased energy to prepare food, inadequate income to purchase food, and other factors, such as loneliness. It is difficult to reach an adequate nutritional intake if the total calories are fewer than 1200 per day. Individuals who are on self-imposed diets of 1000 calories or less per day are inviting malnutrition. Table 10-1 offers some suggestions for common problems elders may experience that interfere with the ability to eat well. Additional resources are listed at the end of the chapter.

Socialization

The social essence ascribed to eating is sharing and providing a feeling of belonging. All of us use food as a means of giving and receiving love, friendship, or belonging. Many older people are forced to remain isolated from the mainstream of life because of impinging factors. When one eats alone, the outcome is often either overindulgence or depression (a common problem of aging and a significant inhibitor of appetite) and disinterest in food. Disinterest in food may also result from the effects of medication or disease processes.

Title VII of the Older Americans Act provides funding for strategically located outreach centers or nutrition sites whose purposes are to provide at least one nutritionally sound meal daily and to facilitate congregate dining to foster social contact and relationships. No one age 60 or over (all spouses are also included) can be denied participation in the nutrition program because of his or her economic situation. Those who are able to pay for their meal do so according to their ability. Meals on Wheels, another community program, encourages both the attainment of good nutrition

Table 10-1 Suggestions for Eating Well as We Age

Problem	Suggestions
Cannot chew	Try fruit juices and soft canned fruits, such as applesauce, peaches, and pears.
	Make a smoothie in the blender using yogurt and fresh fruit.
	Use cooked cereals, rice, bread pudding, and soft cookies.
	Use ground meat, eggs, milk, cheese, yogurt, and foods made with milk, such as pudding and cream soups.
Cannot shop	Ask the local food store to bring groceries to your home. Order groceries over the Internet.
	Ask your church or synagogue for volunteer help.
	Ask a family member or neighbor to shop for you or pay someone to shop.
	Find out about Nutrition Sites or Meals on Wheels in your community.
Cannot cook	Use a microwave oven to cook frozen foods and foods made up ahead of time by the store.
	Take part in group meal programs offered through senior citizen programs or Meals on Wheels.
	Find out about a homemaker service in your community.
Limited income	Buy low-cost foods, such as dried beans and peas, rice, and pasta. Or buy foods that contain these items, such as split pea soup and canned beans and rice.
	Use coupons for money off on foods you like.
	Buy foods on sale and buy store-brand foods.
	Find out if your church or synagogue offers free or low-cost meals.
	Get food stamps. Call the food stamp office listed under your county government.
No appetite	Ask your primary care provider if any of your medications can cause loss of appetite, and ask about changing them.
	Eat with family and friends.
	Take part in group meal programs.
	Could you be depressed? Ask your health care provider for an evaluation.
	Increase the flavor of food by adding spices and herbs.

Adapted from U.S. Food and Drug Administration: *Eating well as we age*, Rockville, Md, 2000, U.S. Department of Health and Human Services, Food and Drug Administration.

and human contact for those who are unable to prepare meals or go out to obtain them. Most cities and rural areas throughout the United States have such programs. Other congregate or group feeding programs exist through church and other community auspices, such as food cooperatives, home grocery delivery services, and chore services for shopping and meal preparation.

Income

There is a strong relationship between poor nutrition and low income (Wakefield, 2000). More older adults live in poverty than younger adults according to the 2000 census (U.S. Bureau of the Census, 2001). Older adults with low incomes need to choose among needs such as food, heat, telephone bills, medications, and health care visits. Some older people eat only once per day in an attempt to make their income last through the month. Medicare began covering nutrition therapy for select diseases, such as diabetes or kidney disease, which creates improved opportunities for older Americans to access information (Pear, 2001).

Older people accustomed to eating meat, fish, and poultry as their main sources of protein have watched the cost climb to heights beyond their purchasing power. Inexpensive alternative protein sources such as tofu (soybean curd) are foreign to the diets of the aged in Western society today but have slowly been making their way into acceptance. At present the development of a taste for alternative protein sources and an understanding of what foods to mix to obtain complete dietary protein require some knowledge and practice to ensure adequate protein intake and to prevent monotony. If at all possible, older adults should be encouraged to use vegetable protein sources to meet daily needs. This is a more economical form of protein that may help the aged conserve their income for other necessities, unexpected bills, or special treats. Combinations such as milk or cheese with bread or pasta; cereal with milk; rice-and-cheese or rice-and-bean casseroles; wheat soy or corn soy bread; wheat bread with baked beans, beans, or pea curry; tortillas and beans; and legume soup with bread are sources of protein.

The food stamp program has the potential for increasing the purchasing power of older adults who qualify, but such programs are vulnerable to federal budget cutting. Many older people may find that the amount of money required to purchase the food stamps is greater than they think they can afford, or they do not see the benefit to them. Transportation may be limited and the distance too far for an older person to travel to acquire the food stamps, which are sold only at designated locations in cities. In addition, many older people, especially those who lived through the depression, are very reluctant to accept "welfare."

Free food programs, such as donated commodities, are also available at distribution centers (food banks) for those with limited incomes. Although this is another valuable option for older people, use of such programs is not always entirely feasible. One takes a chance on the types of food available any particular day or week; quantities distributed are frequently too large for the single older person or the older couple to use or even carry from the distribution site; and the site may be too far away or difficult to reach. The time of distribution of the food may be inconvenient, too. Some cafeterias and restaurants that provide special meal prices for the aged have had to increase their prices as food costs have risen; thus the previous advantages of eating out have diminished, yet many single elders rely on cafeterias and restaurants for most meals.

Transportation

Availability of transportation may be limited for older people. Many small, long-standing neighborhood food stores have been closed in the wake of larger supermarkets, which are located in areas that serve a greater segment of the population. It may become difficult to walk to the market, to reach it by public transportation, or to carry a bag of groceries while using a cane. It is nearly impossible to do this with a walker. Fear is apparent in the elderly's consideration of transportation. They fear not being able to cross the street in the time it takes the traffic light to change and being knocked down or falling as they walk in crowded streets. Despite reduced senior citizen bus fares, older people remain very fearful of attack when using public transportation. Transportation by taxicab for an individual on a limited income is unrealistic, but sharing a taxicab with others who also need to shop may enable the aged to go where food prices are cheaper and to take advantage of sale items. Convenience foods, devoid of many essential nutrients, are lighter to carry or pull along in a cart than fresh fruits and vegetables.

Senior citizen organizations in many parts of the United States have been helpful in providing older adults with van service to shopping areas. In housing complexes it may be possible to schedule group trips to the supermarket. Most communities have multiple sources of transportation available, but the older adult may be unaware of them. In addition, many older adults, particularly widowed men, may have never learned to shop and prepare food. Often, older adults have to rely on others to shop for them, and this may be a cause of concern depending on availability of support and the reluctance to be dependent on someone else, particularly family. For older adults who own a computer, shopping over the Internet and having groceries delivered offer advantages although prices may be higher than in the stores.

Housing

Poor and near-poor older people are likely to reside in substandard housing. Some who live in single rooms lack storage space for food, a means of refrigeration, and a stove for cooking. At certain times of the year some of the single-room dwellers use the window ledges and fire escapes to keep perishables cool for several days' use. It is difficult for the single-room occupant to prepare adequately nutritious meals unless the individual is aware of other alternatives.

Ideally, one meal that consists of protein (generally meat, fish, or poultry), potato, vegetable, salad, and dessert should be eaten out daily. Other meals can be prepared and eaten with a minimum of effort in the older person's room. Pantry-type foods can be safely stored in a heavy cardboard or wooden box with a tight-fitting lid and in the driest, coolest place in the room. This box not only serves as a place of storage but also can be used as a table when one is not available. Cookies and crackers should be placed in plastic bags and then in airtight containers. Screw-top jars or coffee cans will accommodate dried fruit, beans, and sugar. Vacuum-packed foods do not require refrigeration, and a greater variety is available than in the past. Canned food should be purchased in the single-serving size so that there will not be any leftovers. Boxes of edibles should be carefully opened to ensure tight reclosure.

SPECIAL CONCERNS FOR OLDER PEOPLE

Dentition, bowel function, dysphagia, and malnutrition are a few of the factors that affect or are affected by nutritional status and are often encountered by the gerontological nurse in the care of older adults.

Dentition

Dental health of older adults is a basic need that is increasingly neglected with advanced age, debilitation, and limited mobility. One reason for this neglect may be the general assumption that most older people are edentulous (without any teeth). Older people themselves may believe that losing their teeth is a natural consequence of growing old. Tooth loss is not a natural part of the aging process but, rather, is a problem that accrues over time and is most evident in later years. Age-related changes in the buccal cavity are listed in Box 10-2. The major cause of tooth loss in older adults is

---

Box 10-2   Age Changes of the Buccal Cavity

Decrease in the cellular compartment
Loss of submucosal elastin in oral mucosa
Loss of connective tissue (collagen)
Increase in thickness of collagen fibers
Decrease in function of minor salivary glands
Decrease in number and quality of blood vessels and nerves
Attrition on occlusive contact surfaces
Enamel less permeable—teeth more brittle
Tooth color change
Excessive secondary dentin formation
Decrease in rate of cementin deposition
Decrease in size of pulp chamber and root canals
Decrease in size and volume of the tooth pulp
Increase in pulp stones and dystrophic mineralization

---

periodontal disease. Smoking, inadequate oral care techniques and preventive dental care, as well as diseases such as diabetes, osteoporosis, cardiovascular disease, and obesity, have been associated with the development of periodontal disease. Missing teeth or teeth in ill repair affect the type and consistency of food chosen to eat and may also contribute to chewing and swallowing problems. This often leads to limited and monotonous meals. Frequently food eaten by those who are edentulous is inadequate and deficient in nutritive value.

The most prevalent cause of gingivitis (gum inflammation and disease) is inadequate removal of plaque and calculus. This may be exacerbated by partial dentures, overhanging ledges of fillings, and faulty bridges that allow plaque to accumulate between teeth. A predisposition to gingivitis may also occur when the mucous membranes are irritated by dryness of the mouth. Systemic problems, such as endocrine dysfunction, chronic airway limitations, medications, and nutritional deficiencies, may influence the development of the disease (Box 10-3). It is important for the nurse to assess for periodontal disease in the elderly and teach elders the signs to look for (Box 10-4).

Another common oral problem among older adults is dry mouth (xerostomia). Often this is associated with medications. Dry mouth makes

| Box 10-3 | Contributing Factors in Periodontal Problems of Older Adults |

Anatomical
Tooth malalignment
Thinning gingival mucosa

Bacterial
Plaque accumulation
Invasion of organisms at or below gum line
Food impaction

Drugs, Metallic Poisons
Allergic responses
Phenytoin
Cytotoxins
Heavy metals (lead, arsenic, mercury)

Emotional and Psychomotor
Bruxism (grinding of teeth)
Cerebrovascular accident
Mental impairment

Intrinsic (Systemic)
Endocrine
Metabolic
Altered immune system

Mechanical
Calculus
Retention of impacted food
Movable and spreading teeth
Ragged-edged fillings and crown overhangs
Poorly designed or poorly fitting dentures

| Box 10-4 | Signs of Periodontal Disease* |

Gums bleeding when teeth are brushed (Even a little bleeding is not normal. If you have a pink toothbrush, see your dentist.)
Red, swollen, or tender gums
Detachment of the gums from the teeth
Pus that appears from the gum line when the gums are pressed
Teeth that have become loose or change position
Any change in the way your teeth fit together when you bite
Any change in the fit of partial dentures
Chronic bad breath or bad taste

*Not limited to elders alone.

eating, swallowing, tasting, and speaking difficult. Artificial saliva preparations are available, and adequate fluid intake is also important when xerostomia occurs. Miller (2004) reported findings from a study of older people in residential homes involving a sugar-free gum product containing xylitol alone or in combination with chlorhexidine that increased saliva and reduced tooth debris.

The oral health of older people has improved because of improved dental care and techniques. Older adults today are less likely to loose their teeth and become edentulous. Dentures may be considered antiques in the future. However, the increased retention of teeth by today's older adults is creating concern about the increase of periodontal conditions because they affect the tissue supporting the teeth, cementum, periodontal ligaments, alveolar bone, and gingiva. In addition, dental care is expensive and may not be available to some older people, particularly those residing in nursing homes. Kayser-Jones (1997) conducted a comprehensive research study investigating the social, cultural, psychological, environmental, and clinical factors affecting eating in nursing homes. Poor oral health was prevalent among the participants studied; 44% were totally edentulous, and only three of the edentulous residents had upper and lower dentures that fit properly. Poor oral health and lack of attention to oral hygiene are major concerns in institutional settings and contribute significantly to poor nutrition and other negative outcomes, such as aspiration pneumonia (Terpenning et al, 2002). Many reasons exist for this and include lack of access to dental care, difficulty providing oral care to dependent or cognitively impaired elders, and inadequate training and staffing. Many long-term care institutions have implemented programs such as special training of aides for dental care teams, providing visits from mobile dentistry units on a routine basis, or utilizing dental students to perform oral screening and cleaning of teeth (Simons et al, 2001; Coleman, 2002). Cost-effective oral care products that are easy to use will be discussed in the following section.

Oral Health Assessment

Assessment of the oral cavity should be a regular part of nursing assessment. In addition to identifying oral health problems, examination of the mouth can serve as an early warning system for some diseases and many contribute to early diagnosis and treatment (accessed 7/18/04 from http://www.surgeongeneral.gov/library/oral-health/). Assessment instruments such as The Geriatric Oral Health Assessment Index (GOHAI) are available in the Hartford Geriatric Nursing Institute *Try This* Series (http://www.hartford.ign.org). Jones et al (2002) reported on a new dental self-screening measure, the D-E-N-T-A-L, that is being tested to evaluate the need for dental treatment in conjunction with the clinical examination. The instrument queries whether participants experience dry mouth or eating or swallowing problems, have not had a dental examination in the last 2 years, have tooth or mouth problems, have altered eating habits because of teeth or mouth, or have lesions or sores in the mouth.

Interventions

Impaired manual dexterity makes it difficult for elders to adequately maintain their dental routine and remove plaque adequately. The hand grip of manual toothbrushes is too small to grasp and manipulate easily, although enlarging the handle by adding a foam grip or wrapping it with gauze to increase handle size has been effective in facilitating grasp. The ultrasonic toothbrush is an effective method for elders or for those who must brush the teeth of elders to use. The base is large enough for easy grasp, and the ultrasonic movement of the bristles with the usual brushing movement is very effective in plaque removal (Whitmyer et al, 1998).

Therapeutic rinses contain an agent that is beneficial to the surface of the teeth and the oral environment. Some therapeutic rinses require a prescription, such as Peridex (chlorhexidine), which contains alcohol but is also a broad-spectrum antimicrobial agent that helps control plaque. Listerine, which is in this same category, is an over-the-counter product that carries the American Dental Association's approval. Listerine also contains a high volume of alcohol (26.9%). Alcohol, by volume, can be an oral tissue irritant and can exacerbate or create xerostomia. Alco-holism is a problem of many older people, so caution is advised in the use of alcohol-containing rinses.

It is essential to provide oral care daily regardless of whether the elder is severely disabled, physically handicapped, comatose, or mentally incapable of carrying out his or her own oral hygiene. Debilitated elders are at greater risk of developing oral disease. They take more medications; have decreased saliva production; lack resistance to bacterial toxins that cause periodontal disease; and eat softer foods, more liquids, and foods high in sugar, which tend to remain in their mouths longer. Daily removal and cleaning of dentures and brushing of teeth should be a part of the care routines in institutions.

For the homebound elder, daily oral care should be part of general hygiene. Having the proper equipment and using the appropriate technique greatly simplify the task and ensure better results. Box 10-5 provides dental care suggestions for caregivers. Many elders believe that once they have dentures, there is no longer a need for oral care. Older adults with dentures should be taught the proper home care of their dentures and oral tissue to prevent odor, stain, plaque buildup, and oral infections; home care should include removal of debris under dentures to prevent pressure on and shrinkage of underlying support structures. Dentures and other dental appliances, such as bridges, should be cleaned after each meal and any time they are removed (Box 10-6). Dentures should be worn constantly except at night (to allow relief of the compression on the gums) and replaced in the mouth in the morning.

Dentures are very personal and expensive possessions. In communal living situations of nursing homes, hospitals, and other care centers, dentures have often been misplaced or mixed up with others. The utmost care should be taken when handling, cleaning, and storing dentures. Dentures should be marked, and many states require all newly made dentures to contain the client's identification. A commercial denture marking system called Identure, produced by the 3M Company, provides a simple, efficient, and permanent means of marking dentures. Broken or damaged dentures and dentures that no longer fit because of weight loss are a common problem for older adults. Rebasing of dentures is a technique to improve the fit of dentures. Ill-fitting dentures

---

Box 10-5   **Dental Care: Instructions for Caregivers**

1. If the patient is in bed, elevate his or her head by raising the bed or propping it with pillows and have the patient turn his or her head to face you. Place a clean towel across the chest and under the chin, and place a basin under his or her chin.

2. If the patient is sitting in a stationary chair or wheelchair, stand behind the patient and stabilize his or her head by placing one hand under his or her chin and resting his or her head against your body. Place a towel across his or her chest and over the shoulders. (It may be helpful to secure it with a safety pin.) The basin can be kept handy in the patient's lap or on a table placed in front of or at the side of the patient. A wheelchair may be positioned in front of the sink.

3. If the patient's lips are dry or cracked, apply a light coating of petroleum jelly.

4. Brush and floss the patient's teeth as you have been instructed (sulcular brushing, if possible). It may be helpful to retract the patient's lips and cheek with a tongue blade or fingers in order to see the area that is being cleaned. Use a mouth prop as needed if the patient cannot hold his or her mouth open. If manual flossing is too difficult, use a floss holder or interproximal brush to clean the proximal surfaces between the teeth. Use a dentifrice containing fluoride.

5. Provide the conscious patient with fluoride rinses or other rinses as indicated by the dentist or hygienist.

From Papas AS, Niessen LC, Chauncey HH: *Geriatric dentistry: aging and oral health*, St Louis, 1991, Mosby.

Box 10-6   **Instructions for Denture Cleaning**

1. Rinse your denture or dentures after each meal to remove soft debris.

2. Once each day, preferably before retiring, brush your denture according to the method described below. Then place it in a denture-cleaning solution, and allow it to soak overnight or for at least a few hours. (Acrylic denture material must be kept wet at all times to prevent cracking or warping.)

3. Remove your denture from the cleaning solution, and brush it thoroughly.
   a. Although an ordinary *soft* toothbrush is adequate, a specially designed denture brush may clean more effectively. (CAUTION: Acrylic denture material is softer than natural teeth and may be damaged by being brushed with very firm bristles.)
   b. Brush your denture over a sink lined with a facecloth and half-filled with water. This will prevent breakage if the denture is dropped.
   c. Hold the denture *securely* in one hand, but do not squeeze. Hold the brush in the other hand. It is not essential to use a denture paste, particularly if dentures are soaked before being brushed to soften debris. Never use a commercial tooth powder, because it is abrasive and may damage the denture materials. Plain water, mild soap, or sodium bicarbonate may be used.
   d. When cleaning a *removable partial denture*, great care must be taken to remove plaque from the curved metal clasps that hook around the teeth. This can be done with a regular toothbrush or with a specially designed clasp brush.

4. After brushing, rinse your denture thoroughly and insert it into your mouth.

From Papas AS, Niessen LC, Chauncey HH: *Geriatric dentistry: aging and oral health*, St Louis, 1991, Mosby.

or dentures that are not cleaned contribute to oral problems as well as poor nutrition and enjoyment of food. Daily removal and cleaning of dentures and brushing of teeth should be a part of the care routines in institutions. Both nursing students and nursing staff need to be knowledgeable about oral hygiene and techniques to care for teeth and dentures.

Bowel Function

Bowel function of the older adult, although normally only slightly altered by physiological changes of age, can be a source of concern and potentially serious problems. Although it is suggested that older people are known for their concern with bowel function, particularly constipation, knowledge about normal bowel function and lifelong patterns contributes greatly to bowel function concerns of people at many ages. The media places emphasis on specific procedures of eliminating and advertises laxatives. Bowel preoccupation costs millions of dollars in laxative expenditures, mainly to older people. Attention to bowel function occurs when there is a deviation from what is perceived as normal elimination. Whatever the complaint, one needs to know exactly what the individual means when he or she says there is a problem. Bowel function problems that the nurse will encounter among older people are constipation, fecal impaction, irritable bowel syndrome, and fecal incontinence. For the dependent older person, these concerns can become quite serious, and proper assessment and monitoring are important to prevent serious consequences.

Constipation

Constipation has different meanings to different people. Some individuals consider constipation to be infrequent bowel action; others perceive it as difficulty in passing feces. In one study, half the elders who complained of constipation moved their bowels at least once per day (Edwards, 2002). To the health professional, constipation occurs when there are less than three bowel movements per week or there is a decrease in usual stool frequency. It is the most common gastrointestinal complaint to the health care provider, with about 60% of community-based elders reporting laxative use (Beers, Berkow, 2000). About 74% of older adults in long-term care use laxatives daily.

Normal elimination should be an easy passage of feces, without undue straining or a feeling of incomplete evacuation or defecation. The urge to defecate occurs when the distended walls of the sigmoid and rectum, which are filled with feces, stimulate pressure receptors to relax the sphincters for the expulsion of feces through the anus. Evacuation of feces is accomplished by relaxation of the sphincters and contraction of the diaphragm and abdominal muscles, which raises the intra-abdominal pressure.

Constipation appears to be a problem of older people because of age-related physiological changes in addition to reduced activity and diet considerations (Beers, Berkow, 2000). There is impaired rectal sensation so that larger volumes are required to elicit the sensation to defecate. There are also reduced resting anal sphincter pressure and diminished maximum sphincter pressure, predisposing to fecal incontinence. Combined with these changes, the extensive use of laxatives by older people can be considered a cultural habit. During their formative years, weekly doses of rhubarb, cascara, castor oil, and other types of laxatives were consumed to promote health. This belief that cleaning out the colon was paramount to maintaining good health still persists with many elderly people.

Constipation is a symptom. It is a reflection of poor habits, postponed passage of stool, and many chronic illnesses—both physical and psychological. There are numerous precipitating factors for constipation, which can be categorized as physiological, functional, mechanical, psychological, systemic, pharmacological, and others. A list of these factors is provided in Table 10-2.

Assessment. The precipitating factors of constipation need to be included in the assessment of the client to shed light on the possible cause or causes of altered bowel function. A review of these factors will also determine if a client is at risk for altered bowel function. It is recognized that older people at high risk for constipation and subsequent impaction are those who have hypotonic colon function, who are immobilized and debilitated, or who have central nervous system lesions. It is also important to know that alterations in cognitive status, increased agitation, incontinence, increased temperature, poor appetite, or

Table 10-2 Precipitating Factors for Constipation

PHYSIOLOGICAL
Dehydration
Insufficient fiber intake
Poor dietary habits

FUNCTIONAL
Decreased physical activity
Inadequate toileting
Irregular defecation habits
Irritable bowel disease
Weakness

MECHANICAL
Abscess or ulcer
Cerebrovascular disease
Defective electrolyte transfer
Fissures
Hemorrhoids
Hirschsprung's disease
Neurological disease
Parkinson's disease
Postsurgical obstruction
Prostate enlargement
Rectal prolapse
Rectocele
Spinal cord injury
Strictures
Tumors

OTHER
Lack of abdominal muscle tone
Obesity
Poor dentition
Recent environmental changes

PSYCHOLOGICAL
Avoidance of urge to defecate
Cognitive impairment
Depression
Emotional stress

SYSTEMIC
Diabetes mellitus
Hypercalcemia
Hyperparathyroidism
Hypothyroidism
Hypokalemia
Pheochromocytoma
Porphyria
Uremia

PHARMACOLOGICAL
Aluminum-containing antacids
Anticholinergics
Anticonvulsants
Antidepressants
Bismuth salts
Calcium carbonate
Calcium channel blockers
Diuretics
Laxative overuse
Iron salts
Nonsteroidal antiinflammatories
Opiates
Phenothiazines
Sedatives
Sympathomimetics

From Allison OC, Porter ME, Briggs GG: Chronic constipation: assessment and management in the elderly, *J Am Acad Nurse Pract* 6(7):311-317, 1994.

unexplained falls may be the only clinical symptoms of constipation in the cognitively impaired or frail older person. Specific questions for initial assessment of constipation with the rationale for obtaining the assessment data appear in Box 10-7.

A physical examination is needed to rule out systemic causes of constipation. The abdomen is examined for bowel sounds, pain, localized masses (retained stool), distention, and evidence of prior surgery (Edwards, 2002). A rectal examination is important to reveal painful anal disorders, such as hemorrhoids or fissures, that will impede the evacuation of stool and to evaluate sphincter tone, rectal prolapse, stool presence in the vault, strictures, masses, anal reflex, and enlarged prostate (Edwards, 2002). A bowel history is also important to obtain, including usual patterns and any changes. A review of food and fluid intake may be necessary to determine the amount of fiber and fluid ingested. Biochemical tests should include a complete blood count, fasting glucose, chemistry panel, and thyroid studies. If constipation is of

Box 10-7	Constipation Assessment Questions and Rationale

Question	Rationale
When did constipation begin?	Lifelong history of constipation is likely to be a functional disorder; sudden change may be an organic lesion, such as carcinoma.
Has anything in bowel function recently changed?	A sudden change even in constipation may signal an underlying disorder.
How often do bowel movements occur?	Frequency of defecation may actually be normal. The question may also unknowingly let clients describe their cathartic use.
Is the urge to defecate lacking or the stool difficult to expel?	Absent urge may indicate chronic suppression of normal function or neurological disorder. Difficult passage of stool may be due to fiber or fluid deficit, medication use, or thyroid disorder.
Is pain associated with defecation?	Pain implies fecal impaction of rectum, anorectal fissures, or intestinal obstruction.
Is blood evident in bowel movement?	Witnessed, usually is hemorrhoid bleeding, tear, or fissure.
What medications are taken, including over-the-counter drugs?	Multiple drugs are capable of causing constipation.

Modified from Rousseau P: Aging and chronic constipation, *Geriatr Med Today* 9(3):35, 1990.

recent or sudden onset or is accompanied by bleeding, a colonoscopy or other gastrointestinal examination may be warranted. If there is stool seepage and impaction is suspected with an empty vault, abdominal x-ray films will reveal a high impaction, intussusception, or other obstruction (Edwards, 2002).

Interventions. The first intervention is to examine the medications the person is taking and eliminate those that are constipation producing or change to medications that are not constipation producing. Edwards (2002) states that it is better to start a bowel regimen with an empty colon, which may require removal of an impaction manually or with the use of enemas. Any regimen should be started slowly and with the person's preferences included. This will also avoid bloating and cramping gas pains that occur with a faster implementation time.

Nonpharmacological interventions for constipation that have been implemented and evaluated can be grouped into four areas: (1) fluid/fiber, (2) exercise, (3) environmental manipulation, and (4) a combination of these.

FLUIDS AND FIBER. Adequate hydration is the cornerstone of constipation therapy with fluids coming mainly from water (Beers, Berkow, 2000). The use of bran fiber and fruit and vegetable fiber and nuts is recommended. Bran fiber results in a functioning colon with higher fecal bulking action. This may minimize the need for supplemental fibers, such as psyllium and methylcellulose. Individuals who can chew foods well could benefit from eating increased amounts of fresh fruits and vegetables daily or combining unsweetened bran with other types of food. Those who have difficulty chewing could sprinkle unsweetened bran on cereals or in soups, meat loaf, or casseroles. Cooked dried beans are a good source of fiber. Pinto beans, split peas, red beans, and peanuts can be served in casseroles, soups, and dips. These are all relatively inexpensive and nutritious in addition to having high fiber. The quantity of bran used depends on the individual, but generally 1 to 2 tablespoons daily is sufficient to facilitate intestinal motility. Individuals who have not used bran should begin with 1 teaspoon and progressively increase the quantity until the fiber

Box 10-8   Natural Laxative Recipes

Fruit Spread*
2 pounds raisins
2 pounds currants
2 pounds prunes
2 pounds figs
2 pounds dates
2 containers (28 oz each) undiluted prune
  concentrate
  Put fruit through a grinder. Mix with prune concentrate in large mixer (mixture will be very thick). Store in large-mouthed plastic container. Refrigerate. Any dried fruit can be added.

Power Pudding†
$1/2$ cup prune juice
$1/2$ cup applesauce

$1/2$ cup wheat bran flakes
$1/2$ cup whipped topping
$1/2$ cup prunes (canned stewed)
(Diabetics may use no–added sugar applesauce
  and light whipped topping.)
  Blend ingredients, cover, refrigerate, and keep as long as 1 week. Take $1/4$-cup portions of recipe with breakfast. Regulate dose as needed.

Standard Recipe
1 cup bran
1 cup applesauce
1 cup prune juice
  Mix and store in refrigerator. Start with administration of 1 oz per day. Increase or decrease dosage as needed.

*Data from Beverley L, Travis I: Constipation: proposed natural laxative mixtures, *J Gerontol Nurs* 18(10):5-12, 1992.
†Data from Neal LJ: "Power pudding": natural laxative therapy for the elderly who are homebound, *Home Health Nurse* 13(3):66, 1995.

intake is enough to accomplish its purpose. Otherwise, bloating, gas, diarrhea, and other colon discomforts will initially occur and discourage further use of this important dietary ingredient. Box 10-8 provides several recipes for a natural laxative that has been found beneficial for both community-living and institutionalized older people.

EXERCISE. Exercise is important as an intervention to stimulate colon motility and bowel evacuation. Daily walking for 20 to 30 minutes is helpful, especially after a meal. Pelvic tilt exercises, and range-of-motion (passive or active) exercises are beneficial for those who are less mobile or bed bound.

POSITIONING AND ENVIRONMENTAL MANIPULATION. The squatting position facilitates bowel function if the patient is able to squat. A similar position may be obtained by leaning forward and applying firm pressure to the lower abdomen or placing the feet on a stool. Massaging the abdomen may help stimulate the bowel. Establishing a routine for toileting promotes or normalizes bowel function. The gastrocolic reflex occurs after breakfast or supper and may be enhanced by a warm drink. Given privacy and ample time many will have a daily bowel movement. However, any urge to

defecate should be followed by a trip to the bathroom. Older people dependent on others to meet toileting needs should be assisted to maintain normal routines and provided opportunities for routine toilet use.

LAXATIVES AND ENEMAS. Laxatives may be used in addition to fiber, exercise, and environmental manipulation. Senna tea is an effective laxative that is safe for elderly patients and is nontoxic. Cascara is another laxative commonly prescribed. These stimulant-type laxatives should be used on a short term basis because they can cause dependency. They can also cause abdominal cramping and fluid and electrolyte disturbances, especially if impaction is present (Beers, Berkow, 2000). Lactulose and sorbitol increase fluid in the colon and promote soft stools. They work slowly but are effective in frail elders (Edwards, 2002). Emollient laxatives, such as mineral oil or docusate sodium, should not be used because of the risk of oil aspiration and vitamin depletion if used too often. Saline laxatives work by drawing water into the small bowel and stimulating peristalsis; the bowel empties within hours. They should not be used in those elders with poor renal function if they contain magnesium, phosphate, or sulfate salts

(Edwards, 2002). Stool softeners such as docusate sodium can help soften hard stools but do not actually affect constipation. Enemas of any type should be reserved for situations where other methods produce no response or when it is known that there is an impaction. Soapsuds and phosphate enemas irritate the rectal mucosa and should not be used. Normal saline or tap water enema (500 to 1000 ml) at a temperature of about 105° F is the best choice.

Fecal Impaction

Fecal impaction is a major complication of constipation. It is especially common in incapacitated and institutionalized older people. Symptoms of fecal impaction include malaise, urinary retention, elevated temperature, incontinence of bladder or bowel, alterations in cognitive status, fissures, hemorrhoids, and intestinal obstruction. The causes are similar to those of constipation. Unrecognized, unattended, or neglected constipation eventually leads to fecal impaction. Leakage of liquid stool from around the impaction is frequently seen and may be inappropriately diagnosed as diarrhea and treated with antidiarrheal medications, aggravating the problem. When there is oozing liquid stool, the person should have a rectal examination to assess for impaction. Removal of a fecal impaction is at times worse than the misery of the condition. Continued obstruction by a fecal mass may eventually impair sensation, leading to the need for larger stool volume to stimulate the urge to defecate, which contributes to megacolon (Edwards, 2002). Valsalva's maneuvers done during straining at stool defecation can cause transient ischemic attacks and syncope, especially in the frail elderly.

Management of fecal impaction requires the digital removal of the hard, compacted stool from the rectum with use of lubrication containing lidocaine jelly. Generally this is preceded by an oil-retention enema to soften the feces in preparation for manual removal. Use of suppositories is not effective, because their action is blocked by the amount and size of the stool in the rectum. Suppositories do not facilitate the removal of stool in the sigmoid, which may continue to ooze once the rectum is emptied.

Several sessions or days may be required to totally cleanse the sigmoid colon and rectum of

---

Box 10-9	Risk Factors for Dysphagia

Cerebrovascular accident (CVA, stroke)
Parkinson's disease
Neuromuscular disorders, for example, amyotropic lateral sclerosis (ALS), multiple sclerosis (MS), myasthenia gravis, dystonia
Anatomic abnormalities
Cervical osteophytes
Oral and oropharyngeal cancer or surgery
Laryngeal cancer or surgery
Alzheimer's disease and related dementias
Traumatic brain injury
Tracheostomy
Aspiration pneumonia

---

impacted feces. Once this is achieved, attention should be directed to planning a regimen that includes adequate fluid intake, increased dietary fiber, administration of stool softeners if needed, and many of the suggestions presented for prevention of constipation. In acute and long-term care settings, maintenance and monitoring of a bowel record are important since many older people experiencing acute or chronic illness may not be able provide accurate information as to bowel patterns. Fecal impaction is a serious and often dangerous condition for older people and should be prevented.

Dysphagia. The incidence of dysphagia increases with age and the presence of some diseases, including stroke, Parkinson's and Alzheimer's disease, and gastroesophageal reflux disease (GERD). Other factors, such as medications, poor dentition, inadequate feeding techniques, and reduced salivation, may also predispose the older adult to dysphagia. Box 10-9 presents risk factors for dysphagia. Dysphagia is a serious problem and has negative consequences, including weight loss, malnutrition, aspiration pneumonia, and even death. Over half of the 750,000 people affected by stroke each year experience dysphagia at some point. Of these, 50% will be affected by malnutrition, 37% will develop pneumonia, and 4.3% will die of pneumonia (Blackington et al, 2001). Dysphagia can be categorized as transfer or oropharyngeal dysphagia (difficulty moving the food from the mouth to

Box 10-10	Symptoms of Dysphagia

Difficult, labored swallowing
Drooling
Copious oral secretions
Aspiration precautions
Coughing, choking at meals
Holding or pocketing of food in the mouth
Absence of chewing
Absence of swallowing
Excessive throat clearing
Difficulty swallowing medications
Wet or gurgling voice
Discomfort during swallowing
Sensation of something stuck in the throat during swallowing
Food or liquid coming out of the nose during swallowing

Box 10-11	Interventions for Dysphagia

Sit at 90 degrees during all oral (PO) intake.
Maintain 90-degree positioning for at least 1 hour after PO intake.
Keep suction equipment ready at all times.
Supervise all meals.
Monitor temperature.
Observe color of phlegm.
Visually check the mouth for pocketing of food in cheeks.
Provide mouth care every 4 hours.
Follow speech therapist's recommendation for safe swallowing techniques and modified food consistency.

the esophagus), transport dysphagia (difficulty passing the ingested food down the esophagus), or delivery dysphagia (the propulsion of a bolus of food to the stomach is difficult).

ASSESSMENT. It is important to obtain a careful history of the elder's response to dysphagia and to observe the person during mealtime. Symptoms that alert the nurse to possible swallowing problems are presented in Box 10-10. Silent aspiration is common, and a comprehensive evaluation by a speech-language pathologist, usually including a videofluoroscopic recording of a modified barium swallow, should be considered when dysphagia is suspected (Shanley, O'Loughlin, 2000).

INTERVENTIONS. Aspiration is the most profound and dangerous problem for older adults experiencing dysphagia. It is important to have a suction machine available at the bedside or in the dining room in the home or institutional setting. People with dysphagia should have supervision at mealtimes. Other interventions for dysphagia are described in Box 10-11. The gerontological nurse must work closely with other members of the interdisciplinary team, such as speech-language pathologists, in implementing suggested interventions to prevent aspiration. Miceli (1999) presents a comprehensive and practical dysphagia management program for long-term care, including identification of patient help level and corresponding nursing care, supervised dining

methods, staff training, communication, and quality improvement suggestions.

Research on the appropriate management of swallowing disorders in older people, particularly during acute illness and in long-term care facilities, is very limited, and additional study is essential (Robbins et al, 2002). Comprehensive assessment of dysphagia and other factors that influence adequate intake must be conducted before initiating severely restricted diet modifications or considering the use of feeding tubes, particularly in older people with dementia (Chouinard, 2000). A recent study (Mitchell et al, 2003) of nursing home residents with advanced cognitive impairment and the eating and swallowing problems that accompany it reported that 33.8% of the residents had feeding tubes. Short-term enteral feeding may be indicated for some conditions, but the use of tube feeding in patients with advanced dementia to prevent aspiration pneumonia, malnutrition, and infections provides few long-term benefits and may, in fact, contribute to further decline. Tube feeding has never been shown to reduce the risk of regurgitating gastric contents and cannot be expected to prevent aspiration of oral secretions (Finucane et al, 1999). Gerontological nurses play an important role in education of patients and families about appropriate treatments and evidence-based interventions. Careful attention to mealtime ambience, feeding techniques, adequate staffing, assistive devices, dental care, change of body position, use of finger foods, hand-over-hand feeding, enhanced flavor, provision of culturally appropriate food, and special dementia units with trained staff may help minimize nutritional problems associated with dementia. A comprehensive protocol for preventing aspiration in older adults with dysphagia can be found at http://www.hartfordign.org.

Malnutrition. The occurrence of malnutrition among the elderly has been documented in elders in acute care, long-term care, and the community. Protein-calorie malnutrition (PCM), the most common form of malnutrition, results from inadequate intake, digestion, or absorption of protein or calories (Moore, 2001). PCM is characterized by catabolism of fat and muscle tissue, lethargy, generalized weakness, and weight loss. Many of the factors discussed previously contribute to the occurrence of malnutrition in older adults (Box 10-12). The prevalence of PCM varies with the population observed and the definition of malnutrition. In the United States, estimates are that 50% of nursing home patients, 50% of hospitalized patients, and 44% of home health patients over the age of 65 are malnourished (Burger et al, 2000; Crogan, Pasvogel, 2003). A recent study (Thomas et al, 2002) reported that more than 91% of patients admitted to a subacute facility are either malnourished or at risk of malnutrition. The high prevalence of malnutrition in nursing homes and subacute facilities may in part reflect transfer of malnourished patients from acute care to long-term care following an acute illness.

Malnutrition has serious consequences, including infections, pressure ulcers, anemia, hypotension, impaired cognition, hip fractures, and increased mortality and morbidity (Burger et al, 2000). The majority of pathological causes of weight loss are considered reversible. Two mnemonics, MEALS-ON-WHEELS and SCALES (for use in outpatient settings), are helpful in assessing and treating weight loss (Morley, 1991; Morley, Silver, 1995). Depression is frequent in older adults and a common reversible cause of weight loss, accounting for up to 30% of undernutrition in medical outpatients and up to 36% of residents in nursing homes (Morley, Kraenzle, 1994; Blaum et al, 1995; Wilson et al, 1998). Screening for depression using validated tools,

---

Box 10-12	**Factors Potentiating Malnutrition in Older Adults**

Psychosocial Risk Factors
Limited income
Abuse of alcohol and other central nervous system depressants
Bereavement, loneliness, or living alone
Removal from usual cultural patterns
Confusion, forgetfulness, or disorientation
Working toward intentional or subintentional death

Mechanical Risk Factors
Decreased or limited strength and mobility
Neurological deficits, arthritis, handicap, impairment of hand-arm coordination, loss of tongue strength, dysphagia
Decreased or diminished vision or blindness
Inability to feed self and lack of adequate assistance
Pressure ulcers
Loss of teeth, poor-fitting dentures, or chewing problems
Difficult breathing
Polypharmacy
Surgery, nothing by mouth (NPO) for extended periods of time, or intravenous therapy only

---

such as the Geriatric Depression Scale or the Cornell Scale for Depression in Dementia, should be included in assessment of older people with weight loss. In light of current population projections, the number of older adults requiring hospitalization, subacute care, and nursing home care will dramatically increase, leading to increased hospital stays, increased costs, and considerable mortality (Crogan, Pasvogel, 2003). Clearly, malnutrition is a serious challenge for health professionals in all settings.

NUTRITIONAL ASSESSMENT

A nutritional assessment that provides the most conclusive data about a person's actual nutritional state consists of four steps: interview, physical examination, anthropometrical measurements, and biochemical analysis. The collective results can provide the nurse with data needed to identify the immediate and potential nutritional problems of the client. The nurse can then begin to establish plans for supervision, assistance, and education in the attainment of adequate nutrition for the older person. The Nutrition Screening Initiative developed nutritional screening materials to promote nutritional health care in the American health care system (Figure 10-2). The Mini Nutritional Assessment (MNA), developed by Nestle of Geneva, Switzerland, is another tool that can be used to identify older adults at risk of malnutrition (http://www.mna-elderly.com/clinical-practice.htm).

In long-term care, the Minimum Data Set (MDS) includes assessment information that can be used to identify potential nutritional problems, risk factors, and the potential for improved function. The nutrition and dehydration Resident Assessment Protocols (RAPs) guide staff in assessment of nutritionally related problems. Triggers for more thorough investigation of problems include weight loss, alterations in taste, medical therapies, prescription medications, hunger, parenteral or intravenous feedings, mechanically altered or therapeutic diets, percentage of food left uneaten, pressure ulcers, and edema. See Chapter 6 for further information on MDA and RAPs.

Interview

The interview provides background information and clues to the nutritional state and actual and potential problems of the elderly person. Questions about the individual's state of health, social activities, normal patterns, and changes that have occurred should be asked. The nurse must explore the individual's needs, the manner in which food is obtained, and the client's ability to prepare food. Information concerning the relationship of food to daily events will provide clues to the meaning and significance of food to that person. The older person who eats alone is considered a candidate for malnutrition. Information about occupation and daily activities will suggest the degree of energy expenditure and caloric intake most appropriate for the overall activity. One's economic state will have a direct bearing on nutrition. It is there-

fore important to explore the client's financial resources to establish the income available for food. Knowledge of medications taken should be included in the nutrition history. Additional medical information should include the presence or absence of mouth pain or discomfort, visual difficulty, and bowel and bladder function. Food intake patterns should be explored. Frequently a 24-hour diet recall compared with the Food Guide Pyramid can present an estimate of nutritional adequacy. When the older person cannot provide all of the information requested, it may be possible to obtain data from a family member or another source. There will be times, however, when information will not be as complete as one would like, or the older person, too proud to admit that he or she is not eating, will furnish erroneous information. The nurse will still be able to obtain additional data from the other three areas of the nutritional assessment.

Keeping a dietary record for 3 days is another assessment tool. Careful recording of when one ate, what was eaten, and amounts eaten must be made. This approach should be attempted only with dependable elders. Computer analysis of the dietary records provides information on energy and vitamin and mineral intake. Printouts can provide the elderly and the health care professional with a visual graph of their intake.

Physical Examination

The second step of the nutritional assessment, the physical examination, furnishes clinically observable evidence of the existing state of nutrition. Data such as height and weight; vital signs; condition of the tongue, lips, and gums; and skin turgor, texture, and color are assessed, and the general overall appearance is scrutinized for evidence of wasting.

Debate continues in the quest to determine the appropriate weight charts for an older adult. Although weight alone does not indicate the adequacy of diet, unplanned fluctuations in weight are significant and should be evaluated. Accurate weight patterns are sometimes difficult to obtain. One can meet correct weight values for height, but weight changes may be the results of fluid retention, edema, or ascites. However, an unintentional weight loss of more than 5% of body weight in 1

The Warning Signs of poor nutritional health are often overlooked. Use this checklist to find out if you or someone you know is at nutritional risk.

Read the statements below. Circle the number in the yes column for those that apply to you or someone you know. For each yes answer, score the number in the box. Total your nutritional score.

DETERMINE YOUR NUTRITIONAL HEALTH

	YES
I have an illness or condition that made me change the kind and/or amount of food I eat.	2
I eat fewer than 2 meals per day.	3
I eat few fruits or vegetables, or milk products.	2
I have 3 or more drinks of beer, liquor or wine almost everyday.	2
I have tooth or mouth problems that make it hard for me to eat.	2
I don't always have enough money to buy the food I need.	4
I eat alone most of the time.	1
I take 3 or more different prescribed or over-the-counter drugs a day.	1
Without wanting to, I have lost or gained 10 pounds in the last 6 months.	2
I am not always physically able to shop, cook and/or feed myself.	2
TOTAL	

Total Your Nutritional Score. If it's—

0-2   **Good!** Recheck your nutritional score in 6 months.

3-5   **You are at moderate nutritional risk.** See what can be done to improve your eating habits and lifestyle. Your office on aging, senior nutrition program, senior citizens center or health department can help. Recheck your nutritional score in 3 months.

6 or more   You are at high nutritional risk. Bring this checklist the next time you see your doctor, dietitian or other qualified health or social service professional. Talk with them about any problems you may have. Ask for help to improve your nutritional health.

These materials developed and distributed by the Nutrition Screening Initiative, a project of:

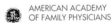
AMERICAN ACADEMY OF FAMILY PHYSICIANS

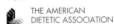
THE AMERICAN DIETETIC ASSOCIATION

NATIONAL COUNCIL ON THE AGING, INC.

Remember that warning signs suggest risk, but do not represent diagnosis of any condition.

Figure 10-2 Warning signs of poor nutrition. (From the Nutrition Screening Initiative, project of the American Academy of Family Physicians, the American Dietetic Association, and the National Council on the Aging, Inc. Funded in part by a grant from Ross Products Division, Abbott Laboratories, Inc.)

month, more than 7.5% in 3 months, or more than 10% in 6 months is considered a significant indicator of poor nutrition as well as an MDS trigger. Burger et al (2000) noted that some older people, particularly those who are small, may be at risk even if they lose slightly less than 5% or 10% of their body weights. These authors recommended that the MDS weight loss trigger be reevaluated or that a special one be developed for residents below a certain body weight or that weight loss should be tracked over a longer period of time. As an example, a resident with a weight loss of 2 or 3 pounds per month may not trigger on the MDS during the specified time frames, but that resident may have lost 25 to 35 pounds over the year, a significant amount (Burger et al, 2000). The adequacy of muscle mass and body fat must also be included in assessment although they rarely are obtained.

Anthropometrical Measurements

Anthropometrical measurements are the third part of the nutritional assessment and should include height, weight, midarm circumference, and triceps skinfold thickness. These include simple body measurement procedures, which take less than 5 minutes to perform. These measurements obtain information about the status of the older person's muscle mass and body fat in relation to height and weight. In some instances an individual is bedridden or confined to a chair, or the individual has a spinal curvature preventing accurate height measurement. An estimation of stature can be made using knee height and a sliding broad-blade calipers, similar to the apparatus used to measure the length of an infant. This device consists of an adjustable blade attached to each end at a 90-degree angle. Unlike stature, knee height changes little with age. It should be noted that blacks have proportionally longer lower extremities and Chinese have shorter extremities than whites (Moore, 2001).

Muscle mass measurements are obtained by measuring the arm circumference of the nondominant upper arm. The arm hangs freely at the side, and a measuring tape is placed around the mid-point of the upper arm, between the acromion of the scapula and the olecranon of the ulna. The centimeter circumference is recorded and compared with standard values.

Body fat and lean muscle mass are assessed by measuring specific skinfolds with Lange or Harpenden calipers. Two areas are accessible for measurement. One area is the mid-point of the upper arm, the triceps area, which is also used to obtain arm circumference. The nondominant arm is again used. The nurse lifts the skin with the thumb and forefinger so that it parallels the humerus. The calipers are placed around the skinfold, 1 cm below where the fingers are grasping the skin. Two

readings are averaged to the nearest half centimeter. If there is a neuropathological condition or hemiplegia following a stroke, the unaffected arm should be used for obtaining measurements.

Biochemical Examination

The final step in a nutritional assessment is the biochemical examination. A decreased albumin may indicate protein deficiency, but albumin is slow to change during malnutrition and may be abnormally elevated in certain disease states and dehydration. Prealbumin levels are more accurate and should be considered when initiating and monitoring interventions for unintentional weight loss in the malnourished person. Transferrin, an iron transport protein, is diminished in protein malnutrition. However, it increases in iron deficiency anemia, which is common in older adults, so it is not a sensitive indicator of PCM. A normocytic red blood cell (RBC) anemia with low hemoglobin and hematocrit indicates protein deficiency, and a microcytic RBC indicates iron or copper deficiency. A macrocytic (large RBC) anemia is caused by vitamin B_{12} or folate deficiency. Serum cholesterol should also be measured. Laboratory test results, although not definitive for malnutrition, provide important clues to nutritional status but should be evaluated in relation to the person's overall health status. Unintentional weight loss remains the most important indicator of potential nutritional deficits. An essential part of any assessment of an older adult should include a current weight and a weight history including usual weight throughout life, as well as recent changes in weight and changes over a period of 1 year.

Interventions

Interventions are formulated around the identified nutritional problem or problems. Perhaps the most significant intervention for the community elder is nutrition education and problem solving with the elder as to how to best resolve the potential or actual nutritional deficit.

Education in the area of reading nutritional information on labels is needed. Since 1994, the U.S. Food and Drug Administration (FDA) has required producers of processed foods to list nutrition information based on daily values. Daily values represent the maximum amounts of nutrients and fiber that are desirable in daily diets of 2000 to 2500 calories. The nutrients were chosen based on evidence suggesting that eating too much or too little of these substances has the greatest impact on one's health. FDA defines a "good source" as a food that contains 10% to 19% of the daily value per serving. The daily totals for fat, cholesterol, and sodium should be less than 100%. Balance should be emphasized as the key to a healthful diet.

FEEDING THE IMPAIRED OLDER ADULT

Older adults experiencing hospitalization and those in institutional settings are more likely to experience a number of the problems that contribute to inadequate nutrition discussed earlier in this chapter. Poor oral health, swallowing disorders, lack of culturally appropriate food, depression, inadequate staffing to provide assistance with meals, and cognitive and physical impairment are some of the factors that contribute to nutritional deficiencies. Polypharmacy is also a common cause of malnutrition, and elders with chronic illnesses consume more medications. Medications most frequently associated with PCM include digoxin, theophylline, nonsteroidal anti-inflammatories, iron supplements, and psychoactive drugs. Weight loss in institutionalized older adults may be the result of a number of circumstances, both physical and emotional.

The incidence of eating disability in long-term care is high. Approximately 50% of all residents cannot eat independently (Burger et al, 2000). Inadequate staffing in nursing homes is associated with poor nutrition and hydration, and as Kayser-Jones (1997, p 19) states: "CNAs have an impossible task trying to feed the number of people who need assistance." She estimated that feeding impaired older adults in nursing homes with inadequate staff could mean that each CNA would be able to spend only about 6 to 10 minutes feeding a resident. Burger et al (2000) called for increases in staffing requirements in nursing homes, recommending the availability of one staff person for every two or three residents who need feeding assistance, thus allowing each resident about 20 to 30 minutes with the CNA. In response to concerns related to the lack of adequate assistance during mealtimes in nursing homes, the Centers for Medicare and Medicaid Services (CMS) implemented a new rule allowing feeding assistants with 8 hours of state-approved training to help nursing home residents with eating. Feeding assistants must be supervised by the registered nurse (RN) or licensed practical nurse (LPN). The new ruling is controversial, and various consumer groups (Alzheimer's Association, National Citizens' Coalition for Nursing Home Reform) have objected to the feeding assistant ruling, stating that the training requirement is inadequate and this is a poor substitute for increasing staffing levels in nursing homes. In the acute care hospital setting, it is equally important to give consideration, care, and attention to the feeding of the dependent older adult. Severely restricted diets, long periods of nothing-by-mouth (NPO) status, and insufficient time and staff for feeding assistance contribute to poor nutrition in this setting as well.

The use of restrictive therapeutic diets for frail elders in long-term care (low cholesterol, low salt, no concentrated sweets) often reduces food intake without significantly helping the clinical status of the resident and should be avoided (Tariq et al, 2001; Morley, 2003). If caloric supplements are used, they should be administered at least 1 hour before meals or they interfere with meal intake. Very little research has been conducted on the outcomes of caloric or "med-pass" nutritional supplements. Studies are warranted since these products are widely used, particularly in hospitals and nursing homes, and can be costly. One study (Kayser-Jones et al, 1998) reported that 75% of supplements ordered were dispensed and only 55% of residents consumed them as ordered.

Attention to the environment in which meals are served is also important. It is not uncommon in long-term care facilities to hear over the public address system at mealtime, "Feeder trays are ready." This reference to the need to feed those unable to feed themselves is, in itself, degrading and erases any trace of dignity the older person is trying to maintain in a controlled environment. It is not malicious intent by nurses or other caregivers but rather a habit of convenience. Feeding the older person who is unable to respond becomes mechanical and devoid of conversation and feeling. The feeding process becomes rapid, and if it bogs down and becomes too slow, the meal may be ended abruptly, depending on the time allotted for feeding. Any pleasure is destroyed that could be derived through socialization and eating, as is any dignity that could be maintained while dependent on others for food (See The Lived Experience at the beginning of this chapter for a poignant description of this by Lustbader [1999]).

In addition to adequate staff, there are many innovative and evidence-based ideas to improve nutritional intake in institutions. Restorative dining programs, homelike dining rooms, individualized menu choices including ethnic foods, cafeteria-style service, kitchens on the nursing unit, availability of food around the clock, choice of mealtimes, liberal diets, finger foods, visually appealing puree foods with texture and shape, music, touch, verbal cueing, hand-over-hand feeding, sitting while assisting a resident to eat, and many other adaptations are found in the literature (Brush et al, 2002; Simons et al, 2002; Roberts, Durnbaugh, 2002). The Council for Nutritional Strategies in Long-Term Care has developed a comprehensive structured approach to improve the management of nutritional problems in long-term care facilities that is a valuable resource for gerontological nurses and other members of the interdisciplinary team (http://www.ltcnutrition.org). A protocol for the assessment and management of eating and feeding difficulties for older people developed by Amella and the NICHE faculty is another valuable resource (Amella, 1998). Other suggestions to improve appetite and increase intake are presented in Box 10-13.

Feeding and nutrition issues are very complex, and the responsibility for ensuring adequate nutrition should not be left to unlicensed personnel. Gerontological nurses are responsible to ensure that patients receive adequate nutrition. Responsibilities of the licensed nurse include assistance and supervision with eating, appropriate delegation of tasks, staff training, assessment, and development of programs to enhance nutritional adequacy and enjoyment. Clearly, there is a need for comprehensive research into issues related to adequate nutrition for older people experiencing hospitalization or institutionalization.

Box 10-13	Suggestions to Improve Intake

- Determine food preferences, including ethnic preferences.
- Ensure that the person has adequate time to eat.
- Provide snacks between meals and at night.
- Do not interrupt meals with medications.
- Encourage family members to share the mealtimes for a heightened social situation.
- If caloric supplements are given, offer between meals or with the medication pass.
- Encourage eating in congregate dining for a more enjoyable social atmosphere.
- Recommend an exercise program that may increase appetite.
- Encourage proper fit of dentures and denture use.
- Wear glasses with meals.
- Sit while feeding a person who needs assistance, use touch, and carry on a social conversation.
- Provide music during dining.
- Use small round tables seating six to eight people; consider tablecloths and centerpieces.
- Seat people with like interests and abilities together, and encourage socialization.
- Utilize restorative dining programs and the use of adaptive equipment.

INTENTIONAL STARVATION

Refusal of food can be an acceptable means of suicide for the older person. Some older persons truly have given up and wish to die. Not eating is one last bastion of control over life and dignity. It is essential for the nurse to differentiate between the individual who is refusing food because it is unpalatable and the person who is depressed and really wishes to die. Assessment of depression and other modifiable factors contributing to refusal to eat is essential. Intentional starvation is easier and more successful when one is not institutionalized. The institutionalized person is often denied this right and is robbed of the option by forced feeding via a nasogastric tube. The American Nurses Association's position statement

NANDA and Wellness Diagnoses

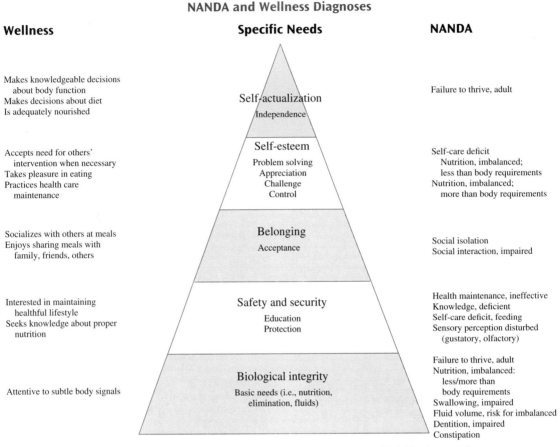

Wellness   **Specific Needs**   **NANDA**

Makes knowledgeable decisions about body function
Makes decisions about diet
Is adequately nourished

Self-actualization
Independence

Failure to thrive, adult

Accepts need for others' intervention when necessary
Takes pleasure in eating
Practices health care maintenance

Self-esteem
Problem solving
Appreciation
Challenge
Control

Self-care deficit
   Nutrition, imbalanced; less than body requirements
Nutrition, imbalanced; more than body requirements

Socializes with others at meals
Enjoys sharing meals with family, friends, others

Belonging
Acceptance

Social isolation
Social interaction, impaired

Interested in maintaining healthful lifestyle
Seeks knowledge about proper nutrition

Safety and security
Education
Protection

Health maintenance, ineffective
Knowledge, deficient
Self-care deficit, feeding
Sensory perception disturbed (gustatory, olfactory)

Attentive to subtle body signals

Biological integrity
Basic needs (i.e., nutrition, elimination, fluids)

Failure to thrive, adult
Nutrition, imbalanced: less/more than body requirements
Swallowing, impaired
Fluid volume, risk for imbalanced
Dentition, impaired
Constipation

These are not all of the possible wellness or NANDA diagnoses that may be identified. The above are frequent examples of nursing diagnoses that should be considered when planning care for the older adult in whatever setting.

on forgoing artificial nutrition and hydration (1992) states: "The decision to withhold artificial nutrition and hydration should be made by the patient or surrogate with the health care team. The nurse continues to provide expert care to patients who are no longer receiving artificial nutrition and hydration."

Watching someone starve is difficult for the nurse, but if intentional starvation is the patient's desire, the nurse should continue to order the tray, take it to the person, and acknowledge that the individual has the right to eat or not eat. It is important to leave the tray so that the person can exercise the option to change his or her mind. If the person is unable to feed himself or herself, the nurse should check shortly after the first offering of food has been refused to see if the person does wish to eat. An empathetic and nonjudgmental approach by the nurse to the older person who demonstrates starvation behavior will convey that the individual is still in control, and if for some reason the individual decides to exercise the option to eat again, that, too, is all right. Either way, the caregiver has provided support and respect for that individual. Professional team conferences are needed to deal with the client's mental status and ethical issues involved in refusal to eat and the right to die. Superficial judgments are not adequate to encompass these profound issues.

IMPLICATIONS FOR GERONTOLOGICAL NURSING AND HEALTHY AGING

Maintenance of adequate nutritional health as one ages is extremely complex. Knowledge of normal nutrition in later years and the many factors contributing to inadequate nutrition is essential for the gerontological nurse and should be a part of every assessment of an older person. Working with members of the interdisciplinary team in appropriate assessment and development of therapeutic interventions is a major role in community, hospital, and long-term care settings. Use of evidence-based practice protocols is important in determining nursing interventions to support and enhance nutritional status and promote adequate bowel function. Ensuring adequate nutrition in aging is a very important role for gerontological nurses and one in which nurses have made significant contributions to the understanding, prevention, treatment, and implementation of best practices. Prevention of undernutrition and malnutrition and the maintenance of dietary needs and food enjoyment until the end of life are also ethical responsibilities. No older person should be hungry or thirsty because he or she cannot shop, cook, or buy food. Nor should any older persons have to suffer because of a lack of assistance with these activities in whatever setting they may reside.

APPLICATION OF MASLOW'S HIERARCHY

Food is a basic human need for people of all ages. Attention must be paid to more than just adequate caloric intake to sustain life. Not only does adequate nutrition satisfy biological needs, but also the experience of eating provides opportunities for belonging. Being able to eat independently and enjoy meals or being provided with kind and competent assistance if unable to be independent promotes self-esteem and a feeling of worth.

▶ KEY CONCEPTS

- Interruption of basic required nutrients may trigger subclinical or chronic disorders.

- Recommended dietary patterns for the older adult are similar to those of younger persons, with some reduction in caloric intake based on decreased metabolic requirements.
- Adequate nutrition is affected by lifelong eating habits and patterns, accessibility of food, mood disorders, capacity for food preparation, and income.
- Medications may interfere with absorption, digestion, and elimination.
- There are many factors affecting adequate nutrition in older adults. A comprehensive nutritional assessment is an essential component of assessment of older adults.
- Making mealtime pleasant and attractive for the older adult who is unable to eat unassisted is a nursing challenge; mealtime *must* be made enjoyable, and there *must* be adequate assistance provided.

▶ Activities and Discussion Questions

1. What are the factors affecting the nutrition of the older adult?
2. How can the nurse intervene to provide better nutrition for elders in the community, in acute care, and in long-term care settings?
3. What are the causes of malnutrition?
4. What is included in the nutritional assessment of an older person?
5. What are the factors contributing to alterations in bowel function as one ages?
6. What proactive measures can the nurse take to promote adequate bowel function for older adults in the community, in acute care, and in long-term care settings?
7. Develop a nursing care plan using wellness and North American Nursing Diagnosis Association (NANDA) diagnoses.

RESOURCES

Websites

Administration on Aging
Washington, DC 20201
(202) 619-0724
website: http://www.aoa.gov

Cooking for One
http://www.eldercare.uniontrib.com/recipes/index.cfm

http://www.solodining.com/cooking4one.html
http://www.microwave cookingfor one.com
http://www.bhg.com

Food and Drug Administration
5600 Fishers Lane
Rockville, MD 20857
(888) 463-6332
website: http://www.fda.gov

Food and Nutrition Information Center
Agricultural Research Service, USDA National
    Agricultural Library, Room 105
10301 Baltimore Avenue
Beltsville, MD 20705-2351
(301) 504-6409
e-mail: fnic@nal.usda.gov
website: http://www.nal.usda.gov/fnic/

General Nutrition Resource List for Seniors
Comprehensive list of information and educational
    materials related to senior nutrition
    http://www.nal.usda/gov/fnic/pubs/old.htm

REFERENCES

Allison OC, Porter ME, Briggs GC: Chronic constipation: assessment and management in the elderly, *J Am Acad Nurse Pract* 6(7):311-317, 1994.

Amella EJ: Assessment and management of eating and feeding difficulties for older people: a NICHE Protocol, *Geriatr Nurs* 19(5):269-274, 1998.

American Nurses Association: *Position statement on forgoing artificial nutrition and hydration,* Washington, DC, 1992, American Nurses Association.

Beers M, Berkow R: *Merck manual of geriatrics,* ed 3, Whitehouse Station, NJ, 2000, Merck Research Laboratories.

Bennett J: Dehydration: Hazards and benefits, *Geriatr Nurs* 21(2):84-88, 2000.

Beverley L, Travis I: Constipation: proposed natural laxative mixtures, *J Gerontol Nurs* 18(10):5-12, 1992.

Blackington E, McCormick, T, Willson B et al: Oropharyngeal dysphagia in the elderly: identifying and managing patients at risk, *Adv Nurse Pract* 9(7):42-49, 2001.

Blaum CS, Fries BE, Fiatarone MA: Factors associated with low body mass index and weight loss in nursing home residents, *J Gerontol A Biol Sci Med Sci* 50(3):M162-M168, 1995.

Brush J, Meehan R, Calkins M: Using the environment to improve intake for people with dementia, *Alzheimer's Care Q* 3(4):330-338, 2002.

Burger S, Kayser-Jones J, Bell J: Malnutrition and dehydration in nursing homes: key issues in prevention and treatment, 2000. Accessed 7/23/04 from http:www.cmwf.org/programs/elders/burger_mal_386.asp.

Chouinard J: Dysphagia in Alzheimer disease: a review, *J Nutr Health Aging* 4(4):214-217, 2000.

Coleman P: Improving oral health care for the frail elderly in nursing homes: a review of widespread problems and best practices, *Geriatr Nurs* 23(4):189-199, 2002.

Crogan NL, Pasvogel A: The influence of protein-calorie malnutrition on quality of life in nursing homes, *J Gerontol* 58:159-164, 2003.

Dawson-Hughes B, Harris SS: Calcium intake influences the association of protein intake with rates of bone loss in elderly men and women, *Am J Clin Nutr* 75(4):773-779, 2002.

Edwards W: Gastrointestinal problems. In Cotter VT, Strumpf NE, editors: *Advanced practice nursing with older adults,* New York, 2002, McGraw-Hill.

Finucane TE, Christmas C, Travis K: Tube feeding in patients with advanced dementia: a review of the evidence. *JAMA* 282(14):1365-1370, 1999.

Grundy SM, Cleeman JI, Merz CN et al: Implications of recent clinical trials for the National Cholesterol Education Program Adult Treatment Panel III Guidelines, *Circulation* 110(2):227-239, 2004.

Ham R, Sloane P, Warshaw G: *Primary care geriatrics,* ed 4, St Louis, 2002, Mosby.

Jensen GL, McGee M, Binkley J: Nutrition in the elderly, *Gastroenterol Clin North Am* 30(2):313-334, 2001.

Johnson KA, Bernard MA, Funderburg K: Vitamin nutrition in older adults, *Clin Geriatr Med* 18(4):773-799, 2002.

Jones JA, Spiro A III, Miller DR et al: Need for dental care in older veterans: assessment of patient-based measures, *J Am Geriatr Soc* 50(1):163-168, 2002.

Kayser-Jones J: Inadequate staffing at mealtime: implications for nursing and health policy, *J Gerontol Nurs* 23(8):14-21, 1997.

Kayser-Jones J, Schell ES, Porter C et al: A prospective study of the use of liquid oral dietary supplements in nursing homes. *J Am Geriatr Soc* 46(11):1378-1386, 1998.

Krebs-Smith SM, Heimendinger J, Patterson BH, et al: Psychosocial factors associated with fruit and vegetable consumption, *Am J Health Promot* 10(2):98-104, 1995.

Lustbader W: Thoughts on the meaning of frailty, *Generations* 13(4):21-22, 1999.

McDowell IF, Lang D: Homocysteine and endothelial dysfunction: a link with cardiovascular disease, *J Nutr* 130(2S, suppl):369S-372S, 2000.

Meydani SN, Meydani M, Blumberg JB et al: Assessment of the safety of supplementation with different amounts of vitamin E in healthy older adults, *Am J Clin Nutr* 68(2):311-318, 1998.

Meyyazhagan S, Palmer RM: Nutritional requirements with aging: prevention of disease, *Clin Geriatr Med* 18(3):557-576, 2002.

Miceli BV: Nursing unit meal management maintenance program: continuation of safe-swallowing and feeding beyond skilled therapeutic intervention, *J Gerontol Nurs* 25(8):22-36, 1999.

Miller C: *Nursing for wellness in older adults*, Philadelphia, 2004, Lippincott Williams & Wilkins.

Mitchell SL, Kiely, DK, Hamel MB et al: Clinical and organizational factors associated with feeding tube use among nursing home residents with advanced cognitive impairment, *JAMA* 290(1):73-80, 2003.

Moore M: *Nutritional care*, St Louis, 2001, Mosby.

Morley JE: Why do physicians fail to recognize and treat malnutrition in older persons? *J Am Geriatr Soc* 39(11):1139-1140, 1991.

Morley JE: Anorexia of aging: physiologic and pathologic, *Am J Clin Nutr* 66(4):760-773, 1997.

Morley JE: Orexigenic and anabolic agents, *Clin Geriatr Med* 18(4):853-66, 2002.

Morley JE: Anorexia and weight loss in older persons, *J Gerontol A Biol Sci Med Sci* 58(2):131-137, 2003.

Morley JE, Kraenzle D: Causes of weight loss in a community nursing home, *J Am Geriatr Soc* 42(2):583-585, 1994.

Morley JE, Silver AJ: Nutritional issues in nursing home care, *Ann Intern Med* 123(11):850-859, 1995.

National Policy and Resource Center of Nutrition and Aging, Issue Panel: Dietary reference intakes and dietary guidelines in Older Americans Act (OAA) Nutrition programs, press release, Jan. 31, 2002.

Neal LJ: Power pudding: natural laxative therapy for the elderly who are homebound, *Home Health Nurse* 13(3):66-71, 1995.

Nutrition Screening Initiative, project of American Academy of Family Physicians, American Dietetic Association, and National Council on Aging, Inc. Grant from Ross-Abbott Laboratories, Inc, 1991.

Papas A, Niessen L, Chauncey H: *Geriatric dentistry: aging and oral health*, St Louis, 1991, Mosby.

Pear R: Nutrition therapy to fall under Medicare umbrella, *New York Times*, Dec. 31, 2001.

Robbins J et al: Dysphagia research in the 21st century and beyond: proceedings from Dysphagia Experts Meeting, 2001, *J Rehabil Res Dev* 39:543-548, 2001.

Roberts S, Durnbaugh T: Enhancing nutrition and eating skills in long-term care, *Alzheimer's Care Q* 3:316-329, 2002.

Rousseau P: Aging and chronic constipation, *Geriatr Med Today* 9(3):35, 1990.

Shanley C, O'Loughlin G: Dysphagia among nursing home residents: An assessment and management protocol, *J Gerontol Soc* 26(8):35-48, 2000.

Simons D, Brailsford S, Kidd E, Beighton D: The effects of medicated chewing gums on oral health in frail older people: a 1-year clinical trial, *J Am Geriatr Soc* 50(8):1348-1353, 2002.

Tariq S, Karcic E, Thomas D et al: The use of a no-concentrated sweets diet in the management of type 2 diabetes in nursing homes, *J Am Diet Assoc* 101(12):1463-1466, 2001.

Terpenning M, Taylor GW, Lopatin DE et al: Aspiration pneumonia: Dental and oral risk factors in an older veteran population, *J Amer Geriatr Soc* 50(3):589-590, 2002.

Thomas D, Zdrowski, Wilson M et al: Malnutrition in subacute care, *Am J Clin Nutr* 75(2):308-313, 2002.

U.S Bureau of the Census: Statistical abstract of the United States, 2000, Washington, DC, 2001. Availabe at www.census.gov/press-release.

U.S. Department of Health and Human Services: *Healthy people 2010*, Hyattsville, Md, 2002, Public Health Service. Available from www.healthypeople.gov.

vanAsselt DZB et al: Role of cobalmin intake and atrophic gastritis in older Dutch subjects, *Am J Clin Nutr* 68:328, 2000.

Wakefield B: A food pyramid for the elderly, *Women's Health Primary Care* 3(1):36, 2000.

Wakimoto, P, Block G: Dietary intake, dietary patterns and changes with age: An epidemiological perspective, *J Geront* 56(A) (Special Issue II):65-80, 2001.

Whitmyer CC, Terezhalmy GT, Miller DL et al: Clinical evaluation of the efficacy and safety of an ultrasonic toothbrush system in an elderly patient population, *Geriatr Nurs* 19(1):29-33, 1998.

Wilson MM, Vaswani S, Liu D et al: Prevalence and causes of undernutrition in medical outpatients, *Am J Med* 104(1):56-63, 1998.

11

Fluids and Continence

▶ LEARNING OBJECTIVES

Upon completion of this chapter, the reader will be able to:

- Identify some manifestations of inadequate fluid intake.
- Discuss interventions to prevent or treat dehydration.
- Define *urinary* and *fecal incontinence.*
- List factors contributing to urinary and fecal incontinence.
- Explain the types of urinary incontinence and their causes.
- Discuss interventions for urinary and fecal incontinence.

▶ GLOSSARY

Detrusor A body part that pushes down, such as the bladder muscle.
Iatrogenic An adverse condition resulting from treatment by a physician or nurse or other health care provider.

Incontinence The inability to control excretory function.
Micturition Urination.
Transient Temporary.

▶ THE LIVED EXPERIENCE

I know I must smell of urine and others don't want to be around me. It has gotten to the point where I don't want to go anywhere. I know Harry gets irritated with me when I need to stop so often to find a bathroom. But, even so, I can't always hold the urine no matter how I try. Beth told me about an incontinence clinic in the city. I guess I really need to find out if they can help me.

Maria, age 60, mother of eight children

It really is too bad so many women think nothing can be done about their problems with incontinence. Just today I met Maria, who has been unable to control her urination for such a long time. I think Kegel exercises may help, but she may need surgery. I'll need to get a consult for her.

Betty, director of an incontinence clinic

*W*ater, an accessible and available commodity to all, is often overlooked as an essential part of nutritional requirements. Water's function in the body includes thermoregulation, dilution of water-soluble medications, facilitation of renal and bowel function, and creating and maintaining metabolic processes.

The percentage of total body water decreases from the time of infancy to old age. By older adulthood, body water composition has decreased to 50% or less of the elder's body weight (Bennett, 2000). This is due to the loss of water content and the increase of body fat, which contains less water. Even small decreases in fluid intake can cause more dehydration in an elder than in a child. The concentrating ability of old kidneys decreases, so urine flow is not diminished with dehydration until late. Thirst decreases in advancing age, resulting in the loss of an important defense against dehydration.

No accepted standard measure to calculate the total body water needs of elders is available at present, but no evidence exists that they need less fluid than younger people (Gaspar, 1999). However, it has been recommended by a number of researchers that 1500 to 2000 ml of noncaffeinated fluids be consumed every 24 hours by the older adult to maintain adequate hydration.

HYDRATION/DEHYDRATION

According to Amella (cited in Peters, 1998), "Old people sit on the edge of dehydration." Dehydration is the most common fluid and electrolyte disorder of frail elders in long-term care and in the community (Burger et al, 2000). Dehydration has serious consequences for older people, including delirium, urinary and respiratory infections, urinary incontinence, constipation and impaction, pressure ulcers, cardiovascular symptoms, increased acute care admissions, and even death (Bennett, 2000; Mentes, 2000). Medications such as diuretics, sedatives, and antipsychotics, alcohol abuse, dementia, inability to feed self, and lack of mobility are additional factors contributing to dehydration in older adults. The incidence of dehydration in long-term care facilities is high, primarily related to the frail status of residents and inadequate fluid intake (Bennett, 2000; Burger et

al, 2000). In hot weather, increased perspiration and evaporation deplete the individual of needed body fluid. Fever, upper respiratory tract infections, and diarrhea also cause dehydration in the aged.

The American Medical Directors Association (AMDA), in the *Clinical Practice Guideline: Dehydration and Fluid Maintenance* (2001) (http://www.amda.com), defines dehydration as the loss of body water causing significant signs and symptoms including physical and/or functional decline from individual baseline. There are three types of dehydration: isotonic, hypertonic, and hypotonic. All of the following elements must be present to diagnose clinical dehydration:

- Suspicion of increased output and/or decreased input
- At least two physiological or functional signs of dehydration (dizziness, dry mucous membranes, functional decline)

  Any of the following must be present:
- Blood urea nitrogen (BUN)/creatinine ratio greater than 25:1
- Orthostasis of systolic blood pressure 20 mm Hg on a change in position
- Pulse greater than 100 beats/min or pulse change of 10 to 20 beats/min more than the patient's baseline pulse on a change in position

Assessment of dehydration is difficult in older people. The clinical signs of dehydration may not appear until dehydration is advanced (Bennett, 2000). Manifestations of dehydration in elders include altered mental status, light-headedness, syncope, orthostatic hypotension, weight loss, and dry mucous membranes, all of which can also be symptoms of other disease entities. Standard indicators for dehydration in older people are unreliable. Skin turgor assessment, if done improperly, is unreliable, and weight alone may not reveal the extent of dehydration in the community and nursing home setting. Dry mucous membranes may be misleading because many elderly persons are mouth breathers and many medications cause dry mouth. Intake and output recordings are generally unreliable because they are not consistently maintained. Urine-specific gravity is poorly correlated with serum biochemical parameters of hydration status because the older kidney has difficulty concentrating urine (Peters, 1998). Laboratory parameters can be used (i.e., BUN and creatinine), but other conditions

Box 11-1	OBRA 1987/1990 Minimum Data Set: Dehydration/Fluid Maintenance Triggers and Additional Risk Factors for Dehydration Among Nursing Home Residents

Dehydration/Fluid Maintenance Triggers
Deterioration in cognitive status, skills, or
    abilities in last 90 days
Failure to eat or take medication(s)
Urinary tract infection in last 30 days
Current diagnosis of dehydration (*ICD-9** code
    276-5)
Diarrhea
Dizziness/vertigo
Fever
Internal bleeding
Vomiting
Weight loss (≥5% in last 30 days; or 10% in last
    180 days)
Insufficient fluid intake (dehydrated)
Did not consume all/almost all liquids provided
    during last 3 days

Leaves ≥25% food uneaten at most meals
Requirement for parenteral (intravenous) fluids

Additional Potential Risk Factors
Hand dexterity/body control problems
Use of diuretics
Abuse of laxatives
Uncontrolled diabetes mellitus
Swallowing problems
Purposeful restriction of fluids
Patients on enteral feedings (need free water in
    addition to feedings)
History of previous episodes of dehydration
Comprehension/communication problems

From Omnibus Budget Reconciliation Act of 1987 and 1990 (federal).
*ICD-9 indicates *International Classification of Diseases*, ed 9.

that can occur in the elderly can alter these laboratory findings. In the nursing home setting, information from the Minimum Data Set (MDS) and the Resident Assessment Protocols (RAP) triggers (see Chapter 5) for dehydration can assist in assessment and identification of dehydration. The indicators are presented in Box 11-1. Malnutrition and dehydration go hand in hand so assessment of both is important. An article entitled "Hydration Management Protocol" (Mentes, 2000) presents a comprehensive guide to assessment, prevention, and treatment of dehydration.

Prevention of dehydration through ensuring adequate fluid intake, preferably water, is essential. Oral hydration is the first treatment approach when dehydration occurs if the patient is able to ingest fluids. Sports drinks, although high in sugar, are often recommended over tap water because they can be easily absorbed by the stomach, are generally palatable to patients, and will more rapidly correct the situation. Other fluids, such as Pedialyte or other commercial fluid-and-electrolyte solutions, are also available. It is suggested that unless contraindicated by a medical condition such as heart failure, renal disease, or liver disease, 30 ml of fluid per kilogram of body weight be consumed to maintain an adequately hydrated state. The last-resort treatment approaches are hypodermoclysis and intravenous therapy (Weinberg, Minaker, 1995). It is also important for gerontological nurses to teach older adults and informal and formal caregivers the symptoms of dehydration, the importance of fluid intake, and ways to increase fluid intake. Interventions to prevent dehydration are presented in Box 11-2.

BLADDER FUNCTION IN OLD AGE

Normal bladder function requires an intact brain and spinal cord, a competent bladder, and active sphincters that will sustain maximum urethral pressure against rising bladder pressure. A full bladder increases pressure and signals the spinal cord and the brainstem center the desire to micturate. Social training then dictates whether mic-

Box 11-2	Measures to Help Prevent Dehydration of Institutionalized Elderly Persons

- Ensure a 24-hour intake of at least 1500 ml of oral fluid unless there are special medical concerns, such as congestive heart failure.
- Offer fluids hourly during the day. Include fluids with an evening snack. Give a full glass of fluid with medications.
- Offer other fluids in addition to water. Find out the types of beverages liked and fluid temperature preferred.
- Provide cups, glasses, and pitchers that are not too big or heavy for the person to handle. (Help those who cannot help themselves to fluids.)
- Allow adequate time and staff for eating or feeding. Meals can provide two thirds of daily fluids.
- Provide beverage carts or a hydration station in accessible areas.
- Encourage family members to participate in feeding and offering fluids.
- Remember that coffee acts as a diuretic. Fluid loss by coffee should be supplemented to compensate for the fluid loss.
- Listen to bowel sounds. Note any change in bowel activity. (Extra soft or loose stool means losing water, and hard stool means dehydration.)

- Be familiar with tests or examinations that the patient may have had. If they involved enemas or laxatives or were NPO (nothing orally) before the tests, there will be a fluid loss.
- Replace fluids when there has been nothing consumed orally or fluids have been lost from test preparation.
- Obtain a drug history to identify medications contributing to poor intake or dehydration.
- Note increases in pulse and respirations and decrease in blood pressure (suggestive of dehydration).
- Check laboratory values for changes: sodium, blood urea nitrogen, hematocrit, hemoglobin, urine and serum osmolarity, and creatinine. Also check for signs of acidosis.
- Weigh the patient daily at the same time, on the same scale, and in the same clothing/chair.
- If a resident develops fever, vomiting, or diarrhea, monitor intake and output.
- Identify residents at risk for dehydration (dysphagia, dependence in feeding, immobile, dementia, malnutrition, depressed).

Adapted from Reedy DF: How can you prevent dehydration? *Geriatr Nurs* 9(4):224-226, 1988; Bennett JA: Dehydration: hazards and benefits, *Geriatr Nurs* 21(2):84-88, 2000.

turition should be attended to or should be postponed until there is an appropriate opportunity to seek out toilet facilities. However, when the bladder contents reach 500 ml or more, the pressure is such that it becomes more difficult to control the urge to void. As volume increases, emptying the bladder becomes an uncontrollable act. The bladder of an older person retains its tonus, but the volume it can hold decreases. If cerebrovascular disease or dementia is present, the changes are exaggerated and bladder control becomes diminished. Nocturnal frequency is common in two thirds of women and men over age 65 who do not take medication and in more than 80% of those elders with three chronic diseases (Wasson, Bruskewitz, 1990).

Many healthy older people are annoyed by frequency and some degree of urgency. The warning period between the desire to void and actual micturition is shortened or lost. In combination with age-related changes, illness, cognitive impairments, difficulty in walking or handling a bedpan or urinal, and problems manipulating clothing may be responsible for some incontinence. Drugs that increase urinary output and sedatives, tranquilizers, and hypnotics, which produce drowsiness, confusion, or limited mobility, promote incontinence by dulling the transmission of the desire to micturate.

URINARY INCONTINENCE

Incontinence, or the loss of ability to control the elimination of urine or feces on an occasional or consistent basis, is one of the most prevalent symptoms encountered in care of older adults. Incontinence causes considerable embarrassment and astronomical costs both socially and economically. The economic costs are $11.2 billion annually in the community and nearly $5.3 billion in long-term care settings (Fourcroy, 2001). Estimates of costs and numbers of individuals enduring incontinence vary widely because many people isolate themselves and keep silent about the problem. Urinary incontinence (UI) affects 12% or more of the older adult population. Estimates are that approximately 10% to 30% of community-living elders, 30% to 35% of elders who are hospitalized, and 50% of elders living in nursing homes experience UI (Ham et al, 2002). Women are at least twice as likely as men to experience UI (Mason et al, 2003). Continence must be routinely addressed in the initial assessment of every older person, yet many older people do not bring up their concerns about incontinence, and many health professionals do not ask. A recent survey of 1400 Americans revealed that despite the prevalence of UI, 64% of those experiencing symptoms were not doing anything to manage their condition. On average, adults waited 6 years after first experiencing symptoms before talking to a health care professional. The common belief that incontinence is inevitable with age leads to inadequate assessment and treatment, and in fact, 38% of those surveyed believed loss of bladder control was just a part of natural aging (accessed 8/5/04 from http://www.nafc.org/NAFCNewsRelease.asp). Incontinence is not a result of advancing age, nor is it a disease. It is a symptom of existing environmental, psychological, drug, or physical disturbances and can become a catastrophic event when it interferes with mobility, sociability, and the ability to remain in one's home. Box 11-3 enumerates risk factors associated with incontinence.

Incontinence ushers in dependence, shame, guilt, and fear. Older people who are aware of a problem of continence are mortified by their state. Psychological consequences of UI include depressive symptoms as a result of anxiety and embarrassment about appearance and odor of urine. This can lead to restricted social activities, isolation, and avoidance of sexual activity. Physical consequences of UI include skin problems (rashes, breakdown, infection), pressure ulcers, urinary tract infections (UTIs), and falls. UI is one of the

| Box 11-3 | **Risk Factors for Urinary Incontinence** |

Immobility of chronic degenerative diseases
Diminished cognitive status, dementia
Delirium
Medications (anticholinergic properties, sedatives, diuretics)
Smoking
Fecal impaction
Low fluid intake
Environmental barriers
High-impact physical exercise
Diabetes
Stroke
Estrogen deficiency
Pelvic muscle weakness
High caffeine intake
Hysterectomy in older women
Childhood enuresis
Pregnancy
Morbid obesity
Environmental barriers

Modified from Fantl JA et al: *Managing acute and chronic urinary incontinence. Clinical practice guideline: quick reference guide for clinicians no. 2, 1996 update, AHCPR pub no. 96-0686*, Rockville, Md, 1996, U.S. Department of Health and Human Services, Public Health Service, Agency for Health Care Policy and Research.

four independent risk factors for institutionalization. Other factors are cognitive impairment, dependence in ambulation, and being unmarried (Ham et al, 2002; Holroyd-Leduc, Straus, 2004).

Health care personnel must begin to change their thinking about incontinence and acknowledge that incontinence can be cured. If it cannot be cured, it can be treated to minimize its detrimental effects. The nurse who cares for the incontinent person either in the community or in other types of facilities needs sensitivity, insight, patience, and understanding. Reassurance rather than guilt should be promoted. The Agency for Health Care Policy and Research (AHCPR) (now AHRQ) increased awareness and knowledge about incontinence and has continued to disseminate factual information through the publication of the Clinical Practice Guideline, *Urinary Inconti-*

nence in Adults, in 1992 and the updated version in 1996 (http://www.guidelines.gov). This information attempts to improve reporting, diagnosis, and treatment of the ambulatory and non-ambulatory individual and to educate health professionals and consumers about urinary incontinence (Fantl et al, 1996). The AMDA (1996) clinical practice guidelines on UI in long-term care are another valuable resource for nurses working in nursing homes (http:www.amda.com), and the "Nursing Standard-of-Practice Protocol: Urinary Incontinence in Older Adults Admitted to Acute Care" (Bradway, Hernly, 1998) is useful for nurses in acute care. Wyman (2003) noted that despite a substantial amount of evidence-based practice protocols, a national clinical practice guideline, identification of competencies for both generalist and specialist practice, and a growing public awareness, UI continues to be underdetected, underdiagnosed, and undertreated across all practice settings. Some who have been diagnosed with UI do not receive treatment, particularly those with cognitive impairments or depression. "Continence remains undervalued, and UI remains underassessed. Even though UI is a basic nursing care issue, nurses are not claiming it as one" (Mason et al, 2003, p 3). Educational competencies for beginning nursing practice in continence care are presented in Box 11-4.

Types of Urinary Incontinence

The types of UI categorized by symptoms are stress, urge, overflow, iatrogenic, mixed, and functional (Dash et al, 2004). Overactive bladder UI, iatrogenic UI, and mixed UI are also commonly cited in the literature. Transient urinary incontinence, the result of functional and iatrogenic causes, can be remembered by the mnemonic *DRIP* (Box 11-5).

Stress incontinence occurs more often in elderly women and occurs when intraabdominal pressure exceeds urethral resistance. Muscles around the urethra become weak so even a small amount of urine may spontaneously pass. It occurs frequently in obese individuals, especially apple-shaped (rather than pear-shaped) individuals (Fourcroy, 2001). It is more common in white women than in African American women but research on UI in minorities is limited. Involuntary urine loss may occur when an individual

sneezes, coughs, bends over, or lifts a heavy object. The amount of urine leakage usually is usually small and the volume is low when postresidual urine is obtained or visualized by ultrasound.

Urge incontinence, or overactive bladder, is more common in younger women and is caused by central nervous system lesions such as stroke, demyelinating diseases, and local irritating factors such as bladder tumors or UTIs. Individuals sense the urge to void but cannot inhibit urination long enough to reach a toilet. The volume of urine lost is moderate, and episodes occur every few hours. Postresidual urine reveals a low volume.

Overflow incontinence is a result of neurological abnormalities of the spinal cord that affect the contractility of the detrusor muscle of the bladder. Any factor disrupting detrusor stability, such as drugs, tumors, strictures, and prostatic hypertrophy, will cause the bladder to become overdistended, leading to frequent or constant loss of urine. Postresidual urine volumes may be high.

Functional incontinence refers to a situation in which the lower urinary tract is intact but the individual is limited by environmental factors, musculoskeletal disability, or severe cognitive impairment. Urine is lost because the individual is unaware of the need to void or is unable to reach a toilet because of arthritis, Parkinson's disease, or, for hospitalized patients, their condition or raised side rails or restraints.

Iatrogenic incontinence is associated with medication side effects. This can be managed by decreasing the dosage of medication to maintain the primary drug effect but eliminate the secondary effects. It may be necessary to change a drug to another class of medication that is not associated with incontinence. Other iatrogenic causes of incontinence include expanded extracellular fluid compartmentalization with the development of nocturia and polyuria, such as occurs in heart failure, in chronic venous insufficiency, and in metabolic states such as polyuria with increased glycosuria or increased calcemia.

In *mixed incontinence,* more than one urinary incontinence problem exists in the same individual. These conditions can be caused by anatomical, physiological, or pathological factors (internal factors) or by outside factors, such as mobility, dexterity, motivation, and environment. Most older adults with UI have the mixed type.

A professional nurse will be able to independently:
1. Obtain a focused health history to include the following:
   A. The presence of risk factors for urinary incontinence (UI) and medical conditions that may be contributing to UI and identifying patients at risk for the development of UI
   B. Confirming the presence and effect of UI subjectively
   C. A detailed exploration of the symptoms of UI and associated factors
   D. Medication review including prescription and nonprescription drugs to identify those patients whose medications may negatively affect urine control
   E. Bowel pattern to include frequency, consistency, and usage of any assistive products (e.g., dietary measures, prescription and nonprescription medications including suppositories and enemas)
   F. Functional, environmental, social, and cognitive factors that may contribute to or result in UI
2. Obtain an intake and output record that includes the following:
   A. Voiding records from patients that include time and onset of incontinent episodes, voiding pattern, 24-hour recording with diurnal and nocturnal frequency, amount voided, amount leaked, activity when leakage
   B. Intake record with 24-hour pattern of fluid intake that includes amount, frequency, and type of oral intake
3. Obtain diagnostic measures to detect evidence of urinary tract infection and other disorders contributing to incontinence that may include the following:
   A. Urinalysis or the use of a chemically treated dipstick to detect hematuria, pyuria, bacteriuria, glycosuria, or proteinuria
   B. Obtaining a clean-catch or catheterized urine specimen for culture and sensitivity if indicated
   C. Obtaining a catheterized urine specimen to detect amount of urine in bladder or postvoid residual (PVR) volume or bladder ultrasound
4. Conduct a physical examination that includes the following:
   A. Focused abdominal examination to estimate suprapubic fullness, to rule out palpable hard stool, and to evaluate bowel sounds
   B. Examination of the genitals, including skin integrity of perineum, appearance of urethral meatus, and presence of prolapse

C. Rectal examination including evaluation of sphincter tone, perineal sensation, and presence or absence of fecal impaction
   D. Confirming the presence of UI objectively and evaluation of the force and character of urine stream during voiding with observation of actual toileting of client
   E. A functional assessment, including mobility, self-care ability, mental status examination, and communication patterns
5. Assess environment
6. Initiate nursing interventions that include the following:
   A. Strategies that promote bladder health (fluid hydration, caffeine reduction, bowel programs, dietary strategies, weight reduction, smoking and alcohol reduction)
   B. Educating and counseling patients and families (e.g., anatomy and physiology of genitourinary system, factors affecting continence, etiological factors related to UI treatment options available to patients who may benefit from scheduled voiding regimens without further testing)
   C. Identifying patients who require further evaluation before therapeutic intervention; collaborating with physicians or advanced practice nurses regarding diagnosis, intervention plan, expected outcomes, and ongoing evaluation
   D. Implementing scheduled toileting programs for functional incontinence and evaluating effectiveness
   E. Supervising nursing staff in the implementation of prompted voiding and scheduled toileting programs and evaluation of effectiveness
   F. Evaluating patients with indwelling catheters for voiding trial and initiation of bladder training
   G. Teaching pelvic muscle exercises to patients at risk for developing stress incontinence
   H. Implementing bladder training programs for early symptoms of stress or urgency
   I. Implementing scheduled toileting programs for patients at risk for developing functional incontinence before UI develops
   J. Identifying patients who would benefit from assistive devices to maintain continence
   K. Recommending appropriate containment devices and topical therapy for prevention and management of skin breakdown

From Jirovec MM, Wyman JF, Wells TJ: Addressing urinary incontinence with educational continence—Care competencies, *Image J Nurs Sch* 30(4):375-378, 1998.

Sample Voiding or Bladder Diary

Name_____   Date_____

Time	Type of intake	Amount of intake	Urge to void	Voided	Leak	Activity

Measured Urine:

Time: Amount:

Figure 11-1 Sample voiding or bladder diary.

Box 11-5 Causes of Acute or Transient Incontinence

D Delirium, depression, dehydration, dementia
R Restricted mobility, retention
I Infection, inflammation, impaction (fecal)
P Polyuria, pharmaceuticals

Modified from Kane RL, Ouslander JG, Abrass IB: *Essentials of clinical geriatrics*, ed 3, New York, 1994, McGraw-Hill.

IMPLICATIONS FOR GERONTOLOGICAL NURSING AND HEALTHY AGING

Assessment

Nurses are often the ones to identify urinary incontinence, but neither nurses nor physicians have been particularly aggressive in management. Assessment is multidimensional. It includes a health history, physical examination, and urinalysis. More extensive examinations are considered after the initial findings are assessed. A thorough health history should focus on the medical, neurological, and genitourinary history; medication review of both prescribed and over-the-counter drugs; a detailed exploration of the symptoms of the urinary incontinence; and associated symptoms and other factors. Nurses, in general, should be able to gather data that will help the physician or the advanced practice nurse in accurate diagnosis and treatment. Box 11-6 presents the assessment of urinary elimination.

One of the best ways to validate and describe incontinence problems is with a voiding diary (Figure 11-1). This is applicable to both community-dwelling and institutionalized elders. Accurate notations should be made of significant burning, itching, or pressure. The character of the urine (color, odor, sediment, or clear) and difficulty starting or stopping the urinary stream should be recorded. Activities of daily living (ADLs) such as ability to reach a toilet and use it and finger dexterity for clothing manipulation should be documented. Older adults in the community can usually do this without much difficulty. Bladder diaries for those in long-term care are usually maintained by the staff. Bladder diaries enable not only identification of problems but also evaluation of the effectiveness of nursing interventions and treatment. Following the MDS requires only a summary of incontinence using the following five categories:

0—Complete control
1—Usually continent (incontinent once per week or less)
2—Occasionally incontinent (two or more times per week but not daily)

Box 11-6   Elements of an Incontinence Assessment

History
1. Onset
   a. Recent onset within past 6 months
   b. Onset within past 3 years
   c. Persistent problem for >3 years
2. Frequency
   a. Once each day or less
   b. At least once and up to twice each day
   c. Three times each day or more
   d. Nighttime only
3. Severity
   a. Small amounts of urine lost
   b. Moderate amount of urine lost
   c. Large amounts of urine lost
4. Risk factors
   a. Smoking
   b. Caffeine intake
   c. Alcohol
   d. Fluid intake inadequate
   e. Chronic constipation
   f. Obesity
5. Psychological impact
   a. Concerned about UI
   b. Not concerned with UI because it is well managed
   c. Unaware of/denies UI
   d. Cost of managing UI burdensome
   e. Major change in lifestyle
   f. Social/family relationships adversely affected
6. Medical history
   a. Stroke
   b. Parkinson's disease
   c. Dementia
   d. CHF
   e. Diabetes
   f. Multiple or difficult vaginal deliveries
   g. Pelvic surgery
   h. Pernicious anemia
   i. Multiple sclerosis
   j. Kidney disease, stones, recurrent infection
   k. Back injury or surgery
7. Current management
   a. Pads/incontinence underwear
   b. Toileting regimen
   c. Catheters or devices
   d. Medication
   e. Skin care
8. Incontinence symptom profile
   a. Stress UI
      (1) Leakage with cough, sneeze, physical activity
      (2) UI lost in small amounts (drops, spurts)
      (3) No nocturia or UI at night
      (4) UI without sensation of urine loss
   b. Urge UI
      (1) Strong, uncontrolled urge before UI
      (2) Moderate/large volume of urine loss (gush)
      (3) Frequency of urination
      (4) Nocturia more than twice nightly
      (5) Enuresis
   c. Overflow UI
      (1) Difficulty starting urine stream
      (2) Weak or intermittent stream (dribbles) with change in position
      (3) Postvoid dribbling
      (4) Feeling of fullness after voiding
      (5) Voiding in small amounts frequently or dribbling
   d. Functional UI
      (1) Mobility or manual dexterity impairments
      (2) Sedative, hypnotic, central nervous system depressant, diuretic, anticholinergic, alpha-adrenergic antagonist
      (3) Depression, delirium, dementia
      (4) Pain

Physical Examination
1. Abdominal examination
   a. Normal
   b. Palpable bladder
   c. Abdominal masses
   d. Distended bowel
2. Genitals
   a. Normal
   b. Reddened, irritated tissue
   c. Discharge
   d. Infection
   e. Odor
   f. Lesions
3. Pelvic examination
   a. Vaginal inspection
      (1) Normal
      (2) Tissue pale, thin, dry
      (3) Pelvic organ descent with Valsalva's maneuver
      (4) Lesions
   b. Pelvic muscle assessment
      (1) Palpable, voluntary contraction, rating 0 to 5
      (2) Unable to elicit voluntary contraction

Box 11-6   Elements of an Incontinence Assessment—*cont'd*

4. Rectal examination
   a. Snug anal sphincter tone and good sensation
   b. Lax or absent anal sphincter tone
   c. Fecal impaction

Functional Assessment
1. Mobility
   a. Can use toilet with assistance
   b. Needs assistance or verbal prompting to toilet
   c. Unable to use toilet
2. Manual dexterity
   a. Independent
   b. Needs assistance
   c. Unable to use toilet
3. Cognitive function
   a. Intact
   b. Impaired Mini-Mental State Exam Score (<24 abnormal)

Environmental Assessment
1. Consider distance to bathroom

2. Assess bathroom for lighting, glare, grab bars, physical barriers
3. Determine caregiver willingness and ability to provide assistance
4. Assess need for toilet substitutes and adaptations (raised toilet seat, grab bars)
5. Consider adaptable clothing and devices to facilitate disrobing for toileting
6. Ensure proper assistive devices (wheelchair, walker, cane)

Bladder Diary
1. Record and review a bladder diary for 3 to 5 days including the following:
   a. Timing of voiding
   b. Volume voided
   c. Circumstances associated with UI episodes

Identify Possible Diagnoses or Clinical Impression
1. Rule out other serious medical problems, assess and treat constipation and fecal impaction, check urine with dipstick

From Yu LC et al: Profile of urinary incontinent elderly in long-term care institutions, *J Am Geriatr* Soc 38(4):433-439, 1990; Fantl JA et al: *Managing acute and chronic urinary incontinence. Clinical practice guideline: quick reference guide for clinicians no. 2, 1996 update, AHCPR pub no. 96-0686*, Rockville, Md, 1996, U.S. Department of Health and Human Services, Public Health Service, Agency for Health Care Policy and Research; Dash ME et al: Urinary incontinence: the Social Health Maintenance Organization's approach, *Geriatr Nurs* 25(2):81-89, 2004.
UI, Urinary incontinence; *CHF*, congestive heart failure.

3—Frequently incontinent (tends to be incontinent daily but has some control)
4—Incontinent (has inadequate control of bladder and multiple daily episodes)

Unfortunately, the MDS does not provide data that are addressed in the bladder diaries; thus its use is limited in the development of a nursing care plan that is beneficial to the patient or that considers the cause of the urinary incontinence.

Use of problematic medications, such as sedatives, hypnotics, anticholinergics, and antidepressants, should be assessed. Diuretics, narcotics, calcium channel blockers, alpha-adrenergic agonists, minor tranquilizers, antispasmodics, and major tranquilizers are among the drugs contributing to UI. Caffeine and alcohol use should

also be assessed. In summary, assessment of urinary incontinence can identify incontinence as either acute/transient (the result of temporary conditions that are amenable to medication, surgery, or psychological intervention) or established (the result of neurological involvement or damage to the urinary system). Transient incontinence is curable; established incontinence is treatable or controllable but not generally curable.

Interventions

When there is sufficient understanding of the problem, various therapeutic modalities and concomitant nursing interventions can be initiated. Selection of a modality and interventions will

---

Box 11-7	**Therapeutic Modalities in the Treatment of Incontinence**

Support Measures
Appropriate attitude
Accessible toilet substitutes (bedpan, urinal, commode)
Avoidance of iatrogenic complications (urinary tract infections, excessive sedation, inaccessible toilets, drugs adversely affecting the bladder or urethral function)
Protective undergarments
Absorbent bed pads
Behavioral techniques (bladder training, toilet scheduling, prompted voiding, conditioning, biofeedback, Kegel exercises)
Good skin care

Drugs
Bladder relaxants
Bladder outlet stimulants

Surgery
Suspension of bladder neck
Prostatectomy
Prosthetic sphincter implants
Urethral sling
Bladder augmentation

Mechanical and Electrical Devices
Catheters
External (condom or "Texas" catheter)
Intermittent
Suprapubic
Indwelling

---

depend on the type of incontinence and its underlying cause and whether the outcome is to cure or to minimize the extent of the incontinence. Box 11-7 lists the numerous modalities available in the treatment of incontinence. Nursing interventions focus primarily on the therapeutic modality of supportive measures and may also be involved in designing restorative therapeutic modalities.

Attitude

An appropriate attitude is most important when providing nursing care to an incontinent individual. Caregivers are often unaware of the many causes of incontinence and passively accept a client's urinary incontinence and believe that it is an inevitable part of aging, which may add to the elder's feelings of low self-worth, dependence, and social isolation. Caregivers who regard incontinence as an unpleasant and demanding hygienic problem emphasize only keeping the patient clean and dry, with little consideration of what causes the problem. The fact that incontinence can be curable and that the nurse and other health care providers will work with the elder to resolve the incontinence is an important idea to foster in the elder who is not cognitively impaired. For those with cognitive impairment who can be routinely taken to the toilet, staying dry and maintaining normal patterns are important to self-esteem and dignity. The role of the nurse in the community is to give the older adult information and tools that will allow the individual to maintain body control.

Toilet Accessibility

Accessibility to the toilet is an intervention that is often not considered in providing assistance for the person with UI. Environmental circumstances can contribute to incontinence. If the distance the older person must either walk or travel by wheelchair to reach the toilet is longer than the time between the onset of the desire to micturate and actual micturition, incontinence is certain to occur. Toilet substitutes for the infirm and ill have been around for hundreds of years. Four types are used: commodes for the bedside; over-toilet chairs for transport; bedpans for beds or commodes; and urinals for both men and women that can be used in bed, in a chair, or in a standing position. The criterion for use of a commode is that the toilet is too far for the elder's mobility or it requires too much energy for the elderly person to get to the toilet. A commode can also substitute for an inadequate number of available toilets. Urinals are generally used by men; however, bottle-shaped urinals have been designed for women and are used on occasion. They can be obtained from a surgical supply store or various mail-order catalogs (see Resources).

Protective Undergarments and Padding

A variety of protective undergarments or adult briefs are available for the incontinent older adult. Disposable types come in several sizes determined by hip and waist measurements, or one size may fit all. Many of these undergarments look like regular underwear and contribute more to dignity than the standard "diaper." The lining of these disposable pants may contain fiberfill or an absorbent polymer or gel substance. Referring to protective undergarments as diapers is demeaning and infantilizing to older people and should be avoided. Polymer and gel substances are more absorbent and tend to keep a protective layer between the skin and wet material. Washable garments with inserts also do a reasonable job of containing urine. However, they tend to be made of plastic or rubber and therefore are hot and cause skin discomfort. If pants are going to leak, they will do so at the groin. It is important to fit them firmly but comfortably around the leg.

A variation of the standard draw sheet is a protective washable pad used along with a plastic sheet. The Australian Kylie pad is a sophisticated version of the draw sheet that is successful in keeping both the bed and the incontinent person dry. It is composed of two layers, with a water-repellent layer next to the individual. Urine is absorbed by the liner. Disposable protective pads are available, but it is important to know the amount and type of fill in the pads. A polymer gel is more economical. It is unwise to purchase pads because they are inexpensive if it means using several more per day than if more expensive and more absorbent pads were bought.

Lifestyle Modifications

Several lifestyle factors are associated with either the development or exacerbation of UI. These include dietary factors (increased fluid, avoidance of caffeine), weight reduction, smoking cessation, bowel management, and physical activity.

Behavioral Techniques

Behavioral techniques such as timed voiding, prompted voiding, bladder training, biofeedback, pelvic floor muscle rehabilitation, and prompted voiding are recommended as first-line treatment of UI. These techniques are usually effective in urge and stress incontinence. In some instances the goal is not to regain a normal voiding pattern but to decrease the number of wetting episodes, to decrease laundry costs and use of absorbent protection, and to improve the person's quality of life and social activity. The methods are free of side effects and do not limit future options. However,

they do require time, effort, practice, motivation, and education for both the patient and the caregiver. Cognitive status, UI and voiding patterns, mobility, and the need for psychological reinforcement to ensure adherence to the regimen determine the choice of program (Lekan-Rutledge, Colling, 2003, p 39), Scheduled voiding regimens may be combined with other interventions such as fluid modification, caffeine reduction, pelvic floor muscle exercises (PFMEs), or drug therapy (Wyman, 2003).

Timed voiding consists of a fixed toilet schedule at 2-hour intervals. This technique may be more useful in stress UI (Wyman, 2003). Bladder training uses an interplay of methods and teaches the individual to void at regular intervals and attempts to lengthen intervals between voidings. Bladder training has been effective in reducing the frequency of urge and stress incontinence in older women and may be even more effective when combined with PFMEs and reduction of caffeine (Wyman, 2003).

Prompted voiding is a scheduled toileting regimen that can be used with cognitively impaired residents who accept toileting. Prompted voiding may improve continence in 25% to 40% of incontinent residents in long-term care facilities. Many factors influence the success of prompted voiding and other toileting regimens in long-term care, including mobility of the residents, staffing ratios, motivation and education of staff, the need for ongoing reinforcement, and a shift in the expectations from incontinence to continence (Lekan-Rutledge, 2000; Schnelle et al, 1998). Suggestions for improved continence care in nursing homes include the use of an advanced practice nurse, restorative programs, and multidisciplinary involvement. This is an area in desperate need of further research, and gerontological nurses can take an active role in design and testing of models of care. Several models of UI management in long-term care that nurses can use in designing programs have been reported in the literature (Remsburg et al, 1999; Lekan-Rutledge, 2000; Dixon, 2002). See Box 11-8 for suggestions for caregivers who are toileting patients with dementia and Box 11-9 for interventions for noninstitutionalized elders.

Pelvic floor muscle rehabilitation includes PFMEs, vaginal weight training, biofeedback-assisted PFMEs, and electrical and magnetic stim-

Box 11-8	Hints for Caregivers Toileting Residents with Dementia

Have the word "bathroom" or "toilet" on the door.

Have a picture of a toilet on the door.

Leave door to bathroom open to visualize toilet.

Decrease clutter in and around the toilet.

Increase environmental safety (i.e., use good lighting, hand rails, elevated toilet).

Use simple verbal or behavioral cues.

Hold out your hand and say pleasantly, "Come with me."

Sing with the resident or use another pleasant distraction if resistant to toileting.

Avoid complicated commands or questions (i.e., "Mr. Jones, is it time for you to go to the bathroom?").

Avoid grabbing the resident's wrist and pulling.

If the resident is nonresponsive, leave alone and return later.

Stay with a routine.

Use a familiar caregiver and only one person working with the resident.

Have residents wear elastic waistbands or other easy-to-remove clothing.

Stay pleasant and avoid confrontation or hurrying.

Use timing with fluids and toileting.

Avoid bladder irritants.

Provide skin care cleanser, moisturizer, and protection.

Keep containment garments simple and similar to regular underpants.

Adapted from Smith DB: A continence care approach for long-term care facilities, *Geriatr Nurs* 19(2):81-86, 1998.

Box 11-9	Helpful Interventions for Noninstitutionalized Elders to Control or Eliminate Incontinence

Empty bladder completely before and after meals and at bedtime.

Urinate whenever the urge arises, never ignore it.

A schedule of urinating every 2 hours during the day and every 4 hours at night is often helpful in retraining the bladder. An alarm clock may be necessary.

Drink 1½ to 2 quarts of fluid day before 8 PM. This helps the kidneys to function properly. Limit fluids after supper to ½ to 1 cup (except in very hot weather).

Drink cranberry juice or take vitamin C to help acidify the urine and lower the chances of bladder infection.

Eliminate or reduce the use of coffee, tea, brown cola, and alcohol since they have a diuretic effect.

Take prescription diuretics in the morning on rising.

Limit the use of sleeping pills, sedatives, and alcohol because they decrease sensation to urinate and can increase incontinence, especially at night.

If overweight, lose weight.

Exercises to strengthen pelvic muscles that help support the bladder are often helpful for women.

Make sure the toilet is nearby with a clear path and good lighting, especially at night. Grab bars or a raised toilet seat may be needed.

Dress protectively with cotton underwear and protective pants or incontinent pads if necessary.

ulation. PFMEs are most effective for stress UI but may also be of benefit in urge and mixed UI in older women. Pelvic floor exercises (also called Kegel exercises) strengthen the periurethral and pelvic floor muscles. The contractions exert a closing force on the urethra. Correct identification of the pelvic floor muscles and adherence to the

exercise regimen are key to success. To help identify the correct muscle groups, it may be helpful to tell the person to try to tighten the anal sphincter (as if to control the passage of flatus or feces) and then tighten the urethral/vaginal muscles (as if to stop the flow of urine). Wyman (2003) recommends 36 to 50 pelvic floor muscle contractions divided into two or three exercise sets performed daily or three times per week for 12 to 16 weeks. Vaginal weight training was introduced in Europe as an alternative for women who have difficulty identifying the pelvic floor muscles. Graded-weight vaginal balls or cones are worn during two 15-minute periods each day or are used in addition to PFMEs. When the weighted cone is placed in the vagina, the pelvic floor muscle contractions keep it from slipping out. Although this technique involves less time and is more easily taught than PFMEs, difficulty inserting the cones and discomfort have been noted as deterrents to use (Wyman, 2003).

Biofeedback uses both visual and auditory instruments to give the individual immediate feedback on how well he or she is controlling the sphincter, the detrusor muscle, and/or the abdominal muscles. Those who are successful learn to contract the sphincter and/or relax the detrusor and abdominal muscles automatically. Further research is indicated as to the effectiveness of this treatment, but women who have weak muscles or difficulty isolating muscles appear to benefit (Wyman, 2003). Table 11-1 provides a summary of behavioral modalities, the type of incontinence, outcomes, and appropriate populations for these approaches.

Skin Care

Skin care maintains the first line of defense against infection. Skin that is in contact with urine should be washed with mild soap and warm water and then dried thoroughly. Application of a skin lubricant or an ointment, such as A & D or skin barrier cream, provides a thin protective layer to skin repeatedly exposed to urine. It is tempting to neglect an individual who is dependent and wears protective undergarments, but it is important that the person be checked every few hours for wetness in order to maintain skin intactness. To minimize the episodes of incontinence, it is prudent to establish the incontinence pattern and place the individual on a toilet or commode before voiding.

Medications

Pharmacological treatment is most often indicated for stress and urge UI and overactive bladder (OAB). OAB symptoms include urgency, frequency, and nocturia with or without urge UI. Drugs for stress UI target the urinary sphincter.

Topical estrogen may be beneficial, particularly when urogenital atrophy or atrophic vaginitis is present. Drugs for urge UI and OAB include anticholinergic (antimuscarinic) agents. The bladder is a smooth muscle that contains muscarinic receptors that are responsible for contractions. Commonly prescribed medications include oxybutynin (Ditropan) and tolterodine (Detrol). Undesirable side effects, such as dry mouth, dry eyes, constipation, confusion, or the precipitation of glaucoma, are problematical, particularly in older people. Tolterodine and the newer forms of oxybutynin (long-acting and topical formulation) have been shown to have fewer side effects (Newman, 2003). Imipramine (Tofranil), a tricyclic antidepressant, exerts both anticholinergic and direct relaxant effects on the detrusor muscle, as well as a contractile effect on the bladder outlet, thus enhancing continence. Two important side effects to be aware of in the elderly are hypotension and sedation.

Surgery

Surgical intervention is appropriate for some conditions of incontinence. Surgical suspension of the bladder neck in women has proved effective in 80% to 95% of persons electing to have this surgical corrective procedure. Outflow obstruction incontinence secondary to prostatic hypertrophy is generally corrected by prostatectomy. Sphincter dysfunction resulting from nerve damage following surgical trauma or radical perineal procedures is 70% to 90% repairable through sphincter implantation. Complications for this type of surgery are greater than 20% and may require an additional surgery. A urethral sling of fascia increases urethral elevation and compression. Continence is restored in approximately 60% to 80% of clients who have this surgery (Newman, Palmer, 2003). Currently periurethral bulking has been added to the number of surgical procedures that address urinary incontinence. Collagen or polytetrafluoroethylene (PTFE) is injected into the periurethral area to increase pressure on the urethra. This adds bulk to the internal sphincter and closes the gap that allowed leakage to occur.

Nonsurgical Devices

The U.S. Food and Drug Administration (FDA) has approved two devices, available through prescription, to manage stress incontinence. The

Table 11-1 Behavioral Intervention Options for Incontinence

Type of Incontinence	Intended Population	Behavioral Intervention	Purpose of Intervention	Expected Outcome
Urge, stress, mixed	Cognitively intact; able to discern urge sensation; able to understand or learn how to inhibit urge; able to toilet with or without assistance	Bladder training	Restore normal pattern of voiding and normal bladder function Inhibit involuntary detrusor contractions	↓ Number of wet episodes ↓ Amount of urine lost ↓ Number of voidings ↑ Bladder capacity ↑ Quality of life
Urge, functional	Cognitively impaired; functionally disabled; incomplete bladder emptying; caregiver dependent	Scheduled toileting	Timed with individual's voiding habits Decrease wet episodes; no attempt to regain normal voiding pattern	↓ Number of wet episodes ↓ Laundry costs and/or use of absorbent devices ↑ Life quality ↑ Social activity
Functional, urge, mixed	Same as above	Habit training Mobility and access to toilet	Develop a pattern for voiding	↓ Frequency of incontinent episodes ↑ Comfort ↑ Quality of life
Urge, functional	Functionally able to use toilet or toileting device; able to feel urge sensation; able to request toileting assistance; caregiver is available	Prompted voiding	Heighten individual awareness of need to void	↑ Interaction between caregiver and individual ↓ Wet episodes
Stress, urge, mixed	Able to identify and contract pelvic muscles; able and willing to follow instructions and committed to actively participate	Pelvic floor training	Strengthen pubococcygeus muscle efficient urethral closure during sudden increases in intravesical pressure	↑ Strength and size of pubococcygeus ↑ Duration of muscle contraction with increased urethral pressure ↓ Urine loss ↑ Ability to stop urine flow once initiated

Stress, urge, mixed	Vaginal weight training	Cognitively intact Compliant with instructions Able to stand Sufficient muscle strength to contract muscle and retain the lightest weight No pelvic organ prolapse	Same as above	Self-report of ↓ urine loss ↑ Self-esteem; enhance quality of life ↓ Reliance on pads, panty liners, or absorbent products
Stress, mixed	Biofeedback	Ability to understand analog or digital signals using auditory or visual display Motivated, able to learn voluntary control through observation of biofeedback A health care provider who can appropriately assess the incontinence problem and provide behavior interventions	Same as above	Same as above
Stress, urge, mixed	Electrical stimulation	Ability to discern stimulation	Reeducation of pelvic muscle; inhibit bladder instability and improve striated sphincter and levator ani contractility and efficiency	↑ Resistance of the pelvic floor; block uninhibited bladder contractions

Adapted and compiled from Anderson MA, Braun JV: *Caring for the elderly client*, Philadelphia, 1995, FA Davis; Fantl JA et al: Managing acute and chronic urinary incontinence. In *Clinical practice guideline: quick reference guide for clinicians*, no. 2, pub no. 96-0686, 1996 update, Rockville, Md, 1996, U.S. Department of Health and Human Services, Agency for Health Care Policy and Research; Palmer MH: *Urinary incontinence*, Gaithersburg, Md, 1996, Aspen; Staab AS, Hodges LC: *Essentials of gerontological nursing*, Philadelphia, 1996, JB Lippincott.

Miniguard is about the size of a postage stamp and fits over the urethral opening. It is contoured with an adhesive foam backing. The other device, the Reliance Urinary Control Insert, is designed for moderate to severe incontinence in women. The device is a balloon-tipped plug, about one fifth the diameter of a tampon, which is inserted by an applicator. The force of the insertion inflates the balloon, so that the neck of the bladder is then obstructed. The device must be removed by pulling a string before urination or intercourse. Trials of both of these devices have been on a limited number of women at present. Women using the devices gained complete or limited continence but also experienced UTIs, particularly with the Reliance Urinary Control Insert. However, it was thought that as the women gained skill in use of the device, the frequency of UTIs and urethral irritation would decline (Harvard Medical School Health Publications, 1996). A third option, the pessary, has been around for many years and has primarily been used to prevent uterine prolapse. The pessary is a device that is fitted into the vagina and that exerts pressure to elevate the urethrovesical junction or the pelvic floor. The patient is taught to insert and remove the pessary much like the insertion and removal of a diaphragm used for contraception. The pessary is removed weekly or monthly for cleaning with soap and water and then reinserted. Adverse effects include vaginal infection, low back pain, and vaginal mucosal erosion. Another concern is forgetting to remove the pessary (Newman, Palmer, 2003).

Catheters

Indwelling catheters may be appropriate for short-term use in hospitalized patients, but clinical guidelines indicate that indwelling catheter use is only appropriate when urethral obstruction or urinary retention is present, with the following conditions:

- Persistent overflow UI, symptomatic infections, or kidney disease
- Surgical or pharmacological interventions inappropriate or unsuccessful
- Contraindications to intermittent catheterization for retention
- When changes of bedding, clothing, and absorbent products may be painful or disruptive for a patient with an irreversible medical condi-

tion, such as metastatic terminal disease, coma, or end-stage congestive heart failure
- For patients with stage 3 or 4 pressure ulcers that are not healing because of continual urine leakage
- For patients who live alone without a caregiver or with a caregiver who is unable to routinely change the person (Fantl et al, 1996; Newman, Palmer, 2003)

Regulatory standards in nursing homes follow these same guidelines, and the use of indwelling catheters must be justified based on medical conditions and failure of other efforts to maintain continence. Long-term catheter use increases the risk of recurrent urinary tract infections leading to urosepsis, urethral damage in men secondary to urethral erosion, urethritis or fistula formation, and bladder stones or cancer (Newman, Palmer, 2003). UTIs are the most common infections in residents in long-term care. Asymptomatic bacteria in the urine are considered a benign disease in older people and should not be treated with antibiotics. Screening urine cultures should also not be performed in patients who are asymptomatic (Midthun et al, 2004). Symptomatic UTIs need antibiotic treatment, but it is important to be observant as to the range of symptoms elderly patients may present. Fever, dysuria, and flank pain may not be present. Changes in mental status, decreased appetite, abdominal pain, new onset of incontinence, or even respiratory distress may signal a possible UTI in older people. Catheter care should consist of washing the meatal area with soap and water daily.

Intermittent catheterization (the periodic insertion of a sterile or clean catheter several times per day to empty the bladder) is frequently used in patients with spinal cord injuries and may be of benefit in other conditions. Complications occur less frequently in patients managed by clean intermittent catheterization than in those with indwelling catheters. The procedure may be problematic for many elders with limited dexterity.

External catheters (condom catheters) are used in male patients who are incontinent and cannot be toileted. Long-term use of external catheters can lead to fungal skin infections, penile skin maceration, edema, fissures, contact burns from urea, phimosis, UTIs, and septicemia (Newman, Palmer, 2003). The catheter should be removed and replaced daily and the penis cleaned, dried, and aired to prevent irritation, maceration, and the development of pressure areas and skin breakdown. If the catheter is not applied and monitored correctly, strangulation of the penile shaft could occur.

Evaluation

The success of interventions in urinary incontinence is measured against phased accomplishment such as the following:

1. The individual voids when placed or sits on the toilet.
2. The individual drinks at least 2000 ml of fluid daily.
3. The individual remains continent 25% of the time.
4. The individual has fewer accidents in each successive phase.
5. The individual is continent all the time.

FECAL OR BOWEL INCONTINENCE

Fecal incontinence is defined as the inability to control the passage of stool or gas via the anus or involuntary loss of stool from the rectum at inappropriate times (Staab, Hodges, 1996). The prevalence of fecal incontinence is approximately 3% to 4% of community-dwelling elders, and approximately 16% to 60% of the institutionalized aged have some fecal incontinence (Richter, 1995). Often fecal incontinence is associated with urinary incontinence. Fecal incontinence, like urinary incontinence, has devastating social ramifications for the individuals and families who experience it. Many factors are similar to urinary incontinence. The factors affecting fecal incontinence include intestinal transit time, rectal factors (sensory), pelvic floor and sphincter tone, pelvic musculature, medications, muscular flaccidity, and the inability to get to the toilet when the urge to eliminate is present. Other factors distinct to bowel evacuation problems are long-term dependence on laxatives, lack of sufficient bulk in the diet, insufficient fluid intake, lack of exercise, hemorrhoids, and depression. Many instances of fecal incontinence result from fecal impaction, or there may be a neurological origin. Serious illness accompanied by delirium and excessive doses of iron, antibiotic, and digitalis preparations may precipitate incontinence. Sedatives, too, can account for incontinence through depression of cerebral awareness and control over sphincter response.

IMPLICATIONS FOR GERONTOLOGICAL NURSING AND HEALTHY AGING

Assessment

Assessment should include a complete client history as in urinary incontinence (described earlier in this chapter) and a bowel record. The following questions should be included in a bowel incontinence assessment:

- What is the availability of the toilet or commode, and what is the time required to get to it?
- What medications, if any, is the older person taking that influence peristaltic action, lucidity, or fluid balance?
- How much bulk is provided in the food? (Pureed food does not help.)
- What is the manual dexterity required to remove clothing once the aged person is in the bathroom?
- Is there any neurological or circulatory impairment of the cerebral cortex?

Interventions

The nurse's attitude in assisting the person who is incontinent of feces should be the same as for the individual with urinary incontinence. Fecal incontinence is a symptom. It requires that the patient be accepted as a person, that the incontinence problem not be advertised or ridiculed, and that the person not be made to feel ashamed or guilty. A great deterrent to successful intervention in incontinence is inconsistency in implementing the planned strategy and unrealistic expectations of rapid, full recovery. Time and patience are essential ingredients of success. Nursing interventions should include several days' surveillance of the patient's bowel function. A chart similar to that used to monitor urinary incontinence can be constructed.

Nursing intervention should work to manage and/or restore bowel continence. Therapies similar to those used in treating urinary incontinence are effective with fecal incontinence, such as environmental manipulation, diet alterations, bowel training, sensory reeducation, sphincter training exercises, biofeedback, electrical stimulation, medication, and/or surgery to correct underlying defects (Wald, 1995). Instituting a diet adequate in dietary fiber (6 to 10 g daily) will add bulk, weight, and form to the stool and improve colon evacuation of the sigmoid and rectum rather than producing a continuous or intermittent oozing of fecal material. This may assist in the attainment of more controlled and complete bowel movements.

When the incontinence has a cerebral or neurological cause, it is often necessary to identify triggers that initiate incontinence. For example, eating a meal stimulates defecation 30 minutes following the completion of the meal, or defecation occurs following the morning cup of coffee. If the fecal incontinence is only once or twice each day, it can be controlled by being prepared. Placing the individual on the toilet, commode, or bedpan at a given time following the trigger event facilitates defecation in the appropriate place at the appropriate time.

When fecal incontinence is continual, it may be necessary to develop a plan that controls the specific time of day when the individual has a bowel movement or movements. Generally, this is accomplished by establishing constipation for several days and evacuating the bowel (e.g., every fourth day) by enema or suppository. Diet plays a role in this also. Creating the proper diet will affect intestinal motility and help evacuation. Bowel training of this type allows for predictability of colon evacuation and more freedom and less embarrassment for the older person (Box 11-10). If protective garments are necessary, they will allow the patient more opportunity to participate actively in events and to be more mobile in the institutional community.

The effectiveness of interventions in fecal incontinence will be self-evident but will take time. As in treatment of urinary incontinence, goals must be realistic. It cannot be stated too often or too strongly that the nurse must always provide immaculate skin care to person with incontinence because self-esteem and skin integrity depend on it.

IMPLICATIONS FOR GERONTOLOGICAL NURSING AND HEALTHY AGING

"Caring for persons with elimination problems has been integral to basic nursing care since Florence Nightingale's time" (Wells, 1994). Gerontological nurses have a pivotal role in continence care. "In all clinical settings, people have the right to be continent" (Mason et al, 2003, p 3). It is important that nurses and other health care providers understand the causes of UI, risk factors, and evidence-based protocols for interventions. Competency in continence care needs to be included in the preparation for beginning nursing practice (Jirovec, 1998). Health promotion education, comprehensive assessments of UI, education of informal and formal caregivers, and use of evidence-based interventions should be part of individualized care for all older people experiencing UI symptoms. Gerontological nurses also need to be knowledgeable about appropriate products and devices as management options.

In the long-term care setting, implementation of UI assessment and establishment of toileting protocols remain problematic (Lekan-Rutledge, Colling, 2003). The establishment of clear policies and procedures, staff training, adequate staffing ratios, restorative programs, and a multidisciplinary approach will contribute to optimum continence care in this setting. Toileting programs in nursing homes are a "powerful multimodal therapeutic activity that positively affects mobility, behavior, skin integrity, urinary tract infection, bowel function, and fluid intake, in addition to continence status" (Lekan-Rutledge, Colling, 2003, p 39). UI leads to excess disability, frailty, and psychological distress. Failure to address continence promotion has enormous consequences for both the individual and society in terms of economics and burden of care. Gerontological nurses have an ethical responsibility to take action. "In all clinical settings, people have the right to be continent" (Mason et al, 2003, p 3).

Further research is needed, and research priorities include the following:
- The prevalence and nature of UI in men, young women, and members of minority groups

Box 11-10	Bowel Training Program

1. Obtain bowel history and establish a schedule for the bowel training program that is normal and comfortable for the patient and conforms to his or her lifestyle.
2. Ensure adequate fiber and fluid intake (normalize stool consistency).
   a. Fiber.
      (1) Add high-fiber foods to diet (dried fruit, dried beans, vegetables, and wheat products).
      (2) Suggest adding 1 to 3 tablespoons bran or Metamucil to diet one or two times each day. (Titrate dosage based on response.)
   b. Fluid.
      (1) Two to three L daily (unless contraindicated).
      (2) Four oz of prune, fig, or pear juice (or a warm fluid) may be given daily as a stimulus (e.g., 30 to 60 minutes before the established time for defecation).
3. Encourage exercise program.
   a. Pelvic tilt, modified sit-ups for abdominal strength.
   b. Walking for general muscle tone and cardiovascular system.
   c. More vigorous program if appropriate.
4. Establish a regular time for the bowel movement.

a. Established time depends on patient's schedule.
b. Best times are 20 to 40 minutes after regularly scheduled meals, when gastrocolic reflex is active.
c. Attempts at evacuation should be made daily within 15 minutes of the established time and whenever the patient senses rectal distention.
d. Instruct patient in normal posture for defecation. (The patient normally sits on the toilet or bedside commode; for the patient who is unable to get out of bed, the left side–lying position is best.)
e. Instruct the patient to contract the abdominal muscles and "bear down."
f. Have patient lean forward to increase the intraabdominal pressure by use of compression against the thighs.
g. Stimulate anorectal reflex and rectal emptying if necessary.
   (1) Insert a rectal suppository or mini-enema into the rectum 15 to 30 minutes before the scheduled bowel movement, placing the suppository against the bowel wall, or
   (2) Insert a gloved, lubricated finger into the anal canal and gently dilate the anal sphincter.

From Basch A, Jensen L: Management of fecal incontinence. In Doughty DB: *Urinary and fecal incontinence: nursing management,* St Louis, 1991, Mosby.

- The effectiveness of various behavioral techniques, devices, and products and pharmacotherapy
- The effectiveness of primary prevention strategies
- Alternative models for educating and using staff in primary and long-term care settings for improved management of incontinence (Mason, Newman, Palmer, 2003, p 53)

Resources listed at the end of this chapter will be valuable to the gerontological nurse as he or she prepares for practice. Gerontological nurses may wish to pursue advanced training and certification through specialty organizations such as The Society of Urologic Nurses and Associates (www.suna.org) and the Wound, Ostomy, and Continence Nurses Society (www.wocncb.org).

APPLICATION OF MASLOW'S HIERARCHY

Meeting elimination needs is basic to the maintenance of biological and physiological integrity, but its importance reaches far higher on the hierarchy. Inadequate attention to this basic need can cause excess disability, cause insecurity, affect safety, cause social isolation and curtailment of meaningful activities and relationships, and interfere with the ability of the older person to achieve

NANDA and Wellness Diagnoses

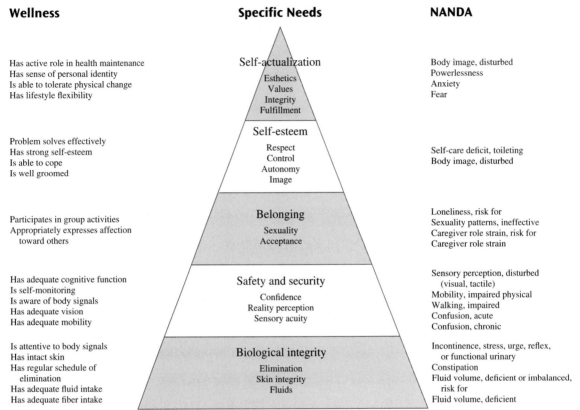

Wellness	Specific Needs	NANDA

Wellness

Has active role in health maintenance
Has sense of personal identity
Is able to tolerate physical change
Has lifestyle flexibility

Problem solves effectively
Has strong self-esteem
Is able to cope
Is well groomed

Participates in group activities
Appropriately expresses affection
    toward others

Has adequate cognitive function
Is self-monitoring
Is aware of body signals
Has adequate vision
Has adequate mobility

Is attentive to body signals
Has intact skin
Has regular schedule of
    elimination
Has adequate fluid intake
Has adequate fiber intake

Specific Needs

Self-actualization
    Esthetics
    Values
    Integrity
    Fulfillment

Self-esteem
    Respect
    Control
    Autonomy
    Image

Belonging
    Sexuality
    Acceptance

Safety and security
    Confidence
    Reality perception
    Sensory acuity

Biological integrity
    Elimination
    Skin integrity
    Fluids

NANDA

Body image, disturbed
Powerlessness
Anxiety
Fear

Self-care deficit, toileting
Body image, disturbed

Loneliness, risk for
Sexuality patterns, ineffective
Caregiver role strain, risk for
Caregiver role strain

Sensory perception, disturbed
    (visual, tactile)
Mobility, impaired physical
Walking, impaired
Confusion, acute
Confusion, chronic

Incontinence, stress, urge, reflex,
    or functional urinary
Constipation
Fluid volume, deficient or imbalanced,
    risk for
Fluid volume, deficient

These are not all of the possible wellness or NANDA diagnoses that may be identified. The above are frequent examples of nursing diagnoses that should be considered when planning care for the older adult in whatever setting.

a meaningful and fulfilling life. Without an adequate knowledge base of continence care, meeting basic elimination needs with basic nursing care will remain mopping up accidents and putting on diapers.

KEY CONCEPTS

- Older adults do not experience thirst and therefore do not drink sufficient fluids to maintain adequate hydration. Certain medications and fluids, such as coffee, tend to abet dehydration.
- Urinary incontinence is not a part of normal aging. It is a symptom, not a disease.

- Urinary incontinence can be minimized or cured.
- Health promotion teaching, identification of risk factors, comprehensive assessments of UI, education of informal and formal caregivers, and use of evidence-based interventions are basic continence competencies for nurses.
- A number of interventions for urinary incontinence are applicable to the management of bowel incontinence.

Activities and Discussion Questions

1. Explain the problems associated with dehydration in the older adult.

2. Identify the signs and symptoms of dehydration in the elderly.
3. Discuss interventions to prevent and treat dehydration.
4. Explain the implications of urinary incontinence for the older adult.
5. What measures can be taken to cure or decrease urinary incontinence in the community and long-term care settings?
6. What interventions can be instituted for managing fecal incontinence?
7. Devise a nursing care plan for an elder with urinary incontinence or fecal incontinence.
8. Conduct a UI history with a partner or with an older adult.

RESOURCES

Publication

Newman D: *Managing and treating incontinence*, Baltimore, 2002, Health Professions Press (book includes useful patient information guides).

Organizations

Association of Women's Health, Obstetric and Neonatal Nurses (continence clinical practice guidelines and UI information)
2000 L Street, NW, Suite 740
Washington, DC 20036
(202) 261-2400
website: http://www.awhonn.org

Home Delivery Incontinent Supplies Co., Inc
1215 Dielman Industrial Court
Olivette, MO 63132
(800)269-4663
website: http://www.hdis.com

International Continence Society
website: http://www.continenceworldwide.org

National Association for Continence (lay and professional education, UI products)
PO Box 1019
Charleston, SC 29402-1019
(800) 252-3337
e-mail: memberservices@nafc.org
website: http://www.nafc.org

Society of Urologic Nurses and Associates
East Holly Avenue, Box 56
Pittman, NJ 08071-0056
(888) 827-7862
website: http://www.suna.org

Wound, Ostomy and Continence Nurses Society
4700 W. Lake Avenue
Glenview, IL 60025
(888) 224-WOCN
website: http://www.wocn.org

REFERENCES

American Medical Directors Association (AMDA): *Clinical practice guideline: urinary incontinence*, Columbia, Md, 1996 (http://www.amda.com). American Medical Directors Association.

American Medical Directors Association (AMDA): *Clinical practice guideline: dehydration and fluid maintenance*, Columbia, Md, 2001, American Medical Directors Association.

Bennett JA: Dehydration: hazards and benefits, *Geriatr Nurs* 21(2):84-88, 2000.

Bradway C, Hernly S: Nursing Standard-of-Practice Protocol: Urinary continence in older adults admitted to acute care, *Geriatr Nurs* 19(2):98-102, 1998.

Burger S, Kayser-Jones J, Bell J: Malnutrition and dehydration in nursing homes: key issues in prevention and treatment, 2000. Accessed 7/23/04 from http:www.cmwf.org/programs/elders/burger_mal_386.asp.

Dash M, Foster E, Smith D, Phillips S: Urinary incontinence: The social health maintenance organization's approach, *Geriatr Nurs* 25:81-89, 2004.

Dixon D: The Wellspring model: implications for LTC, *Caring for the Ages* 3(3):18-21, 2002.

Fantl JA et al: *Managing acute and chronic urinary incontinence. Clinical practice guideline: quick reference guide for clinicians no. 2, 1996 update*, AHCPR pub no. 96-0686, Rockville, Md, 1996, U.S. Department of Health and Human Services, Public Health Service, Agency for Health Care Policy and Research.

Fourcroy JL: Overactive bladder, *Adv Nurse Pract* 9(3):59-62, 2001.

Frantz RA et al: Implementing an incontinence management protocol in long-term care: clinical outcomes and cost, *J Gerontol Nurs* 29(8):46-53, 2003.

Gaspar PM: Water intake of nursing home residents, *J Gerontol Nurs* 25(4):23-29, 1999.

Ham R, Sloane P, Warshaw G: *Primary care geriatrics*, ed 4, St Louis, 2002, Mosby.

Harvard Medical School Health Publications: Strengthening the pelvic floor, *Women's Health Watch* 3(12):2, 1996.

Holroyd-Leduc JM, Straus SE: Management of urinary incontinence in women: clinical applications, *JAMA* 291(8):996-999, 2004.

Jirovec MM et al: Addressing urinary incontinence with educational continence—care competencies, *Image J Nurs Sch* 30(4):375-378, 1998.

Lekan-Rutledge D: Diffusion on innovation: a model for implementation of prompted voiding in long-term care settings, *J Gerontol Nurs* 26(4):25-33, 2000.

Lekan-Rutledge D, Colling J: Urinary incontinence in the frail elderly: even when it's too late to prevent a problem, you can still slow its progress, *Am J Nurs* 3(suppl):36-46, 2003.

Lekan-Rutledge D et al: In their own words; Nursing assistants' perceptions of barriers to implement prompted voiding in long-term care settings, *Gerontologist* 38(3):370-378, 1998.

Mason DJ, Newman DK, Palmer MH: Changing UI practice, *Am J Nurs* 3(suppl):2-3, 2003.

Mentes JC: Iowa-Veterans Affairs Research Consortium: Hydration management protocol, *J Gerontol Nurs* 26(10):6-15, 2000.

Midthun S, Paur R, Lindseth G: Urinary tract infections, *J Gerontol Nurs* 30(6):4-9, 2004.

Newman D: Stress urinary incontinence in women, *Am J Nurs* 103(8):46-56, 2003.

Newman DK, Palmer MH, editors: The state of the science on urinary incontinence, *Am J Nurs* 3(suppl):1-58, 2003 (available at www.NursingCenter.com/UI).

Palmer MH: *Urinary continence assessment and promotion,* Gaithersburg, Md, 1996, Aspen.

Peters S: Helping older adults meet their unique nutrient needs, *Adv Nurse Pract* 6(8):66-68, 1998.

Remsburg RE et al: Two models of restorative nursing care in the nursing home: designated versus integrated restorative nursing assistants, *Geriatr Nurs* 20(6):321-326, 1999.

Richter JE: Functional disorders of the gastrointestinal tract. In Abrams WB, Beers MH, Berkow R, editors: *Merck manual of geriatrics*, ed 2, Whitehouse Station, NJ, 1995, Merck Research Laboratories.

Schnelle JF et al: Developing rehabilitative behavioral interventions for long-term care: technology transfer, acceptance, and maintenance issues, *J Am Geriatr Soc* 46(6):771-777, 1998.

Staab A, Hodges LC: *Essentials of geriatric nursing,* Philadelphia, 1996, Lippincott.

Wald A: Lower gastrointestinal tract disorders. In Abrams WB, Beers MH, Berkow R, editors: *The Merck manual of geriatrics*, ed 2, Whitehouse Station, NJ, 1995, Merck Research Laboratories.

Wasson JH, Bruskewitz RC: Disorders of the lower genitourinary tract: bladder, prostate, testes. In Abrams WB, Beers MH, Berkow R, editors: *The Merck manual of geriatrics*, Rahway, NJ, 1990, Merck Sharpe & Dohme Research Laboratories.

Weinberg AD, Minaker KL: Dehydration: evaluation and management in older adults, *JAMA* 274(19):1552-1556, 1995.

Wells TJ: Nursing research on urinary incontinence, *Urol Nurs* 14(3):109-112, 1994.

Wyman J: Treatment of urinary incontinence in men and older women, *Am J Nurs* 3(suppl):38-45, 2003.

Rest, Sleep, and Activity

Upon completion of this chapter, the reader will be able to:

- Identify age-related changes that affect rest, sleep, and activity.
- List the types of outcomes that occur because of age-related changes in rest, sleep, and activity.
- Describe nursing assessment relevant to rest, sleep, and activity.
- Explain nursing interventions useful in the promotion of rest, sleep, and activity.

Circadian rhythm   Regular recurrence of certain phenomena in cycles of approximately 24 hours.
Insomnia   Inability to fall asleep easily or to remain asleep throughout the night.
Isometrics   Active exercise performed against stable resistance without change in length of the muscle.
Isotonics   Active exercise without appreciable change in force of muscular contraction, with shortening of the muscle.

Non–rapid eye movement (NREM) sleep   First four stages of sleep.
Rapid eye movement (REM) sleep   Wakeful and active form of sleep during which dreaming occurs or tension is discharged.
Sleep apnea   Temporary cessation of breathing during sleep.

You know, I never get a decent night's sleep. I wake up at least four times every night, and I just know I won't get back to sleep. I really don't want to keep taking pills for sleep, but when I lie there awake, I just think of all the difficult times and situations I can't manage. After a while, I'm really in a stew about everything.

Richard, a 67-year-old recent retiree

This is really beginning to tire me out. Richard keeps waking me at night because he can't sleep. I try to tell him to get up and read or something. I really need my sleep if I'm going to get to work on time. I wonder if Richard needs to see a doctor. Maybe he is depressed about being retired and alone while I'm at work. I'll talk to him about it.

Clara, Richard's wife

*R*est, sleep, and activity depend on one another. Inadequacy of rest and sleep affects activity, whether it is strenuous or performing activities of daily living. Activity is necessary to maintain physical and physiological integrity, such as cardiopulmonary endurance and function, musculoskeletal strength, agility, and structure, and it helps a person obtain adequate sleep. Rest, sleep, and activity greatly contribute to overall physical and mental well-being.

REST AND SLEEP

The human organism needs rest and sleep to conserve energy, prevent fatigue, provide organ respite, and relieve tension. Sleep is an extension of rest, and both are physiological and mental necessities for survival. The quality of rest depends on the degree of physical and mental relaxation. It is often assumed that lying in bed constitutes rest, but worries and other related stressors cause muscles throughout the body to continue to contract with tension even though physical activity has ceased. Attainment of rest depends on the interrelationship of psyche and soma. Body functions possess refractory times and rest periods in the continuous cycle of activity (biorhythms). Drastically or continually altered sleep and rest cycles disrupt homeostatic balance and create physical or mental disturbances.

Sleep is a basic need. Rest occurs with sleep in sustained unbroken periods. Sleep is restorative and recuperative and is necessary for the preservation of life.

Biorhythm and Sleep

Our lives are a series of rhythms that influence and regulate physiological function, chemical concentrations, performance, behavioral responses, moods, and the ability to adapt. The most important and obvious biorhythm is the circadian sleep-wake rhythm. Abnormalities of this endogenous cycle may be responsible for some of the difficulties of old age. Gerontologists are beginning to seriously study the relevance of age-related changes in circadian rhythms to health and the process of aging. It is clear that body temperature, pulse, blood pressure, neurotransmitter excretion, and hormonal levels change significantly and predictably in a circadian rhythm. With aging, there is a reduction in the amplitude of all of these circadian endogenous responses. Biological rhythms are synchronized so a disturbance in the sleep cycle can affect the neuroendocrine and immune systems (Hoffman, 2003).

Cycles also exist that are less than 24 hours (infradian) or longer than 24 hours (ultradian). Rhythms can be disrupted by time zone changes, varying work schedules, and physical conditions. Alterations in the usual sleep-wake cycle—sleeping during the day and wakefulness at night—can signal serious illnesses.

Institutions that provide care for older people adhere to specific time schedules, which may not correspond to the biorhythm of the older person and which may place the individual out of synchronization with his or her body functions. Attention to biorhythms can help establish the normal sleep-wake pattern of the older person and identify the best times to introduce activities, periods of rest, and therapeutic measures.

Normal Sleep Pattern

The mystery of sleep has been researched for more than 30 years. The body progresses through the five stages of the normal sleep pattern consisting of rapid eye movement (REM) sleep and non–rapid eye movement (NREM) sleep. Sleep structure is shown in Box 12-1.

Sleep disturbances are common in older people. More than half of community-living elders and approximately two thirds of those in long-term care experience sleep difficulties (Hoffman, 2003). Older people report more time in bed, reduced total sleep time, prolonged sleep latency (time it takes to fall asleep), more frequent awakenings, increased wakefulness after sleep onset, and increased frequency of daytime naps (Cefalu, 2004). Alterations in the phases of sleep also occur with aging. There is a marked increase in stage I sleep and a decrease of stages III and IV sleep. The amount of REM sleep also decreases and has been shown to be related to dementia and altered cerebral blood flow. It is not clear whether these changes in sleep represent normal changes of aging or subtle manifestations of disease (Haponik, McCall, 1999). In addition, melatonin, which is naturally secreted during evening hours

---

Box 12-1   Sleep Structure

Stage I (Light Sleep)
Drops off to sleep
Relaxed
Fleeting thoughts
Easily awakened
Remembers being drowsy but not asleep

Stage II (Medium-Deep Sleep)
Enters within minutes of stage I
More relaxed
Vague, dreamlike thoughts (fragmentary dreams)
Can observe the eyes moving slowly under the eyelids
Unmistakably asleep but easily aroused

Stage III (Medium-Deep Sleep)
About 20 minutes after stage I
Muscles relaxed
Slower pulse
Decreased body temperature
Undisturbed by moderate random stimuli (doors closing, etc.)

Stage IV (Deep Sleep)
Restorative sleep
Very relaxed
Rarely moves
Awakens only with vigorous stimuli
Period during which most sleepwalking, screaming, nightmares, and bedwetting occur
Lasts 10 to 20 minutes

REM Sleep (Active Sleep)
Relieves tensions
Drifts up from stage IV every 90 to 100 minutes (REM sleep resembles stage I by electroencephalogram monitoring)
Rapid eye movement
Head and neck lose tonus, body feels flaccid
Increased and fluctuating pulse, blood pressure, and respirations
Most dreaming and sleep talking occur
When medical crisis occurs (e.g., angina, dyspnea), most often because of anxiety or fear induced by dreams

REM, Rapid eye movement.

---

and promotes sleep, is decreased in older adults. Older people do not sleep less but do seem to be less likely to sleep well or feel rested on awakening, experiencing lighter, more interrupted sleep. The changes that occur with aging are summarized in Box 12-2.

Sleep Disorders

Insomnia

Insomnia is the most common sleep disorder. Insomnia is defined as difficulty falling asleep, difficulty staying asleep, waking up too early in the morning, and/or nonrestorative sleep (Nadolski, 2003). Insomnia can be classified by duration. Transient insomnia (lasting several days to less than 3 weeks) occurs in times of acute stress, which may be due to bereavement, hospitalization, or even retirement. It can also occur with prolonged stress, new medications or stopping a medication, or a psychological disorder. Chronic

Box 12-2   Age-Related Sleep Changes

Total sleep time decreases until age 80, then increases slightly.
Time in bed increases after age 65.
Onset to sleep is lengthened (>30 minutes in about 32% of women and 15% of men).
Awakenings are frequent, increasing after age 50 (>30 minutes of wakefulness after sleep onset in >50% of older subjects).
Naps are more common, although only about 10% of elders report daily napping.
Sleep is subjectively and objectively lighter (more stage I, little stage IV, more disruptions).
REM sleep is short, less intense, and more evenly distributed.
Frequency of abnormal breathing events is increased.
Frequency of leg movements during sleep is increased.

insomnia lasts longer than 3 weeks and may be secondary to changes with age. Additional factors contributing to chronic insomnia include chronic medical illnesses, prescription and nonprescription medications and sleep aids, pain, psychiatric disorders, and other extrinsic causes, such as inadequate sleep hygiene and environmental causes. Older people experiencing institutionalization have additional risk factors for insomnia, and it is estimated that 45% to 75% of nursing home residents have disturbed sleep (Monane et al, 1996; Gentili et al, 1997). Depression is a common cause of insomnia in older adults. Insomnia is more common in women and can be a serious problem to the older person and family. Its effects include mood changes, memory deficits, difficulty with concentration, poor judgment, impaired performance, and changes in the immune system (Fielo, 2001). Insomnia is a symptom. Successful resolution depends on understanding and addressing the individual's special mix of contributing factors, including biological, medical, and emotional factors, as well as bad habits.

Narcolepsy

Narcolepsy is a disorder of unknown etiology and is underdiagnosed (McCullough, 2001). Symptoms include excessive sleepiness and sleep "attacks"; hallucinations or dreamlike perceptions at sleep onset; a sleep paralysis, in which the person does not move at sleep onset and sometimes on awakening; and disturbed nighttime sleep. REM sleep occurs at sleep onset, which is premature, usually occurring later in the sleep cycle. Modafinil (Provigil), a newer drug, promotes daytime alertness and is technically a stimulant (Gorman, 2001). Modafinil has side effects of headache, nausea, and anxiety. This drug is not recommended in patients with a history of cardiac ischemia, arrhythmia, myocardial infarction, or left ventricular hypertrophy.

Sleep Apnea

Sleep apnea syndrome is a disorder characterized by repetitive cessation of respiration during sleep. Obstructive sleep apnea (OSA) is the most common type of sleep apnea, affecting about 10% of those older than 65 and occurring twice as often in men as in women (McCullough, 2001; Drazen, 2002). Identification, evaluation, and appropriate treatment of OSA are goals of *Healthy People 2010*

(U.S. Department of Health and Human Services, 2002). OSA is the involuntary cessation of airflow for 10 seconds or longer, and the occurrence of more than five to eight of these episodes per hour is considered pathological. With OSA, the muscles responsible for holding the throat open relax during sleep, narrowing the throat opening and blocking the passage of air. Symptoms include daytime fatigue, loud periodic snoring, broken sleep with frequent awakenings, gasping and choking on awakenings, unusual nighttime activity such as sitting upright or falling out of bed, morning headache, poor memory and intellectual functioning, and irritability and personality change. Although we usually associate sleep apnea with obesity and it is common in obese elders, obesity is not a risk factor for sleep apnea. After months or years of living with this problem, severe psychological and physiological consequences can occur, including right-sided heart failure, hypertension, cardiac arrhythmias, and death (Drazen, 2002). Other consequences include an increased number of work-related accidents, poor performance, depression, and decreased quality of life (McCullough, 2001).

Assessment. Assessment includes information from the sleeping partner and consideration of a sleep study. The sleeping partner's sleep is often disturbed by this treatment, and the sleeping partner may move to another room to sleep. Therapy will depend on the severity of the sleep apnea. Physical assessment often reveals that the individual is obese, although this is not a specific risk factor. The neck is often short and thick. The uvula is large, and the soft palate hangs low. Tonsils may be enlarged; adenoids are enlarged; and there may be a small or receded chin. It is important to observe for upper airway tumors or cysts.

Interventions. Specific treatment of sleep apnea may involve weight loss, avoidance of alcohol and sedatives, cessation of smoking, and avoiding supine sleep positions. Medical interventions include nasal mask continuous positive airway pressure (CPAP), which presents the difficulty of compliance. Oxygen may be used because it can reduce dysrhythmias; humidifiers, oral appliances, decongestants, nasal steroids, antihistamines, selective serotonin reuptake inhibitor (SSRI) antidepressants, and tricyclic antidepressants may also be used. Surgery to reconstruct the upper airway can be considered; this involves tonsillectomy, uvula surgery, and a number of other procedures.

Nocturnal Myoclonus

The syndrome of periodic limb jerks or movements in sleep (PLMS) is nocturnal myoclonus. The incidence of PLMS increases with age and may occur in up to 45% of community-based elders (Beers, Berkow, 2000). It may occur in up to 80% of those with restless leg syndrome (RLS) (McCullough, 2001). The etiology is unknown, although it has been suggested that the cause may be an age-related decrease in dopamine receptors because carbidopa-levodopa can be used to improve the myoclonus. PLMS occurs only during sleep. Often, the person is unaware of its occurrence; however, it is very disruptive to the sleep partner. It typically manifests as flexion of the big toe, rapid ankle flexion, and some flexion of the knee and hip (Beers, Berkow, 2000). The upper extremities may also move. Carbidopa-levodopa is a preferred treatment, and if this is ineffective, clonazepam (a benzodiazepine) or bromocriptine may be tried. Use of opioids is another option if symptoms are severe and other treatments are ineffective.

Restless Leg Syndrome

RLS is characterized by the uncontrollable need to move the legs. Other symptoms include paresthesias; creeping sensations; crawling sensations; tingling, cramping, burning sensations; pain; or even indescribable sensations (McCullough, 2001). RLS is worse at rest and at night and is relieved by activity. It is a motor restlessness that in daytime is characterized as leg rubbing, stretching, flexing, body rocking, marching in place, and floor pacing. This can occur at any age but most severely affects those in middle to old age. It is often progressive but may have remissions. About 30% of cases report a family history of RLS, but it can occur as a side effect of some medications.

Assessment focuses on the neurological examination, which is usually normal. There may be a peripheral neuropathy or radiculopathy. In secondary RLS, patients usually have one of the following: polyneuropathies, lumbosacral radiculopathy, amyotrophic lateral sclerosis (ALS), Parkinson's disease, multiple sclerosis, or poliomyelitis. It can be caused or precipitated by medications such as SSRIs. Implicated are caffeine, neuroleptics, lithium, calcium channel blockers, and withdrawal of sedatives or narcotics. Diagnosis includes ruling out any medical condition. Walking, stretching, and rubbing the legs usually help. Carbidopa-levodopa or bromocriptine may relieve chronic symptoms. Opioids or benzodiazepines may also be effective for severe symptoms that do not respond to other drugs.

Sleep Disorders Associated with Medical Problems

Many medical problems cause sleep disturbance in the older adult (Table 12-1). These include cardiovascular diseases, diabetes, gastrointestinal reflux, and arthritis. People with chronic obstructive lung disease often experience disrupted sleep because of reduced lung capacity, difficulty breathing, and a buildup of carbon dioxide (McCrae, Lichstein, 2002). Cardiovascular disease can manifest with nocturnal cardiac ischemia and may result in alteration in respiration or transient angina, thus causing frequent awakenings. Diabetes may contribute to nightmares or early-morning awakening as a result of the fluctuation in blood glucose levels. Chronic pain and discomfort, which may be the most common medical cause of insomnia among institutionalized elderly, interfere with sleep and change conventional sleep architecture (Bliwise, Breus, 2000).

Sleep Disorders Associated with Dementia

People with Alzheimer's disease have more arousals and awakenings and spend more time in stage I sleep and less time in stage III and IV NREM sleep than do elders without dementia (McCrae, Lichstein, 2002). This becomes more pronounced with disease progression. The incidence of sleep apnea may also be higher in people with Alzheimer's disease and other dementias. Increased agitation and activity during the late afternoon and evening (often called *sundowner's syndrome*) may also occur. Although the exact causes are not known, the following factors have been suggested: deterioration in the neurological mechanisms controlling the sleep-wake cycle, fatigue, low daytime illumination, and staffing changes that tend to occur in the late afternoon. Before attributing behavior changes to sundowning, it is important to rule out other potential causes of restlessness and agitation, such as pain, depression, infection, fluid and electrolyte imbalances, constipation and impactions, and medication effects, as well as environmental factors, such as noise and changes in routines. Other suggestions for management include medication reviews, providing only short daytime naps, engaging in meaningful activities, exercise, assessment and treatment of pain, calm environments, regular toileting, and adequate daylight or light exposure (McCrae, Lichstein, 2002).

Sleep Disorders Related to Psychiatric Problems

Anxiety and depression also contribute to sleep difficulties, including inability to fall asleep, awaking and not being able to return to sleep, or early-morning awakening (see Table 12-1). Life events of the elderly, such as loss of a spouse, situational disruptions, retirement, and change in living arrangements, often result in anxiety and

Table 12-1 Causes, Reasons/Symptoms, Assessment, and Interventions for Sleep Alterations in Older Adults

Causes	Reasons/symptoms	Assessment	Potential/actual Interventions
Alcoholism	Abnormal EEG pattern results as effects wear off; sleeper may awaken with withdrawal symptoms and a hangover; early-morning awakening	Sleep log and interview with bed partner or caregiver	No alcoholic beverages; explain that reformed alcoholics may experience insomnia 1 yr or so after withdrawal of alcohol; may require temporary medication to relieve symptoms that interfere with sleep
Alzheimer's disease (AD)	AD patients' sleep shows reduction in stage III and stage IV sleep early in disease; late in AD, these stages disappear; daytime sleepiness increases as disease progresses; nighttime wandering; sundowning	Sleep history from family or caregivers	Assist family and/or staff with wandering behavior and sundowning syndrome; be sure person has comfortable chair in which to rest; strict schedule of nighttime bed hours, daytime naps, activity periods, and attendance to needs; for wanderers and behavior problems, stop all drug treatment to see if normal sleep rhythm returns
Anxiety	A feeling of dread, doom, or uneasiness; pacing, irritable, fidgety; stomach or nerve trouble	Psychosocial history; 24-hr sleep diary; Hamilton scale	Supportive care; explain new routines and treatments; encourage decision making; support previous lifestyle
Arthritis	Early-morning awakening secondary to pain of muscle/joint stiffness; wearing off of pain medication	Medical history; sleep history	Sustained-release analgesic 30 min before sleep; provide comfortable pillows to support joints; careful use of electrical blankets for warmth

Table 12-1 Causes, Reasons/Symptoms, Assessment, and Interventions for Sleep Alterations in Older Adults—*Continued*

Causes	Reasons/symptoms	Assessment	Potential/actual Interventions
Cardiovascular	Frequent awakenings, nocturia	Medical history; sleep history	Sustained-release nitroglycerin; nitroglycerin at bedside; take diuretic in morning; restrict fluids close to bedtime; prop up on pillows
Chronic obstructive pulmonary disease (COPD)	Abnormal increase in alveolar tension; decrease in oxygen saturation; prone position causes dyspnea and stasis of mucus	Medical history; sleep history	Patient education regarding self-care; pulmonary toilet before bedtime; use of bronchial dilators; need to prevent fatigue; rest during day; no diuretics in late afternoon; need to avoid cola, coffee, tea, chocolate; need to use caution with sedatives and OTC medication
Depression	Difficulty falling asleep, sustaining sleep, or early-morning awakening; feelings of helplessness, hopelessness, or sadness; decreased energy, low self-esteem; withdrawal; confusion or disorientation; history of recent loss	Psychosocial history; medical history and history of current medication use (prescribed and OTC); Geriatric Depression Scale (GDS)	Counseling; SSRIs or tricyclic antidepressants if depression confirmed; socialization, reminiscence
Diabetes mellitus	Early-morning awakening secondary to hypoglycemia; unpleasant dreams or nightmares; nocturia	Medical history; sleep history; eating schedule; fasting blood glucose levels	Carbohydrate bedtime snack; reevaluate medication regimen (oral hypoglycemic agent or insulin)
Disturbed sensory perception	Early-morning awakening; poor environmental lighting; visual difficulties; nocturnal hallucinations; alteration in REM-NREM cycle	Medical history, check hearing and vision; sleep history	Modify environment; check hearing aid; put glasses nearby; reduce noise in home or hospital; frequent reassurance
Gastrointestinal reflux (GERD)	Difficulty falling asleep or early-morning awakening secondary to abdominal or chest discomfort caused by gastric secretions	Medical history; sleep history	Restrict intake after evening meal; antacid medication 2 hr before bedtime; elevate head and shoulders for sleeping; ensure that medication for reflux is taken appropriately (e.g., H_2 inhibitors, acid pump inhibitors, promotility agents)

Continued

Table 12-1 Causes, Reasons/Symptoms, Assessment, and Interventions for Sleep Alterations in Older Adults—*Continued*

Causes	Reasons/Symptoms	Assessment	Potential/Actual Interventions
Obstructive sleep apnea (OSA)	Frequent awakenings with nocturia; snoring; morning headache; unusual daytime drowsiness or sleepiness; frequent daytime naps	24-hr sleep diary; interview bed partner; clinical sleep studies (polysomnography)	Continuous positive airway pressure via mask; weight loss; surgery
Parkinson's disease	Difficulty with sleep in general; total wake time increases; decreased REM sleep	Medical history; 24-hr sleep diary	Levodopa (L-dopa) at bedtime may help decrease rigidity that occurs during night
Peptic ulcers	Periodic awakenings when in REM sleep (gastric juices increase during REM sleep, causing epigastric pain)	Medical history	Take appropriate prescribed medication
Periodic limb movement disorder	Frequent awakenings; nocturnal restlessness; muscle soreness; daytime fatigue	Interview bed partner; medication history; clinical sleep studies (polysomnography)	Administration of prescribed medications, such as benzodiazepines
Restless leg syndrome	Difficulty falling asleep; crawling, pulling sensation in legs, especially at night when sitting or lying down	Sleep history; medication history	Vitamin E; quinine tablets or capsules or quinine water (tonic water); low-dose narcotic analgesics. Carbidopa-levodopa
Situational insomnia	Difficulty falling asleep and staying asleep on admission to institution; after visiting a relative; after moving to a new residence; after recent loss or death; change in nighttime routine	Usually transient but helpful to get a brief sleep history	Establish a one-to-one relationship; if necessary, use hypnotics for short term only (e.g., 1 wk)
Surgical procedures	Premature arousal related to blood drawn in early morning; anxiety, worry about outcome and pain		Analyze rituals and routines in place; can they be changed? Keep pain free; monitor vital signs frequently and promote rest

Modified from Beck-Little R, Weinrich SP: Assessment and management of sleep disorders in the elderly, *J Gerontol Nurs* 24(4):21-29, 1998; Ebersole P, Hess P: *Toward healthy aging: human needs and nursing response,* ed 5, St Louis, 1998, Mosby.
EEG, Electroencephalogram; *OTC,* over the counter; *SSRIs,* selective serotonin reuptake inhibitors; *REM,* rapid eye movement; *NREM,* non–rapid eye movement.

Table 12-2 Sleep-Related Effects of Commonly Used Medications by the Older Adult

Medication or Chemical	Common Sleep-Related Effect(s)
Antiparkinson agents	Somnolence, insomnia, dizziness, anxiety, confusion, orthostatic hypotension, nightmares
Agents for Alzheimer's disease	Insomnia, fatigue, muscle cramps
Beta blockers (especially the more lipophilic agents, e.g., propranolol)	Nightmares
Diuretics	Awakening for nocturia, somnolence, insomnia, hallucinations
Antidepressants (especially amitriptyline, doxepin, trazodone)	PLMS, suppression of REM sleep, CNS overstimulation, insomnia, sedation
Benzodiazepines	Awakening secondary to apnea, sedation
Anticholinergics	Muscle twitching, urinary retention, dry mouth, hyperreflexia
Psychotropics	CNS depression, drowsiness, paradoxical excitation, somnolence, insomnia, sedation, ataxia
Barbiturates	Nightmares, hallucinations, paradoxical excitation, suppression of REM sleep
Corticosteroids	Sleep disturbances, restlessness
Theophylline, phenytoin	Interfere with sleep onset and sleep stages
Alcohol	Early-morning awakening, suppression of REM sleep
Alcohol or hypnotic withdrawal	Sleep disturbances, rebound insomnia, nightmares
Caffeine	Prolongs sleep latency and interferes with sleep maintenance

PLMS, Periodic limb jerks or movements in sleep; *REM,* rapid eye movement; *CNS,* central nervous system.

depression that interfere with sleep. Depression, dementia, or sensory impairments such as poor hearing and vision may interfere with the person's ability to respond to time and light cues and environmental stimuli (Miller, 2004). The use of SSRIs in the treatment of depression can also have a stimulating effect that disturbs sleep (McCrae, Lichstein, 2002).

Sleep and Drugs

Prescription and nonprescription medications and sleep aids contribute to insomnia in older people. The side effects of many common medications used by older people include sleep disturbances. Table 12-2 presents some of these medications. Caffeine, nicotine, and alcohol also interfere with sleep. Psychotropic medications used in the treatment of behaviors related to Alzheimer's disease or other dementias, especially those with anticholinergic activity, may aggravate or cause insomnia. The use of hypnotics, sedatives, and over-the-counter sleep aids is common among older people. Approximately 40% of sleeping pill prescriptions are written for older people (Hoffman, 2003). However, few hypnotic drugs are compatible with the normal sleep cycle. Instead, these drugs interfere with deep sleep stages and depress the REM sleep necessary for the relief of mental stress, such as tension and anxiety. When medication is discontinued, there may be a rebound period of insomnia before normal sleep patterns return. Dreaming and nightmares are also increased until natural sleep cycles are reestablished. Some researchers believe that this compensates for dreams that have been depressed or obliterated by REM sleep suppression.

Drug tolerance, physical dependence, daytime delirium, drowsiness, and depression of mental alertness also occur with chronic use of bedtime hypnotic agents. Hypnotic drugs often induce night terrors, hallucinations, and such paradoxical responses as agitation instead of relaxation; hangover; depression; changes in memory; and

Box 12-3	OBRA Guidelines for Use of Pharmacological Agents for Sleep in Nursing Homes

- Medications used for sleep induction should be used only if evidence exists that other potential reasons for insomnia have been ruled out (depression, pain, noise, light, caffeine, routine awakenings).
- A drug should only be used if it results in the maintenance or improvement of the resident's functional status.
- If insomnia is assessed, prescribe a short-acting sedative-hypnotic and limit use to less than 10 days unless dosage reduction is unsuccessful.
- Attempt dose reduction three times in 6 months unless harmful to the patient.
- If treatment with a short-acting sedative-hypnotic fails, prescribe a short-acting benzodiazepine and limit use to less than 4 months unless dosage reduction is unsuccessful.
- Attempt dose reduction twice each year unless harmful to the patient.
- Drug doses should be equal to or less than those specified in the dosing guidelines unless higher doses are necessary for improvement or maintenance of the resident's functional status (as evidenced by the resident's response and/or clinical status).
- A gradual dose reduction should be attempted at least three times within 6 months before one can conclude that a gradual dose reduction is contraindicated.

Adapted from Cefalu C: Evaluation and management of insomnia in the institutionalized elderly, *Ann Long-Term Care* 12(6):31, 2004; Appropriate use of psychotropic drugs in nursing homes, *American Family Physician*. Accessed 8/5/04 from http://www.aafp.org.

balance and gait changes leading to falls. If older persons have been taking long-acting benzodiazepines or barbiturates for sleep, they should be tapered over a 1-month period for every year that they have been on continuous therapy. Tapering should be performed with a low dose of a long-acting benzodiazepine rather than a short-acting one to prevent rebound insomnia and withdrawal seizures (Cefalu, 2004).

After a thorough assessment of sleep problems, if medications are indicated, they should be limited to short-term use (7 to 10 days) for the treatment of transient insomnia only and combined with nonpharmacological interventions. The newer nonbenzodiazepines, such as zolpidem (Ambien) and zaleplon (Sonata), should be used since they are short acting and have fewer side effects of sedation or rebound. Trazodone (Desyrel) may be used if there is depression because this antidepressant has a good sleep profile. Many people consider over-the-counter sleep aids a safe substitute for hypnotics. However, most of these preparations contain diphenhydramine hydrochloride with or without acetaminophen. Because of their anticholinergic properties, their use is often associated with reduced quality of sleep, daytime drowsiness, falls, cognitive impairment, blurred vision, constipation, dry mouth, and urinary retention and should be avoided. In the nursing home setting, the use of psychotropic and hypnotic agents (considered chemical restraints) is limited, and their use must comply with the Omnibus Budget Reconciliation Act of 1987 (OBRA '87) (see Box 12-3 for OBRA guidelines). Careful assessment of the causes of sleep disturbances must be conducted before pharmacological treatment is prescribed. Nonpharmacological therapies are discussed later in the chapter.

IMPLICATIONS FOR GERONTOLOGICAL NURSING AND HEALTHY AGING

Assessment

Nurses are in an excellent position to assess sleep, to improve the quality of the aged person's sleep, and to study sleep or assist in sleep research by being available at customary sleep times. Sleep history interviews are important and should be obtained from all elderly clients. The nurse should learn how well the person sleeps at home, how many times the person is awakened at night, what time the person retires, and what rituals occur at bedtime. Rituals include bedtime snacks, watching television, listening to music, or reading—activities that, unless carried out, interfere with the individual's ability to fall asleep. Other assessment data should include the amount and type of daily exercise; favorite position when in bed; room environment, including temperature, ventilation, and illumination; activities engaged in several hours before bedtime; and sleep medications as well as other medications taken routinely. Some medications taken regularly produce side effects that interfere with the ability to sleep. Information about the individual's involvement in hobbies, life satisfaction, and perception of health status is also important in assessing for possible depression. Caregivers and/or family members can also provide valuable information about the person's sleep habits and lifestyle.

Subjective and objective measures of sleep assessment available to nurses include visual analog scales, subjective rating scales (e.g., 0 to 10 or 0 to 100), questionnaires that determine if one's sleep is disturbed, interviews, and daily sleep charts. A self-rating scale, the Pittsburgh Sleep Quality Index (PSQI), can be used to measure the quality and patterns of sleep in the older adult (www.hartfordign.org). Objective measures include polysomnography conducted in sleep laboratories, including electroencephalograms (EEGs), electromyograms (EMGs), and direct observations (Schoenfelder, Culp, 2001).

A nursing standard of practice protocol for sleep disturbances in elderly patients was developed as part of the Nurses Improving Care of the Hospitalized Elderly (NICHE) Project, supported by a grant from the Hartford Foundation. Assessment standards are presented in Table 12-3. The assessment is to elicit information relative to indicators or defining characteristics of sleep disturbance. The sleep diary or log is noted as an important part of assessment. This information will provide an accurate account of the person's sleep problem and identify the sleep disturbance. Usually a family member or the caregiver, if the older person is institutionalized, records specific behaviors on a flow sheet. A period of 2 to 4 weeks

is required to obtain a clear picture of the sleep problem. Important items to record are the following:

1. The number of times a call for assistance to the bathroom or for pain medication or subjective symptoms of inability to sleep (e.g., anxiety) occur
2. If the person is out of bed
3. Whether the person appears to be asleep or awake when the nurse is on rounds
4. Episodes of confusion or disorientation
5. If sleep medication was given and if repeated
6. The time the person awakens in the morning (approximation)
7. Where the person falls asleep in the evening
8. Daytime naps

Interventions

Interventions begin after a thorough sleep history has been recorded and, if possible, a sleep log obtained. Management is directed at identifiable causes. Intervention standards are a part of the nursing standard of practice protocol (see Table 12-3 for sleep disturbances [NICHE Project]). The interventions are based on the principle that to be effective, first, the intervention must be individualized, considering the specific characteristics of the patient and the nature of the sleep disturbance; and second, pharmacological treatment should be considered as an adjuvant treatment to nonpharmacological interventions. A meta-analysis of treatment protocols revealed that 70% to 80% of patients will improve with behavioral therapy (Kirkwood, 2001). Other researchers suggest that the optimal management may be to begin with a hypnotic, followed by behavioral therapy after discontinuing the medication (Griffith, 2002). Behavioral changes have a longer-lasting effect and require more self-direction on the part of the patient. Examples include stimulus control or sleep restriction therapy as well as behavioral routines or other rules of sleep hygiene. Examples of these behavioral treatments are found in Boxes 12-4 and 12-5. Attention to the sleep environment, particularly in institutions, is also important. Limiting noise, light, and frequent awakenings may help promote better sleep. Further research is needed, and gerontological nurses should take an active role in the design of

Table 12-3 Nursing Standard of Practice Protocol: Sleep Disturbance in Elderly Patients

Assessment	Health Promotion and Maintenance Intervention	Evaluation
SLEEP-WAKE PATTERNS Inquire about usual times for retiring and rising, time for falling asleep, frequency and duration of nighttime awakenings; frequency and duration of daytime naps; daytime physical and social activity Have person provide a subjective evaluation of the quality of sleep Have person complete sleep log for 2 wk	MAINTAIN NORMAL SLEEP PATTERN Maintain usual bedtime/ wake time Avoid staying in bed beyond waking hours Encourage to get up at regular time even if did not sleep well Schedule nighttime activities to provide uninterrupted periods of sleep of at least 2-3 hr Balance daytime activity and rest Encourage keeping daytime naps to a minimum Promote social interaction Encourage exercise before evening	OBJECTIVE EVIDENCE Time required to fall asleep; should fall asleep within 30-45 min Time for awakening, at usual reported time Behavior, alertness, attention, ability to concentrate, reaction time Observe duration of sleep: patient should remain asleep for at least 4-hr intervals
BEDTIME ROUTINES/RITUALS Inquire about activities performed by the individual before bedtime (e.g., personal hygiene, prayer, reading, watching TV, listening to music, snacks)	SUPPORT BEDTIME ROUTINES/RITUALS Offer a bedtime snack or beverage Enable bedtime reading or listening to music Assist with aspects of personal hygiene at bedtime (e.g., bath) Encourage prayer or meditation Assist in establishing a relaxing bedtime routine	SUBJECTIVE EVIDENCE Verbalizations about the quality and quantity of sleep (e.g., statements of difficulty falling asleep, of frequent awakenings, of having slept well, of feeling well rested/ refreshed, of an increased sense of well-being)
MEDICATIONS Obtain information relative to all prescribed and self-selected OTC medications used by person, especially sleep aids, diuretics, laxatives Determine types of medications and length of time used by person	AVOID/MINIMIZE DRUGS THAT NEGATIVELY INFLUENCE SLEEP Pharmacological treatment of sleep disturbances is treatment of last resort Discontinue or adjust the dose or dosing schedule of any/all offending medications Consider drug-drug potentiation Administer medications to promote sleep (e.g., give diuretics at least 4 hr before bedtime)	
DIET EFFECTS Obtain information about consumption of caffeinated and alcoholic beverages	MINIMIZE/AVOID FOODS THAT NEGATIVELY INFLUENCE SLEEP Discourage use of beverages containing stimulants (e.g., coffee, tea, sodas) in afternoon and evening Encourage use of food naturally containing L-tryptophan	

Table 12-3 Nursing Standard of Practice Protocol: Sleep Disturbance in Elderly Patients—*Continued*

Assessment	Health Promotion and Maintenance Intervention	Evaluation
	Provide snacks according to patient preference Generally, discourage use of alcoholic beverages Decrease fluid intake 2-4 hr before bedtime Encourage to have lighter meal in evening	
ENVIRONMENTAL FACTORS Evaluate noise, light, temperature, ventilation, bedding Inquire about distance of bathroom from bedroom Inquire about use of night-lights	**CREATE OPTIMAL ENVIRONMENT FOR SLEEP** Keep noise to an absolute minimum Set room temperature according to preference Provide blankets as requested Use night-light as desired Provide soft music or white noise to mask noise Use light exposure during day and evening to maintain wakefulness	
PHYSIOLOGICAL FACTORS Evaluate breathing pattern with sleep, with attention to pauses Observe for periodic movementor jerking during sleep Inquire about sleeping position Note diagnoses of sleep disorders Note diagnoses of specific health problems that adversely affect sleep (e.g., CHF, COPD)	**PROMOTE PHYSIOLOGICAL STABILITY** Elevate head of bed as required Provide extra pillows per preference Administer bronchodilators, if prescribed, before bedtime Use medical therapeutics (e.g., continuous positive airway pressure machine) as prescribed	
ILLNESS FACTORS Inquire about pain, affective disturbances (e.g., depression, anxiety, worry, fatigue, discomfort)	**PROMOTE COMFORT** Provide analgesia as needed 30 min before bedtime (Note that some OTC analgesics may have caffeine.) Massage back or foot to help relax Warm and cool compresses to painful areas as indicated Use relaxation methods—deep breathing, progressive relaxation, mental imagery Encourage to urinate before going to bed Keep path to bathroom clear/provide bedside commode	

Modified from Foreman MD, Wykle M: Nursing standard-of-practice protocol: sleep disturbances in elderly patients, *Geriatr Nurs* 16(5):238-243, 1995.

OTC, Over the counter; *CHF*, congestive heart failure; *COPD*, chronic obstructive pulmonary disease.

Box 12-4	Stimulus Control for Insomnia

- Go to sleep only with the intention of sleep and when sleepy.
- Use the bed only for sleep and sexual activity.
- If you cannot fall asleep, get up and go to another room. Stay up as long as needed to feel sleepy. Return to bed when sleepy. If unable to sleep again after 10 minutes, repeat and get up as long as needed.
- Set the alarm clock and get up at the same time every morning, regardless of how long you slept.
- Do not nap during the day.

Adapted from Kirkwood C: *Treatment of insomnia*, New York, 2001, Power-Pak, CE Publishers. Available at www.powerpak.com.

Box 12-5	Sleep Hygiene Rules

1. Have a regular bedtime and wake-up time even on weekends.
2. Avoid naps. If you must nap, sleep no longer than 30 minutes in early afternoon.
3. Exercise at least 3 hours before bedtime.
4. Wind down during the evening; have a bedtime routine, such as brush teeth, set alarm clock, and read.
5. Limit caffeine (tea, cola, coffee, chocolate), nicotine, and diuretics, especially late in the day.
6. Do not use alcohol to sleep. It maintains a light sleep, not a restful, deep sleep.
7. If you have reflux, eat the evening meal at least 3 to 4 hours before bedtime; have a light snack if needed before bedtime.
8. Give attention to the bed environment (comfortable bed, pillows between the knees, quiet, darkness, warm temperature).
9. Do not watch the clock, which increases anxiety and pressure to sleep; if anxious, take a warm bath.

Adapted from Beers MH, Berkow R: *Merck manual of geriatrics*, ed 3, Whitehouse Station, NJ, 2000, Merck Research Laboratories; Sleep Clinic of San Francisco: *Rules for good sleep hygiene*. Press release 8/30/01.

such studies. Box 12-6 provides suggestions to promote sleep in nursing homes.

Other behavioral techniques include progressive muscle relaxation, meditation, hypnosis, and biofeedback. Bright light therapy helps reset the patient's biological clock. It is also used to treat depression. Bright light therapy is given 30 minutes to 2 hours each day. Duration depends on the brightness of the light (Beers, Berkow, 2000). Outdoor light or a commercially made light box can be used. Room light is inadequate. For older people in moderate climates, time outdoors in the sunlight may be beneficial.

Melatonin, which is classified as a dietary supplement, has been the topic of talk shows and numerous popular magazines over the past several years. It has been cited not only as a sleep aid, but also as an age-reversing, disease-fighting hormone. It is an over-the-counter drug, and its use is controversial. There are no studies known to have been conducted in older adults. The preparations that are available lack control and are unregulated, and quality is unknown. Aromatherapy has also been mentioned as beneficial in sleep promotion. Common essential oils to try for insomnia include *Lavandula angustifolia* (true lavender), *Chamaemelum nobile* (Roman chamomile), *Salvia sclarea* (Clary sage), *Santalum album* (sandalwood),

and *Rosa damascene* (rose). Ethnicity and learned memory of smell influence the choice of essential oil. Hispanics and Latinos prefer *Origanum majorana* (sweet marjoram) to lavender, African Americans prefer *Elettaria cardamomum* (cardamom) to lavender, and Asians prefer *Cananga odorata* (ylang-ylang). Assessment for allergies as well as individual taste is important. The person can place a cotton ball with a few drops of oil under the pillowcase when going to bed, pin a handkerchief with oil to the pajamas, drop oil in a diffuser, or add a few drops to a before-bedtime bath (Buckle, 2002).

Evaluation

The nursing standard of practice protocol presented in Table 12-3 includes an evaluation component. Observation of the person when awake and asleep is necessary. Physiological changes

Box 12-6	Suggestions to Promote Sleep in Nursing Homes

- Limit intake of caffeine and other fluids in excess before bedtime.
- Provide a light snack or warm beverage before bedtime.
- Maintain a quiet environment: soft lights, quiet music, limited noise and staff intrusions when possible.
- Reduce nursing interruptions for resident medication administration by modifying dose schedule if possible.
- Discontinue invasive treatments when possible (Foley catheters, percutaneous gastrostomy tubes (PEG) tubes, intravenous lines).
- Encourage and assist to the bathroom before bed and as needed.
- Give pain medication before bedtime for patients with pain.
- Provide regular exercise or walking programs.
- Allow resident to stay out of bed and out of the room for as long as possible before bed if possible.
- Institute same time for resident to arise and get out of bed every morning.
- Maintain comfortable temperature in room; provide blankets as needed.
- Provide meaningful activities during the daytime.

Adapted from Cefalu C: Evaluation and management of insomnia in the institutionalized elderly, *Ann Long-Term Care* 12(6):25, 2004.

observable for each stage of sleep reviewed previously can be evaluated to give clues to the phases of the sleep cycle experienced. It is essential to obtain subjective evidence of the quality and quantity of sleep.

ACTIVITY

Activity is a direct use of energy in voluntary and involuntary physical and mental ways that alter the microenvironment and macroenvironment of the individual. The focus of this section is on physical activity. Improving individual participation in regular physical activity to improve func-

tional fitness and overall physical and mental health is one of the goals of *Healthy People 2010* (U.S. Department of Health and Human Services, 2002). The Administration on Aging (AOA) at the National Institute on Aging (2002) gives the following facts:

- Exercise may help older people feel better and enjoy life more, even if they think they are too old or too out of shape.
- Most older adults (more than two thirds) do not get enough physical activity.
- The combination of lack of physical activity and poor diet is the second highest underlying cause of death in the United States (smoking is the leading cause).
- Regular exercise can improve function in older people, improve mood, and relieve depression.
- Staying physically active on a regular, permanent basis helps prevent certain diseases, such as cancers, heart disease, diabetes, and disabilities, as we grow older.

Public perceptions of older people and how they spend their time continue to reflect the belief that later life ushers in the pursuit of sedentary, private, isolated activity and the assumption of a passive role in society. Physical activity is often the barometer by which an individual's health and wellness are judged. The inability to exercise, do physical work, or perform activities of daily living is among the first indicators of decline. Research in gerontological exercise physiology is relatively young, but in general, results indicate that maintenance of a physically active lifestyle arrests or significantly delays age changes associated with cardiovascular, respiratory, and musculoskeletal function.

Physical inactivity is a risk factor for many conditions experienced by the elderly, including obesity; diabetes; and cardiovascular, respiratory, and musculoskeletal diseases. These conditions and other changes generally attributed to aging may in fact be due to inactivity. Regular exercise reduces mortality rates even for smokers and obese elders (Beers, Berkow, 2000). Indirect benefits of regular exercise include increased social interaction, increased sense of well-being, and improved quality of sleep.

Direct benefits of exercise include preservation of muscle strength, increased aerobic capacity, greater bone density, and greater mobility and independence (Beers, Berkow, 2000). Regular exercise is known to increase insulin sensitivity and glucose tolerance and therefore is part of the management plan of anyone with diabetes. Exercise, if done on a regular basis, reduces systolic and diastolic blood pressures and can lessen the need for drug therapy. Exercise increases high-density lipoproteins (HDLs) and lowers triglycerides. It is beneficial in mood disorders such as depression, so common in older adults. Other physical benefits include improved cardiac muscle tone, decreased percentage of body fat, improved ability to breathe deeply and effectively, reduced tension, favorable bowel control, and appetite control.

Regular exercise can help prevent falls and injury by improving balance, strength, neuromuscular coordination, joint function, and endurance. Benefits in both physical and psychosocial aspects of function have been found for community-living and institutionalized elderly. All elders, whether frail or healthy, can benefit from various forms of exercise programs.

IMPLICATIONS FOR GERONTOLOGICAL NURSING AND HEALTHY AGING

Assessment

An assessment should be initiated before an older adult begins an exercise program. The assessment needs to include a medical history; knowledge of the individual's physical activity level and/or physical limitations; current medication regimen; and emotional, psychological, and social needs.

In addition to the medical history, a physical examination with emphasis on cardiovascular, pulmonary, musculoskeletal, and neurological systems should be done. The examination should focus on those aspects that may have an impact on functional status and that may give clues to potential risk. Attention should be focused on joint range of motion, flexibility, and strength. Previous injuries and the presence of active inflammation need to be assessed. Conditions that must be stabilized before starting an exercise program include unstable angina, thrombophlebitis, cardiomyopathy, uncontrolled arrhythmias, uncompensated heart failure, and high systolic (>200 mm Hg) and diastolic (>110 mm Hg) blood pressures (Beers, Berkow, 2000).

Fitness Testing

Fitness testing may be warranted in some elders with chronic illnesses. Performance on a 6-minute walk test can help determine the intensity level to start fitness training (Beers, Berkow, 2000). It also provides feedback to the person as he or she improves in performance over time. The American College of Sports Medicine recommends exercise tolerance testing (ETT) for the elderly before they begin a moderately intense or vigorous exercise program. This test provides information regarding metabolic equivalents and the target heart rate of the older person. ETT is not recommended for the frail elderly. A frail elder's functional impairments may hinder the ability to perform an adequate test. The strength required for ETT may exceed the aerobic capacity of a frail elder. ETT is not essential for the elderly who desire to start a simple walking program or perform a level of exercise aimed at improving mobility and performance of activities of daily living.

Exercise Supervision

Some patients should be supervised during exercise testing and the exercise program. This may be done in a rehabilitation center. These patients include those with acquired valvular heart disease, congenital heart disease, angina, ventricular arrhythmias, severe coronary artery disease of three vessels or the main vessel, two previous myocardial infarctions, an ejection fraction of less than 30%, heart disease symptoms at rest or in very low intensity activity, and those that have a drop in systolic blood pressure with exercise (Beers, Berkow, 2000).

The risk of cardiac events in sedentary older women is greater than in younger individuals. Elderly women exercise less than elderly men and are at higher risk for deconditioning. However, a review of randomized, controlled exercise trials confirms a low rate of myocardial infarction and cardiovascular complications (George, Goldberg, 2001). A concern is the increase in blood pressure during resistance exercises. Large changes in blood pressure during exercise can be avoided if older women are educated about avoiding Valsalva's maneuver and maintaining normal breathing patterns.

Laboratory Analysis

Laboratory analysis should include a hematocrit ratio and a hemoglobin level. A low hematocrit ratio and hemoglobin level will increase the workload on the heart to maintain an adequate oxygen supply. In addition, analysis of electrolyte and fluid balance is necessary to evaluate conductivity and contractility of the heart muscle and its ability to function adequately. Lipid levels may be obtained to evaluate positive change, and thyroid studies may be obtained if this is a possible reason for inactivity.

Exercise Prescription

Four types of exercise may be prescribed that will be therapeutic for different people: endurance exercises, muscle strengthening, balance training, and flexibility exercises. The person's level of fitness and medical problems will be considered in choosing the type of exercise. Those who are markedly decompensated should start very slowly. Older adults with difficulty standing can perform seated exercise programs using cuff weights for strength training and those with arthritis can benefit from water exercises. The prescription is most effective if the nurse finds one that consists of activities the person most enjoys or activities the person has selected.

The U.S. Centers for Disease Control and Prevention (CDC) recommends that all adults participate in at least 30 minutes of exercise over a 24-hour period with a goal of 180 minutes of moderate-intensity activity each week. Three 10-minute activities meet the goal and may work best for elders who cannot do 30 minutes at one time. Older people may want to learn to monitor their heart rates during exercise. An exercise stress test will determine the maximum heart rate and target heart rate range. A conservative formula for estimating maximum heart rate is 220 minus age (Beers, Berkow, 2000). Moderate-intensity exercise is that which produces 60% to 79% of maximum heart rate. If the person has a maximum heart rate of 160, the target rate will be 96 to 128 beats/min. A rating of perceived exertion can be used to assess tolerance to exercise. The Borg scale has been used successfully to measure perceived exertion among older adults. The scale ranges from 6 to 20 points, with a rating of 6, 7, or 8 for very, very light intensity; 13 or 14 for somewhat hard intensity; and up to 19 or 20 for very, very hard intensity. It is rec-

ommended that a rating of perceived exertion be used rather than a pulse rate for monitoring exertion during exercise. The ability to talk while exercising suggests how well or how long one can exercise; if one can talk easily while exercising, the exercise intensity level is low or moderate for that person. If talking is difficult, the intensity may be too high.

If the nurse is directing exercise for an older adult, checking the pulse at baseline, during the activity, and following the activity should be done. Careful observation of the person is important during activity and includes observing for dyspnea; flushed cheeks, cyanotic nail beds, or lips. Complaints of fatigue, tiredness, dizziness, and requests to sit down are additional signs of inability to tolerate the activity. Obviously, tightness and heaviness in the chest and tightness in the legs are indicative of diminished capacity for activity. If nothing occurs within the expected tolerance level but the nurse notices that the person is slowing down, shows signs of decreased dexterity or coordination, and needs frequent rests, then the person is not able to tolerate that level of activity.

The older person may be able to integrate activity into daily life rather than doing a specific exercise. Examples are walking to the store instead of driving, golfing, swimming, hiking, raking leaves, and gardening. Where there is a need for especially low-intensity exercise, the person can work for 2 to 3 minutes, rest for 2 to 3 minutes, and continue this pattern for 15 to 20 minutes. Some examples of moderate-intensity activity include washing and waxing the car for 45 to 60 minutes, washing windows or floors for 45 to 60 minutes, gardening for 35 to 40 minutes, wheeling self in wheelchair for 30 to 40 minutes, walking 2 miles in 30 minutes, or swimming laps or water aerobics for 20 minutes (accessed 8/3/04 from http://www.americangeriatrics.org/education/falls.shtml). People who are extremely deconditioned will improve markedly with this program. A sustained brisk walk is one of the most popular and accessible forms of activity for older people. Those who have done little walking are encouraged to start slowly by first walking to the corner of the block and eventually being able to develop the capacity for distance walking of several miles. Those limited to institutional facilities should also be encouraged to increase the amount of walking.

First it may be only from the bed to the bathroom, then with time down the hall, and eventually around the total facility or even outside. Restorative walking programs should be an integral activity in all long-term care institutions.

Intervention and Evaluation

The benefits of activity on the health of elderly persons support the need for incorporation of activity into the plan of care. The nurse's role has implications for knowledge about fitness and approval of exercise programs in which the older person may participate. Attention should be paid to the simplicity, effectiveness, and adaptability of a program for older adults in whatever setting they may live. Acceptable exercise programs for older adults should have realistic objectives and provide for improvement and maintenance of endurance, strength, flexibility, balance, and coordination while minimizing the risk of injury.

Exercise Programs

Participation in exercise programs is influenced by a number of factors. Motivating elders to change behavior is not always easy. A successful exercise program needs to address perceived barriers to exercise (dispel misconceptions about exercise as dangerous, uncomfortable, exhausting, or embarrassing and address poor weather and lack of facilities and transportation); tailor the exercise to the current fitness status and abilities of each individual; provide various forms of social support (leader, class members, family, friends, assigned partners); use a decision balance sheet that has participants contrast potential benefits with barriers to exercise; cue exercise participants to focus on how they feel during exercise; and agree on appropriate exercises. The following variables reflect critical characteristics of exercise programs that improve acceptance into the older person's lifestyle:

1. Low to moderate intensity, duration, and frequency
2. Group participation and social pleasure
3. Emphasis on variety and pleasure, including use of games as exercise
4. Setting of personal goals; contracts
5. Evaluation of response to training and demonstration of improvement

6. Involvement of friends, family, or spouse
7. Use of music
8. Positive feedback
9. Enthusiastic leadership and role models

Barbara Resnick, a leader in gerontological nursing, has done extensive research on the benefits of exercise and ways to motivate older adults to exercise and implement activity and exercise programs for community-living and institutionalized older adults. She suggested a seven-step approach (Resnick, 2004) to implement an exercise program and help older adults stay motivated to continue:

1. Education
2. Exercise prescreening
3. Goal identification
4. Exposure to the exercise behavior
5. Role models
6. Verbal encouragement
7. Verbal reinforcement and rewards

Enjoyment and individualization of the program to meet individual goals and needs are key factors in improving long-term participation. Another consideration for many older adults is the expense associated with the exercise program. Many elderly persons have limited financial reserves for recreational purposes; however, many of today's health, fitness, and recreation centers have low fee rates specifically for those over age 55.

It is also important that individuals who conduct aerobic exercise programs and classes consider differences between the abilities of the young and the old. Classes are generally taught by young and fit persons who become so involved in what they are doing that they are unaware that adults over age 60 may not be able to do the number of repetitions at the intensity they consider necessary for toning muscles. These programs can damage the muscles, tendons, ligaments, and joints of the older adult. Training older fit women or men to lead aerobic exercise programs is helpful; participants can identify and bond with the leaders. The American Senior Fitness Association (http://www.seniorfitness.net) offers information on senior fitness in a variety of settings as well as a senior fitness instructor training program. A variety of exercise programs exist for the elderly. The existing programs need to be evaluated on an individual basis to determine if they are appropriate. Box 12-7 presents guidelines

Box 12-7	Guidelines for Developing or Modifying an Exercise Program

1. Base program on individual assessment data (underlying conditions, medications, present activity level).
2. Establish mutual goals.
3. Teach to use correct body mechanics, wear appropriate clothing (layer so can adapt to environment), wear exercise-specific (supportive) shoes, and maintain sufficient hydration (drink water before, during, and after).
4. Begin at a very low level (40% to 50% of predicted maximal heart rate), and follow very gentle exercise progression.
5. Teach to avoid sudden twisting movements, rapid movements, and rapid transitions from one movement to the next.
6. Avoid exercises that tax vision and balance.
7. Avoid sustained isometric contractions of greater than 10 seconds.
8. Assess ability to tolerate low-level activity without signs and symptoms of muscle fatigue, shortness of breath, angina, dysrhythmias, abnormal blood pressure, or intermittent claudication.
9. Stop exercising if cardiac dysrhythmias, angina, or excessive breathlessness occurs.
10. Instruct to avoid exercise during acute viral infections.
11. Increase activity slowly in relation to intensity (workload), duration (time), and frequency (time interval or length of time).
12. Monitor exercise intensity by perceived exertion and exercise heart rate.
13. Perform a gradual, extended exercise warm-up (i.e., 15 minutes) to maximize flexibility and decrease muscle injury.
14. Perform cool-down until heart rate returns to resting level to decrease postural hypotension and cardiac dysrhythmias.
15. Modify exercise program based on individual's responses.

for developing an exercise program and/or modifying an existing program for older adults. A clinical practice guideline entitled *Exercise Prescription for Older Adults with Osteoarthritic Pain: Consensus Practice Recommendations* is available from http://www.guideline.gov. The National Institutes of Health provides a detailed website on exercise for older adults that includes the benefits of exercise, safety tips, video demonstrations of strength exercises, balance exercises, stretching exercises, and endurance exercises (http://www.nihseniorhealth.gov/exercise/toc.html). Additional resources are listed at the end of the chapter.

Senior Games
Senior centers throughout the United States have instituted physical fitness programs that include Ping-Pong, boccie, golf, horseshoes, and many other activities enjoyed by older people. These activities incorporate rhythmical action and stretching and provide improvement in or maintenance of cardiopulmonary function, muscle tone, and mental stimulation. Nearly all of the 50 states promote "senior games" in collaboration with public service and private corporations. These are Olympic-style competitions for men and women 55 years of age and older. Some companies have established par courses or 1-mile exercise fitness trails for the older adult.

Dancing
For those accustomed to it, ballroom, folk, or square dancing should be encouraged. This form of activity done properly can have as much aerobic benefit as workouts to music videotapes. Dancing is kind to the joints and can burn as many calories as swimming, biking, or walking. However, it should not be done as the only form of activity, since it does not develop upper body strength. To enhance cardiovascular and respiratory fitness, one would have to engage in 20 to 30 minutes of sustained dancing. Dancing provides another means of obtaining pleasant, sociable, vigorous exercise that tones the body and benefits cardiopulmonary and mental health.

Swimming and Water Exercises
Swimming, one of America's most popular sports, or water exercise improves muscle tone, circulation, muscle strength, endurance, flexibility, and weight control, and in addition it can be relaxing and a mood elevator. The benefits of aquatic activ-

ity or exercise therapy are that arm and leg movements against water are less painful and do not seem to require as much effort because of the buoyancy and resistance of the water. A recent study (Takeshima et al, 2002) of 30 older women who participated in a water-based exercise program reported significant improvement in cardiorespiratory status, fitness, muscular strength, body fat, and total cholesterol. The researcher noted that older people who are overweight or mildly disabled find exercising in water hides defects and provides support. Elders with mobility problems move at ease in the water. Some older people maintain a swimming program begun earlier in life; others enjoy this as a relaxing new way to get activity and socialize. Those who are nonswimmers or who do not swim well might benefit from water exercise classes held in the shallow end of the pool. The YMCA, YWCA, American Red Cross, and various health and fitness and recreation centers offer classes in these types of activities. The Arthritis Foundation sponsors water exercise programs, "senior splash" aerobic swim classes, or arthritic aquatic programs that conform to guidelines.

Different Forms of Exercise

Yoga is another form of exercise that can be practiced regardless of one's condition. It can foster mental alacrity, independence, and good health in older adults through simple exercise, relaxation, meditation, and emphasis on nutrition. The National Center for Complementary and Alternative Medicine, part of the National Institutes of Health, is conducting research on the efficacy of yoga. Yoga may be especially appealing to older people who are unable or unwilling to engage in more intense physical activities. These kinds of activities are not just beneficial for active and cognitively intact older people. As part of a therapeutic activity program for older people with memory impairment at Florida Atlantic University, an 84-year-old yoga instructor teaches chair yoga to both the person with the memory impairment and the person's caregiver (see Resources at end of chapter for a videotape of this activity). Another exercise that has met with acceptance is pedaling a bicycle wheel–type device that is put on the floor in front of a chair. When accompanied by music and reminiscing of trips around places where older people grew up, this activity

provides not only exercise but also mental stimulation.

Isotonic exercises train the cardiovascular and skeletal muscles. Isometrics mainly work with the cardiovascular system. Persons who are confined to bed or chair or who are ambulatory can do these rhythmical tasks or calisthenics. The exercises of Tai Chi may be especially helpful for older adults with arthritis or unsteady gait. The American Geriatric Society (http://www.americangeriatrics. org/education/falls.shtml) provides a patient handout on Tai Chi that discusses the potential benefits, such as increased flexibility, muscle strength, and overall fitness. A video, *Tai Chi for Arthritis*, is available from the Arthritis Foundation (http://www.arthritis.org). Tai Chi requires no special equipment, exercises all muscles and joints of the body, is gentle, and may improve one's overall outlook on life by improving the body-mind connection. Numerous other programs have been developed in which simplicity and flexibility of the program make it easily adaptable to a variety of settings.

Special Needs of Older Adults

It is also important to address special needs of older adults when initiating an exercise program. The elderly are less able to adapt to the environment during exercise. They should dress in layers to adjust to different environmental temperatures. Well-fitting footwear and socks are essential to prevent injury because of impaired foot sensation. Blisters and friction injuries may occur without the elderly person knowing it. Maintaining hydration is essential. Total body water is decreased in the elderly. Consumption of fluid before exercising and regularly while exercising is recommended. Environments with poor air quality, including areas near roadways when exercising outside, should be avoided.

Often when one is beginning a physical exercise program, muscles will be sore. Warm, not hot, baths or soaks are excellent. Another way to minimize muscle soreness is to maintain a 5- to 10-minute cool-down period of slow walking or stretching to keep the primary muscle groups active, to decrease venous pooling and increase venous return to the heart, and to prevent vagal responses. When planning activities for the elderly, the age-related changes of the musculoskeletal system need to be considered. Table 12-4 addresses

Table 12-4 Age-Related Musculoskeletal Changes; Outcomes; and Health Prevention, Promotion, and Maintenance Approaches

Age-Related Changes	Outcomes	Health Prevention, Promotion, and Maintenance
Bones become more porous (osteoporosis)	Dowager's hump (kyphosis)	Have good lighting, dry floors, nonskid rugs
Demineralization of vertebral trabecular bone	Risk of hip fracture	Diet high in calcium
Intervertebral disks dehydrate and narrow	Tremors	Calcium supplements as necessary
Reduced height	Back pain	Do moderate exercise: walking or swimming
Erosion of cartilage through exposure and wearing	Joint swelling	Use assistive devices: cane, walker, if needed
Subchondral bone becomes hyperemic and fibrotic	Ankylosis	Do range-of-motion activity
Synovial membranes become fibrotic	Crepitation	Seek medical evaluation of back pain
Synovial fluid thickens	Decreased range of motion	Wear shoes with low heels, nonskid soles, and support
Muscle wasting of hand dorsum	Stiffness	Use leg muscles rather than back muscles when lifting
Diminished protein synthesis in muscle cells	Muscle wasting	Rest joints when pain occurs
Glucose mobilizes slowly in response to exercise	Reduced muscle strength	Lose weight when necessary
Diminished muscle mass decreases glucose stores	Night leg cramps	Develop an appropriate exercise program
Bone and muscle weakness changes the center of gravity	Gait problems	Pace activities
	Smaller steps	Allow for rest periods
	Wider stance base	Break big jobs into small parts
	Poor posture	Adjust activities to periods of day when energy is high
		Remove scatter rugs
		Use nonskid rubber mats in tub and shower
		Take stretch breaks
		Eat more potassium- and calcium-rich foods
		Coordinate and balance exercise

age-related changes of the musculoskeletal system with outcomes and management approaches. Musculoskeletal function is essential to activity.

Nurses should capitalize, more than they do, on activities of daily living, such as providing older persons with bath brushes to wash their own backs in the shower or bathtub and encouraging them to dry body parts or rub the back dry with a towel. Housekeeping activities can be utilized for strength and flexibility. Community-dwelling elders can be taught simple approaches in utiliz-ing household chores for activity. Reaching for objects while cleaning house can be included in an activity program, as can washing dishes in warm water to provide finger exercises. Warm water aids in the relief of stiffness and enables the fingers to move more easily without discomfort. Other activities that can be done while watching television or whenever there are a few spare minutes during the day are rolling a pencil between the hand and a hard surface, exaggerat-ing the chewing motion of the jaw, holding the

Table 12-5   Benefits of Exercise for Chronic Conditions

Condition	Types of Exercise	Benefits
Chronic lung disease	Aerobic	Improves diaphragmatic breathing Reduces reliance on accessory muscles
Cognitive dysfunction	Aerobic	Improves cerebral function Increases cerebral perfusion Increases beta-endorphin secretion
Coronary heart disease	Aerobic Endurance type	Reduces blood pressure Increases HDLs and reduces body fat Increases maximal oxygen consumption
Diabetes mellitus	Aerobic Endurance type	Fat loss Increases insulin sensitivity Decreases glucose intolerance risk
Hypertension	Aerobic Endurance type Leisure-time activity	Decreases systolic blood pressure Decreases total peripheral resistance
Osteoarthritis	Resistance stretching Endurance type	Maintains range of motion; muscle mass Increases muscle strength
Osteoporosis	Resistance Weight bearing	Strengthens postural muscles Stimulates bone growth Decreases rate of bone loss

Data compiled from Elward K, Larson EB: Benefits of exercise for older adults: a review of existing evidence and current recommendations for the general population, *Clin Geriatr Med* 8(1):35-50, 1992; Kligman EW, Pepin E: Prescribing physical activity for older patients, *Geriatrics* 47(8):33-34, 1992; Barry HC, Eathorne SW: Exercise and aging: issues for the practitioner, *Med Clin North Am* 78(2):357-376, 1994.
HDLs, High-density lipoproteins.

stomach in, tightening the buttocks, flexing the fingers, and rotating the head and the ankles. Activity, in general, should be paced and occur regularly every day. Activities that will help eliminate stiffness should be done in the morning, when stiffness is most prevalent. Relaxation exercises should be performed before bedtime to help induce sleep. With any activity in which older adults are involved, sufficient intermittent rest periods should be provided. Various exercises to maintain flexibility are presented in Figure 12-1. Safety is an important consideration in all exercise programs and interventions. Those who are frail should not engage in strenuous activity, nor should their joints be forced past the point of resistance or discomfort. If frail individuals have regularly participated in activity that the nurse deems too stressful to their skeletal systems, it is important to keep in mind that an activity done for many years is not as difficult as it would be if it were just introduced. When the activity is new, serious consideration should be given to the levels of stress produced.

Many older people are fearful of falling because of altered balance or the inability to reach or bend. Many exercises for strength and flexibility can be done from a sitting position if this is a concern. Mental activity should be planned as carefully as physical activity. These activities should be consistent with the individual's interests. New hobbies may develop; involvement in raising or keeping pets may foster caring and affection for others and a rebirth of socialization. Activity should not be thought of as something to keep older adults busy but should be purposeful to enhance their physical and mental well-being. The benefits of exercise for those with chronic conditions appear in Table 12-5.

LYING DOWN

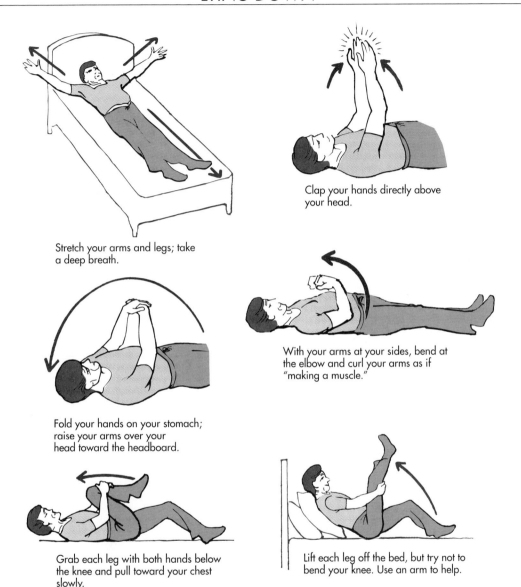

Stretch your arms and legs; take a deep breath.

Clap your hands directly above your head.

Fold your hands on your stomach; raise your arms over your head toward the headboard.

With your arms at your sides, bend at the elbow and curl your arms as if "making a muscle."

Grab each leg with both hands below the knee and pull toward your chest slowly.

Lift each leg off the bed, but try not to bend your knee. Use an arm to help.

Figure 12-1   Exercises: lying down, sitting, standing up, and walking places. (From Johnson-Pawlson JE, Koshes R: Exercise is for everyone, *Geriatr Nurs* 6[6]:322-325, 1985.)

Continued.

SITTING

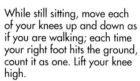

Touch your elbows together in front of you.

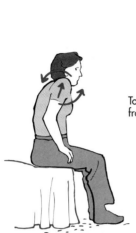

Shrug your shoulders forward, then move them in a circle, raising them high enough to reach your ears.

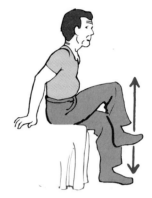

While still sitting, move each of your knees up and down as if you are walking; each time your right foot hits the ground, count it as one. Lift your knee high.

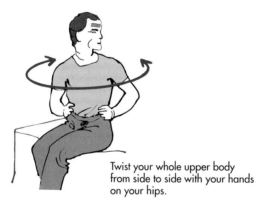

Twist your whole upper body from side to side with your hands on your hips.

Bend forward and let your arms dangle; try to touch the floor with your hands.

Figure 12-1 *Continued.* For legend see p. 231.

STANDING UP

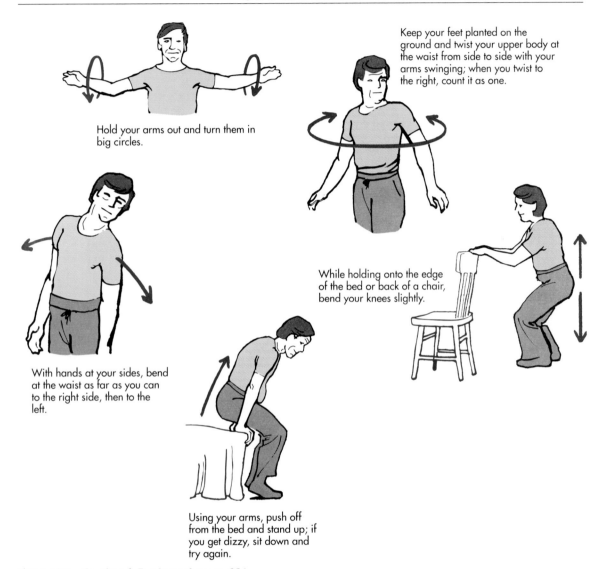

Hold your arms out and turn them in big circles.

Keep your feet planted on the ground and twist your upper body at the waist from side to side with your arms swinging; when you twist to the right, count it as one.

With hands at your sides, bend at the waist as far as you can to the right side, then to the left.

While holding onto the edge of the bed or back of a chair, bend your knees slightly.

Using your arms, push off from the bed and stand up; if you get dizzy, sit down and try again.

Figure 12-1 *Continued*. For legend see p. 231.

Continued.

WALKING PLACES

Walking is good exercise. It helps tone muscles, helps maintaining flexibility of joints, and also is good exercise for the heart and circulatory system. Walking briskly for 20 minutes each day, 3 times each week can be as effective a heart conditioner as jogging, but it does take a longer time to achieve the same effect as jogging. For those who cannot walk rapidly for long periods, walking to the point of muscular fatigue also helps maintain good muscle tone.

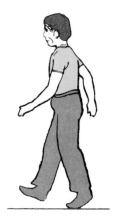

There are signs your body may give you to indicate you are overdoing exercise. Stop, rest, and if necessary call your physician if you experience any of these symptoms:

* SEVERE SHORTNESS OF BREATH
* CHEST PAIN
* SEVERE JOINT PAIN
* DIZZINESS OR FAINT FEELING
* HEART FLUTTERS

In all walking exercises, go only as fast as you are able to walk and still carry on a conversation. If you cannot, slow down.

INSIDE

It is important to maintain walking ability. Determine how far you can walk and each day walk to 3/4 of that distance, building endurance. Wear supportive shoes and use whatever aids are necessary.

OUTSIDE

Wear soft-soled shoes with good support, i.e., jogging shoes. When walking, push off *from* your toes and land on your heels. Swing arms loosely at your sides. Begin with 10-minute walks and build to 20 to 30 minutes.

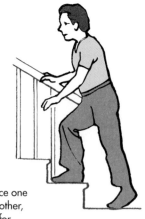

Walking upstairs requires effort. Place one foot flat on a step, push off with the other, and shift your weight. Use a railing for balance if necessary.

Figure 12-1 *Continued.* For legend see p. 231.

NANDA and Wellness Diagnoses

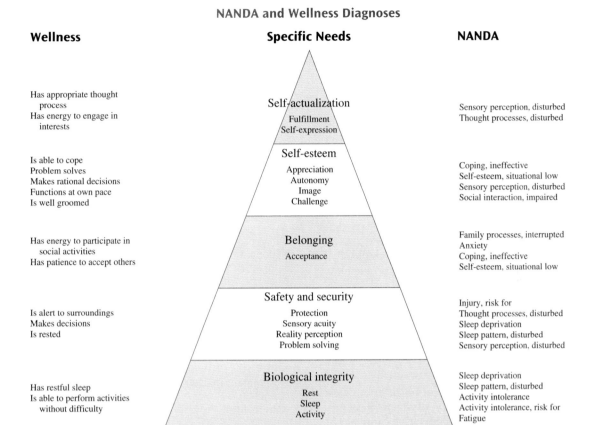

| Wellness | Specific Needs | NANDA |

These are not all of the possible wellness or NANDA diagnoses that may be identified. The above are frequent examples of nursing diagnoses that should be considered when planning care for the older adult in whatever setting.

IMPLICATIONS FOR GERONTOLOGICAL NURSING AND HEALTHY AGING

In summary, this chapter has looked at the need for rest and sleep and the need for activity individually. It is apparent that each area influences the function of the other. The quality and the overall perception of life can be augmented when the nurse monitors these specific functions and provides support or assistance according to identified problems. Gerontological nurses must be knowledgeable about age-related changes in sleep and activity and the effect of lifestyle on these changes. Many older people may have misconceptions about sleep and exercise, and the nurse can assess beliefs and understanding and provide

education to enhance optimal wellness. Assessment of sleep, level of activity, and the design of interventions must be founded in evidence-based knowledge. Common practices such as the use of hypnotics for sleep without a thorough assessment or being confined to a wheelchair because there is no one to help maintain walking skills lead to disabling and preventable problems for older people. Adequate sleep and activity are essential to physical, emotional, and cognitive functioning. Poor sleep and decline in functional capacity affect the ability to perform activities of daily living, compromise independence, and lead to disability and illness. Improvement of function is possible for even the most frail elder, and gerontological nurses need to incorporate the health promotion activities discussed in this chapter into any plan of care for an older adult.

APPLICATION OF MASLOW'S HIERARCHY

Sleep and activity needs must be met not only to maintain biological integrity, but also to meet higher-level needs such as safety and security, belonging and attachment, self-esteem and self-efficacy, and self-actualization and transcendence. The older adult would not survive if these needs were not met independently or with the assistance of others. Ineffective sleep, rest, and activity patterns contribute to depression, loneliness, loss of independence and self-esteem, as well as physical and cognitive illnesses. Maintaining adequate sleep and activity allows the older person to continue to find fulfillment in activities, and in life itself, despite the limitations associated with aging and illness.

▶ KEY CONCEPTS

- Many chronic conditions often interfere with the quality and quantity of sleep. Rest and sleep are restorative, recuperative, and necessary for the preservation of life. Drastic reductions or continually altered or interrupted sleep disrupts homeostatic balance and creates physical and mental aberrations.
- Medication is not always the solution to problems with sleep disturbance.
- Activity is an indication of an individual's health and wellness; inability to exercise, do physical work, or perform activities of daily living is one of the first indicators of decline.
- Lack of physical activity increases the risk for many medical conditions experienced by elders. Exercise can be done by elders who are ambulatory, chair bound, or bedridden and should include an aspect of aerobics, flexibility, and balance (if the elder is ambulatory).
- The benefits of exercise are that it provides maintenance of functional capacity, enhances self-confidence and self-sufficiency, decreases depression, improves one's general lifestyle, maintains mental functional capacity, and decreases the risk of medical problems.

Activities and Discussion Questions

1. What age-related changes affect rest, sleep, and activity in older adults?
2. How would you assess an elder for adequacy or inadequacy of rest, sleep, and activity?
3. Discuss the nursing interventions to promote rest, sleep, and activity.
4. Develop a nursing care plan using wellness and North American Nursing Diagnosis Association (NANDA) diagnoses.

RESOURCES

Sleep

National Center on Sleep Disorders Research
Suite 6022, MSC 7993
6705 Rockledge Drive
Bethesda, MD 20892-7993
(301) 435-0199
e-mail: ncsdr@nih.gov
website: http://www.nhlbi.nih.gov/sleep

National Sleep Foundation
1522 K Street NW, Suite 500
Washington, DC 20005
(202) 347-3471
website: http:///www.sleepfoundation.org

Activity

Active Videos (exercise and dance videos)
10 First Avenue E
Mabridge, SD 57601
(800) 342-4320
e-mail: info@activevideos.com
website: http://www.activevideos.com

American Senior Fitness Association
website: http://www.seniorfitness.net

Armchair Fitness Video Programs (armchair aerobics, strength improvement, gentle exercise, yoga health)
7755 16th Street NW
Washington, DC 20012
(800) 453-6280
e-mail: info@armchairfitness.com
website: http://www.armchairfitness.com

Exercise Prescription for Older Adults with Osteoarthritis Pain: Consensus Practice Recommendations
Available from http://www.guideline.gov

Gentle chair yoga with Veral Paley.
VHS or DVD and companion photo guide.
Available from Memory and Wellness Center.

Memory and Wellness Center
Florida Atlantic University
777 Glades Road
Building AZ-79
Boca Raton, FL 33431
(561) 297-0502
memorylane@fau.edu

International Council on Active Aging
3307 Trutch Street
Vancouver, BC V6L-2T3
(866) 335-9777
website: http://www.icaa.cc

National Center for Chronic Disease Prevention
   and Health Promotion (*Growing Stronger: Strength
   Training for Older Adults,* a downloadable book)
Division of Nutrition and Physical Activity
Centers for Disease Control and Prevention
4770 Buford Highway, NE, MS/K-24
Atlanta, GA 30341-3717
(770) 488-5820
website: http://www.cdc.gov/nccdphp/dnpa/

National Senior Games Association
PO Box 82059
Baton Rouge, LA 70884-2059
(225) 766-6800
website: http://www.nsga.com

NIH Senior Health (exercises for older adults)
website: http://nih.seniorhealth.gov/exercise

REFERENCES

Beers MH, Berkow R: *Merck manual of geriatrics*, ed 3, Whitehouse Station, NJ, 2000, Merck Research Laboratories.

Bliwise DL, Breus MJ: Insomnia in dementia and residential care. In Lichstein KL, Marin CM, editors: *Treatment of late-life insomnia*, Thousand Oaks, Calif, 2000, Sage Publications Inc.

Buckle J: Clinical aromatherapy: therapeutic uses for essential oils, *Adv Nurse Pract* 10(5):67-68, 2002.

Cefalu C: Evaluation and management of insomnia in the institutionalized elderly, *Ann Long-Term Care* 12(6):25-32, 2004.

Drazen JM: Sleep apnea syndrome, *N Engl J Med* 346(6):390, 2002.

Field S: The mystery of sleep: How nurses help the elderly, *Nursing Spectrum* 30, October 2001.

Foreman MD, Wykle M: Nursing standard-of-practice protocol: sleep disturbances in elderly patients, *Geriatr Nurs* 16(5):238-243, 1995.

Gentili A et al: Factors that disturb sleep in nursing home residents, *Aging (Milano)* 9(3):207-213, 1997.

George B, Goldberg N: The benefits of exercise in geriatric women, *Am J Geriatr Cardiol* 10(5):260-263, 2001.

Gorman C: Sleeplessness in America, *Time*, p 43, Dec 17, 2001.

Griffith R: *Treating insomnia in the elderly*, 2002. Available at www.healthandage.com.

Haponik EF, McCall WV: Sleep problems. In Hazzard WR et al, editors: *Principles of geriatric medicine and gerontology*, ed 4, New York, 1999, McGraw-Hill.

Hoffman S: Sleep in the older adult: implications for nurses, *Geriatr Nurs* 24(4):210-214, 2003.

Kirkwood C: *Treatment of insomnia*, New York, 2001, Power-Pak, CE Publishers. Available at www.powerpak.com.

McCrae C, Lichstein K: Managing insomnia in long-term care, *Ann Long-Term Care* 10(4):38-43, 2002.

McCullough P: How well do you sleep? Presentation at the Kentucky Council of Nurse Practitioners and Midwives, Lexington, April 2001.

Miller C: *Nursing for wellness in older adults*, Philadelphia, 2004, Lippincott Williams & Wilkins.

Monane M, Glynn RJ, Avorn J: The impact of sedative-hypnotic use on sleep symptoms in elderly nursing home residents, *Clin Pharmacol Ther* 59(1):83-92, 1996.

Nadolski N: Getting a good night's sleep: diagnosing and treating insomnia, *Am J Nurse Pract*, Special Supplement:S3-S14, Spring 2003.

National Institute on Aging. Available at www.nia.nih.gov/news/pr/2002.

Resnick B: Exercise for older adults: what to prescribe and how to motivate, *Caring for the Ages* 4(1):8-12, 2003. Accessed 8/3/04 from http://www.amda.com/caring/january2003/exercise.htm.

Schoenfelder DP, Culp KR: Sleep pattern disturbance. In Maas ML et al, editors: *Nursing care of older adults: diagnoses, outcomes, and interventions*, St Louis, 2001, Mosby.

Takeshima N, Rogers ME, Watanabe E, et al: Water-based exercise improves health-related aspects of fitness in older women, *Med Sci Sports Exerc* 34(3):544-551, 2002.

U.S. Department of Health and Human Services: *Healthy people 2010*, Hyattsville, Md, 2002, Public Health Service.

Promoting Healthy Skin and Feet

GLOSSARY

Debride To remove dead or infected tissue, usually of a wound.

Emollient An agent that softens and smooths the skin.

Eschar Black, dry, dead tissue.

Hyperemia Redness in a part of the body caused by increased blood flow, such as in area of an infection.

Induration Hardening of tissue as a result of edema or inflammation.

Macerated Tissue that is overhydrated and subject to breakdown.

Slough Dead tissue that has become wet, appearing as yellow to white and fibrous.

Tissue tolerance The amount of pressure a tissue (skin) can endure before it breaks down, as in a pressure sore.

Xerosis Another term for dry ulcer.

THE LIVED EXPERIENCE

I can't thank you enough for helping me with my feet. I have been to the podiatrist, but no one has made them, and me, feel so good. I feel like I can walk forever now—you are an angel.

Tom, age 86

Gerontological nurses have an instrumental role in promoting the health of the skin and feet of the persons who seek their care. Both are sometimes overlooked when dealing with other more immediately life-threatening problems. However, preservation of integrity of the skin and function of the feet is essential to well-being. In order to promote healthy aging, the nurse needs information about common problems encountered by the elderly and skill in developing effective interventions for both acute and chronic conditions.

INTEGUMENT

The skin is the largest organ of the body, and it provides at least seven physiological functions. It protects underlying structures, serves as a heat-regulating mechanism, serves as a sense organ, is involved in the metabolism of salt and water, and stores fat. The skin facilitates two-way gaseous exchange and converts sunshine into vitamin D (Burke, Laramie, 2004). Despite exposure to heat, cold, water trauma, friction, and pressure, the skin maintains a homeostatic environment. The skin is durable, pliable, and strong enough to protect the body by absorbing, reflecting, cushioning, and restricting various substances and forces that might enter and alter its function; yet it is sensitive enough to relay messages to the brain. When the integument malfunctions or is overwhelmed, discomfort, disfigurement, or death may ensue. However, the nurse can both promptly recognize and help to prevent many of the sources of danger to a person's skin.

Photo Damage

One of the most common sources of damage we see to the skin is from the sun. *Solar elastosis*, or photo aging, is a result of environmental damage to the skin from ultraviolet sun rays. Although the amount of sun-induced damage varies with skin type, much of the damage associated with photo aging is preventable. Ideally, preventive measures should begin in childhood, but clinical evidence has shown that some improvement can be achieved through avoidance of sun exposure and the regular use of sunscreens, even after damage has occurred.

Sunscreens offer protection from some harmful ultraviolet rays. All persons who will be exposed to the sun for at least 20 minutes should apply sunscreen approximately 20 minutes before exposure with reapplication after 2 hours. Products used should protect from both A and B type of waves and offer a sun protection factor (SPF)* of 15. Products with an SPF over 15 offer little additional protection (AAD, 2003). Sunscreens protect from sunburns, which in turn decreases one's risk for nonmelanoma-type skin cancers. There is no confirmed evidence that sunscreens prevent melanomas (Vainio et al, 2000). It must be remembered that normal age-related skin changes, such as thinning of the layers and diminished melanocyte activity, can significantly increase the risk for damage.

The development of skin cancer is always a concern, and with the increased number of years of sun exposure, the risk is significantly increased for older adults. Actinic or solar keratoses are often seen as scaly, white, reddish, or brownish patches on an erythematous base on exposed areas, such as the backs of the hands, ears, face, and scalp. Actinic keratosis is a precancerous lesion and should be removed by a dermatologist. Early recognition, treatment, and removal of this lesion are important to prevent serious problems later.

Topical tretinoin (all-*trans*-retinoic acid) has been found to reverse some structural damage caused by excessive sun exposure. The use of tretinoin over a period of 6 to 9 months has been associated with new capillary formation, collagen synthesis, and regulation of epidermal melanin distribution, as well as the disappearance of premalignant actinic keratoses. Prescribed by a health care provider, this topical medication may initially cause erythema and peeling of the treated area. There tends to be more improvement in individuals with slight to moderate sun damage than in those with severe photo aging (Phillips, Gilchrest, 1990).

Skin Cancers

Basal Cell Carcinoma

Basal cell carcinoma is the most common malignant lesion of epidermal tissue and frequently appears around the forties but can occur at any age. It is a slower-growing neoplasm than squamous cell carcinoma (see below). A basal cell lesion can be precipitated by extensive sun exposure, especially burns, chronic irritation, and chronic ulceration of the skin. It is more prevalent in light-skinned persons. This neoplasm begins as a pearly papule with prominent telangiectasis (blood vessels) or as a scarlike area where no history of trauma has occurred. Basal cell carcinoma is also known to ulcerate. Even though metastasis is rare, early detection and treatment are advisable to minimize disfigurement.

Squamous Cell Carcinoma

Squamous cell carcinoma is the second most common skin cancer. However, it is aggressive and has a high incidence of metastasis if it is not identified and treated promptly. Squamous cell cancer is more prevalent in fair-skinned, elderly men who

---

*The effectiveness of sunscreens is measured in terms of the SPF. The equation of minimal erythema dose (MED), the amount of time it takes to cause the skin to become red, times the SPF, provides the length of time, in minutes, that an individual can be in the sun without burning.

live in sunny climates. Individuals in their mid-sixties who have been or are chronically exposed to the sun (e.g., persons who work out-of-doors) are prime candidates for this type of skin cancer. Less common causes include chronic stasis ulcers, scars from injury, chemical carcinogens such as topical hydrocarbons, exposure to arsenic, and radiation exposure. A squamous cell lesion begins as a firm, irregular, fleshy, pink-colored nodule that becomes reddened and scaly, much like actinic keratosis, but it may increase in size rapidly. It may be hard and wartlike with a gray top and horny texture, or it may be ulcerated and indurated with raised, defined borders. Because it can appear so differently, it is often overlooked or thought to be insignificant. The best advice to give an older patient is that if there is any doubt about the type of lesions that he or she has, the lesion should be examined by a skilled dermatologist.

Melanoma

Melanoma, a neoplasm of melanocytes, is the least common skin cancer but has a high mortality rate because of its tendency to metastasize quickly. Blistering sunburns before the age of 18 are thought to damage Langerhans' cells, which affect the immune response of the skin and increase the risk for a later melanoma. The legs and backs of women and backs of men are the most common sites for this neoplasm. Two thirds of melanomas develop from preexisting moles; only one third arise from new moles. Melanoma has a classical, multicolor, raised appearance with an asymmetrical, irregular border. It may appear any size, but the surface diameter is not necessarily reflective of the size beneath the surface, similar in concept to an iceberg. If the nurse finds such a lesion, the individual should be referred to a dermatologist immediately.

Common Skin Problems

Other skin problems seen in older adults are influenced by the normal changes with aging (see Chapter 7) by way of increasing risk, especially for seborrheic keratosis, dry skin, and pruritus. Candidiasis is a pathological condition that is common in persons who are medically fragile, such as those requiring care in nursing home settings.

Keratoses

There are two types of keratoses, actinic as discussed above and seborrheic. Seborrheic keratosis is a benign growth that appears mainly on the trunk, face, and scalp. The etiology of these lesions is unknown; however, they appear almost exclusively in persons over 60. A keratotic lesion is a superficial, circumscribed, raised area that thickens and darkens in color over time with varying shades of brown and skin tone. It may appear greasy or dry and rough, resembling a blob of wax or something that can be peeled off. Multiple keratotic lesions are common. Because the growth gets its coloration from melanin, some individuals fear that it will become malignant, but this is not the case. However, if there is any question as to the type of lesion, a biopsy should be done to rule out melanoma. Generally, if keratoses are cosmetically distressing or in an area of chronic irritation, people will request they be removed by a dermatologist.

Dry Skin

Dry skin (xerosis) is perhaps the most common problem of older adults. The thinner epidermis allows more moisture to escape from the skin. Diminished amounts of available sebum lessen the availability of the protective lipid film that retards the evaporation of water from the stratum corneum (horny layer) in younger persons. Exposure to environmental elements, decreased humidity, use of harsh soaps, frequent hot baths, nutritional deficiencies, smoking, stress, and excessive perspiration all contribute to skin dryness and dehydration. Persons who are cared for in institutions (hospitals, nursing homes) are at greater risk for dry skin through routine bathing, use of soap, prolonged bed rest, and the action of bed linen on the patient's skin. If fluid intake is inadequate the skin is dried further as the body tries to pull needed moisture from the skin.

One of the consequences of xerosis is *pruritus*, otherwise known as itchy skin. It is a symptom, not a diagnosis or a disease, and is a threat to skin integrity because of the attempts to relieve it by scratching. Pruritus is aggravated by heat, sudden temperature changes, sweating, contact with articles of clothing, fatigue, and emotional upheavals. It also may accompany systemic disorders such as chronic renal failure, biliary or hepatic disease,

| Box 13-1 | Causes of Pruritus in the Elderly |

Dermatitis
Eczema
Contact
Seborrhea
Lichen simplex chronicus (neurodermatitis)
Xerosis (dry skin)
Microvascular (stasis dermatitis, erythema)

Papular Scaling Disorders
Psoriasis, lichen planus

Drug Reactions
Drug withdrawal (delirium tremens)
Erythema multiforme
Antidepressants, opiates
Acetylsalicylic acid, idiosyncratic responses

Metabolic Responses
Liver and biliary disorders
Renal failure (uremia)

Diabetes mellitus
Hypothyroidism

Neoplastic Disorders
Benign (seborrheic keratosis)
Malignant (central nervous system tumors)

Hematopoietic Responses
Iron deficiency anemia
Leukemia, lymphoma

Psychogenic Etiologies
Involutional psychoses
Hallucinatory aberrations (dementias)

Infections and Infestations
Bacterial (impetigo, chlamydia)
Viral (herpes zoster)
Yeast infections (candidiasis, monilial intertrigo)
Parasitic (scabies, pediculosis)

and iron deficiency anemia. Box 13-1 lists various causes of pruritus.

Candidiasis (*Candida albicans*)

The fungus *Candida albicans* is present on the skin of healthy persons of any age. However, under certain circumstances and in the right environment it can proliferate into a fungal infection. Persons who are obese, are malnourished, are receiving antibiotic or steroid therapy, or have diabetes are at increased risk. *C. albicans* grows especially well in areas that are moist, warm, and dark, such as in skinfolds, in the axilla, in the groin, and under pendulous breasts. *Candida* can also be found in the corners of the mouth associated with the chronic moisture of angular cheilitis. In the mouth it is called thrush and is associated with poor hygiene and immunocompromise.

In the mouth *Candida* appears as irregular, white, flat to slightly raised patches on an erythematous base that cannot be scraped off. The infection can extend down into the throat and cause painful swallowing. In severely immunocompromised persons the infection can extend down the entire gastrointestinal tract. On the skin,

Candida is usually maculopapular, glazed, and bright red with characteristic satellite lesions, or there may be a centrally affected area and individual lesions a short distance from the center. If the infection is advanced enough, the affected area will be edematous and cause itching or burning.

Implications for Gerontological Nursing and Healthy Aging

The gerontological nurse is in the perfect position to promote the health of the skin in older adults. The first skill is to be knowledgeable about the normal changes with aging and to be able to observe for common lesions. The nurse encourages the use of sun protection, periodic skin screening, and prompt contact with a dermatologist in the appearance of a new or suspicious lesion.

The nurse should be alert to signs of rough, scaly, or flaky skin and accompanying pruritus anywhere on the body. Signs of itching-related skin trauma include linear erosions. Dry skin may be just dry skin, but it may also be a symptom of more serious systemic disease (e.g., diabetes mellitus, hypothyroidism, renal disease).

Because the underlying cause of dry skin is normal aging, it cannot be cured, and treatment is palliative, focusing on the relief of symptoms and the promotion of comfort. The challenge is to find ways to rehydrate the epidermis, especially the keratin, or horny layer. Since the skin is only hydrated with water, substances may be used to enhance water's ability to stay in the skin. Lubricants such as lotions and emollients work by trapping moisture and are most effective when applied to the damp skin immediately after bathing. Bath oils and other hydrophobic preparations may also be used to hold in moisture and retard its escape from the skin. However, bath oil poured into the bathtub creates the potential for falls. It is safer and more effective to apply the oil directly to the moist skin as above. Water-laden emulsions without perfumes are best. Light mineral oil is equally as effective as and more economical than commercial brands.

The application of lotion or emollients to the body several times a day also helps to keep the epidermal layer lubricated and hydrated; vegetable oil is an inexpensive emollient but may smell or stain clothing. Emollients applied to dry (non-moistened) skin trap water rising from the subcutaneous layer if the person is adequately hydrated. In cases of extreme dryness heavy products such as petrolatum and zinc oxide can be applied before bed and the skin will be smoother and moister in the morning. Oils and ointments are designed to coat the skin and replace the skin's natural oil barrier (sebum).

To prevent excessive loss of moisture and natural oil during bathing, only tepid water temperatures and super-fatted soaps or skin cleansers without hexachlorophene or alcohol should be used. Products such as Basis, Dove, Tone, and Caress soaps or Jergens or Neutrogena bath washes are effective in helping to prevent the loss of the protective lipid film to the skin surface. Deodorant soaps and detergents contain alcohol as a drying agent and should be avoided except in places such as the axilla and groin.

Finally, maintaining the environmental humidity at 60% and alleviating mechanical irritation caused by vigorous towel drying, clothing, and bedding will help to control dry skin and consequently pruritus. When rehydration of the stratum corneum is not sufficient to control itching, cool compresses of saline solution, oatmeal, or Epsom salt baths may be indicated. Failure to do so increases the risk for eczema, fissures, and subsequent inflammatory changes. Guidelines for the treatment of pruritus appear in Box 13-2.

The best approach to preventing fungal infections is to limit the conditions that encourage fungal growth. Anyone who is diaphoretic or who sweats profusely should be considered for prevention of candidiasis. In contrast to the treatment of dry skin, attention is given to the adequacy of the drying of target areas of the body after bathing, prompt management of incontinent episodes, and the use of loose-fitting cotton clothing and cotton underwear (and changing it when damp), as well as limiting activity that promotes sweating. Using a hair dryer set on low may help to dry difficult to reach areas. A folded, dry washcloth or cotton sanitary pad can be placed under the breasts or between skinfolds to promote exposure to air and light. Cornstarch should never be used because it promotes the growth of *Candida* organisms. Optimizing nutrition and glycemic control are also important.

The goal of treatment is to eradicate the infection. This includes not only the use of prescribed antifungal medication, but also the active involvement of the nurse to reduce or eliminate the conditions that created the problem. The affected area

---

Box 13-2   Guidelines for Dealing with Pruritus

1. Take tepid baths using bath oil so as not to further dehydrate skin.
2. Minimize use of soaps or soap products.
3. Apply soothing creams or emollients several times daily, especially on hands, feet, and face.
4. Wear soft, absorbent clothing, such as cotton.
5. **Be careful of and use with caution:**
   - Topical steroid creams (unpredictable absorption)
   - Low-dose systemic steroids (likely to result in complications)
   - *Do not use* antihistamines with persons over age 75 (experience sudden, severe side effects)

of the skin must be cleansed carefully and dried thoroughly, and the antifungal must be applied. A mild soap or cleansing agent, such as Cetaphil, should be used. Antifungal preparations come in powders, creams, and lotions. Since the latter two trap moisture, the powder is preferred and the most effective. They are usually needed for 7 to 14 days or until the infection is completely cleared. These antifungal medications include miconazole (Micatin), clotrimazole (Lotrimin), nystatin (Mycostatin), and econazole (Spectazole). Treatment of oral *Candida* infection includes mouth swishing and swallowing with a Mycostatin suspension or sucking on antifungal troches. Angular cheilitis is treated with a topical antifungal ointment to the corners of the mouth. If the *Candida* cannot be eliminated in the usual course of therapy, it may be necessary to use ketoconazole or fluconazole systemically for a prescribed period of time.

Vascular Insufficiency

Because of the high rate of cardiovascular and associated illness in the United States, the gerontological nurse is likely to care for persons with vascular insufficiency that is arterial, venous, or both. Vascular insufficiency often leads to complicated problems for the skin, from mild dermatitis to ulceration or gangrene. In promoting healthy aging, the nurse is aware of the signs of insufficiency and can quickly take steps to minimize the most harmful sequela.

Arterial Insufficiency

Lower extremity arterial disease (LEAD) is most often caused by enlarging atherosclerotic plaques, which lead to ischemia. Most people have no symptoms. For those with symptoms, 80% complain of pain or muscle fatigue with exercise. The remaining 20% have lower extremity pain at rest and ischemic tissue damage. Slight trauma can result in an arterial ulcer, which is very difficult and sometimes impossible to heal. Although only a small number of persons have LEAD, for some, it will lead to the loss of a limb (Woolley, 2002). Risk factors include coronary artery disease, smoking, hyperlipidemia, hypertension, and diabetes or a family history of the same. Treatment includes minimizing risk factors and microvascular surgery.

Venous Insufficiency

The microvascular changes that occur with normal age often leave the vein walls weakened and unable to respond to increased venous pressure. Increased pressure may be due to poor venous flow, vasculitis (inflammation), or thrombophlebitis (venous blood clot). Heredity and obesity are additional factors that contribute to the altered venous integrity of the lower extremities. Weakened veins are responsible for varicosities, foot and ankle edema, and discoloration of the skin in the lower extremity because of leakage of fluid into the tissues. In individuals with dark-pigmented skin, the skin discoloration is darker than the surrounding tissue. If the venous pressure increases, more extensive areas of the lower leg may become involved. Skin tissue becomes vulnerable to insignificant trauma, such as an insect bite or snug elastic-topped ankle socks. Either of these or other events could precipitate the beginning of venous ulcer formation.

Usually symptoms of venous insufficiency begin with pruritus, edema, and stasis dermatitis (also called *varicose* or *gravitational eczema*) or with ulceration from a minor trauma (Friedman, 1995; Gilchrest, 1995). An ulceration will generally appear on the medial aspect of the tibia above the malleolus. Evidence of previously healed ulcers can be identified by brown or tannish discoloration over the skin.

Venous insufficiency affects approximately 500,000 Americans, most of whom are older than 60 years of age ("Leg Ulcers," 1995). Fortunately, venous insufficiency and stasis venous ulcers may respond to conservative treatment, although it takes many weeks and months to resolve, depending on the extent of tissue involvement.

Implications for Gerontological Nursing and Healthy Aging

To promote the health of the lower extremities the nurse stays alert for the signs of potential problems and takes prompt action to minimize tissue damage. The nurse also helps elders reduce risk factors whenever possible, such as encouraging smoking cessation. For LEAD, a complaint of lower extremity pain at rest requires prompt referral to a health care provider. Because the circulation away from the heart and into the periphery is impaired, dangling the feet may at least temporarily relieve pain, and the nurse recalls that

Table 13-1 Comparison of Arterial and Venous Insufficiency of the Lower Extremities

Characteristics	Arterial	Venous
Pain	Sudden onset with acute; gradual onset with chronic pain Exceedingly painful Claudication relieved by rest Rest pain relieved by dependency (with total occlusion, no position will give complete relief)	Deep muscle pain with acute deep vein thrombosis Relieved by elevation
Pulses	Absent or weak	Normal (unless there is also arterial disease)
Associated changes in leg and foot	Thin, shiny, dry skin Thickened toenails Absence of hair growth Temperature variations (cooler if there is no cellulitis) Elevational pallor Dependent rubor Atrophy or no change in limb size	Firm ("brawny") edema Reddish brown discoloration with postphlebitic syndrome Evidence of healed ulcers Dilated and tortuous superficial veins Swollen limb Increased warmth and erythema with acute deep vein thrombosis
Ulcer location	Between toes or at tips of toes Over phalangeal heads On heels Over lateral malleolus or pretibial area (for diabetic patients), over metatarsal heads, on side or sole of foot	"Garter area" around ankles (rich in perforator veins), especially the medial malleolus
Ulcer characteristics	Well-defined edges Black or necrotic tissue Deep, pale base Nonbleeding	Uneven edges Ruddy granulation tissue Superficial Bleeding

elevating the feet may trigger severe pain. Extra efforts are made to prevent injury to the affected tissue, since without adequate arterial support, healing is delayed, if it occurs at all.

Nursing interventions associated with vascular insufficiency are usually focused on maximizing function, relieving edema, and treating the venous stasis ulcers. Treatment usually consists of a combination of therapies, such as leg elevation whenever the person is sitting and elastic support stockings during waking hours. The stocking should be put on before the person gets out of bed for maximal compression. It is sometimes helpful for both men and women with this problem to put on knee-high nylon stockings (not pantyhose) under the elastic hose. The rougher support hose can then be pulled on more easily on top of the hose. This method achieves minimal energy expenditure and promotes independence. Although the stockings are usually considered uncomfortable, they should none-the-less be encouraged.

If ulcers occur, the highest level of care must be given following the standard practices of wound care (see *Pressure Ulcers in Adults: Prediction and Prevention* under Resources). Arterial ulcers are resistant to healing. For venous ulcers to heal, circulation can be increased through the application of compression dressings, such as an Unna boot. Compression dressings cannot be used until the diagnosis of a venous ulcer is confirmed. Table 13-1 compares arterial and venous insufficiency, and Box 13-3 summarizes the treatments used for venous stasis ulcers.

Box 13-3	Treatments for Venous Stasis Ulcers

Conservative Treatment

Dressings
  Wet

  Change daily initially
  (If not infected, an adhesive film or
      absorbent gel or foam is possible.)
Application of fibrinolytic agents
Cleaning

Compression wrap

Elevation of legs

Ambulation

Absorb weeping fluid
Prevent tissue drying out
Decrease risk of infection
Keep clean and protected from bacteria

Mild soap and water
Mechanically removes loose tissue without
    additional trauma
Removes creams/lotions/medications applied
Increases venous flow
Should continue to wear even after lesion is healed
Decreases swelling
Improves venous return
Improves venous return

Treatment for Severe Ulcers

Mechanical pump compression

Elastic stockings or wrap
Surgery
  Skin graft
  Vein stripping

Provides intermittent compression for several
    hours daily

For large ulcers

Treatment for Chronic Recurring Stasis Ulcers

Growth factor from human blood platelets
  applied to ulcer in combination with other
  treatment
Cultured skin grown in laboratory (under
  Food and Drug Administration [FDA] review)

Stimulates new skin formation over ulcer,
    enhances healing

To cover ulcer and enhance healing

Pressure Ulcers (Pressure Sores)

A pressure ulcer is an interruption in the integrity of the skin as a result of compression between a bony prominence and another hard surface, such as a bed, tubing, or chair. As tissue is compressed, blood is diverted, and blood vessels are forcibly constricted by the persistent pressure on the skin and underlying structures; thus cellular respiration is impaired, and cells die from ischemia and anoxia. Pressure sores begin with erythema, which is followed by edema, possible blister formation, and, finally, ulceration. Figure 13-1 illustrates the development of pressure sores. Intervention at any point in the developing process can stop the advancement of the pressure ulcer.

Just how much pressure can be endured by tissue (tissue tolerance) is highly variable from body location to location and person to person. Tissue tolerance is inversely affected by moisture, amount of pressure, friction, shearing, and age and is directly related to poor nutritional status and low arterial pressure.

Pressure ulcers are a concern for huge numbers of persons and therefore nurses. At any one time 1.8 million elders, 10% to 23% of nursing home patients in long-term care settings (Nutrition Screening Initiative, 2001) and 10% to 29% of patients in acute care settings, have at least one pressure ulcer. The prevalence is 41% of critical care patients and about 13% of home care patients

Stage I

Erythema not resolving within thirty (30) minutes of pressure relief. Epidermis remains intact. REVERSIBLE WITH INTERVENTION.

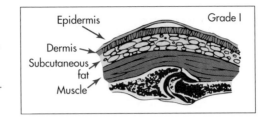

Stage II

Partial-thickness loss of skin layers involving epidermis and possibly penetrating into but not through dermis. May present as blistering with erythema and/or induration; wound base moist and pink; painful; free of necrotic tissue.

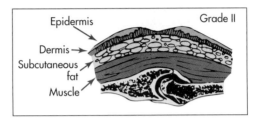

Stage III

Full-thickness tissue loss extending through dermis to involve subcutaneous tissue. Presents as shallow crater unless covered by eschar. May include necrotic tissue, undermining, sinus tract formation, exudate, and/or infection. Wound base is usually not painful.

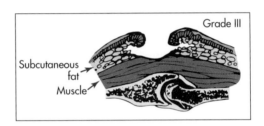

Stage IV

Deep tissue destruction extending through subcutaneous tissue to fascia and may involve muscle layers, joint, and/or bone. Presents as a deep crater. May include necrotic tissue, undermining, sinus tract formation, exudate, and/or infection. Wound base is usually not painful.

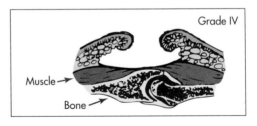

Figure 13-1   Pressure sore development.

(Beers, Berkow, 2000; Cobb, Durfee, 2002). Seventy percent of pressure sores occur in elders older than 70 (Tangalos, 2002).

Pressure ulcers can develop anywhere on the body but are most frequently seen on the posterior aspects, including the occiput, spine, sacrum, ischium, and heels (Ferrell, 2002). Secondary areas of breakdown include the trochanter, lateral condyles of the knee, and ankle. The pinna of the ears is another common lateral aspect for breakdown, as are the elbows and scapulae. If one is lying prone, the knees, shins, and pelvis sustain undue pressure.

Pressure ulcers are costly to treat and may require extended separation from friends and loved ones. For many, it can prolong recovery and extend rehabilitation. An uncomplicated wound in a person over 60 years of age takes approximately 100 days to heal. The acquisition of iatrogenic complications, such as pressure ulcers and complications from them, such as the need for grafting or amputation, sepsis, or even death, may

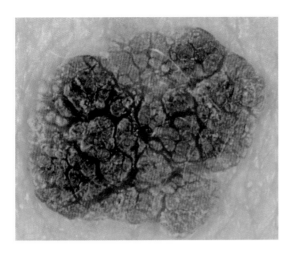

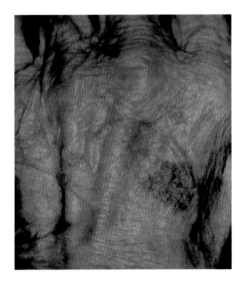

Fig. 1 Seborrheic keratosis in older adult. (From Habif TP: *Clinical dermatology: a color guide to diagnosis and therapy,* ed 3, St Louis, 1996, Mosby.)

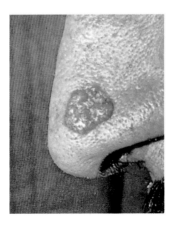

Fig. 2 Lentigo, a brown macule that appears in chronically sun-exposed areas. (From Habif TP: *Clinical dermatology: a color guide to diagnosis and therapy,* ed 3, St Louis, 1996, Mosby.)

Fig. 3 Basal cell carcinoma, the most commonly occurring skin cancer. (Courtesy Gary Monheit, MD, University of Alabama at Birmingham School of Medicine. In Seidel HM et al: *Mosby's guide to physical examination,* ed 4, St Louis, 1999, Mosby.)

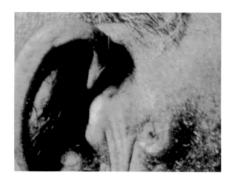

Fig. 4 Squamous cell carcinoma. (Courtesy Gary Monheit, MD, University of Alabama at Birmingham School of Medicine. In Seidel HM et al: *Mosby's guide to physical examination*, ed 4, St Louis, 1999, Mosby.)

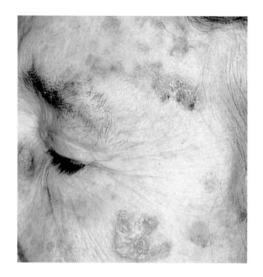

Fig. 5 Actinic keratosis in older adult in area of sun exposure. (From Habif TP: *Clinical dermatology: a color guide to diagnosis and therapy*, ed 3, St Louis, 1996, Mosby.)

Box 13-4	Complications of Pressure Ulcers

Amyloidosis
Endocarditis
Heterotopic bone formation
Maggot infestation
Meningitis
Perineal-urethral fistula
Pseudoaneurysm
Septic arthritis
Sinus tract or abscess
Squamous cell carcinoma in the ulcer
Iodine toxicity or uncover subclinical
   hyperthyroidism (from use of iodine-based
   cleansing)
Hearing loss from use of topical aminoglycosides
Osteomyelitis
Bacteremia
Advanced cellulitis

From Bergstrom N et al: *Treatment of pressure ulcers.*
Clinical practice guideline no. 15, AHCPR pub no. 95-0652,
Rockville, Md, 1994, U.S. Department of Health and
Human Services, Public Health Service, Agency for Health
Care Policy and Research.

lead to legal action by the individual or his or her representative against the caregiver. Box 13-4 lists the associated complications of pressure sores.

Determining Risk for Pressure Ulcers

It is difficult to predict which individuals will develop pressure ulcers, and it is even more difficult to restore skin integrity once they have developed. Anyone can develop pressure sores, but the normal changes to aging skin increase the risk for skin breakdown. The two most important factors are severity of illness and involuntary weight loss because of poor nutritional status, especially dehydration, hypoproteinemia, and vitamin deficiencies. These account for 74% and 42%, respectively, of increased risk (Nutrition Screening Initiative, 2001). Other important indicators of increased risk are impaired sensory feedback systems so that discomfort is not noticed and impaired mobility or immobilization by restraint or sedation. Additional factors include vascular insufficiency, diabetes, anemia, lack of fat padding over bony prominences, incontinence, and some drug therapies, such as corticosteroids. Tissue breakdown

is aggravated by heat, moisture, and irritating substances on the skin. The particularly high-risk groups include those hospitalized for femoral fractures, critical care patients, quadriplegic individuals, and those in skilled nursing facilities.

The development of pressure ulcers is a dynamic process that requires constant vigilance and reassessment. The Braden Scale (Bergstrom et al, 1994) and the Norton Risk Assessment Scale (Norton, 1996) are risk assessment tools used frequently in the clinical setting in predicting individuals at risk for pressure sores. The Braden Scale is probably used most often. The six subscales of the Braden Scale are sensory perception, skin moisture, activity, mobility, friction and shearing, and nutritional status. Each category is rated as 1 (least favorable) to 4 (most favorable). The maximum score possible is 24 points; thus the lower the score, the more at risk a patient is for pressure sores and the greater the need for preventive interventions. The use of either the Braden Scale or another scale provides the means for a systematic evaluation and periodic reevaluation of a person's risk for pressure sores. See the Braden Scale in Appendix 13-B.

Implications for Gerontological Nursing and Healthy Aging

In all settings nurses are the persons who are the most responsible for the prevention and treatment of pressure ulcers. Nurses must be able to identify early signs and initiate appropriate interventions to prevent further skin breakdown and to promote healing. Failure to do this jeopardizes the health and life of the elderly person. In caring for the whole person, the nurse is in a position to ensure that preventive measures are used and that prompt treatment is initiated if needed. The nurse is the person to alert the health care provider of the need for prescribed treatments, and the nurse is the one who recommends and administers treatments as well as evaluates their efficacies.

Care of the person always begins with assessment.

Assessment. Assessment begins with the evaluation of risk as noted above and continues with a brief head to toe examination. Included in this is a review of laboratory values related to anemia and nutritional status. The nurse looks for a lymphocyte count below 1800/mm^3, body weight loss greater than 15%, or serum albumin value below 3.5 g/dl, all indicative of malnutrition and positively correlated with the severity of the pressure sores (Bates-Jensen, 1996).

Visual and tactile inspection of the entire skin surface with special attention to bony prominences is essential. Inspection is best achieved when performed in nonglare daylight or, if that is not possible, under the illumination of a 60-watt light bulb (Jarvis, 1996; Giger, Davidhizar, 1999). Inspection should include actual and potential areas for breakdown, with special attention directed to specific areas when an individual uses orthotic devices such as corsets, braces, prostheses, postural supports, splints, slings, or casts. Heels are a problematic site because they are particularly prone to pressure and are small surfaces that receive a high degree of pressure.

The nurse looks for any interruption of skin integrity, including redness or hyperemia; if pressure is present, it should be relieved and the area reassessed in 1 hour. In darker-pigmented persons, redness may not be present or easily visualized. Instead it is necessary to look for induration, darkening, or a shadowed appearance of the skin and to feel for warmth or a boggy texture to the tissue compared with the surrounding tissue. Blisters or pimples with or without hyperemia and scabs over weight-bearing areas in the absence of trauma should be considered suspicious.

Pressure ulcers are classified according to the stages developed by the National Pressure Ulcer Advisory Panel (www.npuap.org) ranging from a stage I, where the skin is damaged but still intact, to stage IV, where the pressure has caused extensive tissue death from the surface through to the subcutaneous structures (see Figure 13-1). The ulcer is always classified by the highest stage "achieved," and *reverse staging is never used*. This means that the wound is documented at the stage representing the maximal damage and depth that has occurred. As the wound heals, it fills with granulation tissue composed of endothelial cells, fibroblasts, collagen, and an extracellular matrix. Muscle, subcutaneous fat, or dermis is not replaced. A stage IV pressure sore that is healing does not become a stage III and then a stage II. It remains defined as a healing (it is hoped) stage IV. Wounds that are covered in black (eschar) or yellow fibrous (slough) necrosis cannot be staged because it is not possible to see the depth until the dead tissue is removed.

Whereas ulcers are assessed with each dressing change, a detailed assessment is to be done on a weekly or biweekly basis to evaluate the effectiveness of the treatments and nursing interventions. Detailed assessment of each wound should include the following:
1. Location and exact size (width, depth, length)
2. Color of the wound bed
3. Condition of the surrounding tissue
4. Presence, absence, amount, odor, and color of any exudate (fluid) in the wound
5. Condition of the wound edges, for example, smooth and white or irregular and pink, undermined

Finally, careful and detailed documentation of the condition of the skin is required. Bates-Jensen provides a detailed form that covers all aspects of assessment (see Appendix 13-A). Most institutions have special forms or computer screens for the recording of the skin assessment. For those persons with ulcers, photographic documentation is highly recommended both at the onset of the problem and at intervals during its treatment.

Interventions. The goal of nurses is to help maintain skin integrity against the various environmental, mechanical, and chemical assaults that are potential causes of skin breakdown. In promoting healthy aging of all persons, nurses can focus on prevention: actions that eliminate friction and irritation to the skin by lifting, turning, placing, and rolling (using two or more persons) the patient; reduction of moisture so that tissues can breathe and do not macerate; and displacement of body weight from prominent areas to facilitate circulation to the skin. The nurse should be familiar with the types of supportive surfaces so that the most effective surface can be used. The nurse should assess the frequency of position change, adding pillows so that skin surfaces do not touch, and establish a turning schedule. Sitting and activity, skin care, incontinence care, and the use of heel protectors or the use of pillows to keep the heels off the bed, with or without so-called protective booties or blocks, should be assessed. Elevating the heels off the bed with pillows or commercial products is helpful and especially important for individuals with diabetes mellitus and peripheral neuropathy.

Nutritional intake should be monitored, as well as the serum albumin level, hematocrit, and hemoglobin. Diets high in protein, carbohydrates, and vitamins are necessary to maintain and promote tissue growth. If appetite is lacking, appetite stimulants may be prescribed. Supplements of vitamin B help in the metabolism of carbohydrates, and pyridoxine and vitamin C assist in protein use.

Realistically, it is not always possible to prevent interruptions in skin integrity caused by overwhelming conditions, and the nurse is instrumental in both fostering and interfering with the healing process. Fortunately, the state of the science of wound care is well developed. Specific guidelines for the prevention and treatment of pressure ulcers were developed in 1994 and continue to guide practice (Bergstrom et al, 1994). Since that time the products used have grown in numbers, but the guidelines remain in effect. Other sources of information include the National Pressure Ulcer Advisory Panel and the National Association of Wound, Ostomy and Continence Nurses.

Wounds must be kept clean, warm, moist (but not wet) and protected from further injury. Dilute skin cleansers or saline is best and the least caustic. Solutions such as alcohol, certain soaps, hydrogen peroxide, and povidone-iodine (Betadine) are always damaging to newly formed fragile skin (Bergstrom et al, 1994).

Common types of dressing include films, hydrogels, hydrocolloids, alginates, and foams. Enzymes (e.g., Santyl) may be necessary for use in debriding or removing eschar or slough. Dressings are selected based on the amount of exudate that needs to be absorbed and the condition of the wound bed, with the type of dressing changing as the condition of the wound changes. Dressings should be replaced as soon as the wound is cleaned to prevent cooling and slowing down of the healing process. Occlusive dressing cannot be used with infected wounds. Anytime a wound shows worsening the treatment plan must be changed. It is also reevaluated anytime a wound does not show healing during a 2-week interval. Suggestions for interventions for prevention related to risk factors are found in Box 13-5.

Consultation with a wound care specialist is advisable for wounds that do not follow the pattern of healing. Wound care specialists are experienced nurses or nurse practitioners who often work with wound centers or surgeons and may consult in nursing homes, offices, or clinics.

FEET

Socrates is reported to have said, "To him whose feet hurt, everything hurts." If he did say this, most nurses, accustomed to foot strain, would agree. The feet influence the physical, psychological, and social well-being of the individual. The feet carry one's body weight, coordinate and maintain balance in walking, and must be rigid yet loose and adaptable enough to conform to the surfaces underfoot (all the while holding the legs and body in an upright position). Little attention is given to these valuable appendages until the feet interfere with ambulation and the ability to maintain independence. Foot discomfort can cause irritability, fatigue, and chronic complaints.

The feet have a significant effect on one's productivity, and mobility, yet are often overlooked until something is wrong with them. The effect is comparable with that of the automobile. An automobile provides us with freedom and mobility; however, if one is not available or not in working condition the routine of the day is upset and both independence and mobility are hampered. Unlike the automobile, however, the feet do not have easily replaceable parts. Lack of mobility may mean the difference between an independent, active community life, self-respect, motivation, and responsibility for one's health versus institutionalization. Even in an institution, foot problems may mean the difference between confinement to bed or wheelchair and the ability to ambulate in a protected setting.

The feet may also reflect systemic disease conditions or give clues to physical ailments before their actual appearance (Echevarria et al, 1988; "Burning Feet," 1992). Sudden or gradual changes in nail or skin conditions of the feet and/or the appearance of recurring infections may be a precursor of more serious health problems.

Neglect of the feet throughout one's active years results in painful conditions later (Collet, 1995), yet adequate care of the feet can alleviate disability, pain, and the tendency for falling. Through care of a person's feet, the nurse can take an active and well-appreciated step toward fostering both the person's health and his or her well-being.

Box 13-5   Interventions by Risk Factor

Bed or Chair Confinement
Inspect skin at least once daily.
Bathe when needed for comfort or cleanliness.
Prevent dry skin.

Bed confinement
Change position at least every 2 hours.
Use a special mattress that contains foam, air, gel, or water.
Raise head of bed as little and for as short a time as possible.

Chair confinement
Change position every hour.
Use foam, gel, air, or cushion to relieve pressure.

Reduce friction by the following:
    Lifting rather than dragging when repositioning
    Using cornstarch on skin
Avoid use of donut-shaped cushions.
Participate in a rehabilitation program.

Inability to Move

Bed confinement
Place pillow under legs from mid-calf to ankles to keep heels off bed.

Chair confinement
Reposition every hour *if unable* to do by self.
Shift weight and position at least every 15 minutes *if able* to do by self.
Use pillows or wedges to keep knees or ankles from touching one another.

Loss of Bowel and Bladder Control
Clean skin as soon as soiled.
Assess and treat urine leaks.
If moisture cannot be controlled, do the following:
    Use absorbent pads and/or briefs with a
        quick-drying surface.
    Protect skin with a cream or ointment.

Poor Nutrition
Eat a balanced diet.
If a normal diet is not possible, talk to health care provider about nutritional supplements.

Lowered Mental Awareness
Choose preventive action that applies to person with lowered mental awareness. For example, if person chair bound, refer to specific prevention action as outlined in the above risk factors.

From *Preventing pressure ulcers: a patient's guide. Clinical practice guideline*, Rockville, Md, 1992, U.S. Department of Health and Human Services, Public Health Service, Agency for Health Care Policy and Research.

Common Foot Problems

Fifty percent of the general population has foot problems. The number and severity of the problems increase with age. Almost 80% of persons over the age of 50 will have at least one significant foot problem. Three of every four persons 65 years and over complain of foot pain. Individuals over 55 years of age (88% of women and 83% of men) demonstrate arthritic changes in the foot on x-ray examination. Of these older adults, 25% have symptoms of foot problems ("Common Foot Problems," 1993).

Many chronic diseases experienced by older adults also potentially threaten the health of the feet. Osteoarthritis can cause pain in the feet. Rheumatoid arthritis may lead to hammer toes and dislocated toes, pain, and limited function. Peripheral vascular disease can lead to infections of the feet, pain resulting from decreased circulation, and amputation. Gout often affects the great toe and produces swelling, acute pain, and subsequent difficulty in walking. Diabetes, with the development of peripheral neuropathy, predisposes the foot to injury, infection, and in some instances amputation.

Nurses are the ideal persons to significantly promote healthy aging through knowledge of the common problems and skills in care of the feet. Several of the commonly seen foot problems are associated with improperly fitting shoes or those designed with narrow toe spaces.

Corns

Corns, the cone-shaped layers of compacted skin, usually on toes, occur as a result of friction and pressure on the skin rubbing against bony, protuberant areas of the toes, usually from ill-fitting shoes. Corns can interfere with the ability to walk comfortably and wear shoes. Once the small, hard, white corn is established, continued pressure eventually causes pain. Soft corns form in the same manner but occur between opposing surfaces of the toes. Unless the friction and pressure are relieved the corn will continue to enlarge and cause increasing pain.

Most persons with corns have attempted do-it-yourself remedies, following what they have done for years, especially over-the-counter preparations and razor blades or scissors. The use of cutting surfaces could be dangerous if the person has normal age-related vision loss. The over-the-counter preparations dissolve the corn as well as the surrounding healthy tissue, which can lead to chemical burns and ulcerations. For the person with neurological impairments of the lower extremities, peripheral vascular disease, or diabetes, self-treatment can result in the loss of toes or a leg.

Oval corn pads, which seem to provide some pain relief, actually can create greater pressure on the toes and can decrease circulation to the tissue within the oval pad. Oval corn pads can be adapted for effective use. Instead of using the oval pad as it is, the upper or lower section of the corn pad can be cut out so that the pad resembles the letter U. This can be placed around three aspects of the corn, protecting it from pressure without restricting circulation to healthy tissue. Newer gel-type pads are also useful to protect against friction and pressure. Irritation from soft corns between the toes can be eased by loosely wrapping small amounts of lamb's wool around the involved toe, or cotton balls can be placed between the toes.

Mild corns may resolve themselves when pressure is removed and shoes are replaced by those with a better fit. Larger or resistant corns may need surgical removal by a podiatrist. Corns are not usually removed from high-risk persons, such as those with diabetes or peripheral vascular disease (PVD), because of the risk of poor wound healing at the surgical site.

Calluses

Calluses are also layers of dry and compacted skin that usually occur on the soles and heels of the feet because of chronic irritation and friction from shoes. Calluses can be eased by the use of gel pads or with moleskin applied to those areas that receive undue friction. Moleskin is a skin-protective product available in the foot care section of pharmacies and hiking supply stores. Moleskin adheres for several days or longer but should be removed when it becomes wet or excessively soiled. Removing moleskin from the feet should be done slowly to prevent tearing of skin.

For persons prone to calluses, daily lubrication of the feet and intermittent pedicures will help. Again, persons at risk for impaired sensation or circulation of the lower extremity should not use any abrasive measures, such as those received during a pedicure.

Bunions

Bunions (hallux valgus) are bony deformities that develop from long-standing squeezing together of the toes from occupational activity and the wearing of improperly fitting shoes. Bony prominences develop over the medial aspect of the first metatarsal head (the joint of the great toe) and, at times, at the lateral aspect of the fifth metatarsal head (the joint of the little toe and called a *tailor bunion* or a *bunionette).* There also may be a hereditary factor in their development. Once formed, bunions will not go away without surgery.

However, the nurse can promote comfort by working with the person to find shoes that will properly support and protect the foot but not worsen the deformity.

Hammer Toes

A *hammer toe* is a permanently flexed and rotated toe (or toes) with a clawlike appearance; the condition is a result of muscle imbalance and is aggravated by poor-fitting shoes and often seen with bunions. Over time, the toe (usually the second toe) flexes and rotates as a result of pressure of the great toe slanting toward it. The toe then contracts, leaving a bulge on top of the joint. Balance and comfort are affected. Treatment includes professional orthotics or specially designed protective devices; properly fitting, nonconstricting shoes; and/or surgical intervention ("Common Foot Problems," 1993).

Metatarsalgia

Metatarsalgia is pain in the ball of the foot caused by a number of reasons. Usually the arch of the foot in persons with metatarsalgia is narrow and high, which centers pressure on the ball of the foot. It may be seen when the legs are unequal in length, which adds stress to the metatarsal joints of the shorter leg. It can also be seen in the feet of persons with rheumatoid arthritis, stress fractures, fluid accumulation, muscle fatigue, flat feet, or overloaded feet, as in the case of obesity. Relief is often obtained with foot freedom (i.e., when the foot is not restricted by shoes or when shoe length and width are adequate). Orthotics and the use of nonsteroidal antiinflammatory medications are also helpful.

Burning Feet

Burning feet is the term used for the transient sensation of warm or hot feet that is not explained by environmental temperatures. Although usually temporary, it could be a symptom of an underlying systemic problem. This annoyance occurs as a result of irritating fabrics, poorly fitting shoes, fungal infections, or contact with toxic substances, such as poison ivy or poison oak. If one of the aforementioned causes is not found, burning feet may be a more serious indication of underlying diseases such as diabetes, alcoholism, poor nutritional state (folic acid, B_{12} deficiency), chronic kidney failure, or liver disease. In addition, medications and exposure to poisons such as arsenic and lead may cause burning feet.

Self-help measures that can help alleviate burning feet include removing the cause if known, wearing cotton or cotton-blend socks or shoes made of natural materials that breathe, providing a good fit, and having fitted insoles. Cold tap water foot baths 15 minutes twice each day to cool the feet, in conjunction with rest and avoidance of activities that aggravate the problem, can reduce burning. If burning feet are caused by an underlying disease, the treatment must include working with the person to better manage the chronic disease, such as optimizing glycemic control.

Fungal and Bacterial Infections

Fungal and bacterial infections are common in the aged foot. These conditions usually develop because the foot is encased in a warm, dark, and moisture-holding shoe. Fungal infections of the skin, *tinea pedis,* are caused by the same organism that is discussed above as *Candida* under the section on skin. Nail fungus (onychomycosis) is characterized by yellow streaks or total nail discoloration. The nail becomes opaque, scaly, and hypertrophied. A fine powdery substance forms under the center of the nail and pushes it up, causing the sides of the nail to dig into the flesh like an ingrown toenail. Culturing is the only definitive way to identify onychomycosis (Tosti, 1995). Hands should be washed each time the feet of a patient with a fungal infection are handled. Feet, especially between the toes, should be dry and exposed to sun and air. If the feet are prone to fungal and bacterial conditions, a daily dusting with antifungal powder or spray is appropriate.

Tinea pedis is treated similarly to any other fungal skin infection. When nails are involved the treatment is difficult to impossible because of the limited circulation of the nails. Several oral medications are available but all are expensive, have to be taken for long periods of time (3 to 12 months), and are potentially toxic to the liver.

Implications for Gerontological Nursing and Healthy Aging

Foot care is a prime factor in determining mobility and the quality of existence and in retaining

---

Box 13-6   Essential Data of Foot Assessment

Observation of Mobility
Gait
Ambulation
Foot hygiene
Footwear

Past Medical History
Systemic diseases
Musculoskeletal problems
Vascular/ulcerations/peripheral vascular disease
Vision problems
Falls
Trauma
Smoking history
Pain

Bilateral Assessment
Color
Circulation
Pulses
Structures (hammer toe, bunion, overlapping digits)
Temperature
Dermatological aspects
  Skin lesions (fissures, corns, calluses, warts, excoriation)
  Edema
  Itching
  Rash
Toenails
  Long, thick
  Discoloration

---

independence. Elders with painful foot problems often have functional limitations. Nursing care of the foot is directed toward maximizing function while maintaining comfort, removing possible mechanical irritants, and decreasing the likelihood of infection.

The nurse has the important function of assessing the feet of the aged person for clues to well-being and functional ability, not just bathing and applying lotion to the feet. Nurses can identify potential and actual problems and refer or seek podiatric assistance for the foot problems of the patient when it is needed; however, the nurse should not defer the routine care of the foot to the podiatrist.

Assessment

Assessment is the key to maintenance of the person's highest level of function and mobility. For persons with residual foot and leg impairment from strokes; diabetes mellitus; cardiac, hyperthyroid, or kidney conditions; or pernicious anemia, feet should be assessed on a scheduled and regular basis, using a standard format.

King (1978, 1980) developed an assessment tool for the lower extremities that any caregiver can learn to use. As shown in Figure 13-2, the tool provides illustrations of some of the important aspects to look for and evaluate and simple explanations of specific items to ensure uniform evaluation regardless of who performs the assessment.

Until the nurse is familiar with this tool, it will take about 20 minutes or more to complete, but with increased proficiency, the time required can be reduced. The assessment itself includes the essentials of foot care: inspection of the feet for irritation, abrasions, and other lesions; determination of functional and other acquired deviations; checks for hazards to the maintenance of adequate circulation to the lower extremities and the existing circulatory status; and observation of the individual's mobility.

Additional information about foot health can be obtained by examining the shoes. They should be new enough to provide support, and soles should not show signs of excessive wear, especially in any one area. For persons with diabetes or other neurological impairments the shoes should cover and protect the foot entirely. For persons with arthritis, firm soles are more comfortable than soft soles and may decrease the pain.

Box 13-6 lists the essential components of a thorough foot assessment.

Interventions

Care of the toenails. Poor close vision, difficulty bending, obesity, or increased nail thickness makes self-care of the toenails a potential problem. Normal nails that become too long will begin to interfere with stockings, hose, or shoes. Ideally, toenails should be trimmed after the bath or shower when they are softened, but if this is

---

**NURSING ASSESSMENT OF THE
GERIATRIC LOWER EXTREMITY**

Patient Number _____
Date _____
R.N. Number _____

INSTRUCTIONS: FOR EACH ITEM, CIRCLE THE RESPONSE IN THE APPROPRIATE COLUMN, UNLESS DIRECTED OTHERWISE. CLARIFICATION OF ITEMS APPEAR IN THE FAR RIGHT COLUMN.

1. Mobility (check one)
   Walks without assistance ___ Walks with help of equipment ___
   Does not walk—uses wheelchair ___ Bedfast ___
2. Ask the client, "Does the condition of your feet or legs
   limit your activity in any way?"   YES   NO
   If YES, describe. _____
3. ASK THE CLIENT TO WALK APPROXIMATELY 10 FEET.
   Is there any gait disturbance?   YES   NO

REMOVE THE CLIENT'S SHOES AND STOCKINGS

	ACCEP-TABLE	UN-ACCEP-TABLE
4. Cleanliness of feet.		
5. Are the stockings a good fit?	YES	NO
6. Does the client *usually* wear well-fitting, leather (synthetic) shoes that cover the feet completely?	YES	NO
7. Does the client wear garters? (circular)	YES	NO

Fig. 1 — Red, thickness

Dermatologic assessment

8. Skin lesions		
a. Fissure between the toes?	YES	NO
b. Fissure on heel(s)?	YES	NO
c. Excoriation on legs or feet?	YES	NO
d. Corn(s)? (Fig. 1)	YES	NO
e. Callus(es)?	YES	NO
f. Plantar wart?	YES	NO
g. Other, describe _____	YES	NO
9. Itching on legs or feet?	YES	NO
10. Rash on legs or feet?	YES	NO

Corn: painful, circular area of thickened skin, appearing on skin that is normally thin.

Callus: Thickened skin, occurring on skin that is normally thick, i.e., soles.

11. INSPECT PRESSURE AREAS ON THE FEET FOR LOCALIZED
    AREAS OF REDNESS. ARE ANY PRESENT?   YES   NO
    IF YES, WHICH FOOT?   RIGHT   LEFT

12. INSPECT LEGS, FEET, AND TOES FOR LOCALIZED
    SWELLING, WARMTH, TENDERNESS, REDNESS.
    Is any present?   YES   NO
    If YES, specify location.   Rt. leg   Lt. leg
                                                                 Rt. foot   Lt. foot

13. Toenails		
a. Ingrown?	YES	NO
b. Overgrown (long)?	YES	NO
c. Thickened?	YES	NO
d. Yellow discoloration?	YES	NO
e. Black discoloration?	YES	NO

Ingrown toenail: a "tender overhanging nail fold"

Figure 13-2 Nursing assessment of the gerontological lower extremities. (From King PA: Foot assessment of the elderly, *J Gerontol Nurs* 4[6]:47-52, 1978.)

not possible, soaking the feet for 20 to 30 minutes before care is usually sufficient. They should be clipped straight across and even with the top of the toe, with the edges filed slightly to remove the sharpness but not to the point of rounding (Figure 13-3). Diabetic foot care should only be done by the registered nurse (RN) with some experience and with special care to prevent accidental damage to the skin. Diabetic nail care can never be delegated to the licensed practical nurse (LPN) or certified nurse assistant (CNA).

Nails that are neglected or that do not receive treatment may become unusually long and curved. This type of nail is known as *ram's horn* because of its appearance. Hard, thickened nails indicate inadequate nutrition to the nail matrix from trauma or poor circulation. Once the nail becomes thickened, it will remain so. Nails that are hard can easily split, causing trauma to the matrix, pain, and possibly infection. Any attempt by the nurse or other caregiver to cut these nails may result in further damage to the matrix or pre-

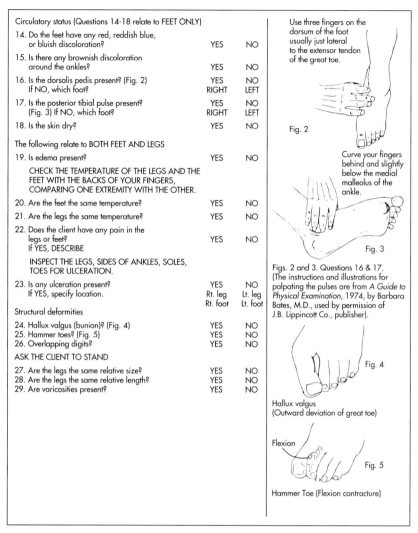

Circulatory status (Questions 14-18 relate to FEET ONLY)

Use three fingers on the dorsum of the foot usually just lateral to the extensor tendon of the great toe.

14. Do the feet have any red, reddish blue, or bluish discoloration?	YES	NO
15. Is there any brownish discoloration around the ankles?	YES	NO
16. Is the dorsalis pedis present? (Fig. 2)	YES	NO
IF NO, which foot?	RIGHT	LEFT
17. Is the posterior tibial pulse present? (Fig. 3) If NO, which foot?	YES	NO
	RIGHT	LEFT
18. Is the skin dry?	YES	NO

Fig. 2

Curve your fingers behind and slightly below the medial malleolus of the ankle.

The following relate to BOTH FEET AND LEGS

19. Is edema present?	YES	NO

CHECK THE TEMPERATURE OF THE LEGS AND THE FEET WITH THE BACKS OF YOUR FINGERS, COMPARING ONE EXTREMITY WITH THE OTHER.

20. Are the feet the same temperature?	YES	NO
21. Are the legs the same temperature?	YES	NO
22. Does the client have any pain in the legs or feet?	YES	NO
IF YES, DESCRIBE		

Fig. 3

Figs. 2 and 3. Questions 16 & 17. (The instructions and illustrations for palpating the pulses are from *A Guide to Physical Examination*, 1974, by Barbara Bates, M.D., used by permission of J.B. Lippincott Co., publisher).

INSPECT THE LEGS, SIDES OF ANKLES, SOLES, TOES FOR ULCERATION.

23. Is any ulceration present?	YES	NO
IF YES, specify location.	Rt. leg	Lt. leg
	Rt. foot	Lt. foot

Structural deformities

24. Hallux valgus (bunion)? (Fig. 4)	YES	NO
25. Hammer toes? (Fig. 5)	YES	NO
26. Overlapping digits?	YES	NO

Fig. 4

ASK THE CLIENT TO STAND

27. Are the legs the same relative size?	YES	NO
28. Are the legs the same relative length?	YES	NO
29. Are varicosities present?	YES	NO

Hallux valgus (Outward deviation of great toe)

Flexion

Fig. 5

Hammer Toe (Flexion contracture)

Figure 13-2 *Continued*

cipitate an infection. These conditions should be brought to the attention of a podiatrist.

An ingrown toenail is a fragment of nail that pierces the skin of the nail lip. Often this problem is a consequence of improper cutting of the nail. An additional cause is pressure exerted on the toes by tight hose or shoes. This problem, too, should be referred to the podiatrist, but as a temporary measure it is simple enough for the nurse to insert a wisp of cotton under the section of the nail that is growing into the nail lip, which will lift it and reduce the pressure and pain.

Shoes. Shoes should be worn that cover, protect, and provide stability for the foot; maximize toe space; and minimize the chance of falls. Shoes should provide enough forefoot space laterally and dorsally with a wide toe box and comfortable fit, such as found in ultralight walking shoes and running shoes. Fabric shoes (not recommended for persons with diabetes or PVD) are perhaps the most comfortable for the aged person with a bunion because fabric stretches more than leather and synthetic materials. Cloth shoes should have a good-quality walking surface.

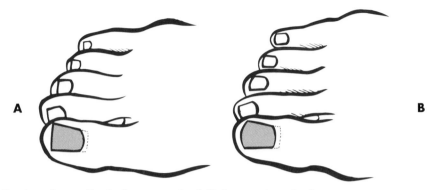

Figure 13-3   Cutting of toenails. **A**, Correct method. **B**, Incorrect method.

Protective pads may be used to cushion bunion joints.

Slip-on shoes are helpful for those aged persons who are unable to bend or lace shoes, but care must be taken that the person will not accidentally "slip out" of the shoe leading to a fall. Velcro closures are also useful to those who have limited finger dexterity. Low-heeled shoes with a wide toe box and a ridged sole minimize falls, place less stress on the legs and back, and are ideal for comfort. The proverbial "thumb's width" is the correct space between the big toe and the toe tip of the shoe. One should also be able to pinch the leather or fabric across the widest part of the upper shoe.

For persons with any of the shoe pressure-related problems noted above, shoe stores have devices that will stretch the shoe at the pressure area, but the customer must purchase the shoe before this easement is made. Shoe repair shops have shoe-stretching devices and charge a reasonable fee for stretching a shoe. At home, leather shoes can be eased while they are being worn by wetting the shoe with alcohol. This allows the leather to stretch to the shape of the foot and will not leave a permanent watermark because the alcohol evaporates. Custom-made shoes, although expensive, are available to the person with bunions or any other deformity or special need.

Orthotics prescribed by a podiatrist and specially designed for the individual foot may be necessary. These come in a broad range of prices. For persons with diabetes, Medicare will cover the cost of one pair of orthotic shoes per year.

Reduction of dependent edema. With age, the circulatory efficiency in the lower extremities, especially the feet, is lessened. Edema of the ankles and feet may be evident after periods of prolonged sitting and standing. It is helpful if the elderly do not wear constricting circular garters, socks with snug bands, or support hose, which constrict the feet, unless the latter are specifically indicated (e.g., Ted Hose). Sitting with the feet elevated on a footstool or hassock is helpful in preventing or reducing edema and facilitating better venous circulation. Foot exercises, too, are a means of reducing edema by encouraging more efficient venous return. Exercises can be done anytime. It would be good to develop the habit of doing foot exercises on rising and going to bed. Other times could be during television commercials.

The exercises are simple, and in addition to helping reduce edema, they facilitate foot flexibility. Toe bends, or curling and relaxing the toes, should be done at least five times on each foot. These can be done one foot at a time or both feet together, followed by rotating the feet at the ankles clockwise and then counterclockwise five to ten times, and, finally, bringing the knees to the chest five to ten times. These exercises can be done consecutively or with short rest periods in between, depending on the stamina of the individual.

Foot massage. Foot massage is another useful means of reducing edema, stimulating circulation, and improving pedal flexibility. Not only does massage aid in accomplishing these things, but also it relaxes the feet and stimulates relax-

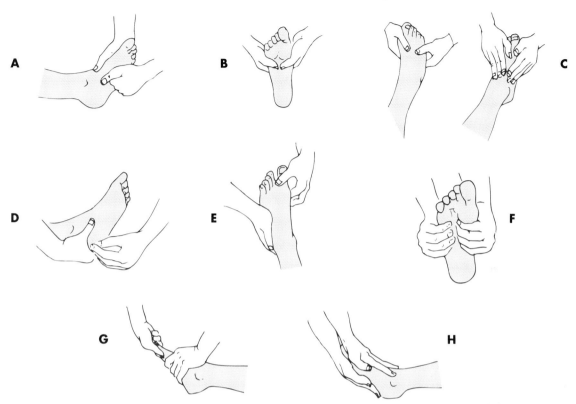

Figure 13-4 Foot massage. **A,** With knuckles make small circles over sole of foot. **B** and **C,** With thumbs and fingers make circles over entire foot. **D,** With tips of fingers make circles on heel. **E,** Gently run thumb between tendon grooves from ankle to toes. **F,** As if breaking a cracker, move the foot back and forth. **G,** Gently stretch and rotate each toe. **H,** End by placing foot between hands.

ation of the rest of the body. However, not all elderly persons are candidates for foot massage. Individuals with foot lesions or vascular problems of the lower extremities should be seen by the physician for a definitive decision before massage is considered.

Foot massage requires little lubrication, and the lotion or oil applied after the bath or shower is sufficient, if done at that time. To give a foot massage, the nurse should be positioned so that the client's feet are easily accessible; sit at the foot of the bed, if the client is reclining, or opposite the client, if the client is seated, sit with the foot to be massaged cradled between the nurse's knees or resting on something comfortable for support.

Steady the foot to be massaged with one hand, and with the knuckles of the other hand make small, firm circles over the entire sole of the foot,

including the heel (Figure 13-4, *A* and *B*). Light touch tends to tickle, whereas firmness does not; however, the feet of the aged may be more sensitive to pressure than those of the young, so the nurse must modulate the firmness of the massage accordingly. Use firm smooth movements. Continue to massage the foot; support the foot with the fingers of both hands while the thumbs repeat the small circles over the entire sole of the foot. As you move your thumbs from the toes you may find that the fingertips are less awkward when you massage around the ankle and the heel (see Figure 13-4, *C* and *D*). When your fingers reach the heel, take one hand and gently lift the foot under the ankle, and with the other hand use the fingertips and thumb to firmly make circles on the heel. More pressure will be required here because of the thicker horny layer of skin (see Figure 13-4, *D*).

NANDA and Wellness Diagnoses

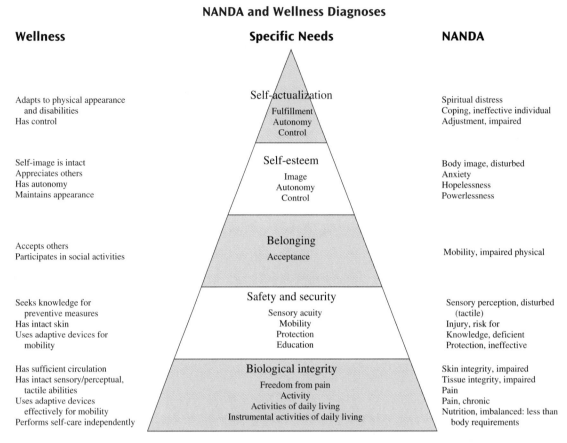

Wellness

Adapts to physical appearance
and disabilities
Has control

Self-image is intact
Appreciates others
Has autonomy
Maintains appearance

Accepts others
Participates in social activities

Seeks knowledge for
preventive measures
Has intact skin
Uses adaptive devices for
mobility

Has sufficient circulation
Has intact sensory/perceptual,
tactile abilities
Uses adaptive devices
effectively for mobility
Performs self-care independently

Specific Needs

Self-actualization
Fulfillment
Autonomy
Control

Self-esteem
Image
Autonomy
Control

Belonging
Acceptance

Safety and security
Sensory acuity
Mobility
Protection
Education

Biological integrity
Freedom from pain
Activity
Activities of daily living
Instrumental activities of daily living

NANDA

Spiritual distress
Coping, ineffective individual
Adjustment, impaired

Body image, disturbed
Anxiety
Hopelessness
Powerlessness

Mobility, impaired physical

Sensory perception, disturbed
(tactile)
Injury, risk for
Knowledge, deficient
Protection, ineffective

Skin integrity, impaired
Tissue integrity, impaired
Pain
Pain, chronic
Nutrition, imbalanced: less than
body requirements

These are not all of the possible wellness or NANDA diagnoses that may be identified. The above are frequent examples of nursing diagnoses that should be considered when planning care for the older adult in whatever setting.

On the top of the foot, starting at the ankle, look at the long tendons that run from the base of the ankle to each toe. Support the heel of the foot with one hand, and with the tip of the thumb on your other hand firmly but gently run your thumb between each tendon groove and off between the toes (see Figure 13-4, *E*). (This can be uncomfortable, so adjust your pressure.) Next grasp the foot between both hands; fingers should be touching on the sole of the foot, heels of the hands touching on the top of the foot (see Figure 13-4, *F*). Press the heels of your hands firmly downward on the foot, and push up on the sole of the foot with your fingers (like breaking a cracker in half). At the same time slide your hands toward the edges of the foot. Repeat this motion

three times. With one hand, steady the foot, and with the thumb and forefinger of the other hand grasp the base of the big toe. Gently stretch and rotate it from side to side, using a corkscrew motion, until your fingers slide off the tip of the toe. Do this to each toe in sequence (see Figure 13-4, *G*). To finish the massage, place the foot between your hands; hold the foot gently for several seconds (see Figure 13-4, *H*); replace it next to the other foot; gently pick up the other foot; and repeat the massage sequence. The nurse will find that foot massage can be easily modified to incorporate range of motion (ROM) exercises for the toes and ankles. In addition to foot massage, lukewarm oil (baby oil, mineral oil) applied to the feet followed by wrapping in warm moist towels and elevation for 10 to 15 minutes not only facilitates a few minutes of relaxation but also aids in improving integrity of the skin of the feet. Feet are then washed in sudsy warm water, dried thoroughly, and dusted with powder, or excess oil can be simply removed with a soft towel. Your patients will be forever grateful for your kindness and skills.

KEY CONCEPTS

- The skin is the largest and most visible organ of the body; it is the direct mediator with the environment.
- The best way to minimize the risk of skin cancer is to avoid prolonged sun exposure.
- The skin and feet often reflect systemic disease.
- Mobility is fundamental to independence; therefore care of the feet and toenails is important and should not be neglected.
- A pressure ulcer is documented by stage, which reflects the greatest degree of tissue damage; and as it heals, back staging is not appropriate.
- A pressure ulcer that is covered in dead tissue (eschar or slough) cannot be staged until it has been debrided.
- Individuals with foot lesions or vascular problems of the extremities should have a qualified podiatrist routinely care for their feet.
- Foot massage with a good lubricating lotion reduces edema, stimulates circulation, improves pedal flexibility, and tends to relax the entire body. Massage should be done only with medical approval if there are foot lesions or vascular problems.

Activities and Discussion Questions

1. Describe the normal age-related changes of the skin.
2. What are the common skin problems of the older adult?
3. Explain what assessment tools are useful to the nurse for skin and foot assessments.
4. List several interventions that apply to skin care; to foot care.
5. Develop a nursing care plan using wellness and North American Nursing Diagnosis Association (NANDA) diagnoses.

RESOURCES

Publications

American Cancer Society publications
The Diagnosis and Management of Common Skin Cancer, no. 2558
Facts on Skin Cancer, no. 825
Fry Now, Pay Later, no. 901
Melanoma/Skin Cancer—Can You Recognize the Signs? no. 904

Krames Communications
312 90th Street
Daly City, CA 94015-1898
Brochure briefly explains how to examine your skin, conditions to look for, prevention of problems, and risk factors.

Pressure Ulcers in Adults: Prediction and Prevention. Clinical Practice Guideline no. 3 Available from AHCPR Publications Clearing House, PO Box 8547, Silver Spring, MD 20907 or www.guidelines.gov

Organizations

Local podiatric college/clinic
Local podiatric society
Local and regional podiatric referral service

REFERENCES

American Academy of Dermatologists (AAD): *Facts about sunscreens, 2003.* Available at www.aad.org. Accessed 7/12/04.

Bates-Jensen BM: *Why and how to assess pressure ulcers.* Presented at the Ninth Annual Symposium on Advanced Wound Care, Atlanta, April 20, 1996.

Bergstrom N et al: *Treatment of pressure ulcers. Clinical practice guideline no. 15,* AHCPR pub no. 95-0652, Rockville, Md, 1994, U.S. Department of Health and Human Services, Public Health Service, Agency for Health Care Policy and Research.

Burke MM, Laramie JA: *Primary care of the older adult: a multidisciplinary approach,* ed 2, St Louis, 2004, Mosby.

Burning feet, *Mayo Clin Health Lett* 10(1):1, 1992.

Cobb DK, Durfee SM: Involuntary weight loss and pressure ulcers: the role of nutrition and anabolic strategies, *Ann Long-Term Care* (suppl), May 2002.

Collet BS: Foot problems. In Abrams WB, Beers MH, Berkow R, editors: *The Merck manual of geriatrics,* ed 2, Whitehouse Station, NJ, 1995, Merck Research Laboratories.

Common foot problems: prevention and treatment, *Perspect Health Promot Aging* 8(2):1, 1993.

Echevarria KH et al: Board and home care: a team approach to foot care, *Geriatr Nurs* 9(6):338-340, 1988.

Ferrell BA: Pressure ulcers. In Ham R, Sloane P, Warshaw G, editors: *Primary care geriatrics,* St Louis, 2002, Mosby.

Friedman SA: Peripheral vascular diseases; aneurysms. In Abrams WB, Beers MH, Berkow R, editors: *The Merck manual of geriatrics,* ed 2, Whitehouse Station, NJ, 1995, Merck Research Laboratories.

Giger JN, Davidhizar RE: *Transcultural nursing: assessment and intervention,* ed 3, St Louis, 1999, Mosby.

Gilchrest BA: Skin changes and disorders. In Abrams WB, Beers MH, Berkow R, editors: *The Merck manual of geriatrics,* ed 2, Whitehouse Station, NJ, 1995, Merck Research Laboratories.

Jarvis C: *Physical examination and health assessment,* ed 2, Philadelphia, 1996, WB Saunders.

King PA: Foot assessment of the elderly, *J Gerontol Nurs* 4(6):47-52, 1978.

King PA: Foot problems and assessment, *Geriatr Nurs* 1(3):182-186, 1980.

Leg ulcers, *Mayo Clin Health Lett* 13:1, 1995.

Norton D: Calculating the risk: reflections on the Norton Scale, *Adv Wound Care* 9(6):38-43, 1996.

Nutrition Screening Initiative: Study shows poor nutrition key cause of pressure ulcers, issue 33, pp 1, 4, Fall/Winter 2001. Available at: www.aafp.org/nsi.xml.

Phillips TJ, Gilchrest BA: Skin changes and disorders. In Abrams WB, Beers MH, Berkow R, editors: *The Merck manual of geriatrics,* Rahway, NJ, 1990, Merck Sharpe & Dohme Research Laboratories.

Tangalos E: *Geriatric pharmaceutical care guidelines,* Covington, Ky, 2002, Omnicare.

Tosti A: Onychomycosis is often misdiagnosed on clinical exam: culture is the key, *Mod Med* 63(12):3, 1995.

Vainio H, Miller AB, Bianchini F: An international evaluation of the cancer-preventive potential of sunscreens, *Int J Cancer* 88(5):838-842, 2000.

Woolley DC: Peripheral vascular disease. In Ham R, Sloane P, Warshaw G, editors: *Primary care geriatrics,* St Louis, 2002, Mosby.

Appendix 13-A *Pressure Sore Status Tool*

INSTRUCTIONS FOR USE

General Guidelines

Fill out the attached rating sheet to assess a pressure sore's status after reading the definitions and methods of assessment described below. Evaluate once per week and whenever a change occurs in the wound. Rate according to each item by picking the response that best describes the wound and entering that score in the item score column for the appropriate date. When you have rated the pressure sore on all items, determine the total score by adding together the 13-item scores. The HIGHER the total score, the more severe the pressure score status. Plot total score on the Pressure Sore Status Continuum to determine progression of the wound.

Specific Instructions

1. Size: Use ruler to measure the longest and widest aspect of the wound surface in centimeters; multiply length X width.
2. Depth: Pick the depth, thickness, most appropriate to the wound using these additional descriptions:
   1 = tissues damaged but no break in skin surface.
   2 = superficial, abrasion, blister, or shallow crater.
   Even with, and/or elevated above skin surface (e.g., hyperplasia).
   3 = deep crater with or without undermining of adjacent tissue.
   4 = visualization of tissue layers not possible due to necrosis.

5 = supporting structures include tendon, joint capsule.
3. Edges: Use this guide:

Indistinct, diffuse	= unable to clearly distinguish wound outline.
Attached	= even or flush with wound base, *no* sides or walls present; flat.
Not attached	= sides or walls *are* present; floor or base of wound is deeper than edge.
Rolled under, thickened	= soft to firm and flexible to touch
Hyperkeratosis	= calluslike tissue formation around wound and at edges.
Fibrotic, scarred	= hard, rigid to touch.

4. Undermining: Assess by inserting a cotton-tipped applicator under the wound edge; advance it as far as it will go without using undue force; raise the tip of the applicator so it may be seen or felt on the surface of the skin; mark the surface with a pen; measure the distance from the mark on the skin to edge of the wound. Continue process around the wound. Then use a transparent metric measuring guide with concentric circles divided into four (25%) pie-shaped quadrants to help determine percent of wound involved.
5. Necrotic Tissue Type: Pick the type of necrotic tissue that is *predominant* in the wound according to color, consistency, and adherence using this guide:

White/gray nonviable tissue	= may appear before wound opening; skin surface is white or gray.
Nonadherent, yellow slough	= thin, mucinous substance; scattered

throughout wound bed; easily separated from wound tissue.

Loosely adherent, yellow slough	=	thick, stringy clumps of debris; attached to wound tissue.
Adherent, soft, black eschar	=	soggy tissue; strongly attached to tissue in center of base of wound.
Firmly adherent, hard, black eschar	=	firm, crusty tissue; strongly attached to wound base and edges (like a hard scab).

6. Necrotic Tissue Amount: Use a transparent metric measuring guide with concentric circles divided into four (25%) pie-shaped quadrants to help determine percent of wound involved.

7. Exudate Type: Some dressings interact with wound drainage to produce a gel or trap liquid. Before assessing exudate type, gently cleanse wound with normal saline or water. Pick the exudate type that is predominant in the wound according to color and consistency, using this guide:

Bloody	=	thin, bright red.
Serosanguineous	=	thin, watery pale red or pink.
Serous	=	thin, watery, clear.
Purulent	=	thin or thick, opaque tan to yellow.
Foul purulent	=	thick, opaque yellow to green with offensive odor.

8. Exudate Amount: Use a transparent metric measuring guide with concentric circles divided into four (25%) pie-shaped quadrants to determine percent of dressing involved with exudate. Use this guide:

None	=	wound tissues dry.
Scant	=	wound tissues moist; no measurable exudate.
Small	=	wound tissues wet; moisture evenly distributed in wound; drainage involves <25% dressing.
Moderate	=	wound tissues saturated; drainage may or may not be evenly distributed in wound; drainage involved >25% to <75% dressing.
Large	=	wound tissues bathed in fluid; drainage freely expressed; may or may not be evenly distributed in wound; drainage involves >75% of dressing.

9. Skin Color Surrounding Wound: Assess tissues with 4 cm of wound edge. Dark-skinned persons show the colors "bright red" and "dark red" as a deepening of normal ethnic skin color or a purple hue. As healing occurs in dark-skinned persons, the new skin is pink and may never darken.

10. Peripheral Tissue Edema: Assess tissues within 4 cm of wound edge. Nonpitting edema appears as skin that is shiny and taut. Identify pitting edema by firmly pressing a finger down into the tissues and waiting for 5 seconds; on release of pressure, tissues fail to resume previous position and an indentation appears. Crepitus is accumulation of air or gas in tissues. Use a transparent metric measuring guide to determine how far edema extends beyond wound.

11. Peripheral Tissue Induration: Assess tissues within 4 cm of wound edge. Induration is abnormal firmness of tissues with margins. Assess by gently pinching the tissues. Induration results in an inability to pinch the tissues. Use a transparent metric measuring guide with concentric circles divided into four (25%) pie-shaped quadrants to determine percent of wound and area involved.

12. Granulation Tissue: Granulation tissue is the growth of small blood vessels and connective tissue to fill in full-thickness wounds. Tissue is healthy when bright, beefy red, shiny, and granular with a velvety appearance. Poor vascular supply appears as pale pink or blanched to dull, dusky red color.

13. Epithelialization: Epithelialization is the process of epidermal resurfacing and appears as pink or red skin. In partial-thickness wounds it can occur throughout the wound bed as well as from the wound edges. In full-thickness wounds it occurs from the edges only. Use a transparent metric measuring guide with concentric circles divided into four (25%) pie-shaped quadrants to help determine percent of wound involved and to measure the distance the epithelial tissue extends into the wound.

PRESSURE SORE STATUS TOOL   NAME _____

Complete the rating sheet to assess pressure sore status. Evaluate each item by picking the response that best describes the wound and entering the score in the item score column for the appropriate date.

Location: Anatomic site. Circle identify right (R) or left (L), and use "X" to mark site on body diagrams
_____ Sacrum and coccyx   _____ Lateral ankle   _____ Trochanter
_____ Medial ankle   _____ Ischial tuberosity   _____ Heel   _____ Other Site

Shape: Overall wound pattern: assess by observing perimeter and depth. Circle and *date* appropriate description:
_____ Irregular   _____ Linear or elongated   _____ Round/oval
_____ Bow/boat   _____ Square/rectangle   _____ Butterfly   _____ Other Site

Item	Assessment	Date/ Score	Date/ Score	Date/ Score
1. Size	1 = Length × width <4 sq cm 2 = Length × width 4–16 sq cm 3 = Length × width 6.1–36 sq cm 4 = Length × width 36.1–80 sq cm 5 = Length × width >80 sq cm			
2. Depth	1 = Nonblanchable erythema on intact skin 2 = Partial-thickness skin loss involving epidermis and/or dermis 3 = Full-thickness skin loss involving damage or necrosis of subcutaneous tissue; may extend down to but not through underlying fascia: and/or mixed partial and full thickness and/or tissue layers obscured by granulation tissue 4 = Obscured by necrosis 5 = Full-thickness skin loss with extensive destruction, tissue necrosis or damage to muscle, bone, or supporting structures			
3. Edges	1 = Indistinct, diffuse, none clearly visible 2 = Distinct, outline clearly visible, attached, even with wound base 3 = Well-defined, not attached to wound base 4 = Well-defined, not attached to base, rolled under, thickened 5 = Well-defined, fibrotic, scarred or hyperkeratotic			
4. Undermining	1 = Undermining <2 cm in any area 2 = Undermining 2–4 cm involving <5% wound margins 3 = Undermining 2–4 cm involving >5% wound margins 4 = Undermining >4 cm in any area 5 = Tunneling and/or sinus tract formation			
5. Necrotic Tissue Type	1 = None visible 2 = White/gray nonviable tissue and/or nonadherent yellow slough 3 = Loosely adherent yellow slough 4 = Adherent, soft, black eschar 5 = Firmly adherent, hard, black eschar			
6. Necrotic Tissue Amount	1 = None visible 2 = <25% of wound bed covered 3 = 25% or 50% of wound covered 4 = >50% and <75% of wound covered 5 = 75%-100% of wound covered			
7. Exudate Type	1 = None or bloody 2 = Serosanguineous: thin, watery, pale red/pink 3 = Serous: thin, water, clear 4 = Purulent: thin or thick, opaque, tan/yellow 5 = Foul purulem; thick, opaque, yellow/green with odor			
8. Exudate Amount	1 = None 2 = Scant 3 = Small 4 = Moderate 5 = Large			
9. Skin Color Surrounding Wound	1 = Pink or normal for ethnic group 2 = Bright red and/or blanches to touch 3 = White or gray pallor or hypopigmented 4 = Dark red or purple and/or nonblanchable 5 = Black or hyperpigmented			
10. Peripheral Tissue Edema	1 = Minimal swelling around wound 2 = Nonpitting edema extends <4 cm around wound 3 = Nonpitting edema extends ≥4 cm around wound 4 = Pitting edema extends <4 cm around wound 5 = Crepitus and/or pitting edema extends ≥4 cm			
11. Peripheral Tissue Induration	1 = Minimal firmness around wound 2 = Induration <2 cm around wound 3 = Induration 2-4 cm extending <50% around wound 4 = Induration 2-4 cm extending ≥50% around wound 5 = Induration >4 cm in any area			
12. Granulation Tissue	1 = Skin intact or partial-thickness wound 2 = Bright, beefy red: 75%-100% of wound filled and/or tissue overgrowth 3 = Bright, beefy red: <75% and >25% of wound filled 4 = Pink and/or dull, dusky red and/or fills ≤25% of wound 5 = No granulation tissue present			
13. Epithelialization	1 = 100% wound covered, surface intact 2 = 75%-<100% wound covered and/or epithelial tissue extends >0.5 cm into wound bed 3 = 50%-<75% wound covered and/or epithelial tissue extends to <0.5 cm into wound bed 4 = 25%-<50% wound covered 5 = <25% wound covered			

TOTAL SCORE

SIGNATURE

PRESSURE SCORE STATUS CONTINUUM

0	10	13	15	20	25	30	35	40	45	50	55	60	65

Tissue   Wound   Wound
Health   Regeneration   Degeneration

Plot the total score on the Pressure Sore Status continuum by putting an "X" on the line and the date beneath the line. Plot multiple scores with their dates to see-at-glance regeneration or degeneration of the wound. © 1990 Barbara Bates-Jensen.

Appendix 13-B *Braden Scale for Predicting Pressure Sore Risk*

Patient's Name _____   Evaluator's Name _____

SENSORY PERCEPTION
Ability to respond meaningfully to pressure-related discomfort

1. COMPLETELY LIMITED:
Unresponsive (does not moan, flinch, or grasp) to painful stimuli, due to diminished level of consciousness or sedation,
OR
limited ability to feel pain over most of body surface.

2. VERY LIMITED:
Responds only to painful stimuli. Cannot communicate discomfort except by moaning or restlessness,
OR
has a sensory impairment that limits the ability to feel pain or discomfort over one half of body.

MOISTURE
Degree to which skin is exposed to moisture

1. CONSTANTLY MOIST:
Skin is kept moist almost constantly by perspiration, urine, etc. Dampness is detected every time patient is moved or turned.

2. MOIST:
Skin is often but not always moist. Linen must be changed at least once per shift.

ACTIVITY
Degree of physical activity

1. BED FAST:
Confined to bed.

2. CHAIR FAST:
Ability to walk severely limited or nonexistent. Cannot bear own weight and/or must be assisted into chair or wheelchair.

MOBILITY
Ability to change and control body position

1. COMPLETELY IMMOBILE:
Does not make even slight changes in body or extremity position without assistance.

2. VERY LIMITED:
Makes occasional slight changes in body or extremity position but unable to make frequent or significant changes independently.

NUTRITION
Usual food intake pattern

1. VERY POOR:
Never eats a complete meal. Rarely eats more than a third of any food offered. Eats 2 servings or less of protein (meat or dairy products) per day. Takes fluids poorly. Does not take a liquid dietary supplement,
OR
is NPO and/or maintained on clear liquids or IV for more than 5 days.

2. PROBABLY INADEQUATE:
Rarely eats a complete meal and generally eats only about half of any food offered. Protein intake includes only 3 servings of meat or dairy products per day. Occasionally will take a dietary supplement,
OR
receives less than optimum amount of liquid diet or tube feeding.

FRICTION AND SHEAR

1. PROBLEM:
Requires moderate to maximum assistance in moving. Complete lifting without sliding against sheets is impossible. Frequently slides down in bed or chair, requiring frequent repositioning with maximum assistance. Spasticity, contractures, or agitation leads to almost constant friction.

2. POTENTIAL PROBLEM:
Moves feebly or requires minimum assistance. During a move skin probably slides to some extent against sheets, chair, restraints, or other devices. Maintains relatively good position in chair or bed most of the time but occasionally slides down.

Copyright © 1988 Barbara Braden and Nancy Bergstrom.
NPO, Nothing by mouth; *IV,* intravenously; *TPN,* total parenteral nutrition.

Appendix 13-B *Braden Scale for Predicting Pressure Sore Risk—cont'd*

Date of Assessment				

3. SLIGHTLY LIMITED:
Responds to verbal commands but cannot always communicate discomfort or need to be turned,
OR
has some sensory impairment that limits ability to feel pain or discomfort in one or two extremities.

4. NO IMPAIRMENT:
Responds to verbal commands. Has no sensory deficit that would limit ability to feel or voice pain or discomfort.

3. OCCASIONALLY MOIST:
Skin is occasionally moist, requiring an extra linen change approximately once per day.

4. RARELY MOIST:
Skin is usually dry; linen requires changing only at routine intervals.

3. WALKS OCCASIONALLY:
Walks occasionally during day but for very short distances, with or without assistance. Spends majority of each shift in bed or chair.

4. WALKS FREQUENTLY:
Walks outside the room at least twice per day and inside room at least once every 2 hours during waking hours.

3. SLIGHTLY LIMITED:
Makes frequent though slight changes in body or extremity position independently.

4. NO LIMITATIONS:
Makes major and frequent changes in position without assistance.

3. ADEQUATE:
Eats over half of most meals. Eats a total of 4 servings of protein (meat, dairy products) each day. Occasionally will refuse a meal, but will usually take a supplement if offered,
OR
is on a tube feeding or TPN regimen, which probably meets most of nutritional needs.

4. EXCELLENT:
Eats most of every meal. Never refuses a meal. Usually eats a total of 4 or more servings of meat and dairy products. Occasionally eats between meals. Does not require supplementation.

3. NO APPARENT PROBLEM:
Moves in bed and in chair independently and has sufficient muscle strength to lift up completely during move. Maintains good position in bed or chair at all times.

Total Score

Assessment Tools in Gerontological Nursing

Upon completion of this chapter, the reader will be able to:

- Discuss the advantages and disadvantages of the use of standardized tools in gerontological assessment.
- Contrast the three types of formats used in the collection of assessment data.
- Describe the range of assessments that may be used in the comprehensive gerontological assessment.
- Begin to develop the skills needed to select an appropriate tool for a specific situation and use it correctly.

ADLs Activities of daily living, those tasks necessary to maintain one's health and basic personal needs.
IADLs Instrumental activities of daily living, those tasks necessary to maintain one's home and live independently at home.

Report-by-proxy One person (the proxy) answering questions or providing information for another person, based on the first person's knowledge of the second person.

ASSESSMENT TOOLS IN GERONTOLOGICAL NURSING

Gerontological nurses conduct skilled and detailed assessments of and with the persons who entrust themselves to their care. The process of assessment of older adults is strikingly different from that of younger adults in that it is more comprehensive, more detailed, and takes much longer to complete. More often, partial or problem-oriented assessments are done. If a comprehensive assessment is needed, this is usually performed by a number of members of the health care team but often led by the nurse.

The health assessment (also called health appraisal, physical examination, and health screening) is composed of a number of parts, which will be reviewed in this chapter. A compre-hensive assessment requires not only physical data but also an integration of the biological, psychosocial, and functional aspects of the older person. Inquiries into physiological and anatomical function, growth and development, family relationships, group involvement, and religious and occupational pursuits are essential in a health assessment interview. Questions regarding genetic background, although important, have less significance for the elderly because genetic consequences usually appear earlier in life.

Assessment of the older adult requires special abilities of the nurse: the ability to listen patiently, to allow for pauses, to ask questions that are not often asked, to observe minute details, to obtain data from all available sources, and to recognize normal changes associated with late life that would be abnormal in one who is younger (see

Chapter 7). Assessment of older adults takes more time due to their increased medical and social complexity than the younger adult. The quality and speed of the assessment are an art born of experience. Novice nurses should neither be expected nor expect themselves to do this proficiently but should expect to see both their skills and the amount of information obtained increase over time. According to Benner (1984), assessment is a task for the expert. However, an expert is not always available. By using assessment tools, reasonably reliable data may be obtained by nurses at all skill levels.

Over the years nurses and others have developed tools to both ease and standardize the collection of data. A number of the tools used in the gerontological setting are presented here. The collection of reliable data is the first step in the nursing process, followed by the analysis of the data or the determination of patient needs or diagnoses. The development of nursing interventions follows the analysis. Taken together, the nurse contributes to the nation's goal of increasing the quality of life lived for all Americans (USDHHS, 2000).

Assessment tools exist that can broadly categorize physical health, motor capacity, manual ability, self-care ability, more complex or instrumental abilities, and cognitive and social function. Assessments are completed in every nursing setting, such as hospitals, nursing facilities, and home health agencies. In most settings standardized formats are used routinely, especially in the switch from written medical records to electronic databases (especially see discussion of MDS and OASIS in chapter 6). Exactly which assessments are done depends both on the setting and the purpose of the evaluation. Sometimes these tools come directly from the gerontological literature, and sometimes they are modified to meet the particular needs of the setting.

There are three major formats of assessment tools: self-report, report-by-proxy, and observational. In the self-report format, elders are asked questions about their health or abilities and the answers are recorded, such as in a health history and in many of the functional assessments. In this format, abilities tend to be overestimated. Report-by-proxy formats are those in which the nurse asks another person, such as a spouse or child, to provide the nurse with the needed data. This format is used extensively with persons who are cognitively impaired and tends to underestimate the person's abilities and health. In the observational format the nurse collects and records the data as she or he has measured and observed the health status to be. The usual physical examination and performance-based functional assessments are examples of observational tools. Observational tools are probably the most accurate but are limited in that they only represent the situation at the time and not the overall situation, which can vary by the time of day and many other factors.

Certain guidelines should be followed regardless of the type or format of tool used:

- Whenever possible, collect the data at a time when the patient is at his or her best.
- If a standard tool is being used, be sure you are familiar with it before you administer it.
- If there is a specific question on the tool it should be asked exactly as written unless directed otherwise.
- To avoid biasing the response, do not direct the way the question is answered.
- Explore for more information only if it is needed to complete the assessment.
- Approach questions that are more personal, such as sexual functioning, in a matter-of-fact but still sensitive manner.
- Record the responses accurately, using the patient's own words where possible; do not analyze at the same time the data are being collected. For example, if the patient says "I have a runny nose" this is not recorded as "patient has a cold."

Ideally, assessment tools should be used to gather baseline data before the older adult has a health crisis. Periodically, the person can be reassessed using the same tools. A person who has an altered mental status as a result of an illness or medication should be reassessed later to determine if his or her status has gotten better or worse. Consider the results of assessment as a yardstick of an individual's status at any given time. Just as children are periodically measured for their weight and height, so, too, should elders be assessed periodically for their physical, functional, social, and mental status in health and illness. When a baseline exists, this allows for a comparison from which care can be planned and resources utilized.

| Box 14-1 | Cultural Assessment Related to Client's Health Problem |

The clinician may need to identify others who can facilitate the discussion of the client's problem(s).

1. How would you describe the problem that has brought you here? (What do you call your problem; does it have a name?)
   a. Who in the community and your family helps you with your problem?
2. How long have you had this problem?
   a. When do you think it started?
   b. What do you think started it?
   c. Do you know anyone else with it?
   d. Tell me what happened to that person when dealing with this problem.
3. What do you think is wrong with you?
   a. What does your sickness do to you?
   b. How severe is it?
   c. What might other people think is wrong with you?
   d. Tell me about people who do not get this problem.
4. Why do you think this happened to you?
   a. Why has it happened to the involved part?
   b. Why do you get sick and not someone else?
   c. Will it have a long or short course?
   d. What do you fear most about your sickness?
5. What are the chief problems your sickness has caused you?
6. What do you think will help clear up this problem? (What treatment should you receive; what are the most important results you hope to receive?)
   a. If specific tests, medications are listed, ask what they are and do.
7. Apart from me, who else do you think can make you feel better?
   a. Are there therapies that make you feel better that I do not know? (may be in another discipline)

Modified from Kleinman A: *Patient and healers in the context of culture: an exploration of the borderland between anthropology, medicine, and psychiatry,* Berkeley, 1980, University of California Press; Pfeifferling JH: A cultural prescription for mediocentrism. In Eisenberg L, Kleinman A, editors: *The relevance of social science for medicine,* Boston, 1981, Reidel.

The Health History

The initiation of the health history marks the beginning of the nurse-client relationship and the assessment process. The health history is collected either verbally in a face-to-face interview or through the clarification of a written history completed by the patient or patient's proxy beforehand. The latter method is usually much faster than the former. If the elder has limited English proficiency a knowledgeable interpreter is needed and the interview will generally take about double the amount of time.

Any health history form or interview should include a patient profile, a past medical history, a review of symptoms and systems, a medication history (prescribed and over-the-counter remedies including herbals and dietary supplements), a family history (especially parents and siblings), and a social history. The social history of the older adult should include the current living arrangements, economic resources to deal with current health issues, amount of family and friend support

if needed, and the types of community resources available if needed. Finally, if functional status is measured by self-report or by proxy, this is also routinely collected at the time of the health history.

In order to meet the needs of our increasingly diverse population of elders, the use of questions related to the explanatory model (see Chapter 4; Kleinman et al, 1980) is recommended to complement the health history (Box 14-1). The responses will better enable the nurse to understand the elder and plan appropriate and effective interventions.

When a more comprehensive assessment is being done, additional components are needed, often with well-established tools. Additional areas are psychological parameters such as cognitive and emotional well-being; caregiver stress or burden; the individual's self-perception; and patterns of health and health care, education, family structure, plans for retirement, and living environment. For those living at home a home safety assessment can be very helpful. Areas or problems not frequently addressed by the care provider or mentioned by the elder but that should be addressed are sexual dysfunction, depression, incontinence, musculoskeletal stiffness, alcoholism, hearing loss, and memory loss or confusion (Ham, 2002).

Physical Assessment

The health assessment is usually followed by the physical assessment or examination process. Tools related to the physical assessment are not included here. Many books provide an essential discussion of examination tools, techniques, and methods. As noted above, most organizations take existing formats and specify them for the needs of the institution and the purposes of the examination.

There is, however, a model that can be applied to the overall assessment with an emphasis on how one's physical health may or may not be affecting functional health; this model is especially useful for the frail elder and less useful for the active and healthy elder. FANCAPES is an assessment model and tool that uses a survival-needs framework with an emphasis on function. The acronym *FANCAPES* represents *F*luids, *A*eration, *N*utrition, *C*ommunication, *A*ctivity, *P*ain, *E*limination, and *S*ocialization and social skills. The information provided is helpful in the appraisal of the older person's ability to meet his or her needs and the extent to which assistance is necessary. FANCAPES can be used in all settings, may be used in part or total (depending on the need), and is easily adaptable to the functional pattern grouping if nursing diagnoses are used in planning care. Assessment data obtained from this method are based on the following considerations in each area.

FANCAPES
Fluids. Evaluation of fluids requires a functional assessment of the client's state of hydration and those physiological, situational, and mental factors that contribute to the maintenance of adequate hydration. Attention is directed to the ability of the client to obtain adequate fluids on his or her own, to express feelings of thirst, to effectively swallow, and to evaluate medications that affect intake and output (see Chapter 11).

Aeration. In considering aeration, one looks at the adequacy of oxygen exchange. Observations include respiratory rate and depth at rest and during activity; talking, walking, and situations requiring added exertion; and the presence or absence of edema in the extremities or abdomen. Breath sounds should be auscultated and medications reviewed to evaluate the effects on aeration.

Nutrition. Nutrition involves mechanical and psychological factors in addition to the type and amount of food consumed. It is necessary to ascertain the client's ability to bite, chew, and swallow. Edentulous clients may have dentures that fit improperly and are not worn. Alterations in diet because of culture, medical restrictions, available economic resources, and living conditions should be considered. Visual and neurological impairment, which might interfere with the client's ability to prepare a meal or feed himself or herself, should be noted (see Chapter 10).

Communication. The sending and receiving of verbal and nonverbal information in the external world and signals in the internal environment of the body require mechanical function of body parts and psychosocial responses from others in the environment. Assessment includes sight and sound acuity; voice quality; and adequate function of the tongue, teeth, pharynx, and larynx. Appraisal of the client's ability to read, write, and understand the spoken language should be ascertained. This is an important issue, since an undetected disability in these skills can lead to erroneous conclusions (see Chapters 3 and 9).

Activity. Activity includes aspects other than exercise. The nurse looks at the ability to feed, toilet, dress, and groom oneself; to prepare meals; to dial the telephone; and to move about with or without assistive devices. Coordination and balance, finger dexterity, grip strength, and other actions necessary to daily life should also be assessed. Ambulation should be considered a major component in activity.

Pain. Pain, both physical and mental, is important to consider. The presence and absence of pressure and discomfort are also aspects of pain assessment. Information about recent losses or visible symptoms of anxiety may help determine manifestations of pain. The manner by which a client customarily attains relief from pain or discomfort will provide further sources of information (see Chapter 17).

Elimination.   Bladder and bowel elimination should be investigated for mechanical factors such as evidence of dribbling or incontinence, for use of assistive devices or altered body structures resulting from surgical intervention, and for medications that affect voiding and intestinal peristalsis. The nurse and patient will need to find words that they both understand when talking about bowel and bladder functioning. The words used in health care, such as stooling or voiding, should be avoided (see chapter 11 for discussion of incontinence).

Socialization and social skills.   Socialization and social skills assess the individual's ability to negotiate in society, to give and receive love and friendship, and to feel self-worth. Attention should focus on the individual's ability to deal with loss and to interact with other people in give-and-take situations.

Functional Assessment

Whereas the emphasis of FANCAPES is on physical functioning, a full functional assessment is broader. A formal functional assessment can be defined as the evaluation of a person's ability to carry out basic tasks for self-care and tasks needed to support independent living. A thorough functional assessment will help the gerontological nurse work toward healthy aging by doing the following:

- Identifying the specific areas in which help is needed or not needed
- Identifying changes in abilities from one period of time to another
- Assisting in the determination of the need for specific service(s)
- Providing information that may be useful in determining the safety of a particular living situation

The major tools used in functional assessment are those that assess the individual's ability to perform the tasks needed for self-care (i.e., those needed to maintain one's health) and separately, those tasks needed for independent living and those to maintain one's home. Self-care activities are known as ADLs or activities of daily living and are international as well as cross-cultural in nature. ADLs are most often listed on tools as eating, toileting, ambulation, bathing, dressing,

and grooming. Three of these tasks (grooming, dressing, bathing) require cognitive function.

The IADLs are tasks needed for independent living, such as cleaning, yard work, shopping, and money management. The successful performance of IADLs requires a higher level of cognitive and physical functioning than the ADLs. For persons with dementia the progression of loss of IADLs begins with those which require the higher cognitive functions, such as handling finances and shopping.

Numerous tools are available that describe, screen, assess, monitor, and predict functional ability. Generally, the assessment does not break down a task into its component parts, such as picking up a spoon or cup or swallowing water, when assessment of eating is done; instead, eating is seen as a total task. Most of the tools result in a score of some kind—a rating of the person's ability to do the task alone, to need assistance, or to not be able to perform the task at all. The ratings are done by self-report, proxy, or observer as noted above. The tools are beneficial in their ability to serve the purposes noted above. However, most are not sensitive to small changes and can only be used as part of a holistic assessment.

The *Katz Index* (Katz et al, 1963) developed in 1963 serves as a basic framework for most of the measures of ADLs since that time. There are several versions of the Katz Index; one is based on a 3-point scale and allows one to score client performance abilities as independent, assistive, dependent, or unable to perform. Another version of the tool assigns 1 point to each ADL that can be completed independently and a zero (0) if it cannot. Scores will range from a maximum of 6 (totally independent) to 0 (totally dependent). A score of 4 indicates moderate impairment, whereas 2 or less indicates severe impairment (Table 14-1). This scoring puts equal weight on all activities, and the determination of a cutoff score is completely subjective. Despite these limitations, the tool is useful because it creates a common language about patient function for all caregivers involved in planning overall care and discharge.

The *Barthel Index* (Mahoney, Barthel, 1965) is probably the tool most commonly used in rehabilitation settings to measure the amount of physical assistance required when a person can no longer carry out ADLs. It has proved especially useful as a method of documenting improvement of a

Table 14-1 Katz Index of Independence in Activities of Daily Living

Activities (0 or 1 point)	Independence (1 point)	Dependence (0 points)
	NO supervision, direction, or personal assistance	WITH supervision, direction, personal assistance, or total care
BATHING	(1 point) Bathes self completely or needs help in bathing only a single part of the body such as the back, genital area, or	(0 points) Needs help with bathing more than one part of the body, getting in or out of the tub or shower. Requires total bathing.
Points: _____	disabled extremity.	
DRESSING	(1 point) Gets clothes from closets and drawers and puts on clothes and outer garments complete with fasteners. May	(0 points) Needs help with dressing self or needs to be completely dressed.
Points: _____	have help tying shoes.	
TOILETING	(1 point) Goes to toilet, gets on and off, arranges clothes, cleans	(0 points) Needs help transferring to the toilet, cleaning self, or
Points: _____	genital area without help.	uses bedpan or commode.
TRANSFERRING	(1 point) Moves in and out of bed or chair unassisted. Mechanical	(0 points) Needs help in moving from bed to chair or requires a
Points: _____	transferring aids are acceptable.	complete transfer.
CONTINENCE	(1 point) Exercises complete self-control over urination and	(0 points) Is partially or totally incontinent of bowel or bladder.
Points: _____	defecation.	
FEEDING	(1 point) Gets food from plate into mouth without help. Preparation of food may be	(0 points) Needs partial or total help with feeding or requires parenteral feeding.
Points: _____	done by another person.	
TOTAL POINTS = _____	6 = High (patient independent)	0 = Low (patient very dependent)

From Katz S et al: Progress in the development of the index of ADL, *Gerontologist* 10(1):20-30, 1970.

patient's ability. The Barthel Index ranks the functional status as either independent or dependent and then allows for further classification of independent into intact or limited and dependent into needing a helper or unable to do the activity at all The nurse should receive instructions in the use and scoring of this tool before implementing it.

The *Functional Independence Measure (FIM)* is a widely used and the most comprehensive functional assessment tool for rehabilitation settings and includes measure of ADLs, mobility, cognition, and social functioning. It was developed through the work of a number of experts and has been thoroughly tested. Ordinarily the tool is completed by the joint efforts of the interdisciplinary team and used for both planning and evaluation of progress. Considerable training is required

to accurately use the FIM (Granger, Hamilton, 1993); however, its use is encouraged.

The IADLs are considered to be more complex activities requiring higher functioning than the ADLs. The original scoring tool was developed by Lawton and Brody (1969). Both the original tool and the subsequent variations again use the self-report, proxy, and observed formats with the three levels of functioning (independent, assisted, and unable to perform). The pros and cons of using these are the same as the measures of ADLs. Box 14-2 gives an example of a self-rated instrument for IADLs.

The ADLs and IADLS can also be measured based on performance tools. These tools overcome the problems associated with self-report and proxy report and yield more objective measurement of

---

Box 14-2   Instrumental Activities of Daily Living

1. Telephone:
   I: Able to look up numbers, dial, receive and make calls without help
   A: Able to answer phone or dial operator in an emergency but needs special phone or help in getting number or dialing
   D: Unable to use telephone
2. Traveling:
   I: Able to drive own car or travel alone on bus or taxi
   A: Able to travel but not alone
   D: Unable to travel
3. Shopping:
   I: Able to take care of all shopping with transportation provided
   A: Able to shop but not alone
   D: Unable to shop
4. Preparing meals:
   I: Able to plan and cook full meals
   A: Able to prepare light foods but unable to cook full meals alone
   D: Unable to prepare any meals
5. Housework:
   I: Able to do heavy housework (e.g., scrub floors)
   A: Able to do light housework but needs help with heavy tasks
   D: Unable to do any housework
6. Medication:
   I: Able to take medications in the right dose at the right time
   A: Able to take medications but needs reminding or someone to prepare them
   D: Unable to take medications
7. Money:
   I: Able to manage buying needs, write checks, pay bills
   A: Able to manage daily buying needs but needs help managing checkbook, paying bills
   D: Unable to manage money

From *Multidimensional Functional Assessment Questionnaire*, ed 2, by Duke University Center for the Study of Aging and Human Development with permission of Duke University, 1978.
I, Independent; *A*, assistance; *D*, dependent.

---

performance. They take longer to conduct, and again the cutoffs are subjective and may be arbitrary. The three performance tests related to mobility are simple and quick: the ability to stand with feet together in a side-by-side manner and in a tandem and semitandem position, a timed walk of 8 feet, and a timed rise from a chair and return to a seated position five times (Box 14-3).

When assessing both functional status and cognitive abilities slightly different tools are indicated. The *Blessed Dementia Score* (Blessed et al, 1968) is based on a 22-item tool that can be scored from 0 to 27. The higher the score, the greater the degree of dementia. This tool incorporates aspects of ADLs, IADLs, memory, recalling events, and finding one's way outdoors. The *Clinical Dementia Rating Scale* (Morris, 1993) and the *Global Deterioration Scale* (Reisberg et al, 1982) also assess both functional and cognitive abilities and are also used to stage dementia. Determining the functional and cognitive stage of the dementia can allow the nurse to provide considerable anticipatory teaching to both the family and other caregivers.

Mental Status Assessment

Older adults are at great risk for impaired mental capacity. With increases in age there is an increased rate of dementing illnesses, such as Alzheimer's. Cognitive ability is also easily threatened by any disturbance in health. Indeed, altered or impaired mental status may be the first sign of anything from a heart attack to a urinary tract infection. The gerontological nurse needs to be aware of the basic tools that are used in the assessment of mental status, especially cognitive abilities and mood.

Cognitive Measures

Mini-Mental State Exam. The tool that is most often seen is probably the *Mini-Mental State Exam (MMSE)* by Folstein et al (1975). The MMSE

Box 14-3   **Functional Performance Tests**

Standing Balance

Instructions: semitandem stand.* The nurse:

a. First demonstrates the task.
   (The heel of one foot is placed to the side of the first toe of the other foot.)
b. Supports one arm of the older adult while he or she positions the feet as demonstrated above. The elder can choose which foot to place forward.
c. Asks if the person is ready, then releases the support and begins timing.
d. Stop timing when the older adult moves the feet or grasps the nurse for support or when 10 seconds have elapsed.

*Start with the semitandem stand. If it cannot be done for 10 seconds, then the **side-by-side** test should be done. If the semitandem can be accomplished for the requisite 10 seconds, follow the same instructions as above, except the **full tandem** requires placing the heel of one foot directly in front of the toes of the other foot.

Scoring	Full tandem	Semitandem	Side-by-side
0	_____	<10 seconds or unable	<10 seconds or unable
1	_____	<10 seconds or unable	10 seconds
2	<3 seconds or unable	10 seconds	_____
3	3 to 9 seconds	10 seconds	_____
4	10 seconds	10 seconds	_____

Standing Balance score: _____

Walking Speed

Instructions: The nurse:

a. Sets up an 8-foot walking course with an additional 2 feet at both ends free of any obstacles.
b. Places an 8-foot rigid carpenter's ruler to the side of the course.
c. Instructs the older adult to "walk to the other end of the course at your normal speed, just like walking down the street to go to the store." Assistive devices should be used if needed.
d. Times two walks. **The fastest of the two is used as the score.**

Scoring

0	Unable
1	>5.6 seconds
2	4.1 to 5.6 seconds
3	3.2 to 4 seconds
4	<3.2 seconds

Walking Speed score: _____

Chair Stands

Instructions: The nurse:

a. Places a straight-backed chair next to a well.
b. Asks the older adult to fold the arms across the chest and stand up from the chair one time. If successful.
c. Asks the older adult to stand and sit five times as quickly as possible.
d. Times from the initial sitting position to the final standing position at the end of the fifth stand.

Scores are for the five rise-and-sits only. If the older adult performs less than five repetitions, the score is 0.

Scoring

0	Unable
1	>16.6 seconds
2	13.7 to 16.5 seconds
3	11.2 to 13.6 seconds
4	<11.2 seconds

Chair Stands score: _____   **Total of all performance tests (0-12)** _____

Modified from Guralnik et al: A short physical performance battery assessment of lower extremity function: association with self-reported disability and prediction of mortality and nursing home admission, *J Gerontol Med Sci* 49(2):M85-M94, 1994; and Bennett JA: Activities of daily living: old-fashioned or still useful? *J Gerontol Nurs* 25(5):22-29, 1999.

is a 30-item instrument that is used to screen for cognitive deficiencies and is one of the factors in the determination of a diagnosis of dementia or delirium. It tests orientation, short-term memory and attention, calculation ability, language, and construction (Table 14-2). To ensure that the results of this test are valid and reliable, it must be administered exactly as it is written. It cannot be given to persons who cannot see or write or who are not proficient in English. A score of 30 suggests no impairment, and a score of 26 or less suggests a potential dementia; however, adjustments are needed for educational level (Osterweil et al, 2000). In the long-term care setting the MMSE is administered by either the nurse or the social worker as part of the collection of period data for the MDS (Minimum Data Set) (see Chapter 6).

Table 14-2   MiniMental LLC

NAME OF SUBJECT _____ Age _____
NAME OF EXAMINER _____ Years of School Completed _____
Approach the patient with respect and encouragement   Date of Examination _____
Ask: Do you have any trouble with your memory?   □ Yes □ No
May I ask you some questions about your memory?   □ Yes □ No

SCORE   ITEM

5 ( )   TIME ORIENTATION
Ask:
What is the year _____ (1), season _____ (1),
month of the year _____ (1), date _____ (1),
day of the week _____ (1)?

5 ( )   PLACE ORIENTATION
Ask:
Where are we now? What is the state _____ (1), city _____ (1),
part of the city _____ (1), building _____ (1),
floor of the building _____ (1)?

3 ( )   REGISTRATION OF THREE WORDS
Say: Listen carefully. I am going to say three words. You say them back after I stop. Ready? Here they are . . . PONY (wait 1 second), QUARTER (wait 1 second), ORANGE (wait 1 second). What were those words?
_____ (1)
_____ (1)
_____ (1)
Give 1 point for each correct answer, then repeat them until the patient learns all three.

5 ( )   SERIAL 7s AS A TEST OF ATTENTION AND CALCULATION
Ask: Subtract 7 from 100 and continue to subtract 7 from each subsequent remainder until I tell you to stop. What is 100 take away 7? _____ (1)
Say:
Keep going _____ (1), _____ (1),
_____ (1), _____ (1).

3 ( )   RECALL OF THREE WORDS
Ask:
What were those three words I asked you to remember?
Give one point for each correct answer _____ (1),
_____ (1), _____ (1).

Table 14-2 MiniMental LLC—*Continued*

For more
information
or additional
copies of this
exam call (617)
587-4215.
©1975, 1998,
MiniMental, LLC

2 ( )   NAMING
Ask:
What is this? (show pencil) _____ (1).
What is this? (show watch) _____ (1).

1 ( )   REPETITION
Say:
Now I am going to ask you to repeat what I say. Ready? No ifs, ands, or buts.
Now you say that _____ (1)

3 ( )   COMPREHENSION
Say:
Listen carefully because I am going to ask you to do something.
Take this paper in your left hand (1), fold it in half (1), and put it on the floor. (1)

1 ( )   READING
Say:
Please read the following and do what it says, but do not say it aloud. (1)
Close your eyes.

1 ( )   WRITING
Say:
Please write a sentence. If patient does not respond, say: Write about the weather. (1)

_____
_____

1 ( )   DRAWING
Say: Please copy this design.

TOTAL SCORE _____ Assess level of consciousness along a continuum

	Alert	Drowsy	Stupor	Coma

	YES	NO		YES	NO	FUNCTION BY PROXY			
Cooperative:	☐	☐	Deterioration from			Please record date when patient was last			
Depressed:	☐	☐	previous level of			able to perform the following tasks.			
Anxious:	☐	☐	functioning:	☐	☐	Ask caregiver if patient independently			
Poor Vision:	☐	☐	Family History of			handles:			
Poor Hearing:	☐	☐	Dementia:	☐	☐		YES	NO	DATE
			Head Trauma:	☐	☐	Money/Bills:	☐	☐	_____
Native Language:			Stroke:	☐	☐	Medication:	☐	☐	_____
			Alcohol Abuse:	☐	☐	Transportation:	☐	☐	_____
_____			Thyroid Disease:	☐	☐	Telephone:	☐	☐	_____

From Folstein MF, Folstein SE, McHugh PR: Mini-mental state: a practical method for grading the cognitive state of patients for the clinician, *J Psychiatr Res* 12(3):189-198, 1975. Copyright 1975, 1998, MiniMental LLC.

Box 14-4 — Short Portable Mental Status Questionnaire (SPMSQ)

1. What is the date today (month/day/year)?
2. What is the day of the week?
3. What is the name of this place?
4. What is your telephone number?
5. How old are you?
6. When were you born (month/day/year)?
7. Who is the current president of the United States?
8. Who was the president just before him?
9. What is your mother's maiden name?
10. Subtract 3 from 20 and keep subtracting each new number you get, all the way down.

Scoring

0-2 errors = intact
3-4 errors = mild intellectual impairment
5-7 errors = moderate intellectual impairment

Source: Pfeiffer E: A short portable mental status questionnaire for the assessment of organic brain deficit in elderly patients, *J Am Geriatr Soc* 23(10):433-441, 1975.

Box 14-5 — Clock Drawing Test

Instructions

On a blank piece of paper:
   Ask the elder to draw a circle.
   Ask the elder to place the numbers inside the circle.
   Ask the elder to place the hands at 3:45.

Scoring

Draws closed circle	Score 1 point
Places numbers in correct position	Score 1 point
Includes all 12 correct numbers	Score 1 point
Places hands in correct position	Score 1 point

Interpretations

Errors such as grossly distorted contour or extraneous markings are rarely produced by cognitively intact persons.

Clinical judgment must be applied, but a low score indicates the need for further evaluation.

Data from Mendez MF, Ala T, Underwood KL: Development of scoring criteria for the clock drawing task in Alzheimer's disease, *J Am Geriatr Soc* 40(11):1095-1099, 1992; Tuokko H et al: The Clock Test: a sensitive measure to differentiate normal elderly from those with Alzheimer disease, *J Am Geriatr Soc* 40(6):579-584, 1992.

Short Portable Mental Status Questionnaire. A second tool that tests cognitive ability is the *Short Portable Mental Status Questionnaire (SPMSQ)* (Pfeiffer, 1975). The tool covers 10 questions that assess the person's orientation, remote memory, concentration, and calculation ability (Box 14-4). The SPMSQ can be used with individuals who have a short attention span and cannot sit long enough for the MMSE to be administered. Its value as an assessment tool is its ease of administration and the fact that it requires no equipment. It can be administered reliably with little preparation, and the established norms take into account educational level. It is difficult to accurately use the normal cutoff points (three wrong answers) for patients with delirium because of its variable presentation.

Clock Drawing Test. The *Clock Drawing Test,* which has been used since 1992 (Mendez et al, 1992; Tuokko et al, 1992), is a screening tool that differentiates normal elders from those with cognitive impairment and that is used as a measure of severity of the impairment. To complete the Clock Drawing Test, the individual needs to be able to adequately hold a pen or pencil, since it does require some manual dexterity. It would not be appropriate to use in individuals with severe arthritis, parkinsonism, or stroke that affects their dominant hand. A person is presented with either a blank piece of paper or a paper with a circle drawn on it. He or she is then asked to draw the face of a clock that says it is 3:45. Scoring is based on both the position of the numbers and the position of the hands (Box 14-5). This tool does not establish criteria for dementia, but if performance on the clock drawing is impaired, it suggests the need for further investigation and analysis.

Mood Measures

The above mentioned tools are measures of cognitive ability. Additional measurements may be needed of affective state or mood, especially the presence or absence of depression, a common and too often unrecognized problem in older adults. Persons with untreated depression are more functionally impaired and will have prolonged hospitalizations and nursing home stays, lowered quality of life, and perhaps shortened length of life (see Chapter 25). Persons with depression may appear as if they have dementia, and many persons with dementia are also depressed. The interconnection between the two calls for skill and sensitivity in the nurse to ensure that elders receive the most appropriate and effective care possible.

Beck Depression Inventory

The *Beck Depression Inventory (BDI;* Beck, 1987) is one of the most widely used self-administered tools in the identification of depression. The 21 items are divided between affective symptoms (e.g., I feel sad) and physical symptoms (e.g., I am having trouble sleeping). The BDI is used for screening, measuring severity of depression, and monitoring changes over time, such as response to treatment.

Zung

The *Zung Self-Rating Depression Scale* (Zung, 1965) has 20 items and is also commonly used in older adults. The items are similar to those in the BDI and are rated on frequency of occurrence from 1 to 4, or "a little of the time" to "most of the time." Elders may score inaccurately higher (indicating more depression) because of the number of physical complaints that are associated with normal aging or frequently used medications rather than true depression.

Geriatric Depression Scale

The *Geriatric Depression Scale (GDS),* developed by Yesavage et al (1983), is a 30-item tool designed for gerontological patients and based almost entirely on psychological discriminators. A short version is also available (Box 14-6). The GDS has been extremely successful in determining depression because it deemphasizes physical complaints, libido, and appetite. It is viewed as a more accurate measure of depression in the elderly than other tools. It cannot be used in persons with dementia or cognitive impairment (Osterweil et al, 2000).

Assessment of Social Supports

A comprehensive assessment of an older adult would be incomplete without an evaluation of social networks and support. Assessment of social supports looks at an individual's surrounding network of intimates, friends, and family. It is an important aspect of one's life and provides the sustenance and comfort often needed to surmount adversity such as a disability resulting from medical conditions. Tools to adequately measure social networks have been in development for a number of years. However, the many nuances and configurations of social support networks make standardized measurements difficult. One tool that has shown some usefulness is the Family APGAR. Although it was designed for younger families, it has potential for use with elders and their families.

Family APGAR

The *Family APGAR* (Smilkstein, 1978; Table 14-3) explores five specific family functions: *A*daptation, *P*artnership, *G*rowth, *A*ffection, and *R*esolution. A score of less than 3 points out of a possible 10 points indicates a highly dysfunctional family (at least as perceived by the person). A 4- to 6-point score suggests moderate family dysfunction. These results alone should not be considered definitive for family dysfunction. The APGAR tool is useful in the following situations:

Interviewing a new patient

Interviewing a person who will be caring for a chronically ill family member

Following adverse events (death, diagnosis of cancer, etc.)

When the patient history suggests family dysfunction

If an elder has more intimate social relationships with friends than with the spouse or family or is without family or spouse, the Friend APGAR should be used. The questions are the same as in the Family APGAR but with the word *Friend* substituted for *Family*.

An additional value of this instrument is the ability to assess the caregiver's perception of emotional support and social supports with a new diagnosis of Alzheimer's disease of a relative. There

Box 14-6	**Geriatric Depression Scale**

Patient _____ Examiner _____ Date _____

Directions to patient: Please choose the best answer for how you have felt over the past week.
Directions to examiner: Present questions VERBALLY. Circle answer given by patient. Do not show to patient.

1. Are you basically satisfied with your life? . . . . yes **no (1)**
2. Have you dropped many of your activities and interests? . . . . **yes (1)** no
3. Do you feel that your life is empty? . . . . **yes (1)** no
4. Do you often get bored? . . . . **yes (1)** no
5. Are you hopeful about the future? . . . . yes **no (1)**
6. Are you bothered by thoughts you can't get out of your head? . . . . **yes (1)** no
7. Are you in good spirits most of the time? . . . . yes **no (1)**
8. Are you afraid that something bad is going to happen to you? . . . . **yes (1)** no
9. Do you feel happy most of the time? . . . . yes **no (1)**
10. Do you often feel helpless? . . . . **yes (1)** no
11. Do you often get restless and fidgety? . . . . **yes (1)** no
12. Do you prefer to stay at home rather than go out and do things? . . . . **yes (1)** no
13. Do you frequently worry about the future? . . . . **yes (1)** no
14. Do you feel you have more problems with memory than most? . . . . **yes (1)** no
15. Do you think it is wonderful to be alive now? . . . . yes **no (1)**
16. Do you feel downhearted and blue? . . . . **yes (1)** no
17. Do you feel pretty worthless the way you are now? . . . . **yes (1)** no
18. Do you worry a lot about the past? . . . . **yes (1)** no
19. Do you find life very exciting? . . . . yes **no (1)**
20. Is it hard for you to get started on new projects? . . . . **yes (1)** no
21. Do you feel full of energy? . . . . yes **no (1)**
22. Do you feel that your situation is hopeless? . . . . **yes (1)** no
23. Do you think that most people are better off than you are? . . . . **yes (1)** no
24. Do you frequently get upset over little things? . . . . **yes (1)** no
25. Do you frequently feel like crying? . . . . **yes (1)** no
26. Do you have trouble concentrating? . . . . **yes (1)** no
27. Do you enjoy getting up in the morning? . . . . yes **no (1)**
28. Do you prefer to avoid social occasions? . . . . **yes (1)** no
29. Is it easy for you to make decisions? . . . . yes **no (1)**
30. Is your mind as clear as it used to be? . . . . yes **no (1)**

Total: Please sum all boldfaced answers (worth one point) for a total score. _____
      Scores: 0-10 Normal   11-20 Moderate depression   21-30 Severe depression

Format modified slightly from original. From Yesavage JA et al: Development and validation of a geriatric depression screening scale: a preliminary report, *J Psychiatr Res* 17(1):37-49, 1982-1983.

are also a number of tools specifically designed to measure the burden of the caregiver role; for example, see Figure 14-1, available at www.hartfordign.org.

Spirituality Assessment

Spirituality, or *spiritual well-being,* whether it is associated with a formal religious practice or non-religious intangible elements, has been recognized as important in the lives of many, including older adults. Spiritual needs are broader and more personal than religion. They transcend the physical and psychosocial elements of the person and are probably an important aspect of self-actualization as defined by Maslow. Nurses tend not to deal with spiritual needs of patients because they are thought to be too personal. However, if nurses are to care for the whole person, spiritual needs must be part of the assessment process. Although a

Table 14-3 The Family APGAR

The following questions have been designed to help us better understand you and your friends. Friends are nonrelatives from your school or community with whom you have a sharing relationship.

The following questions have been designed to help us better understand you and your family. You should feel free to ask questions about any item in the questionnaire.

"Family" is the individual(s) with whom you usually live. If you live alone, consider family as those with whom you now have the strongest emotional ties.

Comment space should be used if you wish to give additional information or if you wish to discuss the way the question applies to your family. Please try to answer all questions.

For each question, check only one box

	Almost always	Some of the time	Hardly ever		Almost always	Some of the time	Hardly ever
I am satisfied that I can turn to my friends for help when something is troubling me.	☐	☐	☐	I am satisfied that I can turn to my family for help when something is troubling me.	☐	☐	☐
Comments:				Comments:			
I am satisfied with the way my friends talk over things with me and share problems with me.	☐	☐	☐	I am satisfied with the way my family talks over things with me and shares problems with me.	☐	☐	☐
Comments:				Comments:			
I am satisfied that my friends accept and support my wishes to take on new activities or directions.	☐	☐	☐	I am satisfied that my family accepts and supports my wishes to take on new activities or directions.	☐	☐	☐
Comments:				Comments:			
I am satisfied with the way my friends express affection, and respond to my emotions, such as anger, sorrow, or love.	☐	☐	☐	I am satisfied with the way my family expresses affection, and responds to my emotions, such as anger, sorrow, or love.	☐	☐	☐
Comments:				Comments:			
I am satisfied with the way my friends and I share time together.	☐	☐	☐	I am satisfied with the way my family and I share time together.	☐	☐	☐
Comments:				Comments:			

Who lives in your home? *List by relationship (e.g., spouse, significant other,†child, or friend).

Please check below the column that best describes how you now get along with each member of the family listed.

Relationship	Age	Sex	Well	Fairly	Poorly
_____	_____	_____	☐	☐	☐
_____	_____	_____	☐	☐	☐
_____	_____	_____	☐	☐	☐

If you don't live with your own family, please list below the individuals to whom you turn for help most frequently. List by relationship (e.g., family member, friend, associate at work, or neighbor).

Please check below the column that best describes how you now get along with each person listed.

Relationship	Age	Sex	Well	Fairly	Poorly
_____	_____	_____	☐	☐	☐
_____	_____	_____	☐	☐	☐
_____	_____	_____	☐	☐	☐

From Smilkstein G, Ashworth C, Montano D: Validity and reliability of the family APGAR as a test of family function, *J Fam Pract* 15(2):303-311, 1982.

*If you have established your own family, consider home to be the place where you live with your spouse, children, or significant other; otherwise, consider home as your place of origin (e.g., the place where your parents or those who raised you live).

†"Significant other" is the partner you live with in a physically and emotionally nurturing relationship, but to whom you are not married.

I am going to read a list of things that other people have found to be difficult. Would you tell me if any of these apply to you? (Give examples.)

	Yes = 1	No = 0
Sleep is disturbed (e.g., because is in and out of bed; wanders around at night)		
It is inconvenient (e.g., because helping takes so much time; it's a long drive over to help)		
It is a physical strain (e.g., because of lifting in and out of a chair; effort or concentration is required)		
It is confining (e.g., helping restricts free time; cannot go visiting)		
There have been family adjustments (e.g., because helping has disrupted routine; there has been no privacy)		
There have been changes in personal plans (e.g., had to turn down a job; could not go on vacation)		
There have been other demands on my time (e.g., from other family members)		
There have been emotional adjustments (e.g., because of severe arguments)		
Some behavior is upsetting (e.g., because of incontinence; has trouble remembering things; accuses people of taking things)		
It is upsetting to find has changed so much from his/her former self (e.g., he/she is a different person than he/she used to be)		
There have been work adjustments (e.g., because of having to take time off)		
It is a financial strain		
Feeling completely overwhelmed (e.g., because of worry about _____; concerns abourt how to manage)		
TOTAL SCORE (Count yes responses. Any positive answer may indicate a need for intervention in that area. A score of 7 or higher indicates a high level of stress.)		

Figure 14-1 Caregiver strain index. (From Robinson BC: Validation of a caregiver strain index, *J Gerontol* 38[3]:344-348, 1983. Copyright The Gerontological Society of America.)

concise tool has yet to be developed, the aspects that would be included in both assessment and subsequent interventions are listed in Box 14-7.

Environmental and Safety Assessment

Environmental safety is an issue for persons at all ages. For persons with limitations in cognition, mobility, vision, or hearing or at risk for a fall-related injury, safety is especially important. Nurses in every setting are responsible for promoting the safety of the persons under their care.

The most commonly used tools related to safety are administered by home health nurses and occupational therapists. In general they consist of lists

Box 14-7	Assessing and Intervening in Spiritual Distress

Assessment
Brief history
  Losses
  Challenged belief, value system
  Separation from religious and cultural ties
  Death
  Personal and family disasters
Symptoms (defining characteristics) such as the
  following:
  Unmet needs
  Threats to self
  Change in environment, health status, self-
    concept, and so on
  Questioning meaning of own existence
  Depression
  Feeling of hopelessness, abandonment, fear
Assessment of the cause of spiritual distress
  Depletion anxiety
  Helplessness, hopelessness
  Perceived powerlessness

Medication reaction
Hormonal imbalances

Interventions
Create a therapeutic environment.
Assess the support system.
Assess past methods of decreasing distress
  (e.g., prayer, imagery, healing, memories-
  reminiscence therapy, medication,
  relaxation).
Determine environmental changes needed to
  enhance function.
Assess and assist implementation of coping
  mechanisms.
Refer to clergy.
Evaluate effects of nursing interventions.
Activate and evaluate appropriate community
  referrals.
Use techniques to assist client and family in
  reducing spiritual distress.

of potential dangers and the status of the danger (present or absent) and provide suggestions or an opportunity for planning to reduce the potential dangers. Often nurses think of safety related to the risk for falling, but fire hazards, poisoning, and problems with temperature (hypothermia or hyperthermia) exist as well. Unfortunately many older persons who have lived in their homes for many years are also in potential danger because of increased crime and victimization. Figure 14-2 provides an example of a tool that could be used in a home safety assessment. See also Chapter 22 for a more detailed discussion of mobility and environmental safety.

Integrated Assessments

In some cases an integrated approach is used rather than a collection of separate tools and assessments. The most well known is the *Older American's Resources and Service (OARS)* developed by Dr. Eric Pfeiffer and colleagues at Duke University (1979). The *Patient Appraisal and Care Evaluation (PACE)* tool was designed particularly for use in long-term care settings but has been used in the home as well (USDHHS, 1978). The *Com-

prehensive Assessment and Referral Evaluation tool* was designed for assessment of functional status and mental health (Gurland et al, 1977). These and other tools were taken into consideration in the development of the MDS currently used in skilled nursing facilities (see Chapters 6 and 14). In the home care setting the *OASIS System (Outcomes and Assessment Information Set)*, a computerized assessment tool, is universally in use at this time. All these tools are quite comprehensive and therefore quite lengthy. Once completed, they serve as a resource for a detailed plan of care. The *Fulmer SPICES Tool* serves as a guide for a much shorter but still comprehensive assessment (Figure 14-3).

Older American's Resources and Service

The *OARS (Older American's Resources and Service) assessment tool* is designed so that each component can be used individually. This enables it to be added to or integrated into self-designed tools. It was designed to evaluate ability, disability, and the capacity level at which the aged person is able to function. Five dimensions are considered for assessment: social resources, economic resources, physical health, mental health, and ADLs. Each

	Okay (y/n)	Plan to improve	
Basic Structure Intact roof Solid floors and stairs Functioning toilet (or outhouse) Source of fresh water Wheelchair ramp **Temperature Control** Fan/air conditioner Proper use of heating pads Proper hot water heater temperature Adequate heat/insulation **Nutrition** Kitchen condition/food storage Evidence of alcohol use Pests **Fire Prevention and Response** Use of kerosene heaters Use of open gas burners on stove for heat Smoking in bed Use of oxygen Dangerous electrical wiring Smoke alarms Exit plans in case of fire **Self-Injury/Violence Prevention** Locks Method of calling for help Proximity of neighbors Surrounding criminal activity Emergency phone numbers by telephone Loaded guns/knives Household toxins Water/bathtub Power tools **Medication Management** Duplicate medicines, outdated drugs, pill box Correct labeling Storage safety, accessibility, refrigeration Caregiver familiarity **Wandering Control (for confused patients)** Doortap latches, special locks Fenced yards with hidden latches Identification bracelets Electronic wandering alarms			|_ client X clinician Clinician's signature _____ Date _____

Figure 14-2   Guidelines for home safety assessment. (Modified from Yoshikawa TT, Cobbs EL, Brummel-Smith K: *Ambulatory geriatric care*, St Louis, 1993, Mosby.)

Patient Name:_____   Date_____

Spices	Evidence
Sleep disorders	
Problems with eating or feeding	
Incontinence	
Confusion	
Evidence of falls	
Skin breakdown	

Figure 14-3   SPICES. (From Fulmer SPICES: an overall assessment tool of older adults. Developed by Meredith Wallace and Terry Fulmer, Hartford Institute for Geriatric Nursing, New York University, New York.)

component uses a quantitative rating scale: 1—excellent, 2—good, 3—mildly impaired, 4—moderately impaired, 5—severely impaired, and 6—completely impaired. At the conclusion of the assessment a cumulative impairment score (CIS) is established, which can range from the most fit (6) to total disability (30). This aids in establishing the degree of need. Information considered in each domain includes the following.

Social resources. The social resources dimension evaluates the social skills and the ability to negotiate and make friends (the number of times friends are seen, the number of telephone conversations). In the assessment interview is the person able to ask for things from friends, family, and strangers? Is there a caregiver around in case of need? Who is it, and how long is the person available? Does the individual belong to any social network or group, such as a special interest or church group?

Economic resources. Data about monthly income and sources (Social Security, Supplemental Security Income, pensions, income generated from capital) are needed to determine the adequacy of income compared with the cost of living and food, shelter, clothing, medications, and small luxury items. This information can provide insight into the client's relative standard of living

and point out areas of need that might be alleviated by use of additional resources unknown to the aged person.

Mental health. Consideration is given to intellectual function, the presence or absence of psychiatric symptoms, and the amount of enjoyment and interaction the person gets from life.

Physical health. Diagnosis of major and common diseases of older persons, the type of prescribed and over-the-counter medications the person is taking, and the person's perception of his or her health status are the basis of evaluation. Excellent physical health includes participation in regular vigorous activity, such as walking, dancing, or biking at least twice each week. Seriously impaired physical health is determined by the presence of one or more illnesses or disabilities that may be severely painful, life threatening, or require extensive care.

Activities of daily living. The ADLs included in the OARS are walking, getting in and out of bed, bathing, combing hair, shaving, dressing, eating, and getting to the bathroom on time by oneself. The IADLs measured include tasks such as dialing the telephone, driving a car, hanging up clothes, obtaining groceries, taking medications, and having correct knowledge of their dosages.

Fulmer SPICES

The *Fulmer SPICES*, an overall assessment tool of older adults (Fulmer, 1991), has proved reliable and valid in use with the elder population whether they are healthy or frail; in acute, skilled nursing, long-term care facilities or at home. The acronym *SPICES* refers to six common syndromes of the elderly that require nursing interventions: *S*leep disorders, *P*roblems with eating or feeding, *I*ncontinence, *C*onfusion, *E*vidence of falls, and *S*kin breakdown. Nurses are encouraged to make a 3 × 5 card with this acronym on it and carry it with them to use as a reference when caring for older adults (see Figure 14-3). It is a system for alerting the nurse of the most common problems that occur in the health and well-being of the older adult, particularly those who have one or more medical conditions.

IMPLICATIONS FOR GERONTOLOGICAL NURSING AND HEALTHY AGING

Whether the nurse is working with a standardized tool or creating one, the goal is always to collect data that are the most accurate and to do so in the most efficient, yet caring manner possible. The use of tools serves as a way to organize the collected data necessary for assessment and to be able to compare the data from time to time. As noted above, each tool has strengths and weaknesses. A number of factors complicate assessment of the older adult. These include the difficulty of differentiating the effects of aging from those originating from disease, the co-existence of multiple diseases, the underreporting of symptoms by older adults, atypical presentation or nonspecific presentation of illness, and the increase in iatrogenic illnesses.

Overdiagnosis or underdiagnosis occurs when the normal age changes are not considered; these include both physical changes and biochemical changes. Underdiagnosis is far more common in the care of the aged. Many symptoms or complaints are ascribed to normal aging rather than to a disease entity that may be developing. Difficulty in assessing the older adult with multiple chronic conditions is also a challenge. Symptoms of one condition can exacerbate or mask symptoms of another. The gerontological nurse is challenged to provide the highest level of excellence in the care of the elderly. If a particular tool will facilitate the achievement of this goal then it should be used. If the tool serves little purpose and is burdensome to either the nurse or the patient, it should be avoided or replaced.

KEY CONCEPTS

- Assessment of the physical, cognitive, psychosocial, and environmental status is essential to meeting the specific needs of the older adult and implementing appropriate interventions.
- Whether the data for an assessment tool are collected by self-report, by report-by-proxy, or through nurse observation will affect the quality and quantity of the data.
- Knowledge of how to use a particular gerontological assessment tool is needed to accurately administer it.
- Co-morbidity of many older adults complicates obtaining and interpreting assessment data.

Activities and Discussion Questions

1. What is the importance of the measurement of ADLs and IADLs in older adults?
2. For each ADL, develop a plan of interventions that you would institute to compensate for ADL deficits and that would still foster an elder's independence as much as is realistic.
3. What makes an assessment tool effective?
4. What tool or tools would be most appropriate for assessing an elder in the community, in the hospital, in long-term care, or in day care? Give your rationale for the choices.

RESOURCES

Publications

Osterweil D, Brummel-Smith K, Beck JC: *Comprehensive geriatric assessment*, New York, 2000, McGraw-Hill (collection of assessment tools).
Teresi JA, Lawton MP, Homles D, Ory M, editors: *Measurement in elderly chronic care populations*, New York, 1997, Springer.

Websites

OASIS: can be downloaded from
www.hcfa.gov/medicare/hsqb/oasis/hhoview/htm
SPICES and other useful tools are available at
www.harfordign.org. in the *Try this: best practice in nursing care to older adults,* series offered by The Hartford Institute for Geriatric Nursing

REFERENCES

Beck AT: *Beck depression inventory: manual,* San Antonio, 1987, Psychological Corporation.

Benner P: *From novice to expert,* Menlo Park, Calif, 1984, Addison-Wesley.

Blessed G, Tomlinson BE, Roth M: The association between qualitative measures of dementia and of senile change in the cerebral grey matter of elderly subjects, *Br J Psychiatry* 114(512):797-811, 1968.

Folstein MF, Folstein SE, McHugh PR: Mini-mental state: a practical method for grading the cognitive state of patients for the clinician, *J Psychiatr Res* 12(3):189-198, 1975.

Fulmer T: The geriatric nurse specialist role: a new model, *Nurs Manage* 22(3):91-93, 1991.

Granger CV, Hamilton BB: The Uniform Data System for Medical Rehabilitation report of first admissions for 1991, *Am J Phys Med Rehabil* 72(1):33-38, 1993.

Gurland B et al: The comprehensive assessment and referral evaluation (CARE), *Int J Aging Hum Dev* 8(1):9-42, 1977-1978.

Ham RJ: Assessment. In Ham RJ, Sloane PD, Warshaw GA, editors: *Primary care geriatrics: a case-based approach,* ed 4, St Louis, 2002, Mosby.

Katz S et al: Studies of illness in the aged: the index of ADL: a standardized measure of biological and psychosocial function, *JAMA* 185:914-919, 1963.

Kleinman A: *Patient and healers in the context of culture: an exploration of the borderland between anthropology, medicine, and psychiatry,* Berkeley, 1980, University of California Press.

Lawton MP, Brody EM: Assessment of older people: self-maintaining and instrumental activities of daily living, *Gerontologist* 9(3):179-186, 1969.

Mahoney FI, Barthel DW: Functional evaluation: the Barthel Index, *Md State Med J* 14:61-65, 1965.

Mendez MF, Ala T, Underwood KL: Development of scoring criteria for the Clock Drawing Task in Alzheimer's disease, *J Am Geriatr Soc* 40(11):1095-1099, 1992.

Morris JC: The clinical dementia rating (CDR): current version and scoring rules, *Neurology* 43(11):2412-2414, 1993.

Osterweil D, Brummel-Smith K, Beck JC: *Comprehensive geriatric assessment,* New York, 2000, McGraw-Hill.

Pfeiffer E: A short portable mental status questionnaire for the assessment of organic brain deficit in elderly patients, *J Am Geriatr Soc* 23(10):433-441, 1975.

Pfeiffer E: *Physical and mental assessment—OARS.* Workshop Intensive, Western Gerontological Society, San Francisco, April 28, 1979.

Reisberg B et al: The global deterioration scale for assessment of primary progressive dementia, *Am J Psychiatry* 139(9):1136-1139, 1982.

Smilkstein G: The Family APGAR: a proposal for a family function test and its use by physicians, *J Fam Pract* 6(6):1231-1239, 1978.

Tuokko H et al: The clock test: a sensitive measure to differentiate normal elderly from those with Alzheimer disease, *J Am Geriatr Soc* 40(6):579-584, 1992.

U.S. Department of Health and Human Services (USDHHS): *Working document on patient care management,* Washington, DC, 1978, U.S. Government Printing Office.

U.S. Department of Health and Human Services (USDHHS): *Healthy people 2010,* Washington, DC, 2000, U.S. Government Printing Office.

Yesavage JA et al: Development and validation of a geriatric depression screening scale: a preliminary report, *J Psychiatr Res* 17(1):37-49, 1982-1983.

Zung WW: A self-rating depression scale, *Arch Gen Psychiatry* 12:63-70, 1965.

Medication Use and Management

▶ GLOSSARY

Adverse reaction A harmful, unintended reaction to a drug.

Anticholinergics A group of drugs that reduce spasms of certain smooth muscles; relax the iris; and decrease gastric, bronchial, and salivary secretions through the blocking of vagal impulses.

Antipsychotics Substances that counteract or diminish symptoms of psychoses. Also called neuroleptics.

Anxiolytics Medications used to treat anxiety.

Bioavailability The amount of drug that becomes available for activity in target tissues.

Biotransformation A series of chemical alterations of a drug occurring in the body.

Chronotherapy Adjustment of medications to coincide with the biological rhythm of the body for therapeutic effect.

Half-life The time it takes to inactivate half of a drug.

Iatrogenic That which is caused by something that is done or given to a person.

Idiosyncratic reaction An abnormal susceptibility to a drug that is peculiar to that individual; hypersensitivity to a particular drug (i.e., an allergy).

Metabolite A substance created in the body during the metabolism of a drug.

Neutraceuticals Substances that are considered dietary supplements but may also have a therapeutic effect on the body.

Potentiation The strengthening of one or more substances when they are used in combination.

Pharmacodynamics The study of the mechanism of action of a drug and the biochemical and physiological effect.

Pharmacokinetics Absorption, distribution, metabolism, and excretion of a drug in the body.

Psychotropic Describes drugs that have a special action on the psyche.

Regimen A systematic course of treatment or behaviors.

Side effect A consequence other than that for which the drug is used (e.g., dry mouth).

Target tissue Tissue or organ intended to receive the greatest concentration of a drug or to be most affected by the drug.

Therapeutic window The range of the plasma concentration of a drug when it is safe and effective.

It is so hard to keep track of my medications. I try arranging them in little cups to take with each meal, but then there are the ones that I take at odd times. Those are the easiest to forget. I get really confused and think sometimes I have taken them twice. I really wish I didn't have to take so many pills, but I'm not sure what would happen if I stopped any of them. I don't even know why I'm taking most of them.

Gerald, hypertensive, diabetic, and having cardiac problems

*I*n the United States, persons 65 years of age and older are the largest users of prescription and over-the-counter (OTC) medications. Making up only 12% of the population, they consume 33% of the prescribed medications (Patel, 2003) and 25% of the OTCs (Besdine et al, 1998). It is estimated that older adults use OTC preparations 69% to 85% of the time for conditions ranging from pain to constipation to fever (Amoako et al, 2003). Because of multiple medical conditions, elders are also more likely to take multiple medications than younger adults. Elders accumulate prescriptions as they accumulate chronic diseases. In a 1999 survey, 53% of older persons took three or more medications, and 33% took eight or more; these included both prescription and OTC medications (*Preventing Medication Errors in the Elderly*, 2002). Elders who reside in long-term care facilities take an average of four to seven different medications (Hogstel, 1992). People are also taking an increasing amount of herbal preparations and supplements referred to as neutraceuticals.

The most commonly prescribed and used drugs in the older population are cardiovascular drugs, antiinfectives, antipsychotic drugs, antidepressants, and diuretics (DeMaagd, 1995). Analgesics, laxatives, and antacids are the most-used OTC medications, followed by cough products, acetaminophen, nonsteroidal topical preparations, milk of magnesia, Pepto-Bismol, eye washes, and vitamins (Hogstel, 1992). Now, with the conversion of many prescription drugs to OTCs, additional categories may appear (Miller, 1996).

How elders use their prescribed medicines and their OTC products depends on many factors related to their own unique characteristics and situations, beliefs and understanding about illness, functional and cognitive status, perception about necessity of the drugs, severity of symptoms, reactions to the medications, finances, access, alternatives, and compatibility with lifestyle.

Many older adults are at risk for adverse drug events, excessive and inappropriate medication use, and nonadherence because of a number of factors, including age-related changes, increase in chronic disease and therefore medications, and varying level of gerontological skills of health care providers. From the perspective of Maslow's hierarchy of needs, drugs impinge on many levels. When they are used appropriately, drugs can enhance one's quality of life at every level. When they are used inappropriately, they threaten all levels of the hierarchy of needs. At times, even when drugs are used appropriately, they may adversely affect the elder's health and well-being.

Gerontological nurses have a responsibility to help minimize the risks of medication use in their clients. A review of the changes in pharmacokinetics, pharmacodynamics, and issues in drug use is presented in this chapter. A special section deals with the use of psychotropic agents. These are frequently prescribed to frail elders with the potential for both great benefit and significant risk.

PHARMACOKINETICS

The term *pharmacokinetics* refers to the movement of a drug in the body from the point of administration through absorption, distribution, metabolism, and finally, excretion. It is important for the gerontological nurse to understand how pharmacokinetics may differ in an older adult (Figure 15-1).

Absorption

In order for a drug to be effective it must be absorbed, or taken into the bloodstream. The

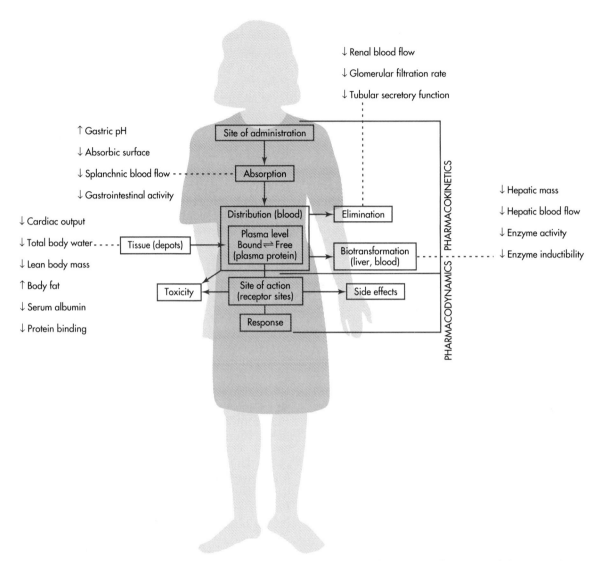

↓ Renal blood flow

↓ Glomerular filtration rate

↓ Tubular secretory function

↑ Gastric pH

↓ Absorbic surface

↓ Splanchnic blood flow

↓ Gastrointestinal activity

↓ Cardiac output

↓ Total body water

↓ Lean body mass

↑ Body fat

↓ Serum albumin

↓ Protein binding

↓ Hepatic mass

↓ Hepatic blood flow

↓ Enzyme activity

↓ Enzyme inductibility

Site of administration

Absorption

Distribution (blood)

Elimination

Plasma level
Bound ⇌ Free
(plasma protein)

Tissue (depots)

Biotransformation
(liver, blood)

Toxicity

Site of action
(receptor sites)

Side effects

Response

PHARMACOKINETICS

PHARMACODYNAMICS

Figure 15-1   Physiological age changes and the pharmacokinetics and pharmacodynamics of drug use. (Data from Kane RL, Ouslander JG, Abrass IB: *Essentials of clinical geriatrics,* New York, 1984, McGraw-Hill; Lamy PP: Hazards of drug use in the elderly: commonsense measures to reduce them, *Postgrad Med* 76[1]:50-53, 1984; Vestal RE, Dawson GW: Pharmacology and aging. In Finch CE, Schneider EL, editors: *Handbook of biology and aging,* New York, 1985, Van Nostrand Reinhold; Roberts J, Tumer N: Pharmacodynamic basis for altered drug action in the elderly, *Clin Geriatr Med* 4[1]:127-149, 1988; Montamat SC, Cusack BJ, Vestal RE: Management of drug therapy in the elderly, *N Engl J Med* 321[5]:303-309, 1989.)

amount of time between the administration of the drug and its absorption depends on a number of factors, including the route of introduction (i.e., intravenous, oral, parenteral, transdermal, or rectal), bioavailability, and the amount of drug that passes through the absorbing surfaces in the body (Lee, 1996). The drug is delivered immediately to the bloodstream with intravenous administration and quickly in the parenteral, transdermal, and rectal routes. Orally administered drugs are absorbed the most slowly and primarily in the small intestine.

There does not seem to be conclusive evidence that there is an appreciable change in the absorption process in older adults. However, we do know that diminished gastric pH, common in the elderly, will retard the action of acid-dependent drugs. The potential changes in gastrointestinal motility may also be important factors that potentially influence absorption. Delayed stomach emptying may diminish or negate the effectiveness of short-lived drugs that could become inactivated before reaching the small intestine. Some enteric-coated medications, which are specifically meant to bypass stomach acidity, may be delayed so long that their action begins in the stomach and may produce undesirable effects, such as gastric irritation or nausea. If there is an increase in the motility of the small intestine, drug effect is diminished because of shortened contact time and therefore decreased absorption. Conversely, slowed intestinal motility can increase the contact time and increase drug effect because of prolonged absorption. This increases the risk for adverse reactions or unpredictable effects.

Medications commonly taken by older adults can also affect the absorption of other drugs. Antispasmodic drugs slow gastric and intestinal motility. In some instances this drug action may be useful, but when there are other medications involved, it is necessary to consider the problem of drug absorption. Antacids or iron preparations affect the availability of some drugs for absorption by binding the drug with elements and forming chemical compounds.

Distribution

Once a drug is absorbed it must be distributed or transported to the receptor site on the target organ. Late life alterations in drug distribution are primarily related to changes in body composition, particularly decreases in lean body mass, increases in body fat, and decreases in total body water. Decreased body water leads to higher serum levels of water-soluble drugs, such as digoxin, ethanol, and aminoglycosides. Adipose tissue, or the fat content of the body, nearly doubles in older men and increases by one half in older women. Drugs that are highly lipid soluble are stored in the fatty tissue, thus extending and possibly elevating the drug effect (Masoro, Austed, 2003; Vestal, 1990; Lee, 1996). This potentially occurs in drugs such as lorazepam, diazepam, chlorpromazine, phenobarbital, and haloperidol (Haldol).

Distribution also depends on the availability of plasma protein in the form of lipoproteins, globulins, and especially albumin. As drugs are absorbed they bind with the protein and are distributed throughout the body. Normally, a predictable percentage of the absorbed drug is inactivated as it is bound to the protein. The remaining free drug is available in the bloodstream for therapeutic effect when an effective concentration is reached in the plasma. In most older adults there is a reduction in the serum albumin, but it is insignificant. However, for others, especially those with prolonged illness or malnutrition, the serum albumin may become dramatically diminished. When this occurs there are unpredictable concentrations of free drug available that may result in toxic levels, especially for highly protein-bound medications with narrow therapeutic windows, such as phenytoin and salicylates.

Metabolism

Metabolism is the process wherein the chemical structure of the drug is converted to a metabolite that is more easily excreted. This process is called *biotransformation*. A drug will continue to exert a therapeutic effect as long as it remains in either the original state or as an active metabolite or metabolites. Active metabolites retain the ability to have a therapeutic effect and have the same or more chance of adverse effects. For example, the metabolites of acetaminophen (Tylenol) can cause liver damage with higher dosages. The duration of drug action is determined by the metabolic rate and measured in terms of half-life, the length of time the drug is active in the body.

The liver is the primary site of drug metabolism. Metabolism occurs in two phases, phase I (oxidative) and phase II (conjugative). With aging, the liver activity, mass, volume, and blood flow are diminished (see Chapter 7). These changes result in the potential for a decrease in the body's ability to metabolize drugs, especially those that are metabolized in phase I, such as benzodiazepines. These changes result in a significant increase in the half-life of these drugs. For example, the half-life of diazepam (Valium) in a younger adult is about 37 hours, but in an older adult this is extended up to 82 hours (Ray et al, 1989). If the dose and timing are not adjusted for the older adult, the accumulation can have significant effects after the administration of a single dose.

Excretion

Drugs and their metabolites are excreted in sweat, saliva, and other secretions but primarily through the kidneys. Since kidney function declines in most older persons, so does the ability to excrete or eliminate drugs in a timely manner. The significantly decreased glomerular filtration rate leads to prolongation of the half-life of drugs eliminated through the renal system, resulting in more opportunities for accumulation and potential toxicity or other adverse events. Although renal function cannot be estimated by the creatinine level, it can be approximated by the calculation of the creatinine clearance (see Chapter 7 for calculation). Reductions in dosages for renally excreted drugs (e.g., allopurinol, vancomycin) are needed when the creatinine clearance is reduced.

PHARMACODYNAMICS

Pharmacodynamics refers to the interaction between a drug and the body (see Figure 15-1). The older the person gets, the more likely there will be an alteration or unreliable response of the body to the drug. Although it is not always possible to explain the alteration, several are known. Older adults tend to have a decreased response to beta-adrenergic receptor stimulators and blockers (Vestal, 2000); decreased baroreceptor sensitivity; and increased sensitivity to a number of medications, especially anticholinergics, benzodiazepines, narcotic analgesics, warfarin (Coumadin), diltiazem, and verapamil (Briggs, 2005).

When anticholinergics are used, beyond the usual dry mouth, confusion may be seen as a side effect (Moore, O'Keefe, 1999). The use of benzodiazepines is associated with an increased risk for accidental injury (Briggs, 2005).

CHRONOPHARMACOLOGY

Another factor that affects both pharmacokinetics and pharmacodynamics is the normal biorhythms of the body. The relationship of biological rhythms to variations in the body's response to drugs is known as chronopharmacology. Chronopharmacology is a developing science that may lead to more effective drug therapy. The best time to administer medications based on biorhythms of various physiological processes is now being considered for therapeutic and toxic effects.

Absorption depends on gastric acid pH, emptying of the gastrointestinal tract, and blood flow. All have been shown to have biorhythmical variations. Distribution of protein-bound drugs depends on albumin and glycoproteins produced by the liver. During the day, albumin levels are high, but they are low in the early-morning hours. Drug metabolism also is influenced by biorhythmical activity. Oxidation, hydrolysis, decarboxylation, and demethylation by liver enzymes demonstrate rhythm variations. Renal elimination depends on kidney perfusion, glomerular filtration, and urine acidity. These also have shown variations in circadian rhythm. The brain, heart, and blood cells have also been found to have varied rhythmicity, resulting in a cyclical response for beta blockers, calcium channel blockers, angiotensin-converting enzyme (ACE) inhibitors, nitrates, and other similar drugs. Table 15-1 shows some of the rhythmical influence on diseases and physiological processes.

The potential for decreasing the dose of medications and/or the frequency of administration for elders is the primary benefit of chronopharmacological therapy. Both decreases may ultimately improve the therapeutic effect and decrease toxic effects for elders, as well as the general population, and they may improve patient adherence to a medication regimen. In addition, chronotherapeutics may provide financial benefit to the patient by reducing the overall medication expense because fewer administrations are needed to achieve a therapeutic effect.

MEDICATION ISSUES AND OLDER ADULTS

Polypharmacy

Polypharmacy simply means the use of multiple medications at the same time. Polypharmacy may be necessary if one has multiple chronic condi-

Table 15-1   Rhythmical Influences on Disease and Physiological Processes

Disease/process	Rhythmical Influence
Allergic rhinitis	Symptoms worse in the morning
Arterial blood pressure	Circadian surge—morning hours
Asthma	Greatest respiratory distress overnight (during sleeping) Symptoms peak in early morning (4:00-5:00)
Blood plasma	Plasma volume falls at night = hematocrit increases
Cancer	Tumor cells proliferate when normal cell miosis is low
Cardiac disease	Angina, myocardial infarction, thrombolytic stroke occur in the first 4 hr after waking (peak 9:00) (through 22:00) (Prinzmetal's angina—during sleep)
Catecholamines	Increase in early morning
Fibrinolytic activity	Increase in early morning
Platelet activation	Increase in early morning
Endogenous depression	May result from abnormality in circadian rhythm, which affects cortisol levels, body temperature, sleep/wake cycle
Gastric system	Gastric acid secretion peaks every morning (2:00-4:00); circannual variability—incidence of gastric ulcers greater in winter
Osteoarthritis	Pain more severe in morning
Potassium excretion	Lowest in morning/highest in late afternoon
Rheumatoid arthritis	Pain more severe in late afternoon
Systemic insulin	Highest in afternoon

From Turkoski BB: Medication timing for the elderly: the impact of biorhythms on effectiveness, *Geriatr Nurs* 19(3):146-151, 1998.

tions, or it may occur "accidentally" if an existing drug regimen is not considered when new prescriptions are given or any number of the thousands of OTC preparations and supplements are added to the prescribed medications. The two major concerns with polypharmacy are the increased risk for drug interactions and the increased risk for adverse events (Gallagher, 2001). The potential for an interaction or adverse drug event is only 6% when two drugs are taken, but the risk increases to 50% with five drugs and reaches 100% with eight or more (Shaughnessy, 1992).

Drug Interactions

The more medications a person takes, the greater the possibility that one or more of them will interact with another one, a nutritional supplement, food, or alcohol. When two or more medications or foods are given at the same time or closely together the drugs may potentiate one another or make one or both stronger; or antagonism may occur, with a drug or a food causes the other one or both to become ineffective. Interactions cause drug-related illness that may account for 15% to 23% of all hospital admissions, 1% to 5% of office visits, and 1 out of 1000 deaths (Torrible, Hogan, 1997).

An interaction may result in altered pharmacokinetic activity or alterations in the absorption, distribution, metabolism, or excretion (Hartshorn, Tatro, 2003). Within the body, absorption can be delayed by drugs exerting an anticholinergic effect. Tricyclic drugs (antidepressants) act in this manner to decrease gastrointestinal motility and interfere with the absorption of other drugs. Several drugs may compete to simultaneously bind and occupy the binding sites needed by the other drug, creating a varied bioavailability of one or both of the drugs. Interaction may be blocked at the receptor site, preventing the drug from reaching the cells. Interference with enzyme activity may alter metabolism and cause drug deficiencies, or toxic and adverse responses may develop from altered renal tubular function. Outside the body, interactions can occur any time that two medications or foods are mixed before administration. An example of this is the improper preparation of more than one type of insulin for injection.

In pharmacodynamic interactions one drug alters the patient's response to another drug without changing the pharmacokinetic properties. This can be especially dangerous for older adults when two or more drugs with the same effect are additive, that is, together they are more potent than they are separately.

Although there is much unknown about the use of herbs and neutraceuticals, some knowledge is building that is important to the gerontological nurse. Persons taking Coumadin (Warfarin) should not take ginkgo biloba, a nutritional supplement touted for maintaining optimal cognitive function in the elderly. It has been found that ginkgo interacts with the warfarin to increase bleeding time as measured by the INR (international normalized ratio) or cause bleeding when it is added to a stable warfarin regimen (Scott, Elmer, 2002; Valli, Giardina, 2002). Glucosamine, a neutraceutical taken for maintaining optimal joint function, can cause decreased glucose tolerance by causing increased insulin resistance and therefore interfere with the treatment of diabetes (Scott, Elmer, 2002).

Adverse Drug Reactions

An adverse drug reaction (ADR) is an unwanted pharmacological effect, ranging from a minor annoyance to death, and includes allergic reactions. ADRs can sometimes be predicted from the pharmacological action of the drug (e.g., bone marrow depression from cancer chemotherapy; bleeding from Counadin). Predictable ADRs can also occur when a patient is started on a drug at a dose that is inappropriately high or one that requires laboratory monitoring that is not done. Other ADRs are unpredictable and have nothing to do with the action of the drug (e.g., hives from penicillin).

An estimated 40% of the elderly in the community have experienced ADRs, 80% of which occurred with well-known drugs given at usual dosages (Lamy, 1990). Among the most common drugs that produce adverse reactions are antipsychotics, warfarin, digoxin, prednisone, diuretics, antihypertensives, insulin, aspirin, and antide-

pressants (Lepkowski, 1992; Willcox et al, 1994). All of these are frequently prescribed to older adults. Because of the large number of medications taken by most older adults and the altered nutritional and fluid status of persons residing in long-term care settings, the risk for adverse reactions is of special concern to nurses. In one study two-thirds of nursing home residents had an adverse drug reaction over a 4-year period, with one out of seven residents requiring hospitalization (Cooper 1999).

ADRs that are extensions of the drug's pharmacology may not always be predictable. An elderly patient who is well controlled on a stable dose of a drug may undergo a change in his or her environment such that the relationship with the drug is altered. Changes in diet can have a profound impact on drug regimens (e.g., decreased salt intake causing lithium toxicity; increased leafy green vegetables countering anticoagulant effects of warfarin) (Lacy et al, 2003). Some drugs interfere with the body's ability to regulate temperature such that hot weather can lead to heat stroke (e.g., antipsychotics, stimulants) (Semla et al, 2003). Some drugs are photosensitizing, and an increase in sun exposure can lead to sunburn much more quickly than expected (e.g., sulfa drugs, antidepressants and many antipsycotics) (Semla et al, 2003). Elderly patients who have decreased fluid intake because of illness or because they cannot get to fluids or who have inadequate intake during hot weather may become volume depleted and develop increased sensitivity to the orthostatic hypotensive effects of alpha blockers (e.g., phenothiazines, terazosin) (Lacy et al, 2003).

One of the most troublesome ADRs for the older adult is drug-induced delirium or confusion. Polypharmacy with several psychoactive drugs exerting anticholinergic action is perhaps the greatest precipitator of the adverse reaction of delirium. Too often it goes unrecognized for what it is and instead is viewed as a worsening of pre-existing dementia or even new-onset dementia. Anytime there is a change in one's cognitive abilities the possibility of drug effect must be thoroughly evaluated. See Box 15-1 for a partial list of drugs with the potential to adversely affect cognitive functioning.

Another common adverse effect seen in older adults is lethargy, especially with the use of a number of the antihypertensives or antidepres-

Box 15-1   Drugs with the Potential to Cause Intellectual Impairment

Alcohol
Analgesics
Anticholinergics
Antidepressants
Antipsychotics
Antihistamines
Antiparkinsonian agents
Beta blockers
Cimetidine
Digitalis
Diuretics
Hypnotics
Muscle relaxants
Sedatives
Sudden withdrawal of benzodiazepines

Data from Lamy PP: Drug interactions and the elderly, *J Gerontol Nurs*, 12(2):36-37, 1986; Nolan L, O'Malley K: Prescribing for the elderly. I. Sensitivity of the elderly to adverse drug reactions, *Am Geriatr Soc* 36(2):142-149, 1988; Lamy PP: Adverse drug effects, *Clin Geriatr Med* 6(2):293-307, 1990.

sants. Like confusion, lethargy can also be misinterpreted as a symptom connected with cardiac, respiratory, or neurological conditions rather than an adverse medication effect.

Among other troublesome adverse effects are those related to vision, especially phototoxicity (Box 15-2), and sexual functioning. Although they are not detailed here, more than 200 medications interfere with or contribute to sexual dysfunction for adults of any age (Butler et al, 1994; Miller, 1995). The categories that are most responsible for sexual dysfunction are cardiovascular drugs (some antihypertensives and ACE inhibitors) and psychotropic drugs (antidepressants, phenothiazines).

Drug toxicity is the most life threatening of the adverse effects. Toxicity or poisoning in the elderly may account for up to 25% of calls to poison control centers (Kroner et al, 1993) and 20-30% of hospitalizations (Cooper, 1999; Zumpano, 2003). The most frequent lethal poisonings from drug toxicity are from analgesics, cardiovascular medications, theophyllines, and tricyclic antidepressants (Haselberger, Kroner, 1995).

Toxicity can occur when the plasma concentration of a drug exceeds that level needed for

Box 15-2   Drugs with Potential for Causing Photosensitivity*

Drug Classes
Anticancer agents
Antidepressants
Antihistamines
Antihyperlipidemics
Antimicrobials
Antiparasitics
Antipsychotics
Antiseizure agents
Diuretics
Hypoglycemics
NSAIDs

Individual Drugs
Amiodarone
Atorvastatin
Benzocaine
Captopril

Chlordiazepoxide
Diltiazem
Disopyramide
Enalapril
Estazolam
Estrogen
Fluvastatin
Gold sodium thiomalate
Hexachlorophene
Lovastatin
PABA
Pravastatin
Quinidine
Saquinavir
Selegiline
Simvastatin
Zolpidem

From Semla TP, Beizer JL, Higbee MD: *Geriatric dosage handbook*, ed 8, Cleveland, 2003, Lexi-Comp, Inc.
*These classes of drugs contain specific medications that can increase sensitivity to ultraviolet light. (For specific drugs under these classes, consult *Geriatric Dosage Handbook*.)
NSAIDs, Nonsteroidal antiinflammatory drugs.

therapeutic effect, especially in those with a narrow therapeutic window, such as phenytoin (Dilantin) or theophylline. This can occur because of alterations in absorption, distribution, or excretion. It is especially common in circumstances such as polypharmacy, slowed metabolism, altered excretion, dehydration, drug overdose because of self-medication errors, or excessive prescribed dosage. Table 15-2 presents several drugs commonly prescribed for the elderly that may result in toxicity.

Misuse of Drugs

The more drugs taken, the more likely misuse will occur. Forms of drug misuse include overuse, underuse, erratic use, and contraindicated use. Misuse can occur for any number of reasons from inadequate skills of the nurse or the prescriber, to misunderstanding of instructions, to inadequate funds to purchase prescribed medications. For the large number of near-poor elders the latter will remain a problem until Medicare includes comprehensive prescription coverage.

As early as 1994 Willcox and others (Willcox et al, 1994) identified 20 drugs that were inappropriately prescribed for elders, including controversial cardiovascular agents (propranolol, methyldopa, reserpine). Since that time Beers (1997) has worked further to identify drugs that have higher than usual risk when used in older adults. These have been now transferred to a "do not use" list for residents in nursing facilities. When one is prescribed without documentation of the overwhelming benefit of its use, it can be considered a form of drug misuse by the prescribing practitioner. See Appendix 15-A for a list of some of the medications that should not be prescribed for or used by the older adult because of their potential for adverse reactions.

Misuse by patients may be accidental, such as with misunderstanding, or deliberate, such as in trying to make a prescription last longer for financial reasons or because of beliefs about drug dosing (Hughes, 2004). Even most health care professionals would admit to having some leftover medications, especially antibiotics, in their medicine cabinet, which is evidence of drug misuse. When the misuse is on the part of the patient, the derogatory terms of noncompliance or nonadherence are used.

When a patient is labeled as noncompliant, the nurse and other health care personnel may become exasperated and angry at the individual for his or her failure to follow the established plan of care. In an attempt to help and do what they think is best for the patient, the nurse and other care providers tend to forget or ignore that one cannot and will not comply with a prescription or treatment plan when there are incompatibilities that interfere with the practicalities of life or are distressful to the individual's well-being or when actual misinformation or disability prevents compliance. For example, the individual cannot follow the instruction to take medication three times per day with meals if he or she eats only two meals each day.

Memory failures associated with nonadherence to medication regimens are of two general types: forgetting the way to correctly take medications and "prospective" recall failure (failure to remember to take medication at the correct times) (Leirer et al, 1991). The more frequently a medication needs to be taken, the less anyone will comply. With more and more medications coming in once daily dosing rather than three or four times each day, we can expect people to more often adhere to the instructions.

Problems with health literacy also limit the older person's ability to correctly follow instructions. Limitations in vision will interfere with reading of instructions, especially of bottle labels. The practice of giving rapid-fire directions is not effective in addressing the person with hearing impairments or the normal age-related need for slightly slower verbalizations; and the use of ambiguous terms such as "slowly increase" or "only in moderation" leads to further difficulties.

It is also common to explain the treatment and give directions concerning medications when the patient is physically uncomfortable or as the person is about to be discharged, to explain in English even when the person has limited English proficiency, or to explain in a noisy or busy place. It is no wonder that a problem of adherence occurs under such circumstances.

Conceptual Framework for Understanding Medication Adherence

Kutzik and Spiers (1993; Spiers, Kutzik, 1995) developed a multidimensional framework for

Table 15-2 Toxic Characteristics of Specific Drugs Prescribed for the Elderly

Drugs	Signs and Symptoms

Benzodiazepines
  Diazepam (Valium)
  Lorazepam (Ativan)
	Ataxia, restlessness, confusion, depression, anticholinergic effect

Cimetidine (Tagamet)	Confusion, depression
Digitalis (Lanoxin)	Confusion, headache, anorexia, vomiting, arrhythmias, blurred vision or visual changes (halos, frost on objects, color blindness), paresthesia
Furosemide (Lasix)	Electrolyte imbalance, hepatic changes, pancreatitis, leukopenia, thrombocytopenia
Gentamycin (Garamycin)	Ototoxicity (impaired hearing and/or balance), nephrotoxicity
Levodopa (L-dopa)	Muscle and eye twitching, disorientation, asterixis, hallucinations, dyskinetic movements, grimacing, depression, delirium, ataxia
Lithium (Eskalith, Lithane)	Confusion, diarrhea, drowsiness, anorexia, slurred speech, tremors, blurred vision, unsteadiness, polyuria, seizures, muscle weakness

Nonsteroidal antiinflammatory drugs (NSAIDs)
  Ibuprofen (Advil, Motrin, Nuprin, Rufen)
  Indomethacin (Indocin)
  Fenoprofen (Nalfon)
  Phenylbutazone (Butazolidin)
  Piroxicam (Feldene)
  Sulindac (Clinoril)
  Tolmetin (Tolectin)
	Photosensitivity, fluid retention, anemia, nephrotoxicity, visual changes
	
	Confusion plus all of the above

Phenothiazide tranquilizers	Tachycardia, dysrhythmias, dyspnea, hyperthermia, postural hypotension, restlessness, anticholinergic effects
Phenytoin (Dilantin)	Ataxia, slurred speech, confusion, nystagmus, diplopia, nausea, vomiting
Procainamide (Pronestyl, Procan, Promine)	Dysrhythmias, depression, hypotension, SLE syndrome, dyspnea, skin rash, nausea, vomiting
Ranitidine (Zantac)	Liver dysfunction, blood dyscrasias

Sulfonylureas—first generation
  Chlorpropamide (Diabinese)
  Tolbutamide (Orinase)
	Hypoglycemia, hepatic changes, HF, bone marrow depression, jaundice

Theophylline (Theo-Dur, Elixophyllin, Slo-Bid)	Anorexia, nausea, vomiting, gastrointestinal bleeding, tachycardia, dysrhythmias, irritability, insomnia, seizures, muscle twitching

Tricyclic antidepressants
  Amitriptyline (Elavil, Endep)
  Doxepin (Sinequan, Adapin)
  Imipramine (Tofranil)
	Confusion, dysrhythmias, seizures, agitation, tachycardia, jaundice, hallucinations, postural hypotension, anticholinergic effects

Data from Semla TP, Beizer JL, Higbee MD: *Geriatric dosage handbook*, ed 8, Cleveland, 2003, Lexi-Comp, Inc.
SLE, Systemic lupus erythematosus; *HF,* heart failure.

Table 15-3 A Multidimensional Framework for Medication Adherence

	Individual	Provider-Treatment	Social Support Network
STAGE 1: INITIAL INSTRUCTIONS	Comprehension Commitment to treatment	Communication effectiveness Number of providers	Community medical education Cultural beliefs
STAGE 2: REGIMEN ESTABLISHMENT			
Attaining medications	Mobility Finances Beliefs (e.g., medication sharing) Motivation	Medication cost Number of medications needed	Accessibility to pharmacies Financial aid
Application	Ability to reconstruct instructions Regimen strategy	Complexity of regimen Container design Label readability	Administration aid
Adjustment	Perception of effectiveness Self-manipulation of dosage/regimen	Rx manipulation Rx monitoring	Level of emotional/functional support
STAGE 3: SELF-MANAGEMENT			
Integration/reintegration	Emotional adjustment to long-term medication dependence Regimen routinization and synthesis Response to challenges/change	Lifestyle change required by regular medication taking Regimen changes	Response to individual change Stability of support network/living situation
Monitoring	Ability to self-monitor for change	Degree of comprehensive Rx review	Support network vigilance

From Spiers MV, Kutzik DM: *A multidimensional framework for understanding medication adherence in the elderly: prescription for rethinking,* Unpublished paper, 1995.

medication use that looks at the barriers to adherence for elders. The framework suggests that there is a simultaneous branching out among the three stages—initial instruction, regimen establishment, and self-management—and the three levels—individual, provider-treatment, and social support network. The integration of the stages and levels provides a reasonable approach to understanding the dynamics of elder adherence (Table 15-3).

The individual must first comprehend and be committed to the treatment. The care provider must be able to communicate the information in a way that compensates for physical-sensory and cognitive changes so that the individual understands and is willing to follow the treatment plan.

The elder must be able to use what has been learned so as to operationalize this information (obtain the medication, apply instructions, adjust to the regimen). The influence of the health professional is relatively strong to this point. Social context has a less direct influence on the drug regimen. However, it is affected by medical knowledge in the elder's cultural/belief system.

Finally, strong social network factors are more important because of the shrinking network that elders have available to them. Success at this level depends on the number of persons in the elder's support network who are able to assist the elder, if necessary, with the integration or reintegration of the regimen and the monitoring of adherence.

IMPLICATIONS FOR GERONTOLOGICAL NURSING AND HEALTHY AGING

The gerontological nurse is a key person in ensuring that the medication use is appropriate, effective, and as safe as possible. The knowledgeable nurse is alert for potential drug interactions and for signs or symptoms of adverse drug effects. The nurse promotes the actions necessary to prevent drugs from becoming toxic and to treat toxicity promptly should it occur. Nurses in the long-term care setting are responsible for monitoring the overall health of the residents, including being alert for the need for laboratory tests and other measures to ensure correct dosage and prompt attention to changes in physiological function that are either the result of the medication regimen or affected by the regimen, such as potassium level. The nurse is often the person to initiate assessment of medication use, evaluate outcomes, and provide the teaching needed for safe drug use and self-administration. In most settings the nurse is also in a position to influence the timing of prescribed doses so residents might more easily benefit from the findings from the field of chronopharmacology (Turkoski, 1998). In all settings, a vital nursing function is to educate patients and to ensure that they understand the purpose and side effects of the medications and to assist the patient and family in adapting the medication regimen to functional ability and lifestyle.

Assessment

The initial step in ensuring that elders use drugs safely and effectively is conducting a comprehensive drug assessment. Although in some settings a clinical pharmacist interviews patients about their medication history, more often it is completed through the combined efforts of the licensed nurse and the health care provider (a physician or a nurse practitioner).

In the ideal situation, it is best to use a "brown bag approach," or to have elders bring to you all medications they are currently taking in a bag, with all OTCs, herbals, and neutraceuticals or dietary supplements included. As each medicine container is removed from the bag the necessary information can be obtained. It is essential to ask the person how he or she actually takes the medicine rather than depending on how the prescription is written to begin to determine possible misunderstandings or misuse. An alternative method is a 24-hour medication history, such as "tell me everything you have taken in the last 24 hours." Two final approaches are associated with the review of systems or problems. These questions will be something like, "What do you take for your heart? circulation? breathing?" Or, if you know the person's major health problems, you may say, for example, "What do you take for headaches?" or "What do you use for indigestion?" Without the bag of medications or a list of some kind patients often answer some of the above questions with descriptions (e.g., "a little blue pill" or "a bad-tasting one"), but it is a start.

As the nurse learns the herbs, supplements, and OTC and prescribed medications that are taken the assessment can continue. There is a great deal of information that is needed, but it is vital to promoting the health of the person and healthy aging. See Box 15-3 for details of the information needed in a comprehensive medication history for all substances taken. Through this assessment the nurse can learn of discrepancies between the prescribed dosage and the actual dosage, potential interactions, and potential or actual ADRs.

Monitoring and Evaluation

A significant part of the responsibilities of the gerontological nurse is to monitor and evaluate the effectiveness of prescribed treatments and observe for signs of problems—either from a change in the condition of the elder or from what are known as iatrogenic complications (problems that are the result of something we have done to the person, including side effects, ADRs, and interactions). Monitoring and evaluating involve making astute observations and documenting those observations, noting changes in physical and functional status (e.g., vital signs, performance of activities of daily living, sleeping, eating, hydrating, eliminating) and mental status (e.g., attention and level of alertness, memory, orientation, behavior, mood, emotional display and

Box 15-3	Components of a Comprehensive Medication Assessment

Medication names, doses and frequency, taken and prescribed

Diagnosis associated with each medication

Belief regarding medications

OTC preparations, with doses, frequency, and reason taken

Herbals, with doses, frequency, and reason taken

Neutraceutical supplements, with doses, frequency, and reason taken

Medication-related problems, such as side effects

Ability to pay for prescription medications

Ability to obtain medications

Persons involved in decision making regarding medications

Use of other drugs, such as tobacco or nicotine in gum, patch, or smoking form

Use of social drugs, such as alcohol and caffeine, and nonprescription drugs

Drugs obtained from others' prescriptions

Recently discontinued drugs

History of allergies, interactions, and adverse drug effects

Strategies used to remember when to take drugs

Identification of malnutrition and hydration status

Recent drug blood levels as appropriate

Recent measurement of liver and kidney functioning

OTC, Over the counter.

affect, content and characteristics of interactions). Monitoring also means ensuring that blood levels are measured as they are needed; such as regular thyroid-stimulating hormone (TSH) levels for all persons taking thyroid replacement, INRs for all persons taking warfarin, or periodic hemoglobin A_{1c} levels for all persons with diabetes. Care of a patient also means that the nurses promptly communicate their findings of potential problems to the patient's nurse practitioner or physician. Accurate monitoring requires that the nurse has information about the treatments and medications that are administered. See Tables 15-4 and 15-5 for monitoring parameters of general and psychiatric drugs more commonly used with older adults or those that are more dangerous to use in this group.

Patient Education

Usually the nurse is responsible for providing patient education for safe drug usage. In a collaborative process, the nurse works with the elder to provide medication information. Ideally, the nurse empowers the person to participate fully in goal setting and treatment planning (Box 15-4). Education relating to the safe use of drugs can be accomplished on an individual basis or in small groups. The elderly should be encouraged to exercise their right to question and know what they are taking, how it will affect them, and the alter-

natives available to them (Higbee, 1994; Delong, 1995). Pamphlets and booklets written in lay terms and in appropriate language and reading level should be available. If there are none that are appropriate, the nurse can be creative and develop a booklet or information sheet that will meet the drug information needs of the patient. Information is best presented in numbered line fashion rather than in paragraph form. Written information should be in large, boldface type. Audiovisual aids are available for health teaching, but if they are too expensive, the nurse should consider devising some.

Because of the complex needs of the older patient, education can be particularly challenging. The following tips may be helpful when the goal of the nurse is to promote healthy aging:

1. Key persons: Find out who, if anyone, manages the person's medications, helps the person, or assists with decision making; and with the elder's permission, make sure that the helper is present when any teaching is done.

2. Environment: Minimize distraction, and avoid competing with television or others demanding the patient's time; make sure the person is comfortable and is not hungry, thirsty, tired, too warm or too cold, in pain, or need of the toilet.

3. Timing: Provide the teaching during the best time of the day for the person, when he or she

Table 15-4 Determining Whether the Drug Is Working: Monitoring Parameters and Common Side Effects of General Drug Categories

Class of Drug	Monitoring Activity	Common Side Effects
Antibiotics and antivirals	Improvement of infection: symptom reduction Take complete prescription	Change in normal flora: yeast infections in mouth or vagina, diarrhea
Antihyperlipidemics	Lipid profile (specific drug is matched to lipid profile) Modify changeable risks: lifestyle changes (exercise, smoking cessation); dietary alterations (decreased fat intake, eliminate trans-fat products); gradual improvement in LDL and HDL levels, see change within 2-4 wk	Statins: muscle weakness, aches Niacin: muscle weakness, aches; flushing (hot flashes); diabetes symptoms
Cardiac medications	Monitor liver function and blood glucose Maintenance of baseline (normal) heart rate and rhythm	Mental status change, visual changes Bradycardia Fever, chills
Anticoagulants	Clotting times (INR, Protime)	Bleeding, bruising, blood in stool
Anticonvulsants	Blood levels Decrease seizure activity	Sedation Mental status changes
Antihypertensives	Maintenance of normal blood pressure Central nervous system effects Intake and output Weight	Diuretics: postural hypotension, bradycardia, hypokalemia Beta blockers: bradycardia, hypotension, chest pain, constipation, diarrhea, nausea, mental status changes (insomnia, confusion, depression, lethargy)
Hypoglycemics	Blood glucose	Hypoglycemia, allergic reactions to beef or pork insulin
Antineoplastics	Cancer activity Bone marrow suppression, laboratory values (e.g., WBC count)	Nausea, vomiting, diarrhea, signs of infection, hair loss, fatigue
Antihistaminics	Relief from allergy symptoms, such as rhinitis	Drowsiness, blurred vision, confusion
Antiarthritics	Relief from arthritis symptoms, such as pain and inflammation	Gastrointestinal problems, depression, personality disturbance, irritability, toxic psychoses
Antiparkinsonians	Improved functional status Less visible immobility; improved mobility	Nausea, hypotension, dyskinesia, agitation, restlessness, insomnia
Cholinergic agents (antidementia medications)	Improved mental status in mildly and moderately demented patients	Nausea, diarrhea, anorexia, weight loss, bradycardia, hypotension, headache, fatigue, depression
Analgesics	Improved symptoms of pain and inflammation	NSAIDs: gastrointestinal distress Opiates: constipation, sedation, confusion, decreased respiration

From Semla TP, Beizer JL, Higbee MD: *Geriatric dosage handbook*, ed 8, Cleveland, 2003, Lexi-Comp, Inc.
LDL, Low-density lipoprotein; *HDL*, high-density lipoprotein; *INR*, international normalized ratio; *WBC*, white blood cell; *NSAIDs*, nonsteroidal antiinflammatory drugs.

Table 15-5 Determining Whether the Drug Is Working: Monitoring Parameters and Common Side Effects of Psychiatric Drug Categories

Class of Drug	Monitoring Activity	Common Side Effects
Anxiolytics	Decreased anxiety Immediate effect May be habit forming	Sedation, confusion, gait disturbances, disinhibition
Mood stabilizers	Blood levels: gradual behavior change based on blood level Lithium: avoid salt restriction; maintain adequate hydration Ensure adequate renal function Decreased hyperactivity, explosive outbursts, mania	Sedation, confusion, tremors
Antidepressants	Dose titration depends on side effects; start with low dose and increase dosage slowly Gradual effect	Tricyclics: dry mouth, blurred vision, constipation, sedation, confusion, urinary retention, orthostatic hypotension SSRIs: restlessness, insomnia, irritability, sexual dysfunction
Antipsychotics	Decreased agitation Immediate response Use lowest possible dose, and eliminate medication as soon as possible	Sedation, confusion, dyskinesia, akathisia, extrapyramidal effects, parkinsonian reactions, somnolence
Hypnotics	Nighttime sleep improvement Habit forming Taper (rebound on withdrawal from these, causing decrease in REM sleep)	Daytime drowsiness, hangover, worsening dementia, confusion, hypotension, delirium, depressed respirations

From Semla TP, Beizer JL, Higbee MD: *Geriatric dosage handbook,* ed 8, Cleveland, 2003, Lexi-Comp, Inc.
SSRIs, Selective serotonin reuptake inhibitors; *REM,* rapid eye movement.

is most engaged and energetic. Keep the education sessions short and succinct.

4. Communication: Ensure that you will be understood. Make sure the elders have their glasses or hearing aids on if they are used. Use simple and direct language, and avoid medical or nursing jargon (e.g., "intake"). Remain respectful at all times, and do not allow negative stereotypes to cloud the communication. Encourage questions. If the person is blind, Braille instructions are available from the pharmacy.

5. Reinforce teaching: Provide memory aids to reinforce teaching. Have actual medications or containers handy to visually illustrate directions. For persons who can read, use written charts and lists with large letters and simple language. For persons who cannot read, charts with pictures of the medications and symbols for times of the day or color coding can be used. If food is required with the medication or must be avoided, this should be indicated on the charts. Weekly calendars with pockets for medications indicating day, time, and date can be used; or a daily tear-off calendar to remind the elder to take daily medication can be used. Clear envelopes or sandwich bags containing the medication can be affixed to the dated square on a daily basis; each envelope or bag should state the name of the drug, dose, and times to be taken that day. Commercial drug boxes are available for single or multiple doses by the day, week, or month, and some have alarms. After discharge from a hospital or

Box 15-4	Empowering the Patient for Safe Medication Practices: What Elders Should Know About Taking Their Medications

- What is the name of each drug?
- What is the purpose of each drug?
- What is the dose per administration?
- What is the number of doses every day?
- What is the best time to take the medication?
- How should the medication be taken?
- Can the medication be taken with other drugs?
- Which medications can and cannot be taken together?
- Are any special techniques, devices, or procedures necessary to administer the medication?
- For how long should the medication be taken?
- What are the common side effects?
- If side effects occur: What should the elder do? What changes in administration are necessary? When should the drug be stopped? When should the physician or pharmacist (or both) be called?
- What can be done at home to monitor for a therapeutic drug response?
- What should be done if a dose is missed?
- How many refills are allowed?
- How should the medication be stored?
- What are the nonprescription (OTC) preparations that should not be used with the present drug therapy?

- Take all medications prescribed unless the physician states otherwise.
- Stop taking the medication and report any new or unusual problems, such as shortness of breath, nausea, diarrhea, vomiting, sleepiness, dizziness, weakness, skin rash, or fever.
- Never take medication prescribed for another person.
- Do not take any medication more than 1 year old or past the expiration date on the container.
- Store medications in a safe place, preferably the kitchen, rather than the bathroom, where moisture from bathing, especially showers, may affect the medicine.
- Do not keep medicines, especially sedatives and hypnotics, on the bedside stand, because when you are sleepy, you may forget that you have already taken the medication earlier.
- Do not place different medicines in the same container.
- Take a sufficient supply of all medicines in their individual containers when traveling away from home.
- Use a chart to keep track of medications.

OTC, Over the counter.

nursing home, a follow-up phone call can help with assessing accurate medication usage or other problems with medications. A nurse's home visit to patients at high risk for problems, such as those with cognitive deficits or those with many medications for new conditions, could reinforce medication information and provide assessment information (Box 15-5).

6. Evaluate teaching: Have the patient repeat back instructions, including names of medications, purposes, side effects, times of administration, and method for remembering to take the medicines and to mark off their ingestion. For example, a strategy is to turn the medication bottle upside down once the dose has been taken for the day. A combination of interventions over an extended period of time has been shown to be the most effective approach (Haynes et al, 1987). Computer-assisted medication teaching has demonstrated effectiveness for improving medication knowledge, adherence, and clinical outcome when given to older patients with osteoarthritis (Edworthy, Devins, 1999).

7. Avoiding interactions: Patients should be taught to obtain all their medications from the same pharmacy if possible. This will allow the pharmacist to monitor for drug duplications and interactions. When elders have no prescription drug coverage, they may need to shop around for the best prices, and this does increase the risk for problems.

Medication Administration

Most elders self-administer their own medications; others receive them from family, friends, or health care professionals. In long-term care settings the

Suggestions to Improve Medication Adherence

Simplify the Medication Administration Process*
Memory aids
Calendars
Day, week, month pill containers
Voice-mail reminders
Convenient medication refills
Easy-to-open medication containers
Reduce number of doses daily when possible
Reduce number of medications when possible
Reduce frequency per day by grouping
  compatible medications together
Tailor medication regimen to lifestyle

*Use lay terms: *twice each day* instead of *bid*.

Disseminate Drug Information
Audiovisual information
Individual or group instruction (including family,
  caregiver, significant other)
Written instructions
Information sheets, leaflets in bold type
Reasonably large print
Periodic review of drug information

Teach Proper Medication Management Skills
Medication administration and training program
Self-care instruction

---

administration of medications to residents occupies nearly all of some nurses' time. Several skills are needed for safe administration.

Because of the high rate of arthritis and other debilitating conditions it may be difficult or impossible for the person to remove a cap or break a tablet. If no children have access to the medications, the patient can request alternative bottle caps that are easier to open. Either the person or nurse can also ask the pharmacist to prebreak the pills or dispense a smaller dose.

Most medications are taken orally. Many tablets and capsules are difficult to swallow because of their size or because they stick to the buccal mucosa. Administration of a drug in liquid form is sometimes preferable and allows flexibility; concentrations can be varied so that quantities of solution can be prepared and taken by the teaspoon, tablespoon, or ounce, simple and commonly used household measurements. Since household spoons vary greatly in actual volume, the nurse should ensure that the client is using an accurate measure. Crushing tablets or emptying the powder from capsules into fluid or food should not be done unless specified by the pharmaceutical company or approved by a pharmacist, because it may interfere with the effectiveness of the drug (either underdose or toxicity) or create problems in administration, as well as injure the mouth or gastrointestinal tract.

Enteric-coated, extended-release, or sustained-released products are all used to allow absorption at different places in the gastrointestinal tract. These should never be crushed, broken, opened, or otherwise altered before administration. See Appendix 15-B for a partial list of medications that cannot be crushed or chewed. When in doubt, the patient or the nurse should refer to a drug book, the package insert, or the pharmacist.

Some people have difficulty swallowing capsules. The person can be advised to place capsules on the front of the tongue and swallow a fluid; this should wash it to the back of the throat and down. Other persons do better with pills or capsules when taken with a semisolid food, such as applesauce, chocolate, or peanut butter—as long as the substances do not interact.

The transdermal patch, also called the transdermal delivery system (TDDS), is one of the newer approaches to medication administration, and more and more fat-soluble medications are being transformed to this method of administration. The TDDS provides for a more constant rate of drug administration and eliminates concern for gastrointestinal absorption variation, gastrointestinal tolerance, and drug interaction. TDDSs are not recommended for persons who are underweight because of unpredictable absorption from the reduced body fat. Box 15-6 provides guidelines for the use of TDDSs.

Box 15-6	Guidelines for Transdermal Delivery Systems

Proper Administration

1. Know the proper place for administration (some require specific anatomical placement).
2. Place on clean surface (if hairy, should be shaved).
3. Press firmly for 10 seconds for secure contact (no wrinkles or raised edges).
4. Wear gloves or wash hands after contact with patch.
5. DO NOT cut patch in half to decrease dose (this can cause evaporation or spill out of medication and decrease adherence to skin).

Site Rotation

1. Do not reapply to same area for at least 7 days.

Rash Management

1. Rash is most common side effect (occurs in about 50% of patients because of active ingredient or adhesive).
2. If ordered, apply topical corticosteroid to site as a pretreatment or after patch is removed.

Proper Disposal

1. Fold sticky edges together.
2. Dispose in a closed garbage can to keep away from pets or children.

Modified from Fischer RG, Clark N: Skin contact: a clinical review of transdermal drug delivery systems, *Adv Nurse Pract* 2(10):15, 1994.

PSYCHIATRIC CONCERNS AND PSYCHOTROPIC MEDICATIONS

The gerontological nurse, especially one working in a long-term care setting, is likely to care for older adults with psychiatric concerns, especially depression, anxiety, and psychosis. The rate of depression for elderly persons living in the community is estimated at about 20%, which increases to about 50% for those living in long-term care settings (Pollock, Reynolds, 2000). Anxiety is also common and when treated with benzodiazepines is always a cause for concern because of the propensity for adverse effects and drug interactions in the elderly. Unfortunately the use of psychotherapy is very limited, first because of the rarity of persons with a specialty training in gerontological psychiatry or counseling, and second because of the very low reimbursement rates established by Medicare.

Finally a small group of elders, especially those with neurological conditions or dementia, may develop psychosis at some time in their illnesses. Psychosis is also seen in delirium from an infection or from an adverse drug effect and in the few elders with schizophrenia (Arunpongpaisal et al, 2004). Persons with psychosis are often treated with antipsychotics that require special attention and skills from the gerontological nurse.

Psychotropic medications are drugs that alter brain chemistry, emotions, and behavior. They include antipsychotics or neuroleptics, antidepressants, mood stabilizers, antianxiety agents, and sedative-hypnotics. This section of the chapter provides an overview of psychotropic medications used to treat symptoms that occur in disorders of behavior, cognition, arousal, and mood in the gerontological population. A section is devoted to treating the movement disorders that may occur as a side effect from the use of neuroleptics. Because each individual experiences symptoms in a unique way, several types of drugs may be prescribed to any one patient.

In 1987 the Health Care Finance Administration mandated that the elderly in long-term care settings may only be prescribed psychotropic drugs for specific diseases or symptoms and that the use be monitored, reduced, or eliminated when possible (OBRA, 1987). Prescribing physicians and nurse practitioners may exceed the recommended doses only if documentation reasonably explains the rationale for the benefit of the higher dose in restoring function or preventing dangerous behavior (Stoudemire, Smith, 1996) (see Chapter 25).

A patient should be prescribed a psychotropic medication only after thorough medical, psychological, and social assessments are done and non-

Table 15-6 Classes and Side Effects of Antidepressants Available in the United States

Class	Examples	Side Effects
Tricyclic antidepressants (TCAs)	Amitriptyline, doxepin, imipramine, clomipramine	Dry mouth, constipation, urinary retention, orthostasis, sedation. Contraindicated for use of depression in the elderly.
	Nortriptyline, desipramine	Less of above side effects
Selective serotonin reuptake inhibitors (SSRIs)	Fluoxetine, sertraline, paroxetine, fluvoxamine, citalopram	Nausea, vomiting, dry mouth, headache, sedation, nervousness, anxiety, dizziness, insomnia, sweating, ejaculatory/orgasmic dysfunction
Nonselective serotonin reuptake inhibitors (SNRIs)	Venlafaxine	Nausea, dry mouth, headache, dizziness, nervousness
Other anti-depressants	Trazodone, bupropion, mirtazapine	Sedation, orthostasis, nausea, dizziness, headache

Data from Kaplan HI, Sadock BJ: *Pocket handbook of psychiatric drug treatment,* ed 2, Baltimore, 1996, Williams & Wilkins; Schatzberg AF: Course of depression in adults: treatment options, *Psychiatr Ann* 26(6):336-341, 1996; Semla TP, Beizer JL, Higbee MD: *Geriatric dosage handbook,* ed 8, Cleveland, 2003, Lexi-Comp, Inc.

pharmacological interventions have been found to be inadequate or ineffective. Nursing assessment before medication intervention contributes knowledge and baseline information that can optimize the patient's medical and psychological improvement. Issues to consider include the patient's medical status (and other medications that might interact with psychotropics), mental status, ability to carry out activities of daily living, ability to participate in social activities and maintain satisfying relationships with others, as well as the potential for patient or caregiver compliance with any pharmacological or nonpharmacological recommendations.

Antidepressants

Antidepressants, as the name implies, are drugs to treat depression. In the past, the major drugs used were monoamine oxidase (MAO) inhibitors and tricyclic antidepressants (TCAs), especially amitriptyline (Elavil) and doxepin (Sinequan). These drugs required high doses to be effective and had a significant number of side effects and adverse effects, especially related to their anticholinergic properties. Since the development of a new class of drugs, the SSRIs (selective serotonin reuptake inhibitors), the MAO inhibitors and TCAs are no longer indicated, nor should they be used for the treatment of depression in older adults.

The SSRIs and the new nonselective serotonin reuptake inhibitors (SRIs) have been found to be highly effective with minimal or manageable side effects and are the drugs of choice for use in older adults. Most of these cause initial problems with nausea or a dry mouth. However, both these and other side effects usually resolve over time (Table 15-6). One side effect of the SSRIs, if experienced, that does not resolve with time is sexual dysfunction. The nonselective SRIs and other antidepressants, such as venlafaxine (Effexor), bupropion (Wellbutrin), and trazodone, are less likely to cause this problem and may be preferred by elders who are sexually active.

Most older adults are sensitive to the SSRIs and may find significant relief from depression at low doses. Although it sometimes takes time to find the most optimal dose, the nurse can help the elder monitor target symptoms and advocate for continued dose adjustments or changes of medication until relief is obtained.

Stimulants

In extreme cases of depression that are resistive to pharmacological intervention, very low doses of stimulants have been found to be effective with some elders who have what are called vegetative symptoms (severe lethargy) or are profoundly withdrawn and apathetic. These symptoms may respond to central nervous system stimulants, such as amphetamine or methylphenidate.

Methylphenidate (Ritalin) and dextroamphetamine (Dexedrine) should be given only in the morning and early afternoon to prevent insomnia at night. Side effects are tachycardia, mild blood pressure increases, agitation, restlessness, and confusion. Methamphetamine (Desoxyn) has similar effects. Patients taking these medications should be encouraged to resume all daily activities. Responses should include motivation, interest, attention, and a sense of well-being.

Antianxiety Agents

Drugs used to treat anxiety are referred to as *anxiolytics* or *antianxiety agents*. These agents include benzodiazepines, buspirone (BuSpar), and beta blockers. Antihistamines, especially diphenhydramine (Benadryl), are often used but are not recommended for use in older adults because of their anticholinergic effects. The decision to treat anxiety pharmacologically is based on the degree to which the anxiety interferes with the person's ability to function and subjective feelings of discomfort.

The most frequently used agents are benzodiazepines. Although benzodiazepines have been available for almost 30 years, only minimal research has been done in the elderly (Madhusoodanan, Bogunovic, 2004). What we do know is that older adults metabolize these drugs slowly so that they persist in the blood stream for long periods of time and can easily reach toxic levels. Side effects include drowsiness, dizziness, ataxia,

mild cognitive deficits, and memory impairment. Signs of toxicity include excessive sedation, unsteady gait, confusion, disorientation, cognitive impairment, memory impairment, agitation, and wandering. Because these symptoms resemble dementia, persons can easily be misdiagnosed once they start taking benzodiazepines.

Benzodiazepines are highly addicting yet very popular because of their quick sedating effects for the person who is experiencing acute anxiety. However, because of the problems noted above they should be avoided except in extreme cases. If necessary, lorazepam (Ativan) appears to be the least problematic when prescribed in very low doses and for short periods of time. It has the shortest half-life of the benzodiazepines and no active metabolites.

Buspirone is a safer alternative. Although a side effect is dizziness, this is often dose related and resolves with time. Buspirone is not addicting and has an additive effect to some of the SSRIs so that lower doses can be used. No effect is felt by the patient or observed by the nurse for 5 to 7 days, and the drug may be mistakenly discontinued for apparent lack of effect. Buspirone is best used for chronic anxiety and is not indicated for acute periods.

Antipsychotics (Neuroleptics)

Psychosis covers a range of thinking and behavioral characteristics that are based on responses of the ill person to a private reality—a reality that may be distressing and problematic for the patient and those around him or her. Characteristically, psychosis occurs in schizophrenia but can also occur in mania, depression, delirium, dementia, and paranoid states. Psychosis manifests itself as delusional thinking and hallucinations, both of which can cause extreme anxiety and bizarre behavior. Antipsychotics, formerly known as *major tranquilizers* and now known as *neuroleptics*, are drugs used to treat psychotic symptoms.

Unfortunately neuroleptics are often misused by caregivers and health care providers in an attempt to control troublesome behaviors, and too often they are used without a careful assessment of the underlying cause of the behavior. Inappropriate use of antipsychotic medications may mask a reversible cause for the psychosis, such as infection, dehydration, fever, electrolyte imbalance, an

Table 15-7 Comparison of Side Effects of Antipsychotics

Generic name	Side Effects			
	Sedative	Anticholinergic	Extrapyramidal	Hypotensive
LOW POTENCY				
Chlorpromazine	High	High	Low	IM: High PO: Low
Thioridazine	High	High	Low	Moderate
INTERMEDIATE POTENCY				
Perphenazine	Moderate	Moderate	Moderate	Low
Loxapine succinate	Moderate	Moderate	Moderate	Low
Molindone HCl	Moderate	Moderate	Moderate	—
HIGH POTENCY				
Haloperidol	Low	Low	High	Low
Thiothixene	Low	Low	High	Moderate
Fluphenazine HCl	Low	Low	High	Low
Trifluoperazine HCl	Moderate	Low	Moderate	Low
NEWER ANTIPSYCHOTICS				
Risperidone	Low	Low	Dose related	Low
Clozapine	High	High	Low	High
Olanzapine	Moderate	Moderate	Low	Moderate

Modified from Jenike MA: *Geriatric psychiatry and psychopharmacology: a clinical approach,* St Louis, 1989, Mosby; Bloom HG, Shlom EA: *Drug prescribing for the elderly,* New York, 1993, Raven; Semla TP, Beizer JL, Higbee MD: *Geriatric dosage handbook,* ed 8, Cleveland, 1998, Lexi-Comp, Inc.

IM, Intramuscularly; *PO,* orally.

adverse drug effect, or a sudden change in the environment (Bullock, Saharan, 2002).

When used appropriately and cautiously in true psychosis, antipsychotics can provide a person with relief from what may be frightening and distressing symptoms. When used, drugs with the lowest side effect profile and at the lowest dose possible should be prescribed by the patient's health care provider. In most states the use of antipsychotics in long-term care settings is carefully monitored.

There are different classes and potencies of antipsychotics. Strong antipsychotics (high potency), such as haloperidol (Haldol), are less sedating but cause more extrapyramidal reactions. The elderly are susceptible to developing extrapyramidal reactions, particularly neuroleptic-induced parkinsonian symptoms. Weak antipsychotics (low potency), such as chlorpromazine (Thorazine), are sedating and cause orthostatic hypotension, thereby precipitating falls. Further,

the anticholinergic properties in the weaker antipsychotics can cause dry mouth, constipation, urinary retention, hypotension, and confusion. Table 15-7 compares sedative, extrapyramidal, anticholinergic, and cardiovascular side effects of the different potencies of antipsychotics. Careful nursing observation is essential for monitoring side effects and drug interactions whenever any of these medications are given (see Chapter 25).

Antipsychotics impair the body's hypothalamic, dopaminergic, thermoregulatory pathways. Hence, patients taking neuroleptics cannot tolerate excess environmental heat. Even mild elevations of core temperature can result in liver damage called *neuroleptic malignant syndrome.* The problem is more likely to occur during hot weather. The nurse or caregiver must protect the elder from hyperthermia by making sure the environment is cool enough. Appropriate interventions include adequate hydration, relocation to a cooler area away from direct sunlight, and use of a fan or sponge bath. The patient may or may not share his or her discomfort about the heat, so assessment of body temperature is essential. Any circumstance resulting in dehydration greatly increases the risk of heatstroke. Diuretics, coffee, alcohol, lithium, and uncontrolled diabetes may decrease vascular volume, thereby decreasing the body's ability to sweat. Anticholinergics inhibit sweating and lead to further heat retention (Lazarus, 1989). Heatstroke in old age is associated with very high mortality and morbidity rates.

Movement Disorders

While neuroleptic malignant syndrome is not commonly seen, the most significant potential side effects of antipsychotics in older adults are movement disorders, also referred to as *extrapyramidal syndrome (EPS)* reactions. These include acute dystonia, akathisia, parkinsonian symptoms, and tardive dyskinesia.

Acute dystonia.   An acute dystonic reaction may occur hours or days following antipsychotic medication administration or after dosage increases, and may last minutes to hours. An acute dystonic reaction is an abnormal involuntary movement consisting of a slow and continuous muscular contraction or spasm. Involuntary muscular contractions of the mouth, jaw, face, and neck are common. The jaw may lock (trismus), the tongue may roll back and block the throat, the neck may arch backward (opisthotonos), or the eyes may close. In an oculogyric crisis, the eyes are fixed in one position. Often this creates a feeling of needing to look up constantly without the ability to make the eyes come down. Dystonias can be painful and frightening.

Akathisia.   Akathisia refers to the compulsion to be in motion and may occur at any time during therapy. Patients describe feeling restless, being unable to be still, having an unrelenting desire to move, and feeling "like crawling out of my skin." Often this symptom is mistaken for worsening psychosis instead of the adverse drug reaction that it is. Pacing, aimless walking, fidgeting, shifting weight from one leg to the other, and marked restlessness are characteristic behaviors for a person experiencing akathisia.

Parkinsonian symptoms.   The use of neuroleptics may cause a collection of symptoms that mimic Parkinson's disease. A bilateral tremor (as opposed to a unilateral tremor in true Parkinson's), bradykinesia, and rigidity may be seen, which may progress to akinesia, or the inability to move. The patient may have an inflexible facial expression and appear bored and apathetic and be mistakenly diagnosed as depressed. More common with the higher-potency antipsychotics, parkinsonian symptoms may occur within weeks to months of initiation of antipsychotic therapy.

Caregivers or others unfamiliar with these EPS reactions often become alarmed. Although frightening, acute dystonia is not usually dangerous and is quickly relieved by anticholinergic medication, such as benztropine (Cogentin), trihexyphenidyl (Artane), or diphenhydramine (Benadryl), providing relief within minutes if given intravenously, within 10 to 15 minutes if given intramuscularly, and within 30 minutes if given orally. These medications should be readily available to treat an EPS reaction for all persons taking antipsychotics. Although they are not recommended for use in the elderly, anticholinergics and amantadine (Symmetrel), a dopamine agonist, are sometimes prescribed to prevent dystonic reactions, but because of slow onset of action, they are not used for acute treatment.

The same drugs are used to counteract akathisia and parkinsonian symptoms; however, their effectiveness is less predictable in these situations. Propranolol and clonidine have also been used for complaints of akathisia. However, hypotension and sedation are often unacceptable side effects and can be dangerous in the elderly.

Tardive dyskinesia.   When neuroleptics have been used continuously for at least 3 to 6 months patients are at risk for the development of the irreversible movement disorder of *tardive dyskinesia (TD)*. Both low- and high-potency agents are implicated (Bullock, Saharan, 2003; Goldberg, 2002). Tardive symptoms usually appear first as wormlike movements of the tongue; other facial movements include grimacing, blinking, and frowning. Slow, maintained, involuntary twisting movements of the limbs, trunk, neck, face, and eyes (involuntary eye closure) have been reported.

There is no treatment that reverses the effect of TD; therefore it is essential that the nurse is attentive for early detection so that the health care provider can make prompt changes to the psychotropic regimen.

Response to treatment is the most important consideration when gerontological patients are

NANDA and Wellness Diagnoses

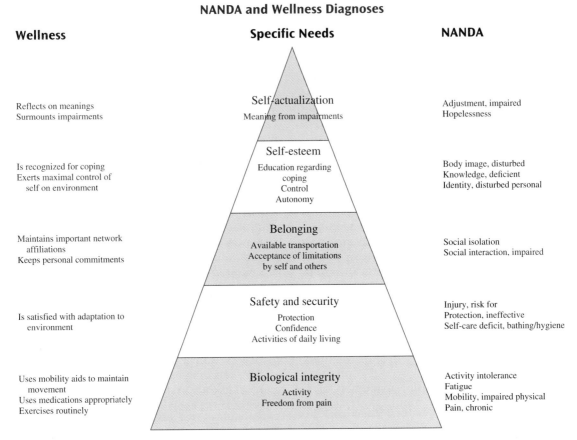

| Wellness | Specific Needs | NANDA |

Wellness

Reflects on meanings
Surmounts impairments

Is recognized for coping
Exerts maximal control of
self on environment

Maintains important network
affiliations
Keeps personal commitments

Is satisfied with adaptation to
environment

Uses mobility aids to maintain
movement
Uses medications appropriately
Exercises routinely

Specific Needs

Self-actualization
Meaning from impairments

Self-esteem
Education regarding
coping
Control
Autonomy

Belonging
Available transportation
Acceptance of limitations
by self and others

Safety and security
Protection
Confidence
Activities of daily living

Biological integrity
Activity
Freedom from pain

NANDA

Adjustment, impaired
Hopelessness

Body image, disturbed
Knowledge, deficient
Identity, disturbed personal

Social isolation
Social interaction, impaired

Injury, risk for
Protection, ineffective
Self-care deficit, bathing/hygiene

Activity intolerance
Fatigue
Mobility, impaired physical
Pain, chronic

These are not all of the possible wellness or NANDA diagnoses that may be identified. The above are frequent examples of nursing diagnoses that should be considered when planning care for the older adult in whatever setting.

taking psychotropics. Subjective patient comments about feelings and symptoms and objective observations about the patient's behavior are important data for evaluating the effectiveness of a drug. Several tools are available to help the nurse monitor the patient taking antipsychotics. The Abnormal Involuntary Movement Scale (AIMS), which was designed by the National Institute of Mental Health (NIMH, 1976), should be used before therapy and after initiation of therapy. For monitoring movement disorders see the Barnes Rating Scale for Drug-Induced Akathisia (Appendix 15-C), the Simpson-Angus Rating Scale for EPS (Appendix 15-D), and the Abnormal Involuntary Movement Scale (AIMS) (Appendix 15-E).

Mood Stabilizers

Although bipolar disorders are not common in the older population, some elders do suffer from them. Often this is something that has been a lifelong problem. Mood stabilizers are the group of agents used for the treatment of bipolar disorders. However, mood stabilizers, especially valproic acid (Depakene), have also been found useful for some persons with depression. Symptoms of the manic phase include confusion, paranoia, labile affect, pressured speech and flight of ideas, morbid or depressive content of thought, increased psychomotor activity resembling agitated depression, a long period between the depressive episode and the appearance of mania, and altered orientation and attention span. In older adults it is essential to combine both non-pharmacological and pharmacological approaches to optimize wellness (Lantz, 2003).

The nurse who is caring for a patient with a bipolar disorder or one who is taking a mood stabilizer should seek guidance from the person's psychiatrist regarding specific strategies to enhance the person's quality of life. The nurse should also be proactive in ensuring that serum concentrations of all mood stabilizers are monitored frequently and correctly.

If the patient is taking lithium, close monitoring by nurses is especially important. Lithium interacts with other medications and certain foods. For example, a low-salt diet will elevate the lithium level, and a high-salt diet will decrease it. Likewise, thiazide diuretics and nonsteroidal anti-inflammatory drugs (NSAIDs) will elevate the serum lithium level. Side effects include the following: confusion, disorientation, and memory loss; flattening of T waves on the electrocardiogram; polyuria and polydipsia; nausea, vomiting, and diarrhea; fine resting tremor; benign goiter; and ataxia.

IMPLICATIONS FOR GERONTOLOGICAL NURSING AND HEALTH AGING

All the medications presented in this chapter have indications, side effects, interactions, and individual patient reactions. The nurse's advocacy role includes education for the patient and family or caregiver. Further, the nurse must determine whether side effects are minimal and tolerable or serious. Asking the patient produces subjective data; and observing the patient's interactions, behavior, mood, emotional responses, and daily habits provides objective data. From this compilation of data, patient problems can be delineated, nursing diagnoses developed, outcome criteria planned, and interventions initiated. Nursing actions for the side effects associated with each drug class are presented in Table 15-8. These actions will help guide care planning for individual elderly persons.

Medications occupy a central place in the lives of many older persons: cost, acceptability, interactions, untoward side effects, and the need to schedule medications appropriately all combine to create many difficulties. Although nurses, with the exception of advance practice nurses, do not prescribe medications, we believe that a full understanding of medications is needed by nurses working with elders.

KEY CONCEPTS

- Individuals over 75 years old cannot be expected to react to medication in the way they did when they were 25 years old.
- Any medication has side effects. The therapeutic goal is to reduce the targeted symptoms without undesirable side effects. Drug-drug and drug-food incompatibilities are an increasing problem of which nurses must be aware.
- Polypharmacy reactions are one of the most serious problems of elders today and are usually the first area to investigate when untoward physiological events occur.
- Drug misuse may be triggered by prescriber practices, individual self-medication, physiological idiosyncrasies, altered biodegradability, nutritional and fluid states, and inadequate assessment before prescribing.
- Nurses must investigate drugs immediately if a change in mental status is observed in an individual who is normally alert and aware. Many drugs cause temporary cognitive impairment in older persons.
- Nonadherence of clients with medication regimens is a constant concern among health professionals. Look for possible reasons. One cannot comply with a prescription or treatment when there are incompatibilities that interfere with the practicalities of life or are distressful to the individual's well-being or when actual misinformation or disability prevents compliance.
- Chronotherapy that uses biorhythms of the body for the most effective medication therapy has the potential to decrease dose, frequency, and cost of medication regimens and to improve adherence to drug therapy.
- Biochemical processes in the brain influence all activities, including behavior, emotion, mood, cognition, and movement.

Table 15-8 Nursing Interventions for Side Effects of Psychotropic Medications

Type of Drug	Common Side Effects	Nursing Interventions
Antipsychotic	Sedation	Reassure patient/family that this side effect subsides in 5-10 days; prevent falls; avoid work requiring alertness, such as driving; dosing only at bedtime may decrease sedation during day.
	Orthostatic hypotension (more pronounced with low-potency medications)	Teach patient to dangle feet at bedside for 1-2 min before rising; rise slowly; support stockings may be helpful; prevent falling or tripping on obstacles.
	Photosensitivity	Protect skin from sun with clothing and sunscreen; sunglasses may be more comfortable because of dilated pupils.
	Photophobia Hyperthermia	Maintain adequately cool environment; teach patient to avoid hot temperatures and to increase water intake; ensure adequate hydration.
	Weight gain	Discuss with patient/family that this is a side effect; consult dietitian for dietary planning; encourage avoidance of fattening foods; sweets may be craved to counteract sedation.
	Acute dystonic reactions (more common with some high-potency medications)	Simpson-Angus testing at regular times of day; benztropine (Cogentin), 0.5 mg IM for immediate relief (may repeat if 0.5 mg ineffective); observe for confusion associated with anticholinergic properties of benztropine; reassure patient of immediate and full recovery with injection; for prevention thereafter, use amantadine; monitor for repeat EPS reactions; assess need for changing medication; assess patient compliance related to EPS.
	Parkinsonism	Same as above; may give benztropine (Cogentin) PO; reassurance needed.
	Tardive dyskinesia (may occur after 3-6 mo of continuous treatment)	Assess for signs using AIMS test; observe for tongue movements and involuntary movement early in treatment; decrease dose of medication, change drug, consider vitamin E; if antipsychotic discontinued, tardive dyskinesia will get worse; if given benztropine (Cogentin), tardive dyskinesia will appear worse. Much support is needed, because this is not always reversible.
	Akathisia	Assess for signs using Barnes scale; decrease dose, change drug, consider propranolol. Reassure patient that this is a side effect and will subside; difficult and uncomfortable to tolerate; monitor for safety and impulsive behavior related to anxiety and distress.

Drug category	Side effect	Nursing intervention
Anticholinergic effects of antipsychotics, antidepressants, antiparkinson agents	Blurred vision	Encourage use of magnifying glass and adequate lighting; reassure that the side effect subsides (up to 2 wk); refer to physician if it continues.
	Urinary hesitancy (particularly in elderly men with benign prostatic hypertrophy)	Consider less anticholinergic drug; encourage patient to report this symptom; provide privacy; run water in the sink, warm water over perineum.
	Urinary retention	Encourage frequent voiding, whenever urge exists; teach patient to monitor output; catheterization may be indicated; observe for discomfort, pain.
	Dry mouth	Give water, ice, sugar-free lozenges or candy or gum; often a disturbing side effect and may be associated with bad breath; provide materials for adequate oral hygiene; explain that this is a side effect.
	Constipation	Often a problem in elderly without medication; add fluids, fruits, vegetables to diet; prune juice at bedtime or in morning (patient preference); stool softener can be helpful. Monitor for bowel movement frequency and bowel sounds to prevent obstruction or ileus.
	Dizziness	Teach patient to change positions slowly, especially from stooping or sitting to standing (tying shoes, lying in bed).
	Tiredness/sedation	Teach to avoid activities requiring alertness and concentration; decrease dose or increase dose more slowly if this occurs with TCAs; give medication at bedtime if possible; teach patient that alcohol and other central nervous system depressants worsen sedative effect.
Anxiolytics	Sedation Confusion Memory loss Amnesia	Prevent accidents by teaching patient and family to avoid activities requiring alertness; keep patient oriented to environment; assess level of confusion by checking mental status daily; use drug with short half-life and no active metabolites (lorazepam); teach patient that sedative effects are worsened with alcohol or other central nervous system depressants.

Data from Keltner NL, Schwecke LH, Bostrom CE: *Psychiatric nursing: a psychotherapeutic approach*, St Louis, 1991, Mosby.

IM, Intramuscularly; *EPS*, extrapyramidal syndrome; *PO*, orally; *TCAs*, tricyclic antidepressants.

- The side effects of psychotropic medications vary significantly; thus these medications must be selected with care when prescribed for the older adult.
- The response of the elder to treatment with psychotropic medications should show reduced distress, clearer thinking, and more appropriate behavior.
- It is always expected that pharmacological approaches augment rather than replace non-pharmacological approaches.
- Older adults are particularly vulnerable to developing movement disorders (extrapyramidal symptoms, parkinsonism symptoms, akathisia, dystonias) with the use of antipsychotics.
- The Health Care Financing Administration and the congressional Omnibus Budget Reconciliation Act (OBRA) have severely restricted the use of psychotropic drugs for the elderly unless they are truly needed for specific disorders and to maintain or improve function. Then they must be carefully monitored.
- Any time a behavior change is noted in a person, reversible causes must be sought and treated before psychotropic medications are used.
- Antidepressant medications must be tailored to the elder with careful observation for side effects.
- Dosage levels of psychotropics must be carefully titrated for elders and their responses accurately and consistently recorded.

► **Activities and Discussion Questions**

1. What are the age-related changes that occur in pharmacokinetics of the older adult?
2. What is meant by *chronotherapeutics,* and how applicable is it to elders? Explain your answer.
3. What are the drug use patterns of the elderly, and what can be done to correct or improve them?
4. Explain the role of the elder, the care provider, and the social network in medication adherence.
5. List a variety of measures that the nurse can suggest to assist older adults with their medication use and adherence to a medication regimen.

6. Develop a nursing care plan using wellness and North American Nursing Diagnosis Association (NANDA) diagnoses.
7. What are the most troublesome side effects of antipsychotic medications?
8. Mrs. J. is calling out repeatedly for a nurse; other patients are complaining, and you simply cannot be available for long periods to quiet her. Considering the setting and the OBRA guidelines, what would you do to manage the situation?

RESOURCES

Websites

www.drugabuse.gov
Detailed drug information as "info facts"

www.nimh.nih.gov
The latest information on the use of psychotropic drugs

www.alzheimers.org
Information about drugs used for Alzheimer's disease

www.hartfordign.org
An excellent review of "Beers' Criteria for Potentially Inappropriate Medication Use in the Elderly" in their "Try This" section

REFERENCES

Amoako EP, Richarson-Cambell L, Kennedy-Malone L: Self-medication with over-the-counter drugs among elderly adults, *J Gerontol Nurs* 29(8):10-15, 2003.

Arunpongpaisal S, Ahmed I, Ageel N, Paholpak S: Antipsychotic use for the treatment of elderly people with late onset schizophrenia, *The Cochrane Library (Oxford)* 2:ID # CD004162, 2004.

Beers MH: Explicit criteria for determining potentially inappropriate medication use by the elderly: an update, *Arch Intern Med* 157(14):1531-1536, 1997.

Besdine R et al: *When medicine hurts instead of helps: preventing medication problems in older persons,* Washington, DC, 1998, Alliance for Aging Research and the American Society of Consultant Pharmacists.

Briggs GC: Geriatric issues. In Younkgin E, Sawin KJ, Kissinger J, Israel D, editors: *Pharmacotherapeutics: a primary care guide,* Upper Saddle River, NJ, 2005, Prentice-Hall.

Bullock R, Saharan A: Atypical antipsychotics: Experience and use in the elderly, *Int J Clinic Prac* 56(7): 515-525, 2002.

Butler RN et al: Love and sex after 60: how physical changes affect intimate expression: a roundtable discussion. Part I, *Geriatrics* 49(9):20-27, 1994.

Cooper JW: Adverse drug reactions related to hospitalization in nursing home patients: A 4-year study, *South Med* 92:485-90, 1999.

Delong MF: Caring for the elderly. IV. Medication use and abuse, *NurseWeek* 8(8):8, 1995.

DeMaagd G: High-risk drugs in the elderly population, *Geriatr Nurs* 16(5):198-207, 1995.

Edworthy SM, Devins GM: Improving medication adherence through patient education distinguishing between appropriate and inappropriate utilization. Patient Education Study Group, *J Rheumatol* 26(8): 1793-1801, 1999.

Gallagher LP: The potential for adverse drug reactions in elderly patients, *Appl Nurs Res* 14(4):221-224, 2001.

Goldberg RJ: Tardive dyskinesia in elderly patients: An update, *J Am Med Dir Assoc* 3(3):152-161, 2002.

Hartshorn E, Tatro D: *Principles of drug interaction, drug interaction facts 2003,* St Louis, 2003, Facts and Comparisons.

Haselberger MB, Kroner BA: Drug poisoning in older patients: preventative and management strategies, *Drugs Aging* 7(4):292-297, 1995.

Haynes RB, Wang E, Gomez MD: A critical review of interventions to improve compliance with prescribed medications, *Patient Educ Couns* 10:155, 1987.

Higbee MD: Consumer guidelines for using medications wisely, *Generations* 18(2):43, 1994.

Hogstel MO, editor: *Clinical manual of gerontological nursing,* St Louis, 1992, Mosby.

Hughes CM: Medication nonadherance in the elderly: How big is the problem, *Drugs Aging* 21(12):793-811, 2004.

Kroner BA et al: Poisoning in the elderly: characteristics of exposures reported to a poison control center, *J Am Geriatr Soc* 41(8):842-846, 1993.

Kutzik D, Spiers M: *Drug therapy adherence among elderly: barriers to successful self management.* Paper presented at the Gerontological Society of America, San Francisco, November 21, 1993.

Lacy C et al: *Drug information handbook 2003-2004,* Cleveland, 2003, Lexi-Comp, Inc.

Lamy PP: Adverse drug effects, *Clin Geriatr Med* 6(2):293-307, 1990.

Lantz MS: Bipolar disorders in the older adult, *Clinical Geriatr* 11(7):18, 20, 21-22, 2003.

Lazarus A: Differentiating neuroleptic-related heatstroke from neuroleptic malignant syndrome, *Psychosomatics* 30(4):454-456, 1989.

Lee M: Drugs and the elderly: do you know the risks? *Am J Nurs* 96(7):24-31, 1996.

Leirer VO et al: Elders' nonadherence: its assessment and medication reminding by voice mail, *Gerontologist* 31(4):514-520, 1991.

Lepkowski MI: General principles of drug therapy in the elderly. In Lantz J, editor: *Nursing care of the elderly,* San Diego, 1992, Western Schools.

Madhusoodanan S, Bogunovic OJ: Safety of benzodiazepine use in the geriatric population, *Expert Opin Drug Saf* 3(5):485-493, 2004.

Masoro EJ, Austed SN (Eds.): *Handbook of biology and aging* ed 5, San Diego, 2003, Academic Press.

Miller CA: Medications and sexual functioning in older adults, *Geriatr Nurs* 16(2):94-95, 1995.

Miller CA: Multiple choices in over-the-counter drugs, *Geriatr Nurs* 17(5):251-252, 1996.

Moore AR, O'Keefe ST: Drug induced cognitive impairment in the elderly, *Drugs Aging* 15(1):15-28, 1999.

National Institute of Mental Health (NIMH), Psychopharmacology Research Branch: Abnormal involuntary movement scale. In Guy W, editor: *ECDEU assessment manual for psychopharmacology,* revised, Rockville, Md, 1976, The Institute.

Omnibus Budget Reconciliation Act (OBRA) of 1987, Washington, DC, 1987, US Government Printing Office. House of Representatives, 100th Congress, 1st Session, Report 100-391.

Patel R: Polypharmacy and the elderly, *J Infusion Nurs* 26(3):166-169, 2003.

Pollock G, Reynolds CF III: Depression in late life. Harvard Mental Health Letter, Harvard Health Online, 2000. Available at www.health.harvard.edu/medline/Mental/M0900b.html.

Preventing medication errors in the elderly, HCPro's Patient Safety Monitor's Pick of the Week, Marblehead, Mass, April 24, 2002, HCPro. Available at www.accreditinfo.com/ptsafety/ptsafety_pick.cfm?content_id=21864.

Ray WA, Griffin WR, Downey W: Benzodiazepines of long and short elimination half-life and the risk of hip fracture, *JAMA* 262(23):3303-3307, 1989.

Scott GN, Elmer GW: Update on natural product-drug interactions, *Am J Health Sys Pharm* 59(4):339, 2002.

Semla TP, Beizer JL, Higbee MD: *Geriatric dosage handbook,* ed 8, Cleveland, 2003, Lexi-Comp, Inc.

Shaughnessy AF: Common drug interactions in the elderly, *Emerg Med* 24(21):21, 1992.

Spiers MV, Kutzik DM: *A multidimensional framework for understanding medication adherence in the elderly: a prescription for rethinking,* Unpublished paper, 1995.

Stoudemire A, Smith DA: OBRA regulations and the use of psychotropic drugs in long-term care facilities: impact and implications for geropsychiatric care, *Gen Hosp Psychiatry* 18(2):77-94, 1996.

Torrible SJ, Hogan DB: Medication use and rural seniors: who really knows what they are taking? *Can Fam Physician* 43:893-898, 1997.

Turkoski BB: Medication timing for the elderly: the impact of biorhythms on effectiveness, *Geriatr Nurs* 19(3):146-151, 1998.

Valli G, Giardina EG: Benefits, adverse effects and drug interactions of herbal therapies with cardiovascular effects, *J Am Coll Cardiol* 39(7):1083-1095, 2002.

Vestal RE: Clinical pharmacology. In Hazzard W et al, editors: *Principles of geriatric medicine and gerontology,* New York, 1990, McGraw-Hill.

Willcox SM, Himmelstein DU, Woolhandler S: Inappropriate drug prescribing for the community-dwelling elderly, *JAMA* 272(4):292-296, 1994.

Zumpano J: Polypharmacy in the elderly patient: A case of hyperkalemia, *Clini Excel Nurse Practit* 7(1-2):9-13, 2003.

Appendix 15-A *Drugs Considered Inappropriate for the Elderly*

Drug	Concern
ANALGESICS	
Propoxyphene and combinations containing propoxyphene	No analgesic advantage over acetaminophen Side effects are similar to narcotics
Indomethacin	Produces the most central nervous system effects of all NSAIDs
Phenylbutazone	Can produce hematological effects
Pentazocine	Produces central nervous system effects more commonly than narcotics, including hallucinations and confusion
Meperidine	Potent metabolite, normeperidine, can accumulate in elderly, causing tremors and seizures
ANTIEMETIC	
Trimethobenzamide	Ineffective as an antiemetic Produces extrapyramidal reactions
MUSCLE RELAXANTS	
Methocarbamol, carisoprodol, oxybutynin, chlorzoxazone, metaxalone, cyclobenzaprine	Side effect profile high: anticholinergic side effects, sedation, weakness Doses of effectiveness not tolerated well in elderly
HYPNOTICS	
Flurazepam, diazepam	Long-acting benzodiazepines produce prolonged sedation, increasing fall risk and confusion risk Small doses of short- and intermediate-acting benzodiazepines may be more appropriate
Barbiturates except phenobarbital	More side effects than other sedative-hypnotics Highly addictive Use only for seizure control
ANTIDEPRESSANTS	
Amitriptyline	Strong anticholinergic and sedating properties
Doxepin	Strong anticholinergic and sedating properties
HYPOGLYCEMIC	
Chlorpropamide	Long lasting, danger of hypoglycemia increased in elderly
ANTIDYSRHYTHMIC	
Disopyramide	May induce heart failure Strongly anticholinergic

Modified from Beers MH: Explicit criteria for determining potentially inappropriate medication use by the elderly, *Arch Intern Med* 157(14):1531-1536, 1997.
NSAIDs, Nonsteroidal antiinflammatory drugs.

Continued.

Appendix 15-A *Drugs Considered Inappropriate for the Elderly—cont'd*

Drug	Concern
ANTIPLATELET Dipyridamole	Causes orthostatic hypotension in elderly Beneficial only in artificial heart valves
ANTICOAGULANT Ticlopidine	No better than aspirin in preventing clots More toxic than aspirin in elderly
ANTIHYPERTENSIVE Methyldopa	May cause bradycardia May exacerbate depression
Reserpine	Poses danger to elderly: depression, impotence, sedation, orthostatic hypotension
CEREBRAL VASODILATORS Ergot mesyloids, cyclandelate (Cyclospasmol)	Not effective; not to be used for dementia or other conditions
GASTROINTESTINAL ANTISPASMODICS Dicyclomine, hyoscyamine, propantheline, belladonna alkaloids, clidinium-chlordiazepoxide	Highly anticholinergic, generally cause toxic effects in elderly Effectiveness at doses tolerated by elderly questionable
TREATMENT/PROPHYLAXIS OF DUODENAL ULCERS Cimetidine	Highly anticholinergic central nervous system effects: confusion, agitation, headache, fatigue
ANTIHISTAMINES (PRESCRIPTION AND NONPRESCRIPTION) Chlorpheniramine, diphenhydramine, hydroxyzine, cyproheptadine, promethazine, tripelennamine, dexchlorpheniramine	Potent anticholinergic properties For elderly, use cold and cough preparations without antihistamines in them Diphenhydramine should not be given for insomnia; only small doses (25 mg) for limited time should be used for allergy

Appendix 15-B *Medications That Should Not Be Chewed or Crushed*

Type	Rationale	Examples
Extended-release products with any of the following abbreviations: CR = controlled release CRT = controlled-release tablet LA = long acting SR = sustained release TR = timed release TD = time delay SA = sustained action XL = extended length XR = extended release	Medication is formulated to be slowly released into the body. The drug may be centered within the core of the tablet, and the multiple layers around it are shed. The outer tablet may be waxed, because this melts in the gastrointestinal tract; this appears as a shiny tablet. An extended-release capsule may have beads within it that will dissolve at different times once ingested.	Potassium chloride: K-Dur, Slow-K Adalat PA, XL Belladenal Spacetab Bellergal Spacetab Bentylol Dospan Wellbutrin SR Tegretol CR Diltiazem CD Choledyl SA Contact C Diamox Sequels Diclofenac tab Dimetapp Extentab Drixoral Tab Duralith Entex LA Inderal LA Indocid SR Macrobid Cap MS Contin Naproxen Nitro-Bid Nitrong SR Norflex Orudis SR Quinidex Entab Theophylline tab
Medications irritating to the stomach or destroyed by stomach acid are enteric coated; these are considered delayed release	Enteric coating delays release of the drug until it reaches the small intestine.	Enteric-coated aspirin Bisacodyl tab Carter's liver pills Divalproic acid Donnazyme Ecotrin Fe sulfate Lansoprazole Mandelamine Phazyme Pyridium Omeprazole
Foul-tasting medication	If a tablet is unpleasant to taste, the manufacturer may coat the tablet in a sugar coating. If crushed, the drug is unpalatable and may lead to noncompliance, but the drug is not altered.	Cefuroxime Chloral hydrate cap Fluoxetine Fluvoxamine Omeprazole Promethazine
Sublingual medication	Absorption is designed for under-the-tongue administration. It is not always easy to distinguish this type of medication; the package should indicate that it is sublingual.	Nitroglycerin SL
Effervescent tablets	Tablets that dissolve in a liquid, yielding a solution. If crushed, the tablets will not dissolve quickly.	

From Spectrum Society for Community Living: Oral drugs that should not be crushed or chewed, 2002. Available at www.spectrumsociety. org/library/SpectrumMedManual.pdf; Semla TP, Beizer JL, Higbee MD: *Geriatric dosage handbook,* ed 8, Cleveland, 2003, Lexi-Comp, Inc.

Appendix 15-C *Barnes Rating Scale for Drug-Induced Akathisia*

For each item circle the number identifying the response that best characterizes the patient:

Patients should be observed while engaged in neutral conversation while they are seated and then standing (for a minimum of 2 minutes in each position). Symptoms observed in other situations (e.g., engaged in activity on the ward) may also be rated. Subsequently, the subjective phenomena should be elicited by direct questioning.

1 OBJECTIVE

0 Normal, occasional fidgety movements of the limbs.
1 Presence of characteristic restless movements: shuffling or tramping movements of the legs/feet, or swinging of one leg, while sitting, and/or rocking from foot to foot or "walking-on-the-spot" when standing, BUT movements present for less than half the time observed.
2 Observed phenomena, as described in (1) above, which are present for at least half the observation period.
3 The patient is constantly engaged in characteristic restless movements and/or has the inability to remain seated or standing without walking or pacing during the time observed.

2 SUBJECTIVE

0 Absence of inner restlessness.
1 Nonspecific sense of inner restlessness.
2 The patient is aware of an inability to keep the legs still, or a desire to move the legs, and/or complains of inner restlessness aggravated specifically by being required to stand still.
3 Awareness of an intense compulsion to move most of the time and/or reports a strong desire to walk or pace most of the time.

3 DISTRESS RELATED TO RESTLESSNESS

0 No distress
1 Mild
2 Moderate
3 Severe

4 GLOBAL CLINICAL ASSESSMENT OF AKATHISIA

0 Absent
No evidence of awareness of restlessness. Observation of characteristic movements of akathisia in the absence of a subjective report of inner restlessness or compulsive desire to move the legs should be classified as pseudoakathisia.
1 Questionable
Nonspecific inner tension and fidgety movements.
2 Mild akathisia
Awareness of restlessness in the legs and/or inner restlessness worse when required to stand still. Fidgety movements present but characteristic restless movements of akathisia not necessarily observed. Condition causes little or no distress.
3 Moderate akathisia
Awareness of restlessness as described for mild akathisia above, combined with characteristic restless movements such as rocking from foot to foot when standing. Patient finds the condition distressing.
4 Marked akathisia
Subjective experience of restlessness includes a compulsive desire to walk or pace. However, the patient is able to remain seated for short periods of at least 5 minutes. The condition is obviously distressing.
5 Severe akathisia
The patient reports a strong compulsion to pace up and down most of the time. Unable to sit or lie down for more than a few minutes. Constant restlessness that is associated with intense distress and insomnia.

From Barnes TR: A rating scale for drug-induced akathisia, *Br J Psychiatry* 154:672-676, 1989.

Appendix 15-D *Simpson-Angus Rating Scale*

For each item circle the number identifying the response that best characterizes the patient:

1. Gait: The patient is examined as he or she walks into the examining room—his gait. The swing of the arms, the general posture all form the basis for an overall score for this item.	0 = Normal 1 = Mild diminution in swing while patient is walking 2 = Obvious diminution in swing suggesting shoulder rigidity 3 = Stiff gait with little or no arm swing noticeable 4 = Rigid gait with arms slightly pronated; this would also include stooped, shuffling gait with propulsion and repropulsion
2. Arm dropping: The patient and the examiner both raise their arms to shoulder height and let them fall to their sides. In a normal subject, a stout slap is heard as the arms hit the sides. In the patient with extreme Parkinson's syndrome, the arms fall very slowly.	0 = Normal, free fall with loud slap and rebound 1 = Fall slowed slightly with less audible contact and little rebound 2 = Fall slowed, no rebound 3 = Marked slowing, no stop at all 4 = Arms fall as though against resistance, as though through glue

Cogwheel rigidity may be palpated when the examination is carried out for items 3, 4, 5, and 6. It is not rated separately and is merely another way to detect rigidity. It would indicate that a minimum score of 1 would be mandatory.

3. Shoulder shaking: The patient's arms are bent at a right angle at the elbow and are taken one at a time by the examiner, who grasps one hand and also clasps the other around the patient's elbow.	0 = Normal 1 = Slight stiffness and resistance 2 = Moderate stiffness and resistance 3 = Marked rigidity with difficulty in passive movement 4 = Extreme stiffness and rigidity with almost a frozen joint
4. Elbow rigidity: The elbow joints are separately bent at right angles and passively extended and flexed with the patient's biceps observed and simultaneously palpated. The resistance to this procedure is rated.	0 = Normal 1 = Slight stiffness and resistance 2 = Moderate stiffness and resistance 3 = Marked rigidity with difficulty in passive movement 4 = Extreme stiffness and rigidity with almost a frozen joint
5. Wrist rigidity: The wrist is held in one hand and the fingers held by the examiner's other hand with the wrist moved to extension, flexion, and ulnar and radial deviation, or the extended wrist is allowed to fall under its own weight, or the arm can be grasped above the wrist and shaken to and fro. A zero score would be a hand that extends easily, falls loosely, or flaps easily upward and downward.	0 = Normal 1 = Slight stiffness and resistance 2 = Moderate stiffness and resistance 3 = Marked rigidity with difficulty in passive movement 4 = Extreme stiffness and rigidity with almost a frozen wrist

From Simpson GM, Angus JWS: A rating scale for extrapyramidal side effects, *Acta Psychiatr Scand* 212:11-18, 1970.

Continued.

Appendix 15-D *Simpson-Angus Rating Scale—cont'd*

6. Head rotation: The patient sits or stands and is told that you are going to move his or her head from side to side; that it will not hurt and that he or she should try to relax. (Questions about pain in the cervical area or difficulty in moving the head should be obtained to avoid causing any pain.) Clasp the patient's head between the two hands with the fingers on the back of the neck. Gently rotate the head in a circular motion three times, and evaluate the muscular resistance to this movement.	0 = Loose, no resistance 1 = Slight resistance to movement although the time to rotate may be normal 2 = Resistance is apparent, and the time of rotation is shortened 3 = Resistance is obvious, and rotation is slowed 4 = Head appears still, and rotation is difficult to carry out
7. Glabellar tap: Patient is told to open eyes wide and not to blink. The globular region is tapped at a steady, rapid speed. The number of times the patient blinks in succession is noted. Care should be taken to stand behind the subject so that he or she does not observe the movement of the tapping finger. A full blink is frequently not observed; more often there will be contraction of the infraorbital muscle producing a twitch each time a stimulus is delivered. Variations in the speed of tapping ensure that the muscle contraction is related to the tap.	0 = 0-5 blinks 1 = 6-10 blinks 2 = 11-15 blinks 3 = 16-20 blinks 4 = 21 or more blinks
8. Tremor: Patient is observed walking into examining room and then is reexamined for this item with arms extended at right angles to the body and the fingers spread out as far as possible.	0 = Normal 1 = Mild finger tremor, obvious to sight and touch 2 = Tremor of hand or arm occurring spasmodically 3 = Persistent tremor of one or more limbs 4 = Whole body tremor
9. Salivation: Patient is observed while talking and then asked to open the mouth and elevate the tongue. (Once the patient has received antiparkinson agents, this sign is unlikely to be present.)	0 = Normal 1 = Excess salivation to the extent that pooling takes place 2 = Excess salivation is present and might occasionally result in difficulty in speaking 3 = Speaking with difficulty because of excess salivation 4 = Frank drooling
10. Akathisia: Patient is observed for the presence of observable restlessness. After a determination of observable restlessness is made, the patient should be assessed by asking, "Do you feel restless or jittery inside; is it difficult to sit still?"	0 = No restlessness reported or observed 1 = Mild restlessness observed during the exam; e.g., occasional jiggling of the foot occurs during the sitting part of the exam 2 = Moderate restlessness observed; e.g., on several occasions, jiggles foot, crosses and uncrosses legs, or twists a part of the body 3 = Restlessness is frequently observed during the exam; e.g., the foot or legs move most of the time 4 = Restlessness persistently observed during the exam; the patient cannot sit still and may get up and walk

Appendix 15-E *Abnormal Involuntary Movement Scale (AIMS)*

Instructions: MOVEMENT RATINGS:	Complete Examination Procedure before making ratings.	Code for #1-7
	Rate highest severity observed. Rate movements that occur upon activation one value less than these observed spontaneously.	0 = None 1 = Minimal, may be extreme normal 2 = Mild 3 = Moderate 4 = Severe
FACIAL AND ORAL MOVEMENTS	1. Muscles of facial expression, e.g., movements of forehead, eyebrows, periorbital area, cheeks; including frowning, blinking, smiling, grimacing. ☐	
	2. Lips and perioral area, e.g., puckering, pouting, smacking. ☐	
	3. Jaw, e.g., biting, clenching, chewing, mouth opening, lateral movement. ☐	
	4. Tongue rate only increases in movement both in and out of mouth. NOT inability to sustain movement. ☐	
EXTREMITY MOVEMENTS	5. Upper (arms, wrists, fingers) Include choreic movements (i.e., rapid, objectively purposeless, irregular, spontaneous) and athetoid movements (i.e., slow, irregular, complex, serpentine). Do NOT include tremor (i.e., repetitive, regular, rhythmic). ☐	
	6. Lower (legs, knees, ankles, toes), e.g., lateral knee movement, foot tapping, heel dropping, foot squirming, inversion and aversion of foot. ☐	
TRUNK MOVEMENTS	7. Neck, shoulders, hips, e.g., rocking, twisting, squirming, pelvic gyrations. ☐	
GLOBAL JUDGEMENTS	8. Severity of abnormal movements: Mark one 0 None 1 Minimal 2 Mild 3 Moderate 4 Severe	
	9. Incapacitation due to abnormal movements: Mark one 0 None 1 Minimal 2 Mild 3 Moderate 4 Severe	
	10. Patient's awareness of abnormal movements (Rate only patient's report) 0 No Awareness 1 Aware, No Distress 2 Aware, Mild Distress 3 Aware, Moderate Distress 4 Aware, Severe Distress	
DENTAL STATUS	11. Current problems with teeth and/or dentures	Yes = 1 No = 0 ☐
	12. Does patient usually wear dentures?	Yes = 1 No = 0 ☐

From Guy W, editor: *ECDEU assessment manual for psychopharmacology, revised,* Rockville, Md, 1976, National Institute of Mental Health.

Continued.

Appendix 15-E *Abnormal Involuntary Movement Scale (AIMS)—cont'd*

AIMS EXAMINATION INSTRUCTION

Step 1:   Ask the patient whether there is anything in his or her mouth (e.g., gum or candy), and if there is, to remove it.

Step 2:   Ask about the current condition of the patient's teeth. Ask if he or she wears dentures. Ask whether teeth or dentures bother the patient now.

Step 3:   Ask whether the patient notices any movements in his or her mouth, face, hands, or feet. If the answer is yes, ask the patient to describe the movements and to what extent they currently bother the patient or interfere with activities.

Step 4:   Have the patient sit in a chair with hands on knees, legs slightly apart, and feet flat on the floor. (Look at the entire body for movements while the patient is in this position.)

Step 5:   Ask the patient to sit with hands hanging unsupported for a male patient, hands hanging between legs, and for a female patient wearing a dress, hands hanging over her knees. (Observe hands and other body areas.)

Step 6:   Ask the patient to open his or her mouth. Observe the tongue at rest within the mouth. Do this twice.

Step 7:   Ask the patient to protrude his or her tongue. (Observe abnormalities of tongue movement.) Do this twice.

Step 8:   Ask the patient to tap his or her thumb with each finger, as rapidly as possible for 10 to 15 seconds, first with the fingers of the right hand, then with the left hand. (Observe facial and leg movements.)

Step 9:   Flex and extend both arms out in front, with palms down. (Observe trunk, legs, and mouth.)

Step 10:   Ask the patient to stand up. (Observe the patient in profile. Observe all body areas again, hips included.)

Step 11:   Ask the patient to extend both arms out in front, with palm down. (Observe trunk, legs, and mouth.)

Step 12:   Have the patient walk a few paces, turn, and walk back to the chair. (Observe hands and gait.) Do this twice.

16

Living with Chronic Illness

LEARNING OBJECTIVES

Upon completion of this chapter, the reader will be able to:

- Explain the concept of wellness in chronic illness.
- Describe various patterns of chronic illness.
- Relate strategies that have been used successfully to maintain maximal function and comfort in the client with a chronic disorder.
- Name the special considerations that influence the experience of chronic illness.
- Describe the essential activities of daily living and the instrumental activities of daily living.
- Discuss strategies that increase an individual's ability for self-care.

GLOSSARY

Accoutrements Equipment necessary to function effectively; originally referring to military equipment.
Exorbitant Exceeding that which is usual or proper.
Rehabilitation The restoration of normal or near-normal function after a disabling disorder.

Restorative Pertaining to the restoration or renewal of a normal state of health or consciousness.
Trajectory The path followed by a body or an event moved along by the action of certain forces.

THE LIVED EXPERIENCE

"Because you understand my disease, you don't understand me. To understand that I am ill does not mean that you understand how I experience my illness. I am unique. I think and feel and behave in a combination that is unique to me. You do not understand me because you have a label for my disease or a plan for my treatment. It is not my disease or treatment that you need to understand. It is me. This could happen to you. . . . You are just a diagnosis away from being a patient. . . . And don't tell me you understand. Even if you have the same disease you couldn't fully understand. I am tired of being told:

* To deal with my feelings by those of you who flee from any intimacy with me and cringe when I confront you;
* To get my life in order by those of you who are obviously cluttered with the unimportant;
* To accept my pain and loss and even face death by those of you who avoid the very topic;
* To live with my limits by those of you who move about freely;
* To accept dependence by those of you who have the resources to assert your rigid safe ways of being."

(Jevne, 1993, p 121)

CHRONIC ILLNESS

Curtin and Lubkin (1995, p 8) offered the following definition of chronic illness from a nursing perspective: "Chronic illness is the irreversible presence, accumulation, or latency of disease states or impairments that involve the total human environment for supportive care and self-care, maintenance of function and prevention of further disability."

Most of the disorders of aging are chronic ones that must be treated within a framework of lifestyle changes, living situation adaptations, and attention to the whole person coping with a disorder (Burggraf, Barry, 1996). Current projections identify a life expectancy of approximately 65 years for men and 71 years for women born in 1950; children born in 2000 will enjoy 73 years and 80 years, respectively (U.S. Department of Health and Human Services, 2000). A longer and healthier life, therefore, requires effective management, if not cure, of chronic illnesses and their antecedent disability risk. This text and particularly this chapter are devoted to those ends.

Chronic disorders and acute illness cannot really be separated, because so many conditions are intricately intertwined; acute disorders have chronic sequelae, and many of the commonly identified chronic disorders tend to intermittently flare up into acute problems and then to go into remission. Many elders have several chronic disorders simultaneously and have great difficulty managing the complexity of the overlapping and often contradictory demands. The management of chronic illness largely relies on the patient and caregiver. Health care coverage is usually limited and available only when a particular improved outcome is expected.

Physical disabilities are often multiple and serious but need not kill the spirit or define the person. Psychological functioning may be more affected than physical or social functioning. The diagnosis, duration of the disease, and economic status are factors influential in psychological adjustment. The challenge to the older adult with multiple disabilities and chronic problems may simply become overwhelming. Women with severe arthritis may be as psychologically distressed as those with breast cancer, and strong social networks will have a more positive effect on both conditions than other factors. In addition, social functioning may mediate psychological adjustment, but that largely depends on education and occupation, as well as age, gender, marital status, and economic status.

One of the earliest nurse pioneers, Eldonna Shields, said: "Old age is a losing game when focused on function" (Shields, 1990). The European-American culture values independence, and winning is among its most revered goals. We, as nurses, are challenged to authenticate necessary dependency and to respect those who have the courage to let go of function when necessary. The things nurses "do" and the order in which they are done are probably far less important in chronic disease management than how they are done and with what attitude.

Carrie (a home health nurse) knelt on the carpet while applying dressings to open, nonhealing leg wounds that were a result of impaired circulation in an elder. She laughed and chatted, sharing some of her own interests and concerns as she worked. She had brought a book of hummingbird photographs for the client to enjoy. She said, "I practice down on my knees." This, from our perspective, is nursing in its highest sense. It is symbolical of much of our practice with elders: conducted "down on our knees," pleading to powers beyond our understanding to maintain the highest levels of health and function.

Wellness in Chronic Illness

The older adult with one or more chronic conditions can be supported toward the achievement of wellness and maximization of life satisfaction by caregivers who ascribe to a holistic philosophy that incorporates efforts directed toward the maintenance of the older person's self-care and self-esteem. Figure 16-1 shows how the wellness continuum and Maslow's hierarchy of needs can complement each other in the attainment of wellness and self-actualization. A reorganization of thinking is needed by many older adults and those associated with them: kin, friends, and caregivers.

Physical manifestations of chronic illness should not be the sole determining factor in the establishment of the elder's state of health or wellness. The greatest factor in establishing wellness is adaptation. To achieve maximization of life satisfaction, adaptation of lifestyle is necessary. What is wellness in the face of chronic illness? Results

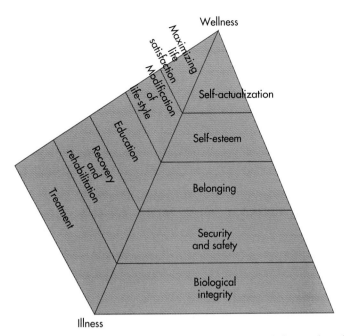

Figure 16-1   Correlation between illness-wellness continuum and Maslow's hierarchy of needs. (Developed by Patricia Hess.)

of a qualitative study (Hodges et al, 2001) using art to explore the perceptions of nurses, students, and the elderly about living with a chronic illness offer insight. Support and safety were considered integral to adaptation. Whereas nurses and students viewed chronic illness negatively, the elderly talked about the importance of hope, a steadfast refusal to give up, and a commitment to going forward in spite of limitations. As one 70-year-old woman stated: "If you stop, you're done" (p 394). Building on the courage of older adults coping with chronic illnesses, disabilities, and other losses is a good starting point for gerontological nurses.

Chronic Illness and Aging

Chronic illnesses tend to be composed of multiple diseases; are long term, unpredictable, and expensive; intrude into the life course and self-concept; and require extensive palliative care. Chronic illness is the accrual of life's earnings, sometimes self-generated, often inherent or a result of imposed lifestyles and environmental hazards. Often treating an acute disorder yields a chronic

residual disability. The thought has been, "It's a small price to pay for staying alive." For years, individuals with strokes or intractable pain of arthritis were simply told, "You must just learn to live with it." But, finally, chronic disorders are being taken seriously as we confront the individual, social, and economic costs of long-term impairment. In this chapter we consider ways in which nurses may assist their clients toward an enriched capacity for living in the shadow of chronic disabilities, so many of which are common to older adults. Arthritis is almost universal but more troublesome for some than others (see Chapter 19); often there is some mild to severe cardiovascular problem (See Chapter 20); breathing becomes more difficult (see Chapter 20); digestive disorders and nutritional problems go hand in hand (see Chapter 10), often including elimination problems (see Chapter 11); and diabetes is common and sometimes out of control (see Chapter 18), creating many other problems. Several of these disorders may intermingle to put a damper on the vitality of all but the most mentally robust. However, a state of wellness may be achieved and maintained consistently if the individual feels capable of managing and is motivated to manage the problem, with or without assistance.

Scope of the Problem

There is a growing recognition that chronic illness is the number one health problem in the United States and that health care professionals and the lay public have inadequate knowledge of chronic illness, its management, and the priorities and economics that have dictated inadequate policies and services. Estimates are that 90 million people in the United States are afflicted by chronic disease and co-morbidities. The incidence of chronic illness triples after 45 years of age but is thought to decrease markedly in relation to higher socioeconomical and educational status. Approximately 80% of older adults experience chronic illnesses that range from those that severely disrupt function to those that cause minor impairments. The most prevalent chronic conditions in individuals over 75 years of age in rank order are arthritis, hypertension, hearing impairments, heart disease, and cataracts (Holden, 2001).

The prevalence of chronic diseases continues to rise with the lengthening of life span for frail elders and highly technical medical care. Estimates are that by 2050, one of every five adults will be 65 years of age or older, and four fifths of them will experience one or more chronic illnesses (Davis, Magilvy, 2000). Chronic illness and its treatment are costly in both financial and personal terms. In 1995 the direct medical cost for treating chronic conditions was $470 billion; it is expected to be as high as $864 billion by 2040 (Holden, 2001). The National Chronic Care Consortium notes that these conditions plunder the personal bank accounts of elders. The average Medicare enrollee spends well over $3000 annually in out-of-pocket expenses on these disorders. Medicare stringently limits home care support for chronic disorders. Verbrugge and Patrick (1995) analyzed seven chronic conditions—three nonfatal (arthritis, visual impairment, hearing impairment) and four fatal (ischemic heart disease, chronic obstructive pulmonary disease, diabetes mellitus, malignant neoplasms)—for their impact on activity levels and use of medical services. The nonfatal conditions limited functioning considerably more than the fatal conditions did but received far fewer health services.

Chronic Illness Trajectory

In considering an appropriate conceptual framework for the study of chronic illness, we have tried to blend Corbin and Strauss with Maslow. The trajectory model of chronic illness, originally conceptualized by Anselm Strauss (Strauss, Glaser, 1975), has aided health care providers to better understand the realities of chronic illness. Later, Corbin and Strauss (1988) presented a view of chronic illness as a trajectory that traces a course of illness through eight phases, which may be upward, downward, or on a plateau. In its entirety, a chronic illness may include a preventive phase, a definitive phase, a crisis phase, an acute phase, a comeback, a stable phase, an unstable phase, deterioration, and death. Key points of the model are based on the theoretical assumptions listed in Box 16-1.

Maslow's concept of five major levels of need that affect function and self-perception fits well with the Corbin/Strauss model (see Figure 16-1). The patient's perceptions of needs met and basic biological functional limitations are paramount to predicting movement within the illness trajectory (Woog, 1992). In this respect, our wellness approach largely hinges on assisting the elder in meeting as many of Maslow's defined needs as possible at any given time. These efforts enhance the individual's potential for remaining on a plateau or gaining ground in any of the trajectory phases (Table 16-1).

The incidence of chronic disease is increasing in proportion to lifesaving technologies. Until the late 1930s, illness was primarily caused by bacteria or parasites. With the advent of antibiotics and immunizations these diseases decreased markedly in the industrialized nations. Instead, cancers, arthritis, and cardiovascular conditions have become the most common health problems. Recently, cancers and cardiovascular conditions have decreased somewhat, and infectious diseases are returning with a vengeance. At present, some restructuring of the health care system is occurring in ways that are beginning to more realistically serve the large numbers of chronically ill persons. In many ways, the acquired immunodeficiency syndrome (AIDS) epidemic has been the catalyst

Box 16-1   Theoretical Assumptions Regarding Chronic Illness Trajectory

- The prevalent form of disease at this time is chronic illness.
- These presumably incurable illnesses may appear at any time in the life span but are most frequent in late life.
- Chronic illnesses are lifelong and entail lifetime adaptations.
- Those with chronic illnesses are likely to experience the trajectory phases identified by Corbin and Strauss (1988).
- The acute phase of illness management is designed to stabilize physiological processes and promote a comeback from the acute phase.
- Other phases of management, except the severely deteriorating, are primarily designed to maximize and extend the period of stability in the home with the help of family and augmented by visits to physicians or clinics.

- Maintaining stable phases is central in the work of managing chronic illness.
- Chronic illness and its management often profoundly affect the lives and identities of the afflicted and the family members.
- The management in the home by the family, self, or significant other is central to care and is not peripheral to medical management (Corbin, Strauss, 1988).
- Recommended actions require appropriate timing and patience of the family and the practitioner.
- A primary care nurse able to coordinate multiple resources may be needed.
- Creativity and ability to use what is available are essential to successful management.

for change. As society becomes less healthy in terms of environment, diet, infectious agents, and stress inducers, more attention is being paid to seeking a healthy lifestyle.

Special Considerations

Regardless of the nature of chronic problems, there are special considerations that almost universally need attention and must be addressed actively by nurses. It is not sufficient to wait until the client brings up the topic.

Gender and Culture in Chronic Illness

Because women typically live longer than men and more frequently live alone, the issues of management of chronic disorders have a large gender component. The Rand Corporation found from a large study of elders (sample of 11,242) hospitalized with congestive heart failure (CHF), heart attack, pneumonia, and stroke that elderly men receive more care and more expensive, highly technical services than do women (Shoben, 1992). Research related to gender and cultural differences in health care access and treatment continues to point out disparities and needs continued attention. We still have much to learn about the experience of chronic illness in

different populations so that we can develop more culturally appropriate nursing responses (Davis, Magilvy, 2000).

Fatigue in Chronic Illness

Fatigue from living with chronic disorders is seldom considered in its full significance. It is a variable and unpredictable condition that is often ignored or relegated to an insignificant and incidental aspect of growing old. It may occur in the presence or absence of any other disorder but cannot be ignored. The lassitude that one experiences is often evidence of depression, as well as chronic illness. Zest for life is gone, and every action seems to involve an inordinate amount of energy that is hardly worth the effort. Nurses confronted by this attitude tend to become either impatient or caught up in the feeling of futility. The most important intervention is undoubtedly to validate the reality and debilitating effects of the disorder. Discussing patterns of fatigue and identifying the precipitants are important. If the elder can be engaged in keeping a log of the low points of energy, it may prove useful. It is also helpful to emphasize the wisdom of the body and the assumption that it is presently necessary for the individual to move in "low gear." Balancing rest and activity within limitations will help con-

Table 16-1 Definitions of Phases and Goals

Phase	Definition
1. Pretrajectory	Before the illness course begins, the preventive phase, no signs or symptoms present
2. Trajectory onset	Signs and symptoms are present, includes diagnostic period
3. Crisis	Life-threatening situation
4. Acute	Active illness or complications that require hospitalization for management
5. Stable	Illness course/symptoms controlled by regimen
6. Unstable	Illness course/symptoms not controlled by regimen but not requiring hospitalization
7. Downward	Progressive deterioration in physical/mental status characterized by increasing disability/symptoms
8. Dying	Immediate weeks, days, hours preceding death

Examples of goals that nurses might establish include the following:

1. To assist the client in overcoming a plateau during a comeback phase by increasing adherence to a regimen so that he or she might reach the highest level of functional ability possible within limits of the disability.

2. To assist a client in making the attitudinal and lifestyle changes needed to promote health and prevent disease.

3. To assist a client who is in a downward trajectory make the adjustments and readjustments in biography and everyday life activities that are necessary to adapt to increasing physical deterioration.

4. To assist the client who is in an unstable phase to gain greater control over symptoms that are interfering with his or her ability to carry out everyday activities.

5. To assist a client in maintaining illness stability by finding a way to blend illness management activities with biographical and everyday life activities.

Goals can be broken down into specific client-oriented objectives. Built into the objectives are the criteria that will be used to evaluate the effectiveness of each intervention. What is important here is to look at what takes place in the process (the steps) of working toward a goal, as well as the end to be reached, and to be realistic about what can be achieved in what time period, taking into consideration the desires, wants, and abilities of the client and family.

From Woog P: *Chronic illness trajectory framework: the Corbin and Strauss nursing model,* New York, 1992, Springer Publishing Co.

serve energy for activities that are most important or necessary.

Energy to enjoy life's activities becomes more precious with advancing age. Chronic problems tax this existing energy level. Direct assistance by caregivers or families may be necessary to aid the older adult in exploring lifestyle adaptations that decrease energy expenditure and permit continued involvement in valued interests. Throughout this process, the older adult with a disability must remain involved in decision making on every level of need. The older adult may have different priorities from the caregiver. Elderly clients may relegate their health needs to a lower priority to fulfill other needs or life demands. One must understand and respect the priorities established by the elder. Nurses should listen carefully to what is most important to the older adult, as well as what responses are most useful. People with chronic illnesses are really the "experts" on managing their illnesses and lifestyle.

Pain and Chronic Illness

The reader is advised to review Chapter 17 thoroughly while keeping in mind that chronic disorders usually involve not only certain painful physical impairments but also frequently depressed moods that exacerbate pain perception. Often an antidepressant is needed in combination with analgesics and nonpharmacological interventions. However, chronic conditions can and often do produce excruciating pain. Chronicity and pain often go hand in hand, and one of the major management issues is the control of pain.

Complementary and Alternative Medicine

Chronic diseases are particularly responsive to complementary therapies of various kinds. Complementary and alternative medicine (CAM) has been used extensively and effectively for centuries, particularly in Asia. Alternative therapies tend to be used by individuals who are more concerned about managing their own health in a holistic manner. Although there is an office of Complementary and Alternative Medicine in the U.S. Department of Health and Human Services, we prefer to consider these holistic alternative therapies more than a branch of medicine. These therapies are particularly effective approaches in the management of chronic conditions such as osteoarthritis and rheumatoid arthritis. Just as the triggers for disease flare-ups are poorly understood, so are the reasons why the alternative, non-medical interventions are often very helpful. Some complementary therapies are now included in Medicaid and Medicare coverage. Although this is an important trend, it places greater responsibility on the client for making wise decisions, sometimes with insufficient information or education. Nursing will be more often called on to assist clients in obtaining background information and seeking out options in health management. Many methods of self-directed care are costly and may actually be ineffectual or actually hazardous. As in all forms of therapy, the consumer is urged to proceed slowly and moderately and to try only one approach at a time to determine effects. Above all, one should listen to one's body signals. Information about complementary and alternative resources can be found at http://www.nccam.nih.gov. Chapter 17 also discusses alternative and complementary therapies.

Chiropractic. Chiropractic is the most widely used of all complementary therapies and is sought chiefly for musculoskeletal pain. Originally, chiropractic therapy involved manipulation of the spine and its effects on the nervous system, but chiropractic has now expanded into a more holistic approach that involves "disease prevention and health promotion through structural integrity and harmony with the environment" (Haldeman, 1992).

Homeopathy. Homeopathy was established as an alternative medical practice by Samuel Hahnemann, a German physician and pharmacist, over 200 years ago. In the late nineteenth century, it was a very popular medical model involving the "law of similars." Homeopathy uses minute doses of substances with properties that resemble the symptoms of the patient and that correctly administered will stimulate the individual's immune reactive system toward self-healing potential. The present model of homeopathic medicine is best seen in immunizations. We still have much to learn about how homeopathy may be effective in chronic and autoimmune disorders.

Acupuncture and acupressure. Acupuncture and acupressure have been used in China since 2500 BC. These therapies are thought to be effective because the techniques balance body, mind, and spirit through manipulation of the universal life-sustaining energy (*chi*). Acupressure exerts pressure at various spots along the 12 meridians, or pathways, through which *chi* flows to nourish the body. Acupuncture uses find-needle twirling at these points. When these points are stimulated, the nervous system releases endorphins and cortisol. Usually 10 to 12 visits with an accredited or certified acupuncturist are sufficient (Lorenzi, 1999). Again, individuals must be cautioned to determine the credentials of alternative care providers.

Reflexology. Reflexology involves pressure on certain zones of the feet or hands that are thought to access the major organs. The thumb or finger is applied with deep pressure to the reflex point on the hand or foot. The goal is similar to that of acupressure in that it is intended to restore the *chi* balance and improve the circulation of blood and lymph. Elders with lower extremity circulatory problems should not use this therapy.

Other therapies. The therapeutic value of massage, therapeutic touch, aromatherapy, crystal therapy, and magnet therapy is not documented as consistently as that of some of the other alternative therapies, but all these therapies are based on some idea of energy exchange, redirection, or enhanced circulation, and all have been found to be effective by some individuals in dealing with chronic illnesses.

We encourage nurses to ask individuals what self-initiated practices they use to manage their chronic disorders more effectively and which therapies have not been helpful. Not only is this often a very interesting and illuminating discussion, but also it opens the topic of alternative therapies for discussion and consideration. People from different cultures may also have many other alternative ways of treating chronic illness and its symptoms. The nurse needs to include discussion of these in assessments as well.

Sexuality and Chronic Illness

Sexual problems and misinformation are pervasive in society in spite of generally high levels of exposure to knowledge about sex and the near-toxic exposure to sexuality in the media, schools, and politics. In spite of this, little attention is paid to those who are living daily with chronic disorders that interfere with sexual satisfaction and the fundamental feelings of sexual attractiveness. Further, older people are not thought of as sexual beings and health professionals often neglect this aspect of human needs when working with older people.

"The centrality and complexity of sexuality continue through the lifespan" (Zeiss, Kasl-Godley, 2001, p 18). Research has shown that older couples report a steady level of interest, activity, and satisfaction with sexual activity. Greater sexual activity and satisfaction are associated with open and positive attitudes toward sexuality, greater sexual knowledge, satisfaction with a relationship, supportive social networks, psychological well-being, and a sense of self-worth (Zeiss, Kasl-Godley, 2001). Much of our information on sexuality is based on research conducted with Caucasian older adults. Further research is needed related to sexuality and sexual behavior of ethnic older adults and older gay, lesbian, and bisexual adults (Zeiss, Kasl-Godley, 2001). The Senior Action in a Gay Environment (SAGE) organization offers many services for older gay and lesbian older adults (http:www/sageusa.org).

Chronic illnesses and medical interventions can have direct and indirect effects on sexual function. Various disorders may produce mechanical problems, erectile problems, decreased libido, and limited mobility. Certain disorders involving ostomies and incontinence may produce revulsion in the partner and sexual anxiety in the afflicted. Discussing and assessing medication regimens, the expected dysfunctions that accompany particular diseases, and the individual's expectations are all important. A sexual history may provide impor-

Box 16-2	**PLISST**

Permission to masturbate, fantasize, and claim feelings
Limited **I**nformation related to problem being experienced
Specific **S**uggestions—only when nurse is clear about the problem
Intensive **T**herapy—referral to professional with advanced training if necessary

tant clues regarding the individual's needs and desires. The nurse's responsibility is toward an open, accepting discussion of the patient's sexuality and the provision of information and resources appropriate to the client's situation. *PLISST* is an acronym that is helpful in reminding us of a useful format for discussing sexuality (Box 16-2). The American Psychological Association's "Aging and Human Sexuality Resource Guide" at http://www.apa.org/pi/aging/sexuality provides valuable resources for health care professionals.

Grieving the Lost Self

Grieving the loss of appearance, function, independence, and comfort may occupy much of one's time initially when adapting to a chronic disorder, particularly if the onset has been abrupt and the loss interferes directly with a major source of one's pleasure. As the mother with a handicapped newborn mourns the loss of the visualized "perfect" infant, the elder may begin to memorialize the "perfect" self that no longer exists. In fact, the perfection of the earlier image of the self may grow far beyond the reality that existed. The nurse's function is to encourage verbalization, talk with the elder about the lost self, and recognize the stages of grief that may be occurring. Clearly, grief reactions will be highly individual, depending on the significance of the loss to the individual and the number of additional losses with which the individual is attempting to cope (see Chapter 26). The number and recent occurrence of other losses in the life of the individual may have depleted psychic reserves.

There often seems to be a subversive sense of failure or weakness in individuals who have developed a chronic disorder, as if they could will it away by strength of mind, determination, and courage. Suffering a chronic illness is compounded by a sense of responsibility for remaining healthy, especially in the current wellness climate (Benner et al, 1994). There is often the persistent thought that hard work and adherence to a strict treatment regimen will bring about cure, and when that does not occur, a sense of shame develops and the person wishes to hide from others (Doolittle, 1994). This is a serious problem that is deeply rooted in the work ethic that has been so cultivated in the older generation, and it may affect an elder's willingness to seek and accept help.

Given these tendencies, it is imperative that the nurse not overtly or covertly reinforce the client's sense of personal failure. It is not helpful to suggest, "Well, have you tried . . .?" Living with a chronic illness is a process that is continually changing as one adapts to the grief of the lost self and learns to embrace the needs of the emerging self. Unfortunately, health care providers often reinforce the notion that the individual is responsible for the illness and is in some way defective in allowing it to occur.

ASSESSMENT

Assessment of the elder with chronic disorders involves selection of appropriate tools, repeated testing, careful observation, periodic monitoring, alert watchfulness, and, most importantly, discussion and corroboration with elders about their perceptions and the meaning their illness has for them. In the case of chronic illness and the great variability in presentation and impact on individual lifestyle, adequate assessment is critical. In chronic illness, assessment focuses on function and how the disease affects function.

Functional assessments strive to identify the quantity and quality of disability in chronic illness. These assessments, although sometimes not specific to the medical treatment regimen, are often a good measure of the patient's response and adaptation to chronic health problems. Disability assessment helps identify the gap between the existing patient self-care abilities and needed self-care resources. The difference between these two (existing abilities and needed resources) identifies areas of nursing care. In this approach to assessment we are embracing the idea of an illness as chronic; patients can achieve various degrees of adaptation, and as nurses we can help maximize their function and therefore their quality of life.

Since many people with chronic illness manage their conditions in a community setting, assessment must also focus on the ability of family or significant others to assist and cope with caregiving. Evaluation of existing resources as well as those needed is also an important component of assessment (see Chapter 14).

Activities of Daily Living

Chronic disorders and the qualifications for home care are defined by the degree of impairment in activities of daily living (ADLs), such as eating, toileting, dressing, bathing, and transferring. The more complex and higher-level functions are categorized as instrumental activities of daily living (IADLs) and include activities such as using the telephone, using transportation, paying bills, planning meals, and managing medications. It is apparent that ADLs are largely mechanical, and IADLs are largely cognitive. To qualify for Medicare coverage of home care, one must be homebound, be expected to improve with treatment, have a signed order from a physician, and require the services of a professional. Impairment in ADLs is not sufficient to receive Medicare reimbursement (Rice, Rappl, 1996). However, it is useful to assess the level of ability of an individual for self-care. Many tools are designed to accomplish this (see Chapter 14).

INTERVENTIONS

Interventions in the care of chronically ill individuals must take into consideration the client's emotional responses, individual needs, motivation for self-care, supports from family and friends, and available resources, as well as the trajectory experience. Chronic illness affects all aspects of a person's life, and interventions must be holistic in focus. Eliopoulos (2001, p 480) states, "The success to which a chronic condition is managed can make the difference between a satisfying lifestyle, in which control of the illness is but one routine component, and a life controlled by the demands of the illness."

Caring

Caring has historically formed the foundation of nursing. The concept of caring has been studied by many nursing scholars. Sister Simone Roach's (1992) 5 C's of caring offer a framework for understanding the meaning of caring. According to Roach, the 5 C's are a way of understanding what the nurse is doing when he or she is caring. The 5 C's are as follows:

Competence: having the ability and skills to provide required nursing care

Compassion: a sensitivity to the pain and brokenness of others

Conscience: moral awareness, practicing within the moral framework, doing what "ought" to be done, and advocating for conditions of justice

Commitment: staying with the person on the journey; nursing as a lifelong commitment and way of life; doing the work of nursing because you want to, not because you have to

Confidence: inspiring trust through the care of the nurse

Older adults with chronic illnesses are not seeking cure; rather, they need care of the highest quality. Practicing within this framework, nurses bring expertise in caring to meet the needs of older adults with chronic illnesses. Nursing's response of caring brings the expertise to assist people in adapting, continuing to grow, and attaining a level of wellness and wholeness despite chronic illnesses and functional limitations. Caring for older people with chronic illnesses requires a different perspective from acute care nursing. "Chronic health problems are not fixable with shiny new technology, and do not promise the suspense, exhilarating hope, and dramatic ending that acute medical crises often do. They simply continue day after day, often invisible or misunderstood" (Hodges et al, 2001, p 390). Gerontological nurses know that understanding and caring for older adults with chronic illnesses and long-term disabilities require close caring relationships and continuing day after day with hope, courage, and joy on the journey. Gerontological nursing offers the opportunity to live caring in daily nursing practice.

Goals of Chronic Care Nursing

Goals of caring for persons with chronic health problems are presented by Eliopoulos (2001) include the following:

- Help clients set realistic goals and expectations
- Encourage verbalization of feelings
- Maintain or improve self-care capacity
- Manage the condition effectively
- Boost the body's healing abilities
- Prevent complications
- Delay deterioration and decline
- Achieve the highest quality of life
- Die with dignity and comfort

An array of nursing interventions can assist clients and families toward accomplishment of goals. Outcomes are always evaluated in terms of quality of life from the perspective of the person. Suggested nursing interventions in chronic illness care include the following:

- Provide education about the illness and its management
- Teach the skills required for effective self-care
- Provide ongoing assessment with a focus on prevention of complications
- Ensure delivery of needed care and support for both the person and the family or significant others
- Assist in helping the chronically ill person balance the effects of treatment on quality of life
- Provide positive reinforcement
- Focus on potential rather than limitations
- Listen to the story and come to know the person and what gives him or her meaning in life
- Relieve symptoms that interfere with function and quality of life
- Maintain hope through development of caring, reciprocal relationships and hopeful environments

Self-Care

In chronic care, self-care is of the greatest importance and must be cultivated beyond all else. The very nature of chronicity demands it. Assessment of self-care abilities is an important part of functional assessment. Self-care deficits are experienced when an individual is unable to carry out basic functions without assistance. These deficits are primarily the result of diseases of the neuromuscular and musculoskeletal systems or deficits in sensory functioning. Deficits in functional abilities may also be a result of situational conditions or treatment sequelae. The convergence of all three of these conditions may require more adaptive capacity than an individual has at that time.

The appropriate approach is highly individual and may involve changing the situation, modifying the treatment, or retraining the individual to compensate for the pathophysiological changes. It may also involve teaching others how to provide the needed care or teaching the person how to direct the provision of care by others. Dorothea Orem's self-care deficit theory provides an excellent nursing model for chronic and rehabilitative care (Orem, 1980).

The impact of chronic illness can be both a devastating event and an opportunity for growth. It is often a great challenge to try to adapt to the changes in lifestyle that an illness may bring. Perhaps even more difficult is learning to accept help from someone else with grace and equanimity. Someone said that a chronic illness is like a grain of sand in an oyster: it irritates and creates a pearl, or it just dies. Part of nursing intervention is to try to help create that pearl.

Maintaining a Health Diary

The health diary has multiple purposes in the assessment and management of chronic disorders. Its most important function is probably to serve as a mechanism by which an elder may develop self-awareness regarding perception and management of a chronic disorder. It has no recommended form or structure and is thus designed according to individual preference. The entries may be lengthy, with much embellishment, or brief, precise descriptions of daily activities and body responses. Some persons make daily entries, whereas others make entries only occasionally. Kept over time, the health diary reveals progression or remission of the condition and provides concrete longitudinal assessment data that may long since have been forgotten by the diarist. It also reveals something of the individual's personality style in the way perceptions are recorded, and it serves as a coping mechanism. A diarist is able to convey, at will, any thoughts or feelings and has full freedom of expression. The act of expressing brings control and solace. The intended, or unintended, recipient of the information becomes incidental to the process when it is considered as a therapeutic mode of self-care, personal integration, and release. Gerontological nurses might encourage clients with prolonged disorders to keep a health diary. It is extremely useful in many ways, the most important being the acute awareness in the nurse of the true meaning of "wellness" and courage.

Disease Management Programs

Disease management is a system of coordinated health care interventions and communications for populations in which patient self-care efforts are significant in disease management (Disease Management Association of America, http://www.dmaa.org). Components of a disease management program include identification of populations, use of evidence-based practice guidelines, interdisciplinary collaboration, patient self-management and education, and process and outcome measurement and feedback. The goals of disease management programs are to improve the health of people with chronic illness and to reduce health care costs and utilization through prevention of avoidable complications. Programs are targeted to individuals with a specific disease and have been most effectively utilized with persons with illnesses such as asthma, diabetes, congestive heart failure, coronary artery disease, end-stage renal disease, hypertension, and arthritis. Such programs are based on the concept that individuals who are better educated about how to manage and control their condition receive better care and avoid complications. Many nurses practice in disease management programs, and the holistic and integrated approach of nurses makes them well suited for these roles. Case management skills are an important component of disease management programs.

Managed health care plans have taken the lead in development of disease management programs although employers are increasingly using these programs to improve the health of employees and contain costs. Many states have implemented Medicaid disease management programs, and the Center for Medicare and Medicaid Services (CMS) is currently conducting disease management demonstration projects for Medicare recipients. Positive outcomes of these programs include improvements in health, satisfaction with care, and enhanced quality of life as well as decreased emergency visits and hospitalization (accessed 9/12/04 from http://ihcrp.georgetown.edu/agingsociety/pubhtml/management/management.html).

Small-Group Approaches to Chronic Illness

Early affiliation with a group confronting similar issues will usually assist in the adaptation to the altered role requirements and provide shared strategies for coping. Group meetings are among the most effective and economical ways of assisting clients in meeting informational and psychosocial needs. They can also be designed to provide family support and counseling. Self-help groups can be seen as support systems, consumer participant systems, expressive-social influence groups, or homogeneously identified therapeutic groups. Support groups provide the opportunity to obtain information and share similar experiences and perspectives. Facilitating adjustment to new roles and activities and facilitating redefinition of self and meanings constitute a large part of working with groups of individuals with chronic illnesses.

The first meeting should set the tone and expectations for the group and also make clear any necessary ground rules. It is important to involve the group in identifying topics and issues that group members wish to focus on during the groups. These ideally should be planned sufficiently in advance to allow the group facilitator to gather information, brochures, and other resources that may be valuable to the group members. In addition to information, there are many psychological issues to be addressed, such as the following:

1. Fears about incapacitation, pain, abandonment, isolation, and death
2. Expressions of low self-esteem and loss of confidence
3. Feelings of helplessness and uselessness; a desire to be whole and well again
4. A desire to fit into the family system once again
5. Willingness to redefine role relationships with significant others
6. A desire to face and handle public situations without fear or embarrassment

Adaptive and Assistive Devices

For the majority of those coping with disabilities, the goal is not just survival but maintaining a quality of life that is gratifying and prolonging independence as long as possible. Disabilities that interfere with the valued activities of one's life must be compensated for to the greatest extent desirable by personal or equipment assistance.

About 71% of all assistive devices are used by individuals over 65 years of age. Assistive devices include mobility aids; vehicle modifications; aids for vision, speech, and hearing impairments; prosthetics and orthotics; bathing devices; environmental control systems; computer access devices; and many others. High technology has been used to provide assistive devices, computerized training programs, programmed pill containers, distance monitoring of patients, and robotic aids for the handicapped. Voice-activated computer programs are now highly developed and can assist elders who are completely disabled in accomplishing many things. Many varieties of adaptive feeding and homemaking devices are available to compensate for deficits in function and encourage self-care and independence. Chapter 22 discusses many assistive devices and home modifications that can be helpful in enhancing function and independence.

Prevention of Iatrogenic Disturbances

In this era of rapid patient turnaround and numerous treatments compressed into a few days, nurses are well aware of the deleterious iatrogenic effects of hospitalization superimposed on the acute illness that required treatment (Box 16-3). Hospitalized individuals with some functional disabilities often rapidly regress into a helpless state. Simple interventions, noted time and again, have proved helpful in retaining functional status during episodic illness. The following interventions are most helpful: staff education regarding special needs of the hospitalized elder; identification of risk factors for delirium and preventive measures; early mobilization; use of speech, physical, and occupational therapy daily for particular therapeutic exercises; environmental modifications and personalization of the environment; minimal use of medications; and interdisciplinary discharge planning with frequent revisions (Box 16-4 includes specifics). Chapter 27 discusses some models to prevent iatrogenesis in hospitalized elders.

Box 16-3 Common Iatrogenic Disorders of Older Adults Caused by Hospitalization

Loss of mobility caused by insufficient ambulation

Temporary incontinence caused by inattention when needed, sometimes becoming a permanent problem

Confusion caused by medications, treatments, anesthesias, translocation

Pressure sores caused by infrequent changes of position

Dehydration caused by limited access to fluids

Fluid overload caused by improper use of intravenous fluids

Nosocomial infections caused by infectious agents in surroundings

Urinary tract infections caused by improper perineal care and catheter usage

Upper respiratory tract infections caused by immobility and shallow breathing; pneumonia

Fluid and electrolyte imbalances caused by medications, treatments

Falls caused by unfamiliar environment and instability

Impaired sleep caused by treatments and environment

Malnutrition caused by anorexia, insufficient assistance in eating

---

Box 16-4 Minimizing the Effects of Hospitalization on Functional Capacity

Staff Education
Mental and functional status assessment
Management of sensoriperceptual function
Mobility
Environmental modifications

Orientation and Communication
Use of cues and repetition
Discussion of condition
Providing anticipatory guidance regarding procedures
Reassurance regarding likelihood of delirium

Mobilization
Getting patients up, out of bed, and out of room
Involving physical and occupational therapy in exercise

Environmental Modifications
Glasses and hearing aids available and working well

Calendars
Favorite programs on radio and television available
Increased lighting, night-lights from dusk until dawn

Caregiver Education and Consultation
Families asked to bring in significant items; photos

Medication Management
Daily medication review; discourage use if not clearly necessary; particularly discourage neuroleptics and anticholinergics, which tend to exacerbate delirium

Discharge Planning
Weekly, or more frequent, case conferences with primary nurse, social worker, physical and occupational therapist, nutritionist, and discharge planner

---

Discharge and Follow-Up

The nursing research of Naylor and her colleagues (1999) demonstrated the effectiveness of a comprehensive discharge planning and follow-up of hospitalized elders implemented by advanced-practice gerontological nurses. Outcomes included reduced hospital readmissions and decreased costs of care. Interventions included visits to the hospitalized patient, home visits, and 24-hour telephone availability. Gerontological nurses can participate in the implementation of effective models such as this and contribute to other innovative models yet to be created that will improve care outcomes for older people with chronic illness.

REHABILITATION AND RESTORATIVE CARE

Restorative care is rehabilitative care within a humanistic framework provided under the guiding assumption that the care and services are thoughtfully designed to capitalize on the individual client's needs and strengths in a manner that will help him or her achieve the "highest practicable level of function" (Klusch, 1995). In gerontological nursing, rehabilitation may not involve a dramatic recovery, but rather many small improvements in functional capacity and independence. The older person with a disabling stroke may not walk independently again but can learn to operate a motorized wheelchair that allows him or her to stay independent and active. Another example would be the older person with Alzheimer's who receives rehabilitative or restorative care and retains ambulatory ability and continence. Unfortunately, with the limitations on Medicare reimbursement for rehabilitation, many older people, particularly those with preexisting functional or cognitive impairments, do not receive needed rehabilitative or restorative care. In the nursing home setting, the existence of restorative nursing programs for ADLs, toileting, range of motion (ROM), ambulation, and feeding contributes to restoration or maintenance of function.

Williams' definition of rehabilitation cited by Lueckenotte (2000) has a great deal of relevance for older adults: "Rehabilitation seeks to improve the individual's quality of life in any way, no matter how small, in relation to physical, emotional, or spiritual well-being; and ultimately return that individual to a residence of his choice and at minimal personal risk. This implies integration into society plus support in and by the community" (Williams, 1993, p 361).

Considerations in Planning Rehabilitation Care

Rehabilitation is long term, but plans for rehabilitation should begin during hospitalization for acute care. The following issues are important to consider:

1. Rehabilitation is not a place but rather a philosophy.
2. Rehabilitation must begin immediately after injury or illness.
3. Rehabilitation focuses on abilities, not disabilities. It maximizes strengths and supports limitations.
4. The person is in a crisis when admitted to the hospital, and personal strengths are not always visible or easily assessed.
5. Multidisciplinary discharge planning must begin on admission, and a nurse/case manager should be assigned to each client who will need rehabilitation.
6. Twenty-four–hour rehabilitative focus is necessary; it is insufficient to consider physical therapy two or three times per day as "rehabilitation." Restorative nursing programs should be available for maintenance of function.

Older adults with skilled rehabilitation needs may be cared for in hospitals, in subacute facilities, in outpatient facilities, or at home. Medicare pays for a limited amount of skilled rehabilitation services provided the patient is making progress toward goals. Conditions and factors that interfere with progress in rehabilitation programs include early discharge from the hospital before acute problems have been resolved, the effects of iatrogenic complications or co-morbidities, and cognitive impairment.

Comprehensive nursing assessment is an essential component of a multidisciplinary assessment. Nurses bring an intimate knowing of the person and their reactions and abilities from a 24 hour/day perspective. Nursing assessment includes a comprehensive biopsychosocial history, functional assessment, and a client care plan with long- and short-term goals. Weekly interdisciplinary team conferences are held to evaluate client progress and revision of goals. Discharge goals and family conferences are a part of these weekly conferences. The following services should be available to patients in acute rehabilitation programs:

1. Rehabilitation nursing
2. Physical therapy
3. Occupational therapy
4. Speech therapy
5. Social services
6. Discharge planning

7. Psychological services
8. Prosthetic and orthotic services
9. Audiology
10. Physician services
11. Consultation with vocational rehabilitation specialists

When assessing individual needs, it is important to focus on loss of function rather than the specific disease because therapeutic treatments will be designed to improve function.

The best of the gerontological rehabilitation units being developed now under various funding mechanisms are specifically designed to foster function and teach individuals how to influence their environment to adapt to whatever their disability may be. These are also the units where health care providers become most acutely aware of the need for interdisciplinary teamwork and planning. Resnick and Fleishell (2002) report on a "restorative care unit" developed by the Department of Medicine at the University of Maryland that is designed to bridge the gap between acute care and home care. In the 6 years of the unit's existence, orthopedic procedures have been the major reason for admission to the unit. Individuals with joint replacements, fractures, stroke, amputations, and arthritis make up most of the clientele. More than 86% of the individuals are discharged to home, and 80% of those are able to remain there for 2 years or longer. We expect many more restorative care units to emerge along the lines of this model. The National Council on the Handicapped recognizes the increasing problems of secondary and iatrogenically induced disabilities, such as pressure ulcers, contractures, and cognitive impairment, as important issues that must be considered in any future rehabilitation models.

Rehabilitation and the Future

Lack of education in rehabilitation among health care professionals in acute care settings results in inadequate care and even further disabilities. Most health care professionals poorly understand the potential of rehabilitative care. Better education, appropriate policies and protocols, and definitions of roles in rehabilitative care for allied health professionals are needed to bring rehabilitative care into the mainstream of the health care system.

In the future, we expect wider acceptance of rehabilitation by all professionals and increased integration of its principles into all medical and social activities. Effective rehabilitation for the older adult with disabilities is consistent with the philosophy that all persons should have the opportunity for optimum personal development and function. The penalty for lack of accessibility to appropriate rehabilitation is increased dependence on family, nursing homes, or other care providers at an even greater cost to society. The agenda for rehabilitation in the twenty-first century includes increased numbers of rehabilitation hospitals, reimbursement, and rehabilitation education programs.

Nurses advocating for the needs of the elderly and disabled, armed with clinical examples, anecdotal evidence, and empirical research findings, have the power to affect the character of public policy, as has been shown by the responsiveness of Congress to the lobbying power of nurses in Washington, DC. Cost effectiveness is the strongest argument in today's political climate. Continued emphasis on prevention of illness and disability, as evidenced by the goals of *Healthy People 2010,* is essential. As a result of such efforts, future generations of older people may not face the consequences of chronic illness to the extent experienced today. However, the increased numbers of disabled older adults who will be alive because of technological advances but will require decades of rehabilitative services is an extremely important issue. How will their care be financed? What will happen to Medicare after 2010, and will exorbitant home care costs be sustainable? Numerous questions need answers very soon.

EFFECTS OF CHRONIC ILLNESS ON THE INDIVIDUAL AND FAMILY

Often the ill individual feels like a burden to the family and engages in numerous compensatory behaviors to reduce this feeling of guilt. Home care is inconsistently provided and financed, and caregiver burdens can be enormous (see Chapter 23 for additional discussion). Most often, families are found to extend themselves far beyond their limits in attempting to deal with a member with a chronic disorder. When we speak of long-term care in the United States, we are speaking of care provided by families.

Caring for chronically ill older adults is caring for two patients, the person with the chronic illness and the family. Nurses are resource persons, advisors, teachers, and at times assistants, but the individual is in control of his or her adaptation. The goal of care of the chronically ill may be to slow decline, relieve discomfort, and support the preferred lifestyle with as few restrictions as possible (Strauss, Glaser, 1975). Not all chronic conditions require nursing service. The ability of the older adult and the family to manage and cope with the problems encountered determines the need. It is necessary for those who care for older adults with chronic conditions to be reoriented and resocialized to care norms and to recognize a different system of rewards.

The basics of the care process emphasize improving function; managing the existing illness; preventing secondary complications; delaying deterioration and disability; and facilitating death with peace, comfort, and dignity. Progress is not measured in attempts to achieve cure but, rather, in maintenance of a steady state or regression of the condition while remembering that the condition does not define the person. This thinking is essential if realistic expectations for the caregiver and the older person are to be achieved.

IMPLICATIONS FOR GERONTOLOGICAL NURSING AND HEALTHY AGING

Nursing care of older people with chronic illnesses and disabilities requires knowledge not only of disease processes but also of the effect of these processes on the function of the individual. Maintaining functional abilities and self-care capacities is the primary goal in caring for those with chronic illness. This kind of nursing requires a different focus from acute care nursing, where the emphasis is on attention to immediate and life-threatening needs and attempts to cure. Chronic illnesses, on the other hand, are illnesses to live with, and nursing's response is one of long-term caring. Living with chronic and disabling conditions often puts a damper on all but the most

mentally robust. Gerontological nurses working with older people experiencing chronic illness use a holistic approach, maximizing strengths, minimizing limitations, facilitating adaptation, and building on their courage to go forward in spite of limitations. Because an illness limits an older person physically, it does not have to limit the person's human potential. Healthy aging does not mean the absence of disease; rather, it means achieving wellness in spite of disease.

APPLICATION OF MASLOW'S HIERARCHY

Chronic illnesses and the consequences of treatment can affect an older adult's ability to fulfill basic physiological needs without assistance or adaptation. Nursing interventions are directed at enhancing self-care abilities as well as providing care to ensure that basic needs can be met with as much independence as possible. A wellness approach centers on assisting elders to meet as many of Maslow's defined needs as possible. Chronic illnesses and disabilities may impair physical function, but a sense of safety, security, belonging, self-esteem, and self-actualization can still be attained. Maintaining integrity and achieving one's maximal potential despite functional limitations and illness may be one of the greater accomplishments of many older people. Our care must support the potential for wellness at all stages in life.

▶ KEY CONCEPTS

- Declines in mortality, increasing medical expertise, and sophisticated technological developments have resulted in a great increase in the survival of the very old with multiple chronic disorders.
- Statistics regarding the extent of chronic disease are suspect because they often reflect only those who have come for medical care. In addition, decreased function without incapacitation is rarely reported.
- Women live longer than men and for that and other unknown reasons tend to have a higher incidence of chronic disease.

NANDA and Wellness Diagnoses

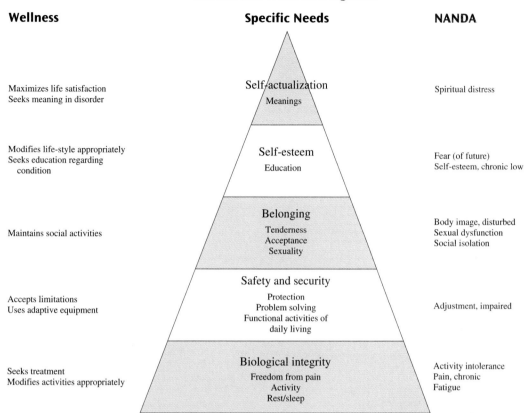

Wellness	Specific Needs	NANDA

Self-actualization
Meanings

Maximizes life satisfaction
Seeks meaning in disorder

Spiritual distress

Self-esteem
Education

Modifies life-style appropriately
Seeks education regarding
    condition

Fear (of future)
Self-esteem, chronic low

Belonging
Tenderness
Acceptance
Sexuality

Maintains social activities

Body image, disturbed
Sexual dysfunction
Social isolation

Safety and security
Protection
Problem solving
Functional activities of
daily living

Accepts limitations
Uses adaptive equipment

Adjustment, impaired

Biological integrity
Freedom from pain
Activity
Rest/sleep

Seeks treatment
Modifies activities appropriately

Activity intolerance
Pain, chronic
Fatigue

These are not all of the possible wellness or NANDA diagnoses that may be identified. The above are frequent examples of nursing diagnoses that should be considered when planning care for the older adult in whatever setting.

- One of the most difficult aspects of chronic disease is the unpredictability of the trajectory.
- The management in the home by the family, self, or significant other is central to care and should not be considered peripheral to medical management.
- Adaptations and assistance with activities of daily living (ADLs) and instrumental activities of daily living (IADLs) are the crux of chronic disease management.
- The most prevalent chronic problems of the aged are arthritis, hearing impairment, heart conditions, and hypertension.
- The most frequent assistance needed by those with chronic disorders is with bathing, dressing, and ambulation.

- The goal of rehabilitation for the older adult is to ensure opportunity for optimal personal development and function.

Activities and Discussion Questions

1. What are some of the patterns of chronic illness that cause great distress?
2. Discuss ways that one might modify a living situation to accommodate an individual with limited energy as a result of chronic disorders.
3. What are the special considerations that nurses should address when counseling an individual with a chronic disorder? Practice or role-play various ways that these issues can be addressed.

4. What do you think would be the most devastating loss in activities of daily living?
5. How would you encourage an individual toward maximal participation in self-care?
6. What would be the measures of wellness during chronic illness?

RESOURCES

Organizations

Association of Rehabilitation Nurses
4700 West Lake Road
Glenview, IL 60025-1485
(800) 229-7530 or (708) 375-4710
website: http://www.rehabnurse.org

National Center on Complementary and Alternative Medicine
PO Box 7923
Gaithersburg, MD 20898
(888) 644-6226
website: http://www.mccam.nih.gov

National Chronic Pain Outreach Association
PO Box 274
Milboro, VA 24460
(540) 862-9437
website: http://www.chronicpain.org

National Council on Disability
1331 F Street NW, Suite 850
Washington, DC 20004
(202) 272-2004
website: http://www.ncd.gov

Rehabilitation Institute of Chicago
345 Superior Street
Chicago, IL 60611
(312) 908-6000
website: http://ric.org

Senior Action in a Gay Environment
208 W. 13th Street
New York, NY 10011
(212) 741-2247
website: http://www.sageusa.org

Websites

American Psychological Association
"Aging and Human Sexuality Resource Guide"
Available from:
http://www.apa.org/pi/aging/sexuality

Center for Medicare and Medicaid Services
(information on disease management programs for Medicare beneficiaries)

Available from:
http://www.cms.hhs.gov/media/press/release.asp?Counter=967

Disease Management Association of America
website: http://dmaa.org

REFERENCES

Benner P et al: Moral dimensions of living with a chronic illness: autonomy, responsibility, and the limits of control. In Benner P, editor: *Interpretive phenomenology: embodiment, caring and ethics in health and illness,* Thousand Oaks, Calif, 1994, Sage.

Burggraf V, Barry R: *Gerontological nursing: current practice and research,* Thorofare, NJ, 1996, Slack.

Corbin JM, Strauss A: *Unending work and care: managing chronic illness at home,* San Francisco, 1988, Jossey-Bass.

Curtin M, Lubkin I: What is chronicity? In Lubkin I, editor: *Chronic illness: impact and interventions,* ed 3, Sudbury, Mass, 1995, Jones & Bartlett.

Davis R, Magilvy JK: Quiet pride: the experience of chronic illness by rural older adults, *Image J Nurs Sch* 32(4):385-390, 2000.

Doolittle ND: A clinical ethnography of stroke recovery. In Benner P, editor: *Interpretive phenomenology: embodiment, caring and ethics in health and illness,* Thousand Oaks, Calif, 1994, Sage.

Eliopoulos C: *Gerontological nursing,* ed 6, Philadelphia, 2001, Lippincott Williams & Wilkins.

Haldeman S: *Principles and practice of chiropractic,* ed, Norwalk, Conn, 1992, Appleton and Lange.

Hodges HF, Keeley AC, Grier EC: Masterworks of art and chronic illness experiences in the elderly, *J Adv Nurs* 36(3):389-398, 2001.

Holden K: Chronic and disabling conditions: the economic cost to individuals and society, *Public Policy and Aging Report* 11(2):1, 2001.

Jevne R: Enhancing hope in the chronically ill, *Humane Med* 9(2):121-130, 1993.

Klusch L: *Solutions in restorative caregiving,* Des Moines, 1995, Briggs Health Care Products.

Lorenzi EA: Complementary/alternative therapies: so many choices, *Geriatr Nurs* 20(3):125-133, 1999.

Lubkin IM, Larsen P: *Chronic illness: impact and interventions,* ed 5, Sudbury, Mass, 2002, Jones and Bartlett.

Lueckenotte A: *Gerontological nursing,* St Louis, 2000, Mosby.

Naylor MD et al: Comprehensive discharge planning and home follow-up of hospitalized elders: a randomized clinical trial, *JAMA* 281(7):613-620, 1999.

Orem D: *Nursing: concepts of practice,* ed 2, New York, 1980, McGraw-Hill.

Resnick B, Fleishell A: Developing a restorative nursing program, *Am J Nurs* 102(7):91-95, 2002.

Rice R, Rappl L: The patient receiving rehabilitation services. In Rice R, editor: *Home health nursing practice: concepts and application,* ed 2, St Louis, 1996, Mosby.

Roach S: *The human act of caring,* Ottawa, 1992, Canadian Hospital Association.

Shields E: Personal communication, Sept. 23, 1990, Vermillion, Ohio.

Shoben: Hospitals provide similar care to elderly women and men: Rand study finds differences in quality very small. Rand news release, October 14, 1992.

Strauss A, Glaser B: *Chronic illness and the quality of life,* St Louis, 1975, Mosby.

U.S. Department of Health and Human Services: *Healthy people 2010,* Sudbury, Mass, 2000, Jones and Bartlett.

Verbrugge LM, Patrick DL: Seven chronic conditions: their impact on US adults' activity levels and use of medical services, *Am J Public Health* 85(2):173-182, 1995.

Williams J: Rehabilitation challenge, *Nurs Times* 18(31):66-70, 1993.

Woog P: *Chronic illness trajectory framework: the Corbin and Strauss nursing model,* New York, 1992, Springer Publishing Co.

Zeiss A, Kasl-Godley J.: Sexuality in older adults' relationships, *Generations* 25(2):18-25, 2001.

17

Pain and Comfort

LEARNING OBJECTIVES

Upon completion of this chapter, the reader will be able to:

- Define the concept of pain.
- Differentiate acute from persistent pain.
- Identify data to include in a pain assessment.
- Discuss comfort measures.
- Discuss pharmacological and non-pharmacological management of pain.
- Identify factors that affect elders' pain experience.
- Discuss the goals of pain management for the elderly.
- Develop a nursing care plan for an elder in acute pain and chronic pain.

GLOSSARY

Adjuvant A drug that has a primary use other than pain (antidepressant, anticonvulsant) but also provides analgesia for some painful conditions.

Endorphins Opiate-like substances produced naturally by the body that modulate the transmission of pain and raise the pain threshold.

Equianalgesic The dosage and route of administration of one drug that produce approximately the same degree of analgesia as the dosage of another drug.

Iatrogenic Caused by medical personnel or procedures or through exposure to the environment of a health care facility.

Intractable Having a disease or symptom that remains unrelieved by treatment.

Nociceptors Afferent nerve receptors particularly sensitive to a noxious (harmful, injurious, toxic) stimulus.

Titration The adjustment of a given medication until the desired effect is established.

THE LIVED EXPERIENCE

Pain
Pain isolates
No matter how many friends you have
Or how devoted
Well-meaning, they sit beside your bed,
And press your hand,
You slip away,

Though your fingers stay entwined.
I have gone into the pain, deep and far,
How cold, how desolate it is here,
Starting at every sound,
Half-hoping, half in fear,
Death, is that you?
Now, are you here?

From Maclay E: Green winter: celebrations of old age, *New York, 1977.*
Copyright © 1977 by Elise Maclay.

Comfort seems to be an intrinsic balance of the physiological, emotional, social, and spiritual essence of an individual and can be perceived as an integral component of wellness. Experiencing comfort is a basic human need at the bottom of Maslow's hierarchy of needs. This does not mean that the need is the least important; quite the contrary—it is fundamental, and all higher levels of needs become insignificant to the person in pain. By definition, comfort is "a state of ease and satisfaction of the bodily wants and freedom from pain and anxiety." The absence of physical pain is not always sufficient to provide comfort. Elders and others may have their biological or body needs satisfied but still have emotional or spiritual pain. Conversely, physical needs may be the priority, and no comfort is possible until that need fulfillment is accomplished.

The International Association for the Study of Pain (1979, 1992) and the American Pain Society (1992) define *pain* as "an unpleasant sensory and emotional experience associated with actual or potential tissue damage, or described in terms of such damage." Pain is a subjective response and therefore difficult to objectively assess. McCaffery and Beebe's (1989) classic definition is the one most commonly used in nursing: "Pain is whatever the person experiencing pain says it is."

Pain is a multidimensional and totally pervasive phenomenon with sensory, physical, psychosocial, emotional, and spiritual components (Lynch, 2001). Pain, whatever its source, is one of the most common complaints of the elderly. It erodes personality, saps energy, and manifests itself in an ever-intensifying cycle of pain, anxiety, and anguish until the cycle is broken. Pain can evoke depression, sleep disorders, decreased socialization, impaired mobility, and increased health care costs (Morley, 2001; Thernstrom, 2001; Fine, 2002; Jeffery, Lubkin, 2002).

Pain is now considered the fifth vital sign. It is just as important as the other vital signs and should receive as much attention. The Joint Commission on Accreditation of Healthcare Organizations (JCAHO) has published standards for pain assessment and management in hospitals ambulatory care, home care, and nursing home settings. This accrediting body expects health care professionals working in health care settings to (1) recognize and treat pain properly, (2) make infor-

mation about both pharmacological and non-pharmacological interventions readily available, (3) promise patients attentive analgesic care, (4) define policies for using analgesic technology, and (5) continuously monitor and improve the quality of pain management (Pasero et al, 1999a). In the nursing home setting, pain is one of the quality indicators and the nurse is required to determine the presence or absence of pain when completing the Minimum Data Set (MDS) assessment (see Chapter 6). Patients have a right to have their pain adequately controlled (Box 17-1).

The nurse has a definition or interpretation of pain, as does the patient for whom the nurse cares. These interpretations are formulated from experiences and are influenced by the unique history of the individual and the meaning ascribed to the pain. It is also important to realize that an individual responds in a way that reflects cultural expectations and acceptable behavior. Values, experience with pain, and myths and stereotypes also influence both the perception of and the response to pain. Ethnically diverse responses to pain are based on years of social modeling, group-pressure influence on pain tolerance, and the observation of the family when in pain (Jeffery, Lubkin, 2002) (Box 17-2).

Nurses, caregivers, and elders themselves persist with and act on their misconceptions about pain. Despite increased education about pain and effective methods of pain management, many people, especially older adults, suffer from unrelieved pain. Myths about pain and the elderly contribute to the underdiagnosis and undertreatment of pain (Box 17-3).

ACUTE AND PERSISTENT PAIN

Acute pain is temporary and includes postoperative, procedural, and traumatic pain. It is easily controlled by analgesic medications. Almost everyone has experienced this type of pain and knows that it is a time-limited situation with attainable relief. Persistent pain, also called chronic pain, is not that simple. It has no time frame; it is continually persistent at varying levels of intensity. The guidelines of the American Geriatrics Society (AGS, 2002) suggest the use of the term *persistent pain* to overcome the negative images associated with the term *chronic pain*.

Box 17-1	Pain Patient's Bill of Rights

I have the right to:
- Have my pain prevented or controlled adequately
- Have my pain and pain medication history taken
- Have my pain questions answered freely
- Develop a pain plan with my health care provider
- Know the risks, benefits, and side effects of treatment
- Know what alternative pain treatments may be available
- Sign a statement of informed consent before any treatment
- Be believed when I say I have pain

- Have my pain assessed on an individual basis
- Have my pain assessed using the 0 = no pain, 10 = worst pain scale
- Ask for changes in treatment if my pain persists
- Receive compassionate and sympathetic care
- Refuse treatment without prejudice from my health care provider
- Seek a second opinion or request a pain care specialist
- Be given my records on request
- Include my family in decision making
- Remind those who care for me that my pain management is part of my diagnostic, medical, or surgical care

Modified from Cowles J: *Pain relief,* New York, 1994, MasterMedia.

Box 17-2	Culturally Oriented Responses to Pain

- Minimizes pain with significant others
  or
  Uses pain to elicit sympathy and support from others
- Carefully controls the expression of pain (calm and unemotional)
  or
  Is vocal about pain (cries and moans, complains)
- Withdraws and wants to be alone when pain is severe
  or
  Seeks attention and presence of others
- Willingly accepts pain relief measures
  or
  Avoids pain relief measures in the belief that they indicate weakness
- Wants and expects quick pain relief
  or
  Accepts pain for long periods before requesting help

Modified from Kozier B et al: *Fundamentals of nursing,* Redwood City, Calif, 1995, Addison-Wesley; Bates MS: *Biocultural dimensions of chronic pain,* Albany, 1996, State University of New York Press; Salerno E, Willens JS: *Pain management handbook,* St Louis, 1996, Mosby.

The term *chronic pain* may conjure up images of malingering, psychiatric problems, drug-seeking behavior, and futility in treatment in the minds of providers. Persistent pain is multifactorial in nature. Lipman and Jackson (2000) note that persistent pain can manifest as depression, eating and sleeping disturbances, and impaired function. The effects of persistent pain affect physical, psychological, social, and spiritual well-being (McElhaney, 2001). Chronic, persistent pain is categorized as either of nonmalignant origin or of malignant origin. Intractable, nonmalignant pain is the most common pain in elders and erodes an individual's coping ability. Table 17-1 compares the many facets of acute and chronic or persistent pain.

Persistent pain is further classified as follows:
- Nociceptive pain is associated with injury to the skin, mucosa, muscle, or bone and is most often the result of stimulation of pain receptors. This type of pain arises from tissue inflammation, trauma, burns, infection, ischemia, arthropathies (rheumatoid arthritis, osteoarthritis, gout), nonarticular inflammatory disorders, skin and mucosal ulcerations, and internal organ and visceral pain from distention, obstruction, inflammation, compression, or ischemia of organs. Pancreatitis, appendicitis, and tumor infiltration are common causes of visceral pain.

| Box 17-3 | Fact and Fiction About Pain in the Elderly |

MYTH: Pain is expected with aging.

FACT: Pain is not normal with aging. The presence of pain in the elderly necessitates aggressive assessment, diagnosis, and management similar to that of younger patients.

MYTH: Pain sensitivity and perception decrease with aging.

FACT: This assumption is dangerous! Data are conflicting regarding age-associated changes in pain perception, sensitivity, and tolerance. Consequences of this assumption are needless suffering and undertreatment of both pain and underlying cause.

MYTH: If a patient doesn't complain of pain, there must not be much pain.

FACT: This is erroneous in all ages but particularly in the elderly. Older patients may not report pain for a variety of reasons. They may fear the meaning of pain, diagnostic workups, or pain treatments. They may think pain is normal.

MYTH: A person who has no functional impairment, appears occupied, or is otherwise distracted from pain must not have significant pain.

FACT: Patients have a variety of reactions to pain. Many patients are stoic and refuse to "give in" to their pain. Over extended periods of time, the elderly may mask any outward signs of pain.

MYTH: Narcotic medications are inappropriate for patients with chronic nonmalignant pain.

FACT: Opioid analgesics are often indicated in nonmalignant pain.

MYTH: Potential side effects of narcotic medication make them too dangerous to use in the elderly.

FACT: Narcotics may be used safely in the elderly. Although elderly patients may be more sensitive to narcotics, this does not justify withholding narcotics and failing to relieve pain.

From Ferrell BR, Ferrell BA: Pain in the elderly. In Watt-Watson JH, Donovan MI, editors: *Pain management: nursing perspective*, St Louis, 1992, Mosby.

Nociceptive mechanisms usually respond well to common analgesic medications and non-pharmacological interventions (Lynch, 2001; AGS, 2002).

- Neuropathic pain involves a pathophysiological process of the peripheral or central nervous system and presents as altered sensation and discomfort. Conditions causing this type of pain include postherpetic or trigeminal neuralgia, poststroke or postamputation pain (phantom pain), diabetic neuropathy, or radiculopathies (e.g., spinal stenosis). This type of pain may be described as stabbing, tingling, burning, or shooting. These pain syndromes do not respond as well as nociceptive pain to conventional analgesic therapy. Use of antidepressant medications and anticonvulsants has been effective (Lynch, 2001; AGS, 2002).

- Mixed or unspecified pain usually has mixed or unknown causes. Examples include recurrent headaches and vasculitis. A compression fracture causing nerve root irritation, common in older people with osteoporosis (see Chapter 19), is an example of a mix of nociceptive and neuropathic pain (Lynch, 2001; McElhaney, 2001; AGS, 2002).

PAIN IN THE OLDER ADULT

The prevalence of pain in community-dwelling elderly persons is known to be twice that of the young and is considered to be extremely high in the long-term care setting. Fine (2002) and Herr (2002) suggest that the incidence of pain in community-dwelling elders is 25% to 50%. In the nursing home setting, estimates are that 45% to 80% of older adults have substantial pain that is undertreated (Teno et al, 2001). Multiple chronic conditions and the high prevalence of cognitive impairment in this setting make recognition, assessment, and treatment of pain problematic (AGS, 2002).

Table 17-1 Comparison of Acute and Persistent Pain

	Acute Pain	Persistent Pain (Nonmalignant Origin)	Persistent Pain (Malignant Origin)
Source	An event, external agent, or internal disease	A situation, state of existence Unknown or if known, changes cannot occur or treatment is prolonged or ineffective	Usually associated with terminal disease
Onset	Usually sudden	May be sudden or insidious	Unpredictable
Duration	Hours, days, usually transient, lasting no more than 3-6 mo	Prolonged for months or years	Prolonged, often for the course of the disease or in its later stages
Pain identification	Pain vs. lack of pain Areas generally well defined	Pain vs. lack of pain Areas are less well defined Intensity becomes more difficult to evaluate (change in sensation); intensity varies, may be constant or intermittent	Areas(s) may be well defined or diffuse; pain may be more constant than intermittent
Associated pathological conditions	Present	Often unknown	Usually present
Associated problems	Uncommon	Depression, anxiety, secondary pain issues	Many of the same as chronic nonmalignant pain
Behavior	Typical response patterns with more visible signs: Facial expressions Crying, guarding Guarding, moaning Clenching teeth	Response patterns vary, few overt signs (adaptation): Sleeping Sleep disturbances Confusion Rubbing	Response pattern similar to chronic nonmalignant pain: Sleep disturbance Withdrawal Depression Inactivity

	Biting lower lip Tightly shut eyes Open, somber eyes Involuntary movements Immobility of body part Purposeless body movement Rhythmical body movements, rocking, rubbing Change in speech and vocal pitch (anxiety) Slow monotone (severe pain) Fetal position	Stoicism Depression Inactivity Combativeness Inactivity Immobilizing body part or assuming an awkward body position	Slow moving Anger Anxiety Fearful Short tempered or passive
Nerve conduction	Rapid	Slow	Slow
Autonomic system involvement (clinical signs)	Present Elevation of blood pressure Tachycardia Diaphoresis	Generally absent No change in vital signs	May be present or absent
Meaning pattern	Meaningful: informs person something is wrong; self-limiting or readily corrected	Meaningless: person looks for meaning	May have meaning or be meaningless
Treatment	Primary—analgesic drugs	Multimodal: primary behavioral and physical therapy; drugs may be primarily adjunctive	Multimodal: analgesics usually play a major role

Compiled and modified from Karb V: Pain. In Phipps W, Long B, Woods N, editors: *Medical-surgical nursing: concepts and clinical practice*, ed 4, St Louis, 1991, Mosby; Forrest J: Assessment of acute and chronic pain in older adults, *J Gerontol Nurs* 21:10, 1995; Lipman AG, Jackson KC: *Use of opioids in chronic noncancer pain*, Stamford, Conn, 2000, Power-Pak Communications, Inc., Purdue Pharma LP.

Older people are at high risk for pain-inducing situations. They have lived longer and have a greater chance of developing degenerative and pathological conditions through disease or injury. Several conditions may be present simultaneously, so a single pain-producing condition may be overlooked in the complexity of health management. Increased susceptibility to accidents because of medications, cognitive function, or illness impacts functional abilities, which further contributes to accidents such as falls. The resultant hip fractures, sprains, and hematomas require longer periods of time to heal and prolong the pain experience. Loneliness and emotional pain from loss of a spouse, a job, independence, and friends and the presence of boredom and depression decrease the ability to cope with physical pain. These psychosocial aspects of an elder's life are rarely self-reported because of the associated stigma.

Persistent pain experienced by a number of elders often results in dramatic lifestyle changes, such as altered family relationships and the inability to visit friends. In a study by Ferrell and Ferrell (1990) of 65 elderly patients, 54% experienced impairment of enjoyable activities; 53% experienced impaired ambulation; 49% experienced impaired posture; and 45% and 32% experienced sleep disorders and depression, respectively. It is estimated that the prevalence of persistent pain is twice as high among older people as among younger individuals (Leo, Singh, 2002).

Behavioral changes or manifestations such as confusion and restlessness have been cited as possible indicators of painful stimuli in the cognitively intact and cognitively impaired aged (Davis, 1997; Feldt et al, 1998; Herr, 2002). The older person may suffer in silence or attempt to relieve pain with inadequate measures because of the high cost of medical care, consultation, equipment, diagnostic tests, hospitalization, and medications. In addition, older adults often underreport pain because they consider it a normal part of the aging process. Fear of addiction is another reason why older people may not report pain or ask for medication.

Common Causes of Persistent Pain

The majority of those over the age of 65 have chronic pain. The most common pain in elders is probably musculoskeletal, but a significant number also have neuropathic pain. Among com-

Box 17-4	**Common Nonmalignant Pain Conditions in the Elderly**

Temporal arteritis
Osteoarthritis of neck, shoulders, lumbar area, hips, knees, or hands
Rheumatoid arthritis
Lumbar disk disease
Lumbar stenosis
Osteoporosis
Peripheral vascular disease
Trigeminal neuralgia
Herpes zoster
Postsurgical intercostal neuralgia
Postherpetic neuralgia
Peripheral neuropathy
Diabetic neuropathy
Reflex sympathetic dystrophy
Phantom limb pain
Angina
Postmastectomy pain
Hiatal hernia
Irritable bowel syndrome
Chronic constipation
Acute cholecystitis

munity-dwelling elders, 66% have joint pain and 28% have back pain; among elders in long-term care facilities, 70% have joint pain, 13% have pain from old fracture sites, and 10% have neuropathic pain, much of this from postherpetic neuralgia (Ferrell, 2000). Box 17-4 lists common nonmalignant pain conditions in elders.

Osteoarthritis

By age 50, nearly 90% of adults have degenerative abnormalities of the lower spine (see Chapter 19). One of the most typical is thinning of the intervertebral disks, which can eventually lead to arthritis and other painful conditions. Osteoarthritis, or the destruction of the inner joint surfaces, is one of the most common forms of joint disease and the most disabling for those persons over age 65. Joint pain and stiffness are initially intermittent and then can become constant. Pain is characterized by aching in the joints, surrounding muscles, and soft tissue, usually relieved by rest and exacerbated by activity. The knees, hips, spine, and hands are most commonly affected.

Relief from arthritic pain requires the skillful use of both pharmacological and nonpharmacological measures. Since osteoarthritis is a noninflammatory condition, acetaminophen (Tylenol) remains the drug of choice for mild chronic pain. However, most people report increased relief with the nonsteroidal antiinflammatory drugs (NSAIDs), and they are quiet frequently used by older adults. As noted earlier, the use of NSAIDs in the elderly carries a considerable risk of interactions and adverse events (Durrance, 2003). Topical capsaicin may reduce osteoarthritis pain; however, it is necessary to warn patients to wash their hands after application and to keep their hands away from their eyes. It is also important to tell patients to expect a strong sensation of burning. Severe arthritis with unrelieved pain and extensive disability may require local anesthetics and corticosteroid injections into joints or epidural spaces for lumbar pain; surgical intervention, such as joint replacement, for intractable pain; or narcotic pain relievers.

Nonpharmacological pain management includes application of moist heat to relieve pain, spasm, and stiffness and joint care. Joint care may include orthotic devices such as braces and splints to support painful joints, weight reduction if the patient is overweight, avoiding stress to the joints, and occupational and physical therapy. Cognitive-behavioral measures are directed at coping skills and self-efficacy and feeling safe with activity.

Postherpetic Neuralgia

Nearly 1 million cases of herpes zoster (shingles) occur each year, most often in those between ages 60 and 79. It has been estimated that about 50% of people who live to age 80 will have an attack of shingles (Diamond, Urban, 2002). This may be due to the decrease in cellular immune response to the varicella zoster antigen, which is undetected in up to 30% of previously immune healthy elders over 60 (Chiu, 2000). An attack of shingles can occur when there is reactivation of the varicella virus through immunosuppression, malignancy, trauma, surgery, or local radiation (Gilchrest, 1995). Postherpetic neuralgia is a complication that is experienced because of irritation of the nerve roots that leave the spinal cord. Ophthalmic zoster causes postherpetic neuralgia when the trigeminal nerve is involved. The stinging, burning pain with or without an underlying

sharp, jabbing sensation continues for weeks, months, and for some elderly indefinitely after the initial skin lesions have healed. Once postherpetic neuralgia is established it is hard to treat. Analgesics provide limited relief from the pain; codeine is often prescribed. More effective in providing relief is a combination of antiviral medications, steroids, aspirin, and topical anesthetics for pain. The U.S. Food and Drug Administration (FDA) has approved prescription medications such as acyclovir and famciclovir, which shorten the duration of chronic shingle pain but may not prevent postherpetic neuralgia. Capsaicin cream (Zostrix), an over-the-counter topical anesthetic, or the anesthetic EMLA patch (Reyes, 1994; Chiu, 2000) may be helpful in relieving postherpetic neuralgia pain. Low doses of tricyclic antidepressants (e.g., desipramine) or the newer neuropathic drugs, such as gabapentin, and nerve blocks are considered in resistant cases.

Pain and the Impaired Elder

In nursing the accepted standard used in both the assessment and the response to the person is through the subjective report; as noted earlier, pain is "whatever the experiencing person says it is." For persons who have lost verbal skills through a condition such as a stroke or advanced Parkinson's disease or for those who are cognitively impaired to the point that the changes in mental function greatly interfere with their ability to report pain, this standard becomes unrealistic (Kovach et al, 1999).

For older adults with physical or psychological impairments, many things may interfere with the communication of pain. Hearing loss, depression, aphasia, and chemical and physical restraints may interfere with communicating pain. The nurse cannot assume that those individuals who cannot verbalize their pain clearly for whatever reason do not have pain or as much pain as others who are not impaired but the nurse must be alert to the cues that suggest that pain and discomfort are present. If a condition causes pain in a person who can self-report the pain, the condition is also painful to one who is impaired and the nurse must therefore treat the pain. Understanding what the person is trying to communicate through his or her behavior is an essential skill in caring for older people with cognitive impairment. Chapter 21 discusses this in more detail.

IMPLICATIONS FOR GERONTOLOGICAL NURSING AND HEALTHY AGING

As always, care of the elder in pain begins with assessment and continues through to the application of interventions and finally the evaluation of the interventions. The nurse is usually the person most attuned to the needs of patients, and through the nursing record, the nurse is in a key position to work with the elder in the management of pain, be it acute or persistent. The nurse is the person who works with the whole person to find a solution to the problem of pain.

Assessment

A comprehensive assessment of pain includes a complete history and physical, as well as a specific assessment of pain. Special attention is given to the musculoskeletal and nervous systems as the sites of common pain producing conditions in older people. Assessment begins with a patient's self-report of pain. According to Frampton (2004), "the guiding principle in pain assessment is simple and straightforward: The patient is the most important source of information about their pain. Therefore, you must regularly ask about their pain and assess it systematically" (http://www.amda.com/caring/may2004/pain.htm). Many times older people will not relate pain complaints unless directly asked specific questions such as "Do you have pain now?" "Where is your pain?" "Do you have pain everyday?" "Does pain keep you from sleeping at night or doing your daily activities?" (Frampton, 2004). In addition, older people may not use the word *pain*, so words such as *achy, hurt,* and *discomfort* should also be used in assessments (Frampton, 2004). See Box 17-5 for additional cues in the assessment of pain in older adults especially

---

Box 17-5   Pain Cues in Older Adults

Overt Behavior

Aggressive
Striking out: pinching; hitting; biting; or scratching

Physical movements
Restlessness/agitation
Drawing legs up or fetal position
Stretches
Repetitive movements
Clenched fists
Slow movements, cautious movements
Guarding
Trying to get someone's attention

Activities of daily living
Resists care
Change in appetite (decrease)
Altered sleep (decreased)

Sounds

Verbalizations
Says has pain
Antisocial behavior
Complains
Critical

Blames
Silence—does not speak

Vocalizations
Groans
Moans
Screams
Cries
Babbles
Noisy breathing

Appearance

Facial expression
Expressionless; stares or looks past you
Winces
Pleading
Grimaces: eyes—tighten up or light up; mouth—open or pinched; brows—wrinkled or folded

Body language
Complexion—flushed look

Other
Tense
Lacks concentration
Perspires

Modified from Parke B: Gerontologic nurses' way of knowing, *J Gerontol Nurs* 24(6):21, 1998; McCaffery M, Pasero C: *Pain: clinical manual*, ed 2, St Louis, 1999, Mosby.

Box 17-6	Additional Factors to Consider when Assessing Pain in the Elderly

Function: How is the pain affecting the elder's ability to participate in usual activities, perform activities of daily living and instrumental activities of daily living?

Alternative expression of pain: Have there been recent changes in cognitive ability or behavior, such as increased pacing, grimacing, or irritability? Is there an increase in the number of complaints? Are they vague and difficult to respond to? Has there been a change in sleep-wake patterns? Is the person resisting certain activities, movements, or positions?

Social support: What are the resources available to the elder in pain? What is the role of the elder in the social system, and how is pain affecting this role? How is pain affecting the elder's relationship with others?

Pain history: How has the elder managed previous experiences with pain? What is the perceived meaning of the past and present pain? What are the cultural factors that affect the elder's ability to express pain and receive relief?

Box 17-7	Mnemonics for Pain Assessment

Pain is real (Believe the patient!)
Ask about pain regularly
Isolation (psychological and social problems)
Notice nonverbal pain signs
Evaluate pain characteristics
Does pain impair function?

Onset
Location
Duration

Characteristics
Aggravating factors
Relieving factors
Treatment previously tried

From *Aging Successfully* (newsletter of the Division of Geriatric Medicine, St Louis University School of Medicine; Geriatric Research, Education and Clinical Centers, St Louis Veterans Administration Medical Center; the Gateway Geriatric Education Center of Missouri and Illinois) 11(3):6, 2001.

helpful when working with those with cognitive limitations.

Assessment then moves to a detailed description of pain intensity, frequency, quality, location, and aggravating and alleviating factors (AGS, 2002) (Box 17-6). This information requires careful evaluation since treatment may differ based on the etiology of the complaint (Herr, 2002). The McGill Pain Assessment Questionnaire (Melzack, 1975) is a comprehensive tool that is useful for initial pain assessment and is used as a standard in many settings. However, the tool is lengthy, relies heavily on verbal and cognitive capacity, and may not be useful for some older people. Figure 17-1 presents an alternative initial pain assessment instrument that would cover all the essential components. Medication history, including over-the-counter drugs, is also part of assessment. Screening for cognitive impairment (dementia, delirium), depression, and assessment of other quality of life indicators, such as functional assessment, nutrition, sleep, and involvement and enjoyment of social activities, should

also be included (AGS, 2002; Herr, 2002). Box 17-7 presents a mnemonic for pain assessment that nurses may find helpful.

There should also be an assessment of pain that may occur during activity, such as in the physical therapy during a period of rehabilitation or in day-to-day nursing activities. Travis et al (2003) use the term *iatrogenic disturbance pain (IDP)* to describe a type of pain that can be caused by the care provider. The authors suggest that in some circumstances, tasks such as application of a blood pressure cuff, transfers out of bed, bathing, and moving and repositioning patients in the bed may cause levels of discomfort. Patients with severe physical limitations such as contractures or significant cognitive impairment and persons at the end of life may be particularly likely to experience IDP. Travis et al (2003) suggest the use of a 5-day IDP Tracking Sheet for assessment and monitoring of IDP. Other suggestions provided include gentle handling, adequate staffing, appropriate lifting devices and techniques, medication before care or treatments that may cause discomfort, and

INITIAL PAIN ASSESSMENT TOOL   Date _____

Patient's name _____ Age _____ Room _____

Diagnosis _____ Physician _____

Nurse _____

I. LOCATION: Patient or nurse mark drawing.

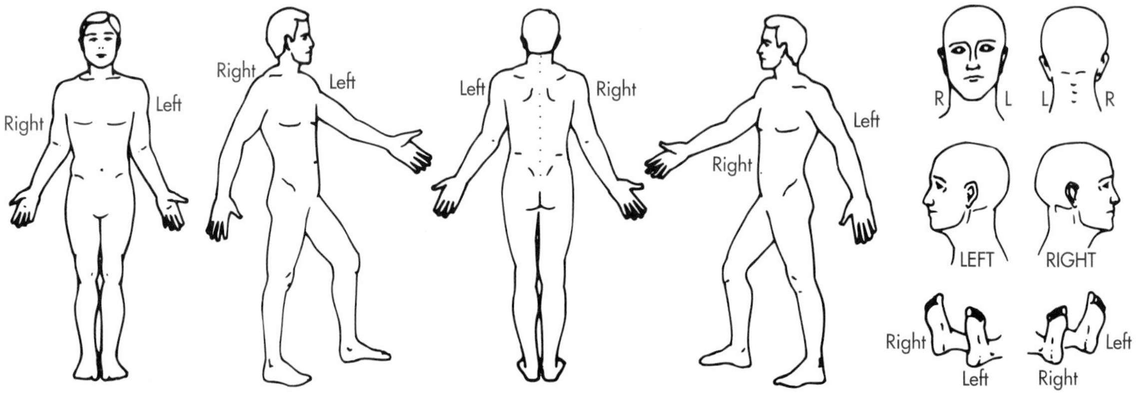

II. INTENSITY: Patient rates the pain. Scale used _____

    Present: _____
    Worst pain gets: _____
    Best pain gets: _____
    Acceptable level of pain: _____

III. QUALITY: (Use patient's own words, e.g., *prick, ache, burn, throb, pull, sharp.*) _____

IV. ONSET, DURATION VARIATIONS, RHYTHMS: _____

V. MANNER OF EXPRESSING PAIN: _____

VI. WHAT RELIEVES THE PAIN? _____

VII. WHAT CAUSES OR INCREASES THE PAIN? _____

VIII. EFFECTS OF PAIN: (Note decreased function, decreased quality of life.) _____
    Accompanying symptoms (e.g., nausea) _____
    Sleep _____
    Appetite _____
    Physical activity _____
    Relationship with others (e.g., irritability) _____
    Emotions (e.g., anger, suicidal, crying) _____
    Concentration _____
    Other _____

IX. OTHER COMMENTS: _____

X. PLAN: _____

Figure 17-1 Pain assessment. (From McCaffery M, Bebee A: *Pain: clinical manual of nursing practice,* St Louis, 1989, Mosby.)

education of staff on lifting and moving techniques and assessment of discomfort during care provision.

Pain Rating Scales

A key component to pain assessment is the individual's rating of the intensity of pain. This rating can be used to determine the patient's level of pain at the time of the assessment and the worst, the best, and the desired level (Figure 17-2). When the same scale is used over time, it provides a reliable measure of the effectiveness of the pain-relieving interventions; thus use of the same scale is highly recommended. A variety of scales have been developed with variations for persons with or without cognitive impairment. For cognitively intact older adults, the Verbal Descriptor Scale (VDS), the Pain Thermometer, an adaptation of the VDS, and the Numeric Rating Scale are the best choices and have been shown to be effective in the older adult population (Herr, 2002). Verbal descriptor scales include adjectives describing pain, such as mild, moderate, severe, worst pain imaginable. The Pain Thermometer is a diagram of a thermometer with word descriptions that show increasing pain intensities. The FACES Pain Scale (FPS), a series of faces each depicting a different facial expression indicating level of pain, was originally developed for children but may be effective for older adults as well, especially for persons with poorer verbal skills. The Painometer, a handheld tool developed by Dr. Fannie Gaston-Johanson, incorporates many of the features of existing scales to make it a multidimensional approach. It has been clinically tested and meets the current practice guidelines. JCAHO approved its use in May 2000 with implementation beginning in 2001 (Mattson, 2000). Sample pain rating scales are presented in Figure 17-3.

Special Considerations for Older People with Cognitive Impairments

For the nurse to conduct an adequate assessment of pain in persons with cognitive impairments he or she usually will need to engage the persons who are most familiar with the patient on a relatively intimate basis, either informal (family) or formal (nursing assistants) caregivers. They can be asked about their observations of potentially pain-related behaviors. Some of the nonspecific symptoms that may indicate pain in cognitively impaired older adults or those who are very frail may include the following:

- Frowning, grimacing, fidgeting, crying
- Disruptive vocalizations, striking out
- Withdrawal, refusal to participate in activities
- Eating and sleeping poorly
- Exiting behavior, pacing

Careful observation of nonverbal pain behaviors and changes in behavior patterns is important in assessment of pain in cognitively impaired elders. However, nurses should also ask the person, regardless of assessed cognitive function, about his or her experience of pain. Several studies have found that older people with mild to moderate cognitive impairment can respond to pain scales with some adaptation and simple questions about pain (Herr, 2002). Once behaviors that appear to indicate pain and pain relief are identified, these should be recorded clearly in the plan of care for use by all care providers.

Too often, cognitively impaired elders are medicated with antipsychotic or anxiolytic medications for aggressive behaviors when the underlying problem is pain. Since the use of these medications significantly increases the risk to the patient, they should be avoided (see Chapter 15). Kovach et al (1999) designed a protocol related to pain and discomfort in people with dementia. The Assessment of Discomfort in Dementia (ADD) protocol is designed to more effectively assess both physical pain and affective discomfort and guide its appropriate treatment, which will in turn decrease the inappropriate use of psychotropic medications. This instrument is unique in that it also assesses affective discomfort, defined by Kovach et al (1999) as an unpleasant internal state resulting from nonphysiological stimuli. Kovach et al state: "For the person with late stage dementia, a good deal of their discomfort comes from non-physiological sources, for example, from difficulty sorting out and negotiating everyday life activities" (p 412). The ADD protocol directs nurses to look first for physical causes of discomfort (infection, illness, chronic conditions causing pain, noise, uncomfortable positioning, poorly fitting clothing or shoes) if behavior is unusual, review the patient's history for potentially painful conditions (compression fractures, old fractures), utilize comfort measures (music,

Brief Pain Inventory

Date _____ / _____ / _____   Time: _____
Name: _____ _____ _____
        Last   First   Middle Initial

1) Throughout our lives, most of us have had pain from time to time (such as minor headaches, sprains, and toothaches). Have you had pain other than these everyday kinds of pain today?
   1. Yes   2. No

2) On the diagram, shade in the areas where you feel pain. Put an X on the area that hurts the most.

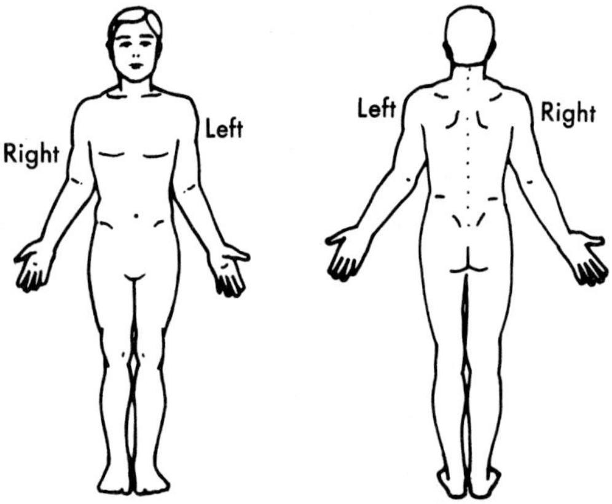

3) Please rate your pain by circling the one number that best describes your pain at its **worst** in the past 24 hours.

0 1 2 3 4 5 6 7 8 9 10
No   Pain as bad as
pain   you can imagine

4) Please rate your pain by circling the one number that best describes your pain at its **least** in the past 24 hours.

0 1 2 3 4 5 6 7 8 9 10
No   Pain as bad as
pain   you can imagine

5) Please rate your pain by circling the one number that best describes your pain on the **average.**

0 1 2 3 4 5 6 7 8 9 10
No   Pain as bad as
pain   you can imagine

6) Please rate your pain by circling the one number that tells how much pain you have **right now.**

0 1 2 3 4 5 6 7 8 9 10
No   Pain as bad as
pain   you can imagine

7) What treatments or medications are you receiving for your pain?

_____

_____

8) In the past 24 hours, how much **relief** have pain treatments or medications provided? Please circle the one percentage that most shows how much relief you have received.

0% 10 20 30 40 50 60 70 80 90 100%
No   Complete
relief   relief

9) Circle the one number that describes how, during the past 24 hours, pain has **interfered** with your:
   A. General activity

0 1 2 3 4 5 6 7 8 9 10
Does not   Completely
interfere   interferes

   B. Mood

0 1 2 3 4 5 6 7 8 9 10
Does not   Completely
interfere   interferes

   C. Walking ability

0 1 2 3 4 5 6 7 8 9 10
Does not   Completely
interfere   interferes

   D. Normal work (includes both work outside the home and housework)

0 1 2 3 4 5 6 7 8 9 10
Does not   Completely
interfere   interferes

   E. Relations with other people

0 1 2 3 4 5 6 7 8 9 10
Does not   Completely
interfere   interferes

   F. Sleep

0 1 2 3 4 5 6 7 8 9 10
Does not   Completely
interfere   interferes

   G. Enjoyment of life

0 1 2 3 4 5 6 7 8 9 10
Does not   Completely
interfere   interferes

May be duplicated for use in clinical practice.

Figure 17-2 Brief pain inventory. (Copyright Charles S. Cleeland, PhD, Houston.)

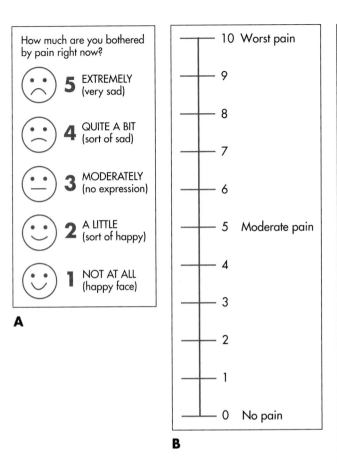

A

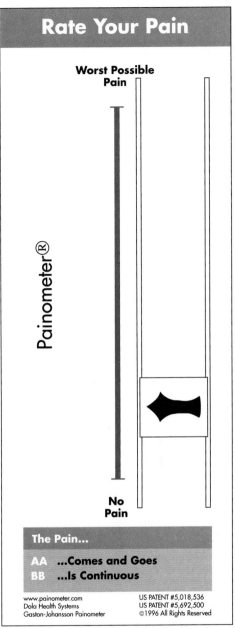

B

C

May be duplicated for use in clinical practice.

Figure 17-3 Examples of commonly used pain assessment scales. **A**, Example of a visual analog scale (VAS), these are either a series of faces or colors of varying intensities. **B**, Example of a numeric rating scale (NRS), length, direction (horizontal or vertical), and number of choices varies. Sometimes the VAS and NRS are combined on one instrument. **C**, is a hand-held slide device measure as a variation of the above. **C**, Copyright © 1996, Fannie Gaston-Johansson, Dr. Med Sc., RN, FAAN, Baltimore. For more scale examples see: www.stat.washington.edu/TALARIA/attachb3.html and www.va.gov/oaa/pocketcard/section4.asp.

massage, therapeutic communication, fluid or food, repositioning, changing incontinence products or toileting). If no source of pain can be found, administer a prescribed nonopioid pain reliever if comfort measures have no effect on behavior, and consult with the health care provider if the pain medication does not improve behavior. Other scales to assist with behavioral observation of pain in cognitively impaired older people include the Checklist on Nonverbal Pain Indicators (Feldt, 2000) and the Discomfort Scale (Hurley et al, 1992).

Interventions

Pharmacological, nonpharmacological, and other comfort measures can relieve or minimize pain. An awareness of the totally pervasive nature of pain, as well as the multifactorial components influencing pain, requires a holistic approach in nursing interventions. Interventions include appropriate administration of pharmacological agents and use of nonpharmacological interventions with careful and systematic evaluation of response. An appreciation of the psychological and social consequences of pain includes careful listening, unconditional positive regard, and ongoing support and mobilization of resources. Pain can be minimized through gentle handling, touch, and careful observation of the person's reaction to procedures. Use of pillows for support or body positioning, appropriate and comfortable seating and mattresses, frequent rest periods, and pacing of activities to balance activity and rest are important.

The nurse should encourage the patient to stay as active as possible. Gaumer (1974) found that the less active an individual was, the less tolerable activity became. Anyone who becomes inactive will feel more aches and pain than the active person. Distraction through the use of activity may help to change the behavior of the individual who uses pain to gain attention and sympathy. Some people have pain with a specific activity (e.g., in rehabilitation); they may become very anxious in anticipation of pain. In this case the plan of care should include both pharmacological and nonpharmacological interventions before the recommended activity. Administering an effective medication 20 to 30 minutes before the specific activity may eventually lessen or eliminate the

fear of discomfort and can greatly enhance the individual's capacity for that activity. The nurse should learn the patient's body potential for coping with pain and work within those parameters.

The nurse encourages elders to have a role in the management of their pain. The patient can be involved by keeping a weekly journal that includes an account of pain during the day; the times, type, and dose of medication taken; its effect; and the duration of its benefit. This type of information helps establish patterns that may be useful in improving pain management by adjusting activity, providing medications appropriately, and helping the patient feel useful and in control of some aspect of care. An example of a symptom severity log can be found at http://www.amda.com/clinical/chronicpain. The diary should be reviewed with the care provider to assess the relationship among pain, medication use, and activity. The pain graph provides a visual picture of the highs and lows of the pain. The caregiver can assist in the plotting of the pain experience when necessary.

Pharmacological Measures

Generally, pain relief is accomplished by medication aimed at altering sensory transmission to the cerebral cortex. Various analgesics (nonnarcotic and narcotic agents) as well as adjuvant medications (antidepressants, anticonvulsants) are currently available for use and may be prescribed to the older adult. The general principles of pain control for older adults are the same as for younger adults; however, older adults may experience more adverse drug reactions related to age-associated changes in drug absorption, distribution, metabolism, and excretion. Older adults with multiple chronic illnesses requiring a number of medications are also more susceptible to drug reactions and interactions. Some products used in younger adults, for example, meperidine (Demerol), is contraindicated in the older adult (see Chapter 15). General principles of appropriate pain management in older adults are presented in Box 17-8. Two essential guidelines for the management of pain in older people are provided by the AGS's publication *The Management of Persistent Pain in Older Persons* (AGS, 2002) and the American Medical Directors Association's publication *Pain Management in the Long-Term*

| Box 17-8 | Principles of Pain Management in the Elderly |

- Always ask elderly patients about pain.
- Accept the patient's word about pain and its intensity.
- Never underestimate the potential effects of chronic pain on the patient's overall condition and quality of life.
- Be compulsive about pain assessment. An accurate diagnosis will lead to more effective treatment.
- Treat pain to facilitate diagnostic procedures or uncomfortable care routines. Do not wait for a diagnosis to relieve pain and needless suffering.
- Carefully observe behavior and reactions of older adults with cognitive impairment for pain. Consider pain first with a change in behavior. Involve family and caregivers in assessment of pain for cognitively impaired elders.
- Use verbal descriptor scales for rating of pain intensity. Ensure that the scale is large enough for an older adult with vision impairment to read. Explain fully.
- Use a combination of pharmacological and nonpharmacological measures whenever possible.
- Give adequate amounts of drug at the appropriate frequency to control pain based on constant assessment.
- Use analgesic drugs correctly. With opioids, start with a low dosage and increase slowly. Titrate to the desired effect or to intolerable side effects. Use around-the-clock dosing whenever possible.
- Use noninvasive route first, and try to make drug regimen as simple as possible, avoiding multiple medications and frequent dosing. Choose medications with the fewest side effects. Assess all medications, including over-the-counter drugs, for interactions.
- Anticipate and prevent side effects common in elders:
  - Give antiinflammatory drugs with food.
  - Begin bowel regimen early to prevent constipation.
  - Be prepared to give an antinausea medication with narcotic analgesic drugs.
  - Anticipate some impaired balance and cognitive function with narcotic analgesic drugs.
- Consult an equianalgesic potency table when changing medication.
- There is no role for placebos in assessment or management of pain.
- Mobilize the patient physically and psychologically. Involve the patient in his or her own care.
- Anticipate and attend to anxiety and depression.
- Reassess responses to treatment at regular intervals. Alter therapy to maximize pain relief and improve functional status and quality of life.

Modified from Ferrell BA: Pain management in elderly people, *J Am Geriatr Soc* 39:64-73, 1991; Glickstein JK, editor: Managing chronic pain, *Focus Geriatr Care Rehabil* 10(3):6, 1996.

Care Setting (American Medical Directors Association, 2003). Information about these documents can be found on the organizations' respective websites (http://www.americangeriatrics.org and http://www.amda.com).

Most nurses should be familiar with the essential principles of pain control as described by the World Health Organization's three-step ladder approach of pharmacological pain control (WHO, 1990), starting with the use of nonopioid analgesics (acetaminophen) and progressing to antiinflammatory drugs (NSAIDs) and finally opioids (Figure 17-4). The use of this approach is also rec-

ommended for the elderly (AGS, 2002). In addition, adjuvant analgesic drugs, such as low doses of anticonvulsants and antidepressants, are particularly useful for neuropathic pain. Effective management of pain may require a combination of all of these medications as indicated in the WHO ladder. For persistent pain, around-the-clock dosing is recommended because it provides a more stable therapeutic plasma level of drug and eliminates the extremes of overmedication and undermedication. The goal of pain management therapy, particularly for persistent pain, is to prevent the pain, not simply relieve it. As-needed

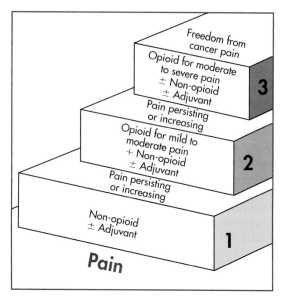

Freedom from
cancer pain

Opioid for moderate
to severe pain
± Non-opioid
± Adjuvant

3

Pain persisting
or increasing

Opioid for mild to
moderate pain
+ Non-opioid
± Adjuvant

2

Pain persisting
or increasing

Non-opioid
± Adjuvant

1

Pain

Figure 17-4 World Health Organization (WHO) three-step analgesic ladder. (Redrawn from World Health Organization: *Cancer pain relief,* ed 2, Geneva, 1996, WHO.)

the-counter NSAIDs is common to relieve pain associated with osteoarthritis and degenerative joint disease. Often, older people, and some nurses, think that these medications may not be harmful. However, acetaminophen and NSAIDs must be used with caution because of increased risk of adverse effects, especially gastrointestinal bleeding and renal and hepatic impairments.

NSAIDs can potentiate and increase or decrease the effect of many prescription medications that older people are likely to be taking. The most problematic interactions are with anticoagulants, oral hypoglycemics, diuretics, and antihypertensives. It is estimated that over 16,000 NSAID-related deaths occur each year among patients with osteoarthritis and rheumatoid arthritis, making it the fifteenth most common cause of death in the United States (Durrance, 2003). As cited in Durrance (2003), Mercola (2002) reported that older people taking over-the-counter medications twice per week for 2 months were more likely to have beginning stages of chronic kidney failure. Risk for gastrointestinal bleeding is high, particularly in frail older adults with multisystem disease.

Alternatives include topical therapies (e.g., capsaicin, lidocaine patch) for persons with intact skin.

Clearly, the use of medications, even the nonopioids, requires careful review for potential drug interactions, monitoring for side effects and interactions, and patient teaching about safety when using over-the-counter NSAIDs (Durrance, 2003). If long-term management of pain is necessary, the opioids may be preferred because of their lower rate of adverse reactions.

Opioid analgesics. Opioid medications are used for acute pain as well as both malignant (cancer) and nonmalignant persistent pain. Opiates produce a greater analgesic effect, a higher peak, and a longer duration of effect in older adults. Recommendations are to start with the lowest anticipated effective dose, monitor response frequently, and titrate slowly to desired effect. Generally, an initial dose should be one-half to two-thirds the usual dose given to a younger person and, as needed, increased in increments of 25% (Pasero et al, 1999b; Portenoy et al, 1999; Young, 1999). Long-acting or sustained-release analgesics should be used for continuous pain, and breakthrough pain should be treated with fast-onset, short-acting preparations.

or prn medications should be used freely for intermittent pain that "breaks through" the around-the-clock management (ATC) (Fine, 2002; Herr, 2002). Use of opioids for long-term chronic pain control in older people should be convenient, easy to administer, and short acting for ease of dose adjustment. The simplest drug regimen is more likely to be effective and to be followed more easily.

Nonopioid analgesics. Acetaminophen (Tylenol) is often adequate for mild to moderate pain relief; if used for persistent pain, around-the-clock dosing may provide adequate relief. The maximum dose of 4 g (4000 mg) is reduced for people with renal or hepatic dysfunction or who drink alcohol. Although this seems like a high dose, with the availability of products such as Extra-Strength Tylenol at 500 mg per tablet, it may be reached quickly.

If acetaminophen is not effective or is not tolerated, nonacetylated salicylates (trisalicylate, choline magnesium) may also be effective or one of the many NSAIDs that are available (e.g., aspirin, ibuprofen [Advil, Motrin]), may be used (AGS, 2002). Among older people, the use of over-

Side effects of opioids include gait disturbance, dizziness, sedation, falls, nausea, pruritus (rash), and constipation. Several of these will resolve on their own as the body becomes adjusted to the drug (tolerance). The side effects may be prevented when the prescribing provider works closely with the patient and the nurse to slowly increase (titrate) the dose of the drug to a point where the best relief can be obtained with the fewest side effects. The nurse provides close observation of the person's response and prevention and prompt treatment of side effects. Since constipation is almost universal when opioids are used in older patients, the nurse should ensure that an appropriate bowel regimen is ordered at the same time as the opioids. A daily dose of a combination stool softener and mild laxative may be very helpful, and adequate fluid intake is needed. Prophylactic use of antiemetics may be helpful for nausea until tolerance develops. Lynch (2001) suggests that if nausea or vomiting continues, the provider may be asked about switching to a different drug or brand.

All opioid treatment should begin with "as needed" doses of short-acting medications and should be titrated based on response and side effects (Lynch, 2001). Sedation and impaired cognition do occur when opioid analgesics are started or doses increased. This often causes great concern from patients, families, and nurses. The AGS guidelines state that this is to be expected and patients and caregivers should be cautioned about the potential for falls and appropriate safety precautions instituted. Starting with low doses of short-acting opioids and titrating slowly can help to avoid these effects. Once an effective dose has been reached, conversion is made to long-acting opioids to achieve a steady-state, round-the-clock effect. As needed, opioids are then used for break-through, PRN treatment. Sedation usually resolves with the development of tolerance, and if it is persistent, use of psychostimulant medications (e.g., methylphenidate [Ritalin]) might be helpful (Lynch, 2001; AGS, 2002). Respiratory depression is uncommon in patients taking opioids, and sedation always precedes respiratory depression. Profound sedation or respiratory depression requires use of naloxone (Narcan) (AGS, 2002).

Opioids that can safely be used with the older adult are morphine, oxycodone, hydrocodone, hydromorphone, and transdermal fentanyl. Most are available in multiple forms. Fentanyl is available in a transdermal delivery system (Duragesic) as well as an oral transmucosal lozenge (Actiq). The transdermal form depends on absorption through body fat and should not be used in persons who are underweight.

Most of the other opioids are not recommended for use in older adults because of problems with the toxicity of metabolites that are produced as they are metabolized. The use of meperidine (Demerol) is absolutely contraindicated. The metabolites of meperidine can quickly produce confusion, psychotic behavior, and seizure activity. The same can be said for pentazocine (Talwin), Tramadol (Ultram), and methadone. Propoxyphene (Darvon) has a long half-life and a metabolite that has been associated with cardiac irregularities and pulmonary edema and is not recommended (Lynch, 2001). The nurse can refer to the Agency for Healthcare Research and Quality (formerly AHCPR) guidelines for acute and chronic pain management as well as the latest equianalgesic charts if they are needed (http://www.ahrq.gov).

Adjuvant drugs. Adjuvant medications have been developed for purposes other than analgesia (tricyclic antidepressants, anticonvulsants) but are thought to alter or modulate the perception of pain. They may be used alone or in combination with nonopioid or opioid analgesics and are particularly effective for sharp, shooting, dull, aching, or burning pain associated with neuropathic conditions. Used in combination with analgesics, they may potentiate (enhance) the overall analgesic effects. Elders frequently respond well to adjuvant pain regimens. However, it is important to remember that many adjuvant drugs have a very long half-life, which increases the plasma concentration in elders. When this group of medications is used the nurse has to be especially diligent to watch for adverse effects or early signs of toxicity (see Chapter 15).

Nonpharmacological Measures

Nurses have a long history of comforting patients through nonpharmacological measures and the psychological modulation of pain by providing understanding and support as well as specific techniques either performed by the nurse or at the recommendation of the nurse. Nurses are also responsible for meeting patients' education needs regarding pain management in their work with older adults, their families, and other caregivers. Excellent patient brochures about persistent pain as well as assessment of pain in cognitively impaired older people are available from the AGS (http://www.americangeriatrics.org).

It has now been shown that a combination of pharmacological and nonpharmacological interventions appears to be most effective in the relief of both acute and chronic pain. The basic approach to pain control is one that considers that whatever has worked in the past and been effective without causing harm; these should be encouraged. This is particularly applicable for older adults with a lifetime of experience at managing pain with both the approaches used in Western medicine and those learned through their cultural heritages. More and more of the nonpharmacological measures are gaining acceptance by both patients and insurers such as Medicare. Several methods that elders use are briefly reviewed here but acknowledged as far from inclusive of all of those used. Table 17-2 compares several of the nonpharmacological pain relief measures.

Cutaneous nerve stimulation. Deep and superficial stimulation of nerves for the purpose of pain relief has been practiced for centuries. Nurses have long provided massage, vibration, heat, cold, and ointments. Heat and cold temporarily interrupt the transmission of pain impulses to the cerebral pain center; however, caution must be used in consideration of the pathological cause of the pain. Heat is effective for some disorders, such as the deep pain of inflammatory musculoskeletal conditions such as rheumatic conditions. Heat will increase the circulation to the area and therefore is contraindicated in occlusive vascular disease and in nonexpansive tissue such as bursae (some joints), where it may increase pain. At the same time intermittent application of cold packs is helpful in low back pain and some situations of nerve irritation. Care must be taken when applying heat and cold to the skin of the aged to prevent skin damage from extended periods of heat and cold applications.

Transcutaneous electrical nerve stimulation. Another method of cutaneous stimulation is transcutaneous electrical nerve stimulation (TENS) or another form, namely, PENS (percuta-neous electrical nerve stimulation). Electrodes taped to the skin over the pain site or on the spine emit a mild electrical current that is felt as a tingling, buzzing, or vibrating sensation. The patient operates the stimulator and starts the electrical impulses, which then activate the large nerve fibers that transmit impulses to close the hypothetical gate in the spinal cord and prevent pain signals from reaching the brain. PENS and TENS have been helpful in phantom limb pain, postherpetic neuralgia, and low back pain (Resnick, 2003). In many cases Medicare will pay for the use of a prescribed TENS unit. Units are often available through the physical therapy department of skilled nursing facilities.

Touch. Touch is a natural form of providing comfort, although its therapeutic properties are still not clearly understood. Sometimes touch is considered a cutaneous stimulation technique, such as the specific techniques of "therapeutic touch." In this technique, developed by nurse Delores Kreiger (1992), hands placed on or near the body with the concentrated intention of healing has been found to be effective in some cases but not in others (Mackey, 1995). When combined with purposeful relaxation touch has also been found to decrease anxiety, reduce muscle tension, and help relieve pain.

Perceptual tendencies and sensory dimensions influence pain reactions and tolerance. Persons who were sensory deprived exhibited low pain tolerance, but those who received adequate or a high degree of sensory stimulation possessed a high pain tolerance. Fakouri and Jones (1987) demonstrated the positive effects of a 3-minute, slow-stroke back rub on both sides of the spinous processes from the crown of the head to the sacrum as a means of promoting relaxation in the aged. The back rub resulted in a decrease in heart rate and blood pressure and an increase in skin temperature. Meek (1993) found that slow-stroking back massage increased relaxation, decreased blood pressure and heart rate, and increased body temperature of hospice patients. No mention was made of its effect on pain. However, it is known that tension and anxiety reduction can contribute to an increase in pain tolerance.

Acupuncture and acupressure. Acute pain is registered as pain impulses pass through the gate of the spine and register the sensation in

Table 17-2 Advantages and Disadvantages of Nonpharmacological Measures

Therapy	Advantages	Disadvantages
Cutaneous nerve stimulation TENS PENS Touch Acupuncture, acupressure	Pleasurable sensations make them popular with elders Pain decreases during and after stimulation Requires little patient participation Good for those with limited mobility Relaxation and distraction from pain May be feasible for elders with limited income Requires limited energy expenditure Self-administration provides a sense of control	Some elders perceive stimulation as objectionable; odors from creams and ointments intolerable, such as menthol Improper use of heat, cold, etc. may do tissue damage Choice may be limited by cognitive and sensory impairment TENS requires special education and learning
Distraction: tactile, auditory, visual, kinesthetic	Improved mood Easy to learn Relaxation Increased pain tolerance	Lasts only as long as stimulus present
Relaxation	Decreases skeletal muscle tension Decreases anxiety Useful with chronic pain, muscle spasms, sleep loss caused by pain	Must be able to understand instructions Takes time and energy to learn Ineffective with depressed or very fatigued person Must be practiced daily
Biofeedback	Decreases chronic pain	Requires equipment (moderate to expensive), time, and energy to learn Must be cognitively intact
Imagery	Very simple, uses elder's imagination: may enhance relaxation and distraction; may feel control over pain; may perceive an escape from pain; always available Little or no economic or social impact for elderly	Must be cognitively intact Not all health professionals able to teach it
Hypnosis	Pain relief on a long-term basis without side effects Useful for elders unable to tolerate pharmacological measures Does not alter mental function (a fear of the elderly)	Feel loss of mental control Must be cognitively intact Requires trained personnel May not be available in remote or small settings May be too expensive

Developed by Patricia Hess.

TENS, Trancutaneous electrical nerve stimulation; *PENS*, percutaneous electrical nerve stimulation.

the brain, which in turn signals the central mechanism of the brain to return counterimpulses, which close the gate. It is thought that acupuncture and acupressure stimulate nerves clusters that cause the gate to close more quickly or that they trigger the release of the body's own opiate substances, enkephalins (endorphins). Acupuncture and acupressure are therapies with growing scientific evidence of their effectiveness for chronic pain (National Institutes of Health, 1990; Berman, Swyer, 1999; Lee, 2000). In some cases Medicare and some private insurance companies will pay for the cost of acupuncture treatment from a licensed acupuncturist.

Biofeedback. Biofeedback is a cognitive behavioral strategy. An individual can learn voluntary control over some body processes and alter them by changing the physiological correlates appropriate to them. Response to certain types of pain can be controlled. Boczkowski (1984) found that biofeedback decreased the chronic pain of rheumatoid arthritis. Other studies demonstrated no appreciable effect of biofeedback on migraine headaches in the elderly (Hamm, King, 1984). Training and often time and equipment of some type are needed to learn how to alter one's body response.

Distraction. Distraction is a behavioral strategy that lessens the perception of pain by drawing the person's attention away from the pain and relegating it to peripheral awareness. In some instances the individual is completely unaware of the pain; in other instances the intensity of pain is significantly diminished. The success of distraction can be explained by the gate theory (see Acupuncture and Acupressure above). Pain messages are slower than diversional messages; therefore the gate closes before the pain signal arrives, and less pain is felt.

Mild to moderate pain responds well to distraction. At times, if an individual concentrates intently on another subject, the acute pain may be relieved. The most common forms of distraction include slow rhythmical breathing, slow rhythmical massage, rhythmical singing or tapping, active listening, guided imagery, and humor (Kosier et al, 1995; Jeffery, Lubkin, 2002). McCaffrey and Freeman (2003) found music as a form of distraction to be helpful when dealing with pain from osteoarthritis.

Relaxation, meditation, and imagery. As a behavioral strategy, relaxation enables the quieting of the mind and muscles, providing the release of tension and anxiety. Relaxation should be adjunctive to all pharmacological interventions. Meditation and imagery are two methods of promoting relaxation. Imagery uses the client's imagination to focus on settings full of happiness and relaxation rather than on stressful situations. Several studies using guided imagery have shown that there was a decrease in pain perception in foot pain and abdominal pain. It was suggested that a strong image of a pain-free state effectively alters the autonomic nervous system's responses to pain (Hamm, King, 1984; Griffin, 1986; Pearson, 1987; McCaffery, Pasero, 1999).

Hypnosis. Hypnosis, another behavioral strategy, can be used to alter pain perception, thus blocking pain awareness; to substitute another feeling for a painful one; to displace pain sensation to a smaller body area; or to alter the meaning of pain so that it is viewed as less important and less debilitating (Thomas, 1990; Sarvis, 1995). Research has demonstrated that hypnotic analgesia reduces what are called "overreactions" to pain when apprehension and stress are apparent. Most of the population has some capacity for hypnosis and with training can increase their control in this area.

Pain Clinics

Pain clinics provide a specialized, often comprehensive and multidisciplinary approach to the management of pain which has not responded to the usual, more standard approaches as described herein. The use of such pain clinics by the elderly has been limited. However their use should be encouraged when appropriate. The number and types of pain clinics and programs have increased as a response to continued poor pain management by general medical practice. Pain center programs may be inpatient, outpatient, or both. Pain clinics are generally one of three types: syndrome oriented, modality oriented, or comprehensive. Syndrome-oriented centers focus on a specific chronic pain problem, such as headache or arthritis pain. Modality-oriented centers focus on a specific treatment technique, such as relaxation or acupuncture/acupressure. The comprehensive centers tend to be larger and associated with medical centers. These centers include many services that require a thorough initial assessment (physical, mental, psychosocial). Only then can a comprehensive treatment plan with follow-up be developed. Staff members are usually part of a coordinated, multidisciplinary team consisting of physician, nurse, physical therapist, occupational therapist, massage therapist, rehabilitation specialist, and social worker.

The goals of pain management centers are to decrease pain intensity to a tolerable limit or eliminate it, if possible; improve functionality and activities of daily living (ADLs); increase involvement in family and social activities; decrease depression; and improve mood. This is accomplished by improving quality and frequency of

Box 17-9	Pain Control Plan

Pain Control Plan for _____

At home, I will take the following medications for pain control:

Medication	How to take	How many	How often	Comments
_____	_____	_____	_____	_____
_____	_____	_____	_____	_____

Medicines that I may take to help side effects:

Side effect	Medicine	How to take	How many	How often	Comments
_____	_____	_____	_____	_____	_____
_____	_____	_____	_____	_____	_____

Constipation is a very common problem when taking opioid medication. When this happens, do the following:

_____ Increase fluid intake (8 to 10 glasses of fluid per day)
_____ Exercise regularly
_____ Increase fiber in diet (bran, fresh fruit, vegetables)
_____ Use a mild laxative, such as milk of magnesia, if no nondrug pain control methods

_____
_____

If you do not have a bowel movement in 3 days:

_____ Take _____ every day at _____ (time) with a full glass of water.
_____ Use a glycerin suppository every morning (this may help make a bowel movement less painful).

Additional instructions:

_____
_____

Important phone numbers:

Your doctor _____   Your nurse _____
Your pharmacy _____   Emergencies _____

Call your doctor or nurse immediately if your pain increases or if you have new pain. Also call your doctor early for a refill of pain medication. Do not let your medication get below 3 or 4 days' supply.

From *Managing cancer pain*, consumer version. Clinical Practice Guideline, AHCPR pub no. 9, Rockville, Md, 1994, U.S. Department of Health and Human Services, Public Health Service, Agency for Health Care Policy and Research.

assessment, improving optimal use of analgesics, assisting in minimizing analgesic adverse reactions, and documenting outcomes associated with treatment. Physiological and cognitive-behavioral modalities are used to reduce or alleviate pain. The nurse should be familiar with the types of pain management clinics to provide the patient and family with necessary information to make a knowledgeable decision in selecting a center.

Evaluation

Evaluation of pain relief outcomes requires reassessment of the patient's status. Reevaluation

of the frequency and intensity of pain, behavioral signs and symptoms that suggest pain, response to pharmacological and nonpharmacological interventions, and the impact of pain on mood, ADLs, sleep, and other quality of life measures are all included in ongoing reassessment. Adjustments of treatment regimens and interventions are based on reassessment findings. Active involvement of the patient, family, and all caregivers is essential for comprehensive pain assessment, management, and evaluation. Box 17-9 presents a pain control plan.

A comprehensive article discussing pain assessment and management and nursing responsibilities (Hanks-Bell et al, 2003) can be found at

NANDA and Wellness Diagnoses

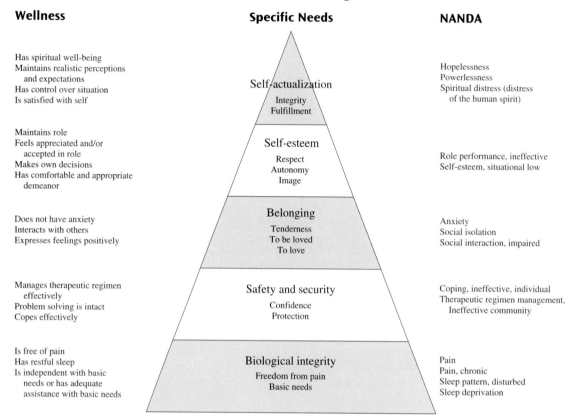

Wellness	Specific Needs	NANDA
Has spiritual well-being Maintains realistic perceptions and expectations Has control over situation Is satisfied with self	**Self-actualization** Integrity Fulfillment	Hopelessness Powerlessness Spiritual distress (distress of the human spirit)
Maintains role Feels appreciated and/or accepted in role Makes own decisions Has comfortable and appropriate demeanor	**Self-esteem** Respect Autonomy Image	Role performance, ineffective Self-esteem, situational low
Does not have anxiety Interacts with others Expresses feelings positively	**Belonging** Tenderness To be loved To love	Anxiety Social isolation Social interaction, impaired
Manages therapeutic regimen effectively Problem solving is intact Copes effectively	**Safety and security** Confidence Protection	Coping, ineffective, individual Therapeutic regimen management, Ineffective community
Is free of pain Has restful sleep Is independent with basic needs or has adequate assistance with basic needs	**Biological integrity** Freedom from pain Basic needs	Pain Pain, chronic Sleep pattern, disturbed Sleep deprivation

These are not all of the possible wellness or NANDA diagnoses that may be identified. The above are frequent examples of nursing diagnoses that should be considered when planning care for the older adult in whatever setting.

http://www.nurisngworld.org/ojin/topic21/tpc21_6.htm. Links to many references and descriptions of assessment tools and interventions are included in this reference. See also the work of Fulmer et al (1996) for a comprehensive protocol for management of acute pain in older adults.

▶ KEY CONCEPTS

- The absence of pain does not necessarily imply comfort. Comfort is a state of ease and satisfaction of body needs, as well as freedom from pain and anxiety.
- Assessment of pain is influenced by many misconceptions and myths and stereotypes about pain. Inadequate treatment of pain is a major concern in health care today.
- Culture, ethnicity, family, and individual characteristics all influence one's tolerance and expression of pain.
- Older people with various degrees of cognitive impairment may demonstrate pain by increased levels of confusion, restlessness, or withdrawal.
- Although it is sometimes assumed, it has not been shown that pain sensitivity and perception decrease with age.
- Pain is whatever the elder says it is. The nursing goal is to assist in pain relief. Some pain medications are more appropriate than others for use with elders.

- Acute pain and persistent pain require different therapeutic approaches. Persistent pain predominates in the lives of many older adults.
- Various combinations of pharmacological and nonpharmacological pain control can be effective but must be individually designed with the elder involved in the decision making.
- Giving a placebo is never justified.

Activities and Discussion Questions

1. What is pain?
2. Compare the features of acute and persistent pain.
3. List data necessary for an accurate pain assessment.
4. What are the barriers that interfere with assessment and treatment of pain for all patients? What barriers are associated with pain management in older people?
5. How might pain be expressed in cognitively impaired older people? How does assessment of pain differ in cognitively impaired older people?
6. What pharmacological and nonpharmacological therapy is available, and how can each type work with the other to relieve pain?
7. Develop a nursing care plan using wellness and North American Nursing Diagnosis Association (NANDA) diagnoses.

RESOURCES

Organizations

American Academy of Pain Management
13947 Mono Way #A
Sonora, CA 95370
(209) 533-9744
website: http://www.aapainmanage.org

American Chronic Pain Association
PO Box 850
Rocklin, CA 95677
(800) 533-3231
website: http://www.theacpa.org

American Pain Foundation
201 N. Charles Street, Suite 710
Baltimore, MD 21201
website: http://www.painfoundation.org

American Pain Society
4700 W. Lake Avenue
Glenview, IL 60025
(847) 375-4715
website: http://www.ampainsoc.org

American Society of Pain Management Nursing
7794 Grow Drive
Pensacola, FL 32514
(850) 484-7766
website: http://www.aspmn.org

International Association for the Study of Pain
909 NE 43rd Street, Suite 306
Seattle, WA 98105
(206) 547-6409
website: http://www.iasp-pain.org

National Center on Complementary and Alternative Medicine
PO Box 7923
Gaithersburg, MD 20898
(888) 644-6226
website: http://www.mccam.nih.gov

The National Chronic Pain Outreach Association, Inc.
7979 Old Georgetown Road, Suite 100
Bethesda, MD 20814
(301) 652-4948
website: http://www.chronicpain.org

Nurse Healers—Professional Associates International
Alamo Plaza, Suite 111R
4550 W. Oakey Boulevard
Las Vegas, NV 89102
(702) 870-5507
website: http://www.therapeutic-touch.org

REFERENCES

American Geriatrics Society (AGS): The management of persistent pain in older persons, *J Am Geriatr Soc* 50(6, suppl):S205-S224, 2002.

American Medical Directors Association: *Pain management in the long-term care setting, American Medical Directors Practice Guideline,* 2003. Available at http://www.amda.com.

American Pain Society: *Principles of analgesic use in the treatment of acute and cancer pain,* ed 3, Skokie, Ill, 1992, The Society.

Berman BM, Swyer JP: Complementary medicine treatments for fibromyalgia syndrome, *Baillieres Best Prac Res Clin Rheumatol* 13(3):487-492, 1999.

Boczkowski JA: Biofeedback training for the treatment of chronic pain in the elderly arthritic female, *Clin Gerontol* 2:39, 1984.

Chiu N: Herpes zoster. In Beers MH, Berkow R, editors: *The Merck manual of geriatrics,* ed 3, Whitehouse Station, NJ, 2000, Merck Research Laboratories.

Davis GC: Chronic pain management of older adults in residential settings, *J Gerontol Nurs* 23(6):16-22, 1997.

Diamond S, Urban G: Coping with postherpetic neuralgia, *Consultant* 42(5):639, 2002.

Durrance SA: Older adults and NSAIDs: avoiding adverse reactions, *Geriatr Nurs* 24(6):349-352, 2003.

Fakouri C, Jones P: Relaxation Rx: slow stroke back rub, *J Gerontol Nurs* 13(2):32-35, 1987.

Feldt KS: The checklist of nonverbal pain indicators, *Pain Manage Nurs* 1(1):13-21, 2000.

Feldt KS, Warne MA, Ryden MB: Examining pain in aggressive cognitively impaired older adults, *J Gerontol Nurs* 24(11):14-22, 1998.

Ferrell BA: Pain. In Beers MH, Berkow R, editors: *The Merck manual of geriatrics,* ed 3, Whitehouse Station, NJ, 2000, Merck Research Laboratories.

Ferrell BR, Ferrell BA: Easing the pain, *Geriatr Nurs* 11(4):175-178, 1990.

Fine PG: Chronic pain in long-term care: assessment, management, and improvement of quality indicators, Elder Care Summit Conference, San Francisco, April 24, 2002.

Frampton K: Vital sign #5: pain assessment and management in LTC requires a thorough, team-oriented care plan, *Caring for the Ages* 5(5), 2004. Available at http://www.amda.com/caring/may2004/pain.htm.

Fulmer TT, Mion LC, Bottrell MM: Pain management protocol, *Geriatr Nurs* 17(5):222-226, 1996.

Gaumer WC: Psychological potentials of chronic pain, *J Psychiatr Nurs* 12:23, 1974.

Gilchrest BA: Skin changes and disorders. In Abrams WB, Beers MH, Berkow R, editors: *The Merck manual of geriatrics,* ed 2, Whitehouse Station, NJ, 1995, Merck Research Laboratories.

Griffin M: In the mind's eye, *Am J Nurs* 86(7):804-806, 1986.

Hamm BH, King V: A holistic approach to pain control with geriatric clients, *J Holist Nurs* 11:32, 1984.

Hanks-Bell M, Halvey K, Paice J: Pain assessment and management in aging, *Online J Issues Nurs,* Aug 31, 2003. Available at www.nursingworld.org/ojin/topic21_6.htm.

Health news, NBC TV, Channel 4, Aug 5, 1999.

Herr K: Chronic pain challenges and assessment strategies, *J Gerontol Nurs* 28(1):20-27, 2002.

Hurley AC et al: Assessment of discomfort in advanced Alzheimer's patients, *Res Nurs Health* 15(5):369-377, 1992.

International Association for the Study of Pain: Position Statement, *Pain* 6:249, 1979.

International Association for the Study of Pain: Position Statement, *Pain* 1992.

Jeffery JE, Lubkin IM: Chronic pain. In Lubkin IM, Larsen PD, editors: *Chronic illness,* ed 5, Sudbury, Mass, 2002, Jones & Bartlett.

Kosier B et al: *Fundamentals of nursing: comfort and pain,* Redwood City, Calif, 1995, Addison-Wesley.

Kovach CR et al: Assessment and treatment of discomfort for people with late-stage dementia, *J Pain Symptom Manage* 18(6):412-419, 1999.

Kreiger D: *The therapeutic touch: how to use your hands to help or heal,* New York, 1992, Prentice-Hall.

Lee TL: Acupuncture and chronic pain management, *Ann Acad Med Singapore* 29(1):17-21, 2000.

Leo R, Singh A: Pain management in the elderly: use of psychopharmacologic agents, *Ann Long-Term Care* 10(2):37, 2002.

Lipman AG, Jackson KC: *Use of opioids in chronic noncancer pain,* Stamford, Conn, 2000, Purdue Pharm LP, Power-Pak, Inc.

Lynch M: Pain: the fifth vital sign: comprehensive assessment leads to proper treatment, *Adv Nurse Pract* 9(11):28-36, 2001.

Mackey RB: Discover the healing power of therapeutic touch, *Am J Nurs* 95(4):27, 1995.

Mattson JE: The language of pain, *Reflect Nurs Leadersh* 26(4):10-14, 2000.

McCaffery M, Beebe A: *Pain: clinical manual for nursing practice,* St Louis, 1989, Mosby.

McCaffery M, Pasero C: *Pain: clinical manual,* ed 2, St Louis, 1999, Mosby.

McCaffrey R, Freeman E: Effect of music on chronic osteoarthritic pain in older people, *Journ Adv Nsg,* 44(5):517-24, 2003.

McElhaney J: Chronic pain in older adults, *Consultant,* p 337, March 2001.

Meek SS: Effects of slow stroke back massage on relaxation in hospice clients, *Image J Nurs Sch* 25(1):17-21, 1993.

Melzack R: The McGill Pain Questionnaire: major properties and scoring method, *Pain* 1(3):277-299, 1975.

Mercola J: NSAIDs may harm kidneys of elderly, Sept 14, 2002. Available at www.mercola.com/1999/may9/nsaids_may_harm_elderly_kidneys.htm.

Morley JE: Aging successfully. I, *Aging Successfully* (Division of Geriatric Medicine, St Louis University School of Medicine) 11(3):1, 2001.

National Institutes of Health: *Special report on aging,* Bethesda, Md, 1990, Department of Health and Human Services, National Institutes of Health.

Pasero C, Gordon DB, McCaffery M: JCAHO on assessing and managing pain, *Am J Nurs* 99(7):22, 1999a.

Pasero C, Reed BA, McCaffery M: Pain in the elderly. In McCaffery M, Pasero C, editors: *Pain: clinical manual,* ed 2, St Louis, 1999b, Mosby.

Pearson BD: Pain control: an experiment with imagery, *Geriatr Nurs* 8(1):28-30, 1987.

Portenoy RK, Pasero C, McCaffery M: Opioid analgesics. In McCaffery M, Pasero C, editors: *Pain: clinical manual,* ed 2, St Louis, 1999, Mosby.

Resnick B: Managing chronic pain in the older patient, *Geriatr Nurs* 24(6):373, 2003.

Reyes KW: Early treatment makes shingles easier to bear, *Mod Maturity* 36(6):79, 1994.

Sarvis CM: *Pain management in the elderly,* Sacramento, Calif, 1995, CME Resources.

Teno JM et al: Persistent pain in nursing home residents, *JAMA* 285(16):2081, 2001.

Thernstrom M: Pain, the disease, *New York Times Magazine,* Dec 16, 2001, p 66.

Thomas BL: Pain management for the elderly: alternative interventions. I, *AORN J* 52(6):1268-1272, 1990.

Travis S, Dixon S, Turner M, Thornton M: Assessing and managing iatrogenic disturbance pain for frail, dependent adults in long-term care situations, *Ann Long-Term Care* 11(5):33, 2003.

World Health Organization (WHO): *Management of cancer pain: adults. Quick Reference Guide for Clinicians no. 9, AHCPR pub no. 94-0593,* Rockville, Md, 1994, U.S. Department of Health and Human Services, Public Health Service, Agency for Health Care Policy and Research.

Young DM: Pain in older adults: assessment, intervention, and outcomes, *Old News, Gerontological Nursing at the University of Iowa* 1(2):5, 1999.

18

Diabetes Mellitus in Late Life

Upon completion of this chapter, the reader will be able to:

- Explain the risks for and complications of diabetes mellitus in the older adult.
- State the assessment necessary in the screening and monitoring of persons with diabetes mellitus
- Explain the important components of diabetes management.
- Discuss the nurse's role in diabetes management.
- Develop a nursing care plan for elders with diabetes.

Autoimmune Term applied to the condition where the body sees a part of itself as a foreign object and works to destroy it.

Hgb A_{1c} Glycosylated hemoglobin; a blood test that measures the amount of glucose in the hemoglobin of red blood cells averaged over the three month life span of the cell. Provides an accurate picture of the average blood glucose.

Insulin resistance A condition in which body cells are insensitive to the insulin produced by the pancreas, thus impairing glucose metabolism.

Postprandial After a meal.

I can see that Anna is going to need a lot of help learning to manage her diabetes. I know now that I overwhelmed her with brochures and information right off. She just looked frightened to death, and she really just has a mild elevation in blood sugar; it should be controlled with diet and exercise. I will call her tomorrow and see if she is less anxious.

Anna's gerontological clinical nurse specialist

DIABETES

Diabetes mellitus (DM) is a syndrome of disorders of glucose metabolism resulting in hyperglycemia, either from the inadequate secretion of insulin (type 1) or from both inadequate secretion and the development of resistance of tissues to insulin (type 2). Persons with diabetes often have other health problems as well, including problems with the metabolism of lipids and proteins. Diabetes is the leading cause of end-stage renal disease and blindness.

Diabetes affects approximately 8.7% of the adults in the United States, with this number more that doubling to 18.3% for persons over 60. However, there is considerable variation in the prevalence of diabetes for all adults by ethnic group and region of residence. The lowest rate (8.2%) is seen in persons who identify themselves as Hispanic, yet for Mexican-Americans this number is 16.8% and for Puerto Ricans, 15.1%. Caucasian Americans have the next highest overall rate of 8.4% with significant elevations in persons of Scandinavian descent. Native

Americans have the highest rate of diabetes in the world: 14.9% overall but increasing to 27.8% for those living in the southeastern United States and Arizona (NIDDK, 2003). The national rate is equal between men and women.

The question remains whether diabetes is a primary or secondary event when there is a co-existing illness. The increase in cases of diabetes after about 60 may be influenced by a number of predisposing factors, including age-related insulin decrease, obesity, decreased physical activity, drugs, and co-existing illnesses. However, any acute illness can precipitate an elevation of glucose attributable to stress on hormones. Co-existing illnesses, such as hypertension and hyperlipidemia, are associated with a decrease in insulin sensitivity. Drugs such as diuretics, glucocorticoids, nonsteroidal antiinflammatory drugs (NSAIDs), and alcohol may also contribute to insulin resistance or the body's failure to utilize the insulin that is present.

Diabetes type 1 (formerly called insulin-dependent diabetes mellitus [IDDM]) usually develops in early life and is a result of autoimmune destruction of the insulin-producing beta cells of the pancreas. The resulting absence of insulin is incompatible with life; without replacement of the insulin, the person will soon die. It is very rare that someone with DM type 1 lives to late life, and it is seen in only 5% to 10% of adults.

The overwhelming number of older persons with diabetes have type 2 (formerly called non–insulin dependent diabetes mellitus [NIDDM]). In this case, the pancreas is making insulin but not enough to keep up with the needs of the body. This lack of adequate supplies of naturally occurring insulin is combined with insulin resistance which is characteristic of DM type 2. The onset is usually insidious, and up to one half of all persons with DM type 2 may be undiagnosed. They may go a number of years without treatment while they are developing serious complications.

Other persons develop conditions that may advance to diabetes if left untreated; these are impaired glucose tolerance (IGT) or impaired fasting glucose (IFG). A fasting plasma glucose between 110 and 125 is considered IFG, and a glucose between 141 and 199 mg/dl 2 hours after a glucose challenge is considered IGT. Diabetes is diagnosed after two tests indicate a fasting plasma glucose of more than 125. The numbers used to make these decisions do not change with age.

Aside from ethnicity (discussed above), a number of factors increase one's risk of developing diabetes, including the following:
- Blood pressure $\geq$ 140/90 mm Hg
- First-degree relative (parent, sibling, child) with diabetes
- History of impaired glucose tolerance or impaired fasting plasma glucose
- Obesity $\geq$ 120% of desirable weight or body mass index (BMI) $\geq$ 30 kg/m^2
- Previous gestational DM or having had a child with a birth weight of >9 pounds
- Undesirable lipid levels: high-density lipoproteins (HDLs) $\geq$ 35 mg/dl or triglycerides $\geq$ 250 mg/dl

The national goals for the year 2010 include diagnosing at least 80% of all persons over 65 who have diabetes. For the person with diabetes the goals are related to minimizing the damage caused by complications, at least biannual measurement of glycosylated hemoglobin (Hgb A$_{1c}$), annual dilated eye and foot examinations, daily self-monitoring of glucose, and taking one aspirin at least 15 days per month (USDHHS, 2000).

Complications

Complications occur over the long course of the disease and are microvascular, macrovascular, or both. Macrovascular complications include myocardial infarction, stroke, peripheral vascular disease, and neuropathy. The most common cause of death for persons with diabetes is heart disease. The microvascular problems are loss of vision (diabetic retinopathy) and end-stage renal failure from diabetic nephropathy. The advancement of retinopathy also correlates with neuropathy and peripheral neuropathy (Delcourt et al., 1996). There is also delayed wound healing that, when combined with peripheral neuropathy, may lead to amputation.

Combined macrovascular and microvascular damages also lead to sexual impotence. Impotence in men is a result of reduction in vascular flow, peripheral neuropathy, and uncontrolled circulating blood glucose. Sexual dysfunction is two to five times greater in this group than in the general population, even though interest and desire are still present.

Persons with diabetes commonly have problems with their feet which can have a considerable impact on their functional status. Warning signs of foot problems include cold feet and intermittent claudication (vascular); burning, tingling, hypersensitivity, or numbness (neurological); gradual change in shape or sudden painless change without trauma (musculoskeletal); and infections, skin color and texture changes, and slow-healing, exquisitely painful or painless wounds (dermatological) (Scardina, 1983).

Goals

Diabetes is truly a chronic disease that, even in the best of circumstances, causes damage to the organs. When diabetes is untreated or undertreated the complications develop faster and more severely. Therefore, holding back progression of the disease is the major goal. The first step is to maintain glycemic control the majority of the time. The measurements indicative of ideal glycemic control are given in Table 18-1. Good control of the blood sugar leads to significant prevention of microvascular complications and slows the progression of the disorder (Fonseca, Wall, 1995; Hernandez, 1998). As might be expected, poor perceptions of one's health, anxiety, and depression are frequent accompaniments of a diagnosis of diabetes (Bailey, 1996), and these may dishearten and discourage the individual from consistent self-management. Social support, mastery, and self-esteem have been found to be the chief ameliorators of depression and anxiety surrounding the diagnosis of diabetes and living with diabetes (Bailey, 1996). A holistic, qualitative approach to diabetes and more depth and breadth in nursing practice related to the care of the diabetic patient can facilitate improved health maintenance and adherence to recommended therapies.

IMPLICATIONS FOR GERONTOLOGICAL NURSING AND HEALTHY AGING

Gerontological nurses have great potential for helping individuals and the nation reach the goals set forth in *Healthy People 2010* (USDHHS, 2000), from conducting screenings to patient education and coaching. The nurse can participate in public screenings or pay attention to the need for screening of persons residing in communal settings such as nursing homes and assistive living centers. The nurse can promote healthy aging by helping people do what they can do to reduce their risk, such as obtaining or maintaining an ideal body weight, eating a healthy diet that provides for adequate protein without excessive carbohydrates, exercising, and keeping their cholesterol and blood pressure under control.

For persons at higher risk for diabetes, especially those with IFG or IGT, attention should be directed at reducing the risk for both diabetes and heart disease. This means education and interventions to help the person reach the following goals (ADA, 2003):

No smoking
Blood pressure ≤ 130/80 mm Hg
Cholesterol <200 mg/dl
Low-density lipoprotein (LDL) <100 mg/dl
HDL >40 mg/dl
Triglycerides <150 mg/dl
Blood glucose <126 mg/dl
BMI <25

Table 18-1 Measuring Glycemic Control			
	Normal	Goal	Action Needed
Whole blood	Preprandial <100	80-140	<80 or >140
(mg/dl)	Postprandial <100	100-160	<100 or >160
Plasma	Preprandial <110	90-130	<90 or >150
(mg/dl)	Postprandial <102	110-150	<110 or >180
Hemoglobin A$_{1c}$	<6 %	<7 %	>8 %

Box 18-1   Signs and Symptoms Suggestive of Diabetes in the Elderly

1. General symptoms such as polyphagia, polyuria, polydipsia, and weight loss
2. Recurrent infections, particularly of bacterial or fungal origin, that involve the skin, intertriginous areas, or urinary tract and sores or wounds that tend to heal slowly
3. Neurological dysfunction, including paresthesia, dysesthesia, or hyperesthesia; muscle weakness and pain (amyotrophy); cranial nerve palsies; and autonomic dysfunction of the gastrointestinal tract (diarrhea); cardiovascular system (orthostatic hypotension, dysrhythmias); reproductive system (impotence); and bladder (atony, overflow incontinence)
4. Arterial disease (macroangiopathy) involving the cardiovascular, cerebrovascular, or peripheral vasculature structures
5. Small-vessel disease (microangiopathy) involving the kidneys (proteinuria, glomerulopathy, uremia) and eyes (macular disease, exudates, hemorrhages)
6. Lesions of the skin, such as Dupuytren's contractures, facial rubeosis, and diabetic dermopathy
7. Endocrine-metabolic complications, including hyperlipidemia, obesity, and a history of thyroid or adrenal insufficiency (Schmidt's syndrome)
8. A family history of type 1 or type 2 diabetes and a poor obstetrical history (miscarriages, stillbirths, large babies)

Data from Andres R, Bierman E, Hazzard W: *Principles of geriatric medicine,* New York, 1985, McGraw-Hill; Davidson MB: Diabetes mellitus and other disorders of carbohydrate metabolism. In Abrams WB, Beers MH, Berkow R, editors: *The Merck manual of geriatrics,* ed 2, Whitehouse Station, NJ, 1995, Merck Research Laboratories.

Screening for diabetes by fasting plasma and random blood glucose testing is important for early identification of potential or actual disease. Annual screening fasting plasma glucose measurements are recommended for all persons in high-risk groups, which includes all persons over 65. The overall health and financial benefits of early screening could save $100 billion in direct medical costs and indirect costs of premature death and disability (Genuth et al, 1998). Two thirds of all medical costs for DM occur with older adults with the disease.

Assessment

After the consideration of risk factors, the nurse begins the assessment with a subjective report, including the evaluation of the presence or absence of symptoms of hyperglycemia: polydipsia, polyuria, or polyphagia, even though these are rarely seen in older adults. It is more common to find more vague symptoms, such as fatigue, change in weight, and varied or recurrent infections (Box 18-1). When there are symptoms, the duration and character of the symptoms should be described. Family history is important because of the genetic influence. Nutrition, weight, and exercise history is important to identify eating patterns, an active or sedentary lifestyle, and weight control measures, all of which can provide clues for realistic education and better adherence to a therapy regimen. Assessing economic resources helps establish the ability to purchase equipment, materials, and foods that may be needed to maintain diabetes control. Medication history of over-the-counter and prescription drugs (Box 18-2) and use of alcohol and tobacco are also factors that provide important information in the assessment of the elder. All have a direct or indirect effect on renal, circulatory, neurological, and nutritional function.

The objective data (the physical examination) should include the measurement of height, weight, waist and hip circumferences. From the height and weight a BMI can be calculated (Figure 18-1). The greater the BMI over 25 (>25 is overweight; >30 is obese), the higher the risk for both diabetes and heart disease. For the very aged, BMI is less useful because of the replacement of muscle mass with adipose tissue. Waist and hip circumferences are used to determine the presence of central obesity even in the persons with a lower

BMI. The person is measured (in centimeters) at his or her natural waistline and also around the hips at the superior iliac crests. The hip measurement is divided into the waist measurement in centimeters. A normal measurement is ≤0.8 for women and ≤1.0 for men. The greater the figure above the norm, the higher the cardiac and diabetes risk for the individual.

The nursing assessment also includes careful measurement of blood pressure, visual acuity, and gross neurological function. Distant vision can be checked with a Snellen chart and near vision with a newspaper. The skin and feet should be meticulously inspected for any breach of skin integrity, such as corns, calluses, blisters, fissures, or fungal infections. Clinical guidelines suggest that the best means of testing neurological and sensory intactness is the use of the Semmes-Weinstein mono-

filament instrument. These tests should be performed at least once per year.

Management

Promoting healthy aging in the person with diabetes requires an array of interventions and usually involves persons from a number of disciplines working together with the patient. Management of such a disease requires expertise in medication use, diet, exercise, counseling, and support. The persons involved may include the usual care nurses as well as nutritionists, pharmacists, podiatrists, ophthalmologists, physicians or nurse practitioners, certified diabetic educators, and counselors. If the person's disease is hard to control, endocrinologists are involved, and as complications develop, more specialists are called

---

Box 18-2	Medications that May Affect Blood Glucose Levels

Increase Blood Glucose Levels
Corticosteroids
Diazoxide
Estrogens
Furosemide and thiazide diuretics
Glucagon
Lithium
Phenytoin
Rifampin
Sympathomimetics (antihistamines, decongestants, bronchodilators)
Thyroid replacement preparations

Decrease Blood Glucose Levels
Alcohol
Anabolic steroids
Beta blockers (antihypertensives)
Salicylates (high doses)

Interactions with Sulfonylureas (Oral Hypoglycemics)

Increased Effects (Lower Blood Glucose Levels Further)
Allopurinol
Beta blockers

Clofibrate
Histamine antagonists
Imidazole antifungals
Low-dose salicylates
Monamine oxidase inhibitors
Probenecid
Tricyclic antidepressants

Drugs Not to Be Taken in Combination with Sulfonylureas
Azapropazone
Chloramphenicol
Dicumarol
Oxyphenbutazone
Phenylbutazone
Salicylates (high dose)
Sulfonamides

Decreased Effects (Hinder Hypoglycemic Action)
Barbiturates
Corticosteroids
Diuretics
Estrogens
Rifampin

Summarized from an unidentified source: handout at workshop, Chronic Disorders of the Aged, sponsored by Arizona State School of Nursing, Phoenix, Sept 1992.

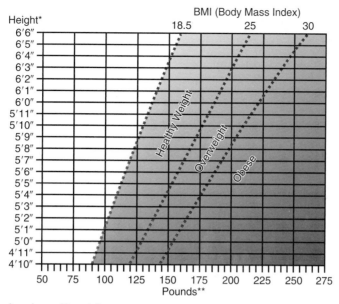

Figure 18-1   Determination of body mass index.
NOTE: For the very aged this is not useful because of the replacement of muscle mass with adipose tissue. (Source: National Institute of Diabetes and Digestive and Kidney Diseases: *Weight and waist measurement: tools for adults.* National Institutes of Health Pub No. 03-5282, Washington, DC, 2003, National Institutes of Health [NIH].)

in, such as nephrologists, cardiologists, and wound care specialists.

The essential components of management include nutrition, exercise, medications, self-health skills, and attention to the psychological aspects of dealing with a chronic illness. This requires the cooperation of the nurse, the patient, and the health care provider, at a minimum. However, good glucose control is of primary importance. Monitoring the blood glucose, especially with the Hgb A_{1c}, is the best measure of the effectiveness of the interventions. The goal is an Hgb A_{1c} measurement of ≤7% at all times (ADA, 2003). We know that the risk of complications is high even with mild hyperglycemia. Experiential teaching, encouragement, and reinforcement of mastery are important factors that promote successful self-management. Some of the factors affecting diabetes control in older adults are identified in Box 18-3.

Nutrition

Adequate and appropriate nutrition is a key factor in the control of diabetes. An initial nutrition

assessment with a 24-hour recall will provide some clues to the patient's dietary habits, intake, and style of eating. If a recall is not possible, have the person bring in his or her grocery list for the past week. If the elder is from an ethnic group different from the nurse, the nurse will need to learn more about the usual ingredients and methods of food preparation to be able to give reasonable instructions. Ideally, all persons with diabetes should have medical nutrition therapy by a registered dietitian on an annual basis. At the time of this writing their services were covered by Medicare.

The new ADA guidelines focus on controlling glucose without restricting foods (ADA, 2002). A healthful diet is a good diabetes diet. Again, the goal is keeping the glucose level under control through regular exercise; losing weight (if obese); limiting saturated fats in the diet; and eating carbohydrates that are whole grains, fruits and vegetables, and low-fat milk. Foods high in monounsaturated fats (e.g. nuts; avocados; and olive, canola, and peanut oils) are thought to be good for people with diabetes. The ADA (2002)

Box 18-3	Summary of Factors Affecting Diabetes Control in Older Adults

1. A decline in visual acuity could affect the individual's ability to see printed educational material, medication labels, markings on a syringe, and blood glucose monitoring devices.
2. Auditory impairments could lead to difficulty hearing instructions.
3. Altered taste could affect food choices and nutritional status.
4. Poor dentition or changes in the gastrointestinal system could lead to difficulties with food ingestion and digestion.
5. Altered ability to recognize hunger and thirst may lead to weight loss, dehydration, and increased risk for hyperosmolar nonketotic syndrome.
6. Changes in hepatic or renal function could affect ability to self-administer medications.
7. Arthritis or tremors could affect ability to self-administer medications and use monitoring devices.
8. Polypharmacy complicates medication choices.
9. Depression affects motivation for self-management.
10. Cognitive impairment and dementia decrease self-care ability.
11. Inadequate education and poor literacy call for modifications in the method of teaching about diabetes care.
12. The level of income can affect the level of care sought or obtained.
13. Living alone without a resource person for help with management can have a negative effect on the person with diabetes.
14. A sedentary lifestyle and obesity can result in decreased tissue sensitivity to insulin.

reports a study from the University of Texas in the mid-1990s that found that patients with diabetes "thrived" on this diet.

If the person is overweight or obese, a weight loss plan is important. Reductions of as little as 10% in weight may mean the difference in developing or not developing diabetes or the difference between taking oral antihyperglycemic agents or insulin and controlling the diabetes by diet and exercise alone (Armetta, Molony, 1999; Halter, 1999).

It is part of the nurse's responsibility to learn if there is difficulty with access to food, including food preparation and shopping for food. Working with elders' dietary habits that have been formed over a lifetime may be difficult but not impossible.

Exercise

Exercise is an important aspect of therapy for type 2 diabetes because exercise increases insulin production. Walking is an inexpensive and beneficial way to exercise. Exercise in conjunction with an appropriate diet may be sufficient to maintain blood glucose levels within normal levels in some cases. A more intensive exercise program should not be started until the older adult has had a phys-

ical examination, including a stress test and electrocardiogram (ECG). Results will govern the type and extent of an exercise program that would be safe. Exercise is usually recommended to be performed for 30 minutes at least three times per week to achieve the benefit of increased carbohydrate metabolism, increased insulin sensitivity, prevention of cardiovascular disease, decreased triglyceride levels, weight loss or maintenance, and lowered blood pressure. Those who have limited mobility can still do chair exercises or if possible use exercise machines that enable sitting and holding on for support. The pace of exercise is slower for most older adults than it is for younger persons.

Exercise decreases blood sugar. If the person is using insulin, exercise needs to be done on a regular rather than an erratic basis and blood glucose should be tested before and after exercise to avoid hypoglycemia.

Medications

Antihyperglycemics include oral agents and insulin. The mainstay of treatment of type 2 DM in elders is oral medication (Whitehead, 2002). Oral medications are prescribed according to the insulin deficit identified: no secretion of insulin,

Table 18-2 Oral Agents in Diabetes Management

Generic Name	Brand Name	Purpose
SULFONYLUREAS		Enhance insulin secretion
Chlorpropamide	Diabinese	
Glimepiride	Amaryl	
Glipizide	Glucotrol	
Glyburide	Micronase	
Glyburide, micronized	Glynase	
MEGLITINIDES		Enhance insulin secretion
Nateglinide	Starlix	
Repaglinide	Prandin	
ALPHA-GLUCOSIDASE INHIBITOR		Decreases glucose absorption
Acarbose	Precose	
BIGUANIDE		Decreases hepatic glucose production
Metformin	Glucophage	
THIAZOLIDINEDIONES		Enhance insulin sensitivity
Rosiglitazone	Avandia	
Pioglitazone	Actos	

insulin resistance, or inadequate secretion of insulin. The sulfonylureas and meglitinides increase insulin secretion. Enhanced insulin sensitivity occurs with the biguanides or thiazolidinediones which decrease insulin resistance. One can delay or reduce the intestinal absorption of carbohydrates with alpha-glucosidase inhibitors and reduce absorption of fats with lipase inhibitors. These agents may be used alone or in combination to achieve the desired blood glucose control. Table 18-2 describes the action of various oral antihyperglycemic agents prescribed in the treatment of DM.

Insulin is used for type 2 diabetes when oral agents, exercise and diet do not adequately control the blood sugar. It is important to note that the use of insulin by someone with diabetes type 2 does not convert them to diabetes type 1, since the diagnosis is made on the type of disorder rather than on the treatment. Insulin has been used to treat diabetes for many years, and there are many advantages and some disadvantages to its use. Box 18-4 lists the advantages and disadvantages of this drug.

In addition to the antiglycemics used by the person with diabetes, it is now recommended that all persons with diabetes type 2 be prescribed an angiotensin-converting enzyme (ACE) inhibitor (e.g., enalapril [Vasotec], lisinopril) and in most cases, a daily aspirin as well (ADA, 2003). The ACE is prescribed regardless of whether the person has hypertension or not, although caution must be used to be alert for hypotension. Both of these adjuvant interventions have been demonstrated to improve outcomes in persons with diabetes.

If other medications are prescribed, they must be carefully reviewed. The effects of drugs on blood glucose must be given serious consideration because a number of medications commonly used for elders adversely affect blood glucose levels. Therefore older adults should be advised to ask if the particular drug prescribed affects their therapy and should check with their primary care provider before taking any over-the-counter medications.

Self-Care
The nurse is often the professional who is responsible for working with the elder in the develop-

Box 18-4	Advantages and Disadvantages of Insulin Therapy

Advantages
- No known drug interaction
- Proven effective for 75 years
- Safe for patients with renal and hepatic insufficiency who cannot eat during major illness
- Encourages self-care
- Adequate dosage can effectively and quickly lower glucose in any patient

Disadvantages
- Injections necessary
- Hypoglycemia a risk
- Treatment program can be complex

Box 18-5	Questions to Ascertain Ability of Elders for Diabetes Self-Management

1. What is the individual's lifestyle?
2. How will diabetes impact his or her lifestyle?
3. What is the individual's functional status? How well can he or she perform ADLs, IADLs, and activities involved in glucose monitoring and in preparing and self-administering medications?
4. What is the individual's mental and psychosocial status?
5. What is the individual's overall health status?

ADLs, Activities of daily living; *IADLs,* instrumental activities of daily living.

ment of the self-care skills needed for the management of chronic illnesses. For the person with diabetes this is especially important. In addition to diet, exercise, and medication use already discussed, self-care skills include the use of personal glucose monitors, optimal care of the feet, and knowledge about the disease. Questions that the nurse can ask to help determine if elders are able to manage their own diabetes care are given in Box 18-5.

Demonstration of techniques for self-monitoring blood glucose (SMBG) include teaching how to obtain a blood sample, use of the glucose monitoring equipment, troubleshooting when there are results indicating an error, and recording the values from the machine. Education includes helping to determine the timing and frequency of the self-monitoring, the adjustment in the schedule when ill , and what to do with the results. Self-care includes bringing the results to each medical visit to review them with the nurse or health care provider.

Where appropriate, demonstration and return demonstration should be given for drawing up insulin, selecting the injection site, injecting and storing insulin, and disposing of the used needle and syringes. Safely transporting insulin for travel is also important (Brown et al, 1999).

Daily foot care and foot examination should be discussed and demonstrated. If the person is not particularly flexible, he or she will have difficulty reaching and inspecting his or her feet and a family member or friend can be asked to do this or checking can be done by placing a mirror on the floor. Box 18-6 details the essential components of daily foot care, and Table 18-3 presents the warning signs and symptoms of diabetic foot problems. Attention to foot care can reduce the risk of amputation. Awareness of the need for good shoes that fit well is essential. Elders who have Medicare are eligible for one pair of specially made shoes annually.

Knowledge about the disease and its effects includes knowing what affects the blood sugar level and knowing that eating and drinking increases blood sugar. Skipping a meal decreases blood sugar. The elder should have a list of warning signs for high and low blood sugar levels (Box 18-7), and know that extra SMBG should be done any time the person feels clammy or cold, sweaty, shaky, or confused, all signs of low blood sugar. Hypoglycemia is the most common problem for elderly diabetics, especially for those taking sulfonylureas. An identification bracelet is a consideration because confusion may be a manifestation of low blood sugar.

Box 18-6	Essentials of Daily Foot Care to Reduce the Risk of Amputation for Persons with Diabetes

- Inspect the feet daily for blisters, cuts, reddened areas, and scratches. Use a magnifying glass or mirror to inspect the feet or have someone else do it if you cannot reach or see well enough.
- Wash feet daily, but *do not* soak feet daily (causes excessive dryness).
- Blot dry rather than rub dry to avoid injury to sensitive skin. Pay particular attention to between the toes.
- Use emollient lotion, cocoa butter, lanolin lotion, mineral oil, or vegetable oil to soften dry skin and to help retain moisture and prevent cracking. *Do not* put between toes; it may contribute to fungal infections.
- If nails are thick and difficult to trim, consult a podiatrist to cut them.
- If you are doing your own nails, soak them in warm water 10 to 15 minutes to soften them before cutting. Cut straight across using toenail clipper. *Do not* cut corns and calluses; have the podiatrist treat them. *Do not* apply harsh chemicals or corn or wart products to toes or feet. These can remove skin, as well as the corn or wart. *Do not* apply heating pads—chemical or battery operated—to feet.
- Wear clean socks, hose, or stockings daily. Cotton socks absorb perspiration for feet that sweat. Keep feet warm with thick fleecy insoles inside slippers to protect from cold, or wear cotton socks with comfortable slippers.
- *Do not* walk barefooted at any time. Sandals for the beach protect feet from hot sand, sharp objects, and so on. At home or in a care facility, wear shoes or slippers, even at night when going to the bathroom.
- Wear comfortable, well-fitting shoes with broad toe space and low heels. Good-quality athletic shoes, although expensive, outlast regular shoes and are less expensive in the long run. Carefully break in new shoes. Begin by wearing shoes 1 hour each day, gradually increasing the time worn.
- Shake out shoes before putting them on to remove foreign objects that might cause injury.
- *Do not* pop blisters. Infection can occur. See health care provider immediately.
- Avoid wearing tight-fitting hose, tight stockings, or stockings with garters; *do not* sit with legs crossed. All of these things constrict blood flow to the lower extremities.
- Stop smoking. Smoking constricts blood vessels, reducing blood flow to the lower extremities.
- Call health care provider for any problems such as tenderness, redness, warmth, drainage, an ingrown toenail, athlete's foot, or pain in the feet or calf.

Modified from Jarvik L, Small G: *Patient,* New York, 1988, Crown; Helfand AE, issue editor: The aging foot, *Focus Geriatr Care Rehabil* 2(10):1, 1989; Dellasega C, Yonushonis MEH: Diabetes mellitus in the elderly. In Stanley M, Beare PG: *Gerontological nursing,* Philadelphia, 1995, Davis.

Box 18-7	Signs and Symptoms of Hyperglycemia and Hypoglycemia

Hyperglycemia	Hypoglycemia
Frequent urination	Shaking
Extreme thirst	Fast heartbeat
Hunger	Sweating
Blurred vision	Anxiety
Drowsiness	Dizziness
Nausea	Hunger
Dry and itchy skin	Impaired vision
	Weakness or fatigue
	Headache
	Irritability

Table 18-3 Warning Signs and Symptoms of Diabetic Foot Problems

Signs	Symptoms
VASCULAR	
Absence of pedal, popliteal, or femoral pulses	Cold feet
Femoral bruits	Intermittent claudication involving calf or foot
Dependent rubor, plantar pallor on elevation	Pain at rest, especially nocturnal, relieved by
Prolonged capillary filling time (>3-4 sec)	dependency
Decreased skin temperature	
NEUROLOGICAL	
Sensory: deficits in perception of vibration, proprioception, pain, and temperature	
MUSCULOSKELETAL	
Claw toes on feet	Gradual change in foot shape
Foot drop	Sudden, painless change in foot shape, with
"Rocker bottom" foot (Charcot's joint)	swelling, without history of trauma
Neuropathic arthropathy	
DERMATOLOGICAL	
Abnormal dryness	
Chronic tinea infections	
Keratotic lesions with or without hemorrhage (plantar or digital)	
Trophic ulcer	
Hair diminished or absent	
Nails: trophic changes	
Onychomycosis	
Subungual ulceration or abscess	
Ingrown nails with paronychia	

Standards of Care

The three most important evaluations recommended by the ADA (2003) are regular medical visits (at least two office visits per year), annual lipid profiles, biannual Hgb A_{1c} levels for persons in good control (quarterly until then), and annual dilated eye and foot examinations. Nurses must advocate for elders and encourage them to demand quality care to prevent the devastating end results of poor management. The following evaluation is recommended:

- History should include dietary habits, weight patterns, previous treatment programs, current treatment regimen, exercise and activity levels, infections, illnesses, and complications of diabetes.
- Physical examination should include blood pressure; dilated eye examination; thyroid palpation; auscultation of pulses; foot, periodontal, and skin examination; and neurological examination.
- Laboratory tests should include fasting plasma glucose; glycosylated hemoglobin (A1C); fasting lipid profile; serum creatinine if proteinuria is present; urinalysis, including microalbuminuria, urine culture if indicated, and thyroid function (T_4 or thyroid-stimulating hormone [TSH]); and ECG.

Long-Term Care and the Elder with Diabetes

Many of the persons cared for by gerontological nurses in long-term care facilities have diabetes. In this setting the nurse may be responsible for many

NANDA and Wellness Diagnoses

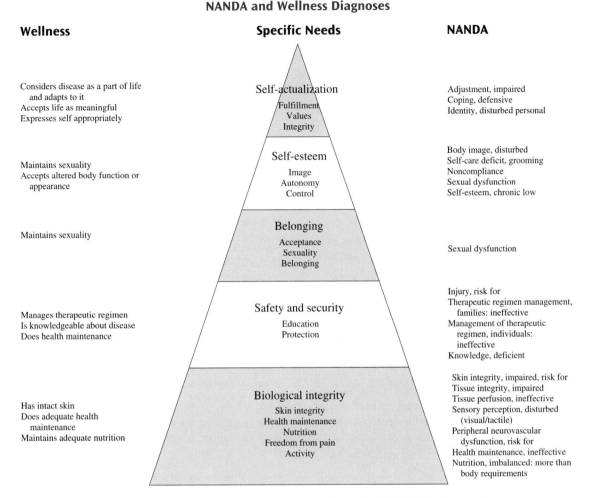

Wellness	Specific Needs	NANDA

Wellness

Considers disease as a part of life and adapts to it
Accepts life as meaningful
Expresses self appropriately

Maintains sexuality
Accepts altered body function or appearance

Maintains sexuality

Manages therapeutic regimen
Is knowledgeable about disease
Does health maintenance

Has intact skin
Does adequate health maintenance
Maintains adequate nutrition

Specific Needs

Self-actualization
Fulfillment
Values
Integrity

Self-esteem
Image
Autonomy
Control

Belonging
Acceptance
Sexuality
Belonging

Safety and security
Education
Protection

Biological integrity
Skin integrity
Health maintenance
Nutrition
Freedom from pain
Activity

NANDA

Adjustment, impaired
Coping, defensive
Identity, disturbed personal

Body image, disturbed
Self-care deficit, grooming
Noncompliance
Sexual dysfunction
Self-esteem, chronic low

Sexual dysfunction

Injury, risk for
Therapeutic regimen management, families: ineffective
Management of therapeutic regimen, individuals: ineffective
Knowledge, deficient

Skin integrity, impaired, risk for
Tissue integrity, impaired
Tissue perfusion, ineffective
Sensory perception, disturbed (visual/tactile)
Peripheral neurovascular dysfunction, risk for
Health maintenance, ineffective
Nutrition, imbalanced: more than body requirements

These are not all of the possible wellness or NANDA diagnoses that may be identified. The above are frequent examples of nursing diagnoses that should be considered when planning care for the older adult in whatever setting.

of the activities that would otherwise fall on the patient or a home caregiver in addition to those as a professional. Meals, nutritional status, intake and output, and exercise/activity are monitored. The nurse assesses the person for signs of hypoglycemia and hyperglycemia as well as evidence of complications. The nurse ensures that the standards of care for the person with diabetes are met. The nurse monitors the effect and side effects of diet, exercise, and medication use. The nurse administers or supervises the administration of

medications. If the person requires what is called sliding scale insulin wherein the dosage depends on the current glucose reading, it is the nurse who must make the determination of the dosage under "sliding scale" guidelines.

The goals of nursing care are to maintain the older adult with diabetes in the best health that is realistically possible. Maintaining the older adult's health is a team effort. The nurse as part of the team serves as an educator, care provider, advocate, supporter, and guide for the older person.

KEY CONCEPTS

- Signs and symptoms of diabetes in the older adult may be vague or suggestive of other medical conditions or considered as part of "old age" rather than being the usual expected symptoms of polyuria, polydipsia, and polyphagia.
- Close monitoring of blood glucose levels is the most effective way to prevent, delay, or slow the progression of macrovascular, microvascular, and neurological complications of the disease.
- Management of diabetes is a comprehensive team effort and should include the elder as much as he or she can realistically participate as part of the team. If this is not possible, the caregiver, if not the nurse, will need to ensure that the medical regimen is effective.
- Preventive foot care is essential for prevention of the possibility of future problems.

Activities and Discussion Questions

1. What are the risks and complications of diabetes for the older adult?
2. State the components of diabetes management, and explain what each component requires.
3. Describe the nurse's role in the management of diabetes.
4. Develop a nursing care plan for an elder in the community, in an acute care hospital, and in long-term care using wellness and North American Nursing Diagnosis Association (NANDA) diagnoses.

RESOURCES

Organizations

American Diabetes Association
National Center
PO Box 25757
1660 Duke Street
Arlington, VA 22314-3427
www.diabetes.org

National Diabetes Information Clearing House
1 Information Way
Bethesda, MD 20892-3560
NDIC@info.niddk.nih.gov

Websites

CDC Diabetes Public Health Resource
www.cdc.gov/diabetes

National Institute of Diabetes and Digestive and Kidney Disorders
www.niddk.nih.gov

REFERENCES

American Diabetes Association (ADA): 2002 guidelines. 60th Annual Scientic Sessions, 2002, American Diabetes Association. Available at www.advancefornp.com/npfeatures.

American Diabetes Association (ADA): Standards of medical care for patients with diabetes, *Diabetes Care* 26(suppl 1):S33-S50, 2003.

Armetta M, Molony SL: Topics in endocrine and hematologic care. In Molony SL et al, editors: *Gerontological nursing: an advanced practice approach,* Stamford, Conn, 1999, Appleton-Lange.

Bailey BJ: Mediators of depression in adults with diabetes, *Clin Nurs Res* 5(1):28-42, 1996.

Brown JB, Bedford NK, White SJ: *Gerontological protocols for nurse practitioners,* Philadelphia, 1999, Lippincott.

Delcourt C et al: Clinical correlates of advanced retinopathy in type II diabetic patients: implications for screening, *J Clin Epidemiol* 49(6):679-685, 1996.

Fonseca V, Wall J: Diet and diabetes in the elderly, *Nutr Aging Age Depend Dis* 11(4):613, 1995.

Genuth S, Palmer J, Zimmerman BR: Diabetes: new criteria for diagnosis, screening, and classification, *Patient Care Nurse Pract* 1(1):12, 1998.

Halter JB: Diabetes mellitus. In Hazzard WR et al, editors: *Principles of geriatric medicine and gerontology,* ed 4, New York, 1999, McGraw-Hill.

Hernandez D: Microvascular complications of diabetes, *Am J Nutr* 98(6):26, 1998.

National Institute of Diabetes and Digestive and Kidney Diseases (NIDDK): *National diabetes statistics fact sheet: general information and national estimates on diabetes in the United States,* Bethesda, Md, 2003, National Institutes of Health (NIH). Available at www.niddk.nih.gov.

Scardina RJ: Diabetic foot problems: assessment and prevention, *Clin Diabet* 1(2):42, 1983.

U.S. Department of Health and Human Services (USDHHS): *Healthy people 2010,* vol 1, ed 2, Washington, DC, 2000, U.S. Government Printing Office. Available at www.healthypeople.gov.

Whitehead JB: An overview of the management of diabetes in the elderly, *Ann Long-Term Care* (suppl), 1-7, March 2002.

19

Bone and Joint Problems in the Elderly

Upon completion of this chapter, the reader will be able to:

- Discuss the potential dangers of osteoporosis.
- Recognize postural changes that suggest the presence of osteoporosis.
- Discuss the factors that lead to osteoporosis.
- Explain some effective ways of preventing or slowing the progression of osteoporosis.
- Relate the differences in osteoarthritis and rheumatoid arthritis.
- Describe the nurse's responsibility in care for the person with gout.
- Name several methods of dealing with pain and disability resulting from joint and bone disorders.

GLOSSARY

Crepitus The sound or feel of bone rubbing on bone.
Resorption The loss of a substance or bone by physiological or pathological processes.

Sarcopenia Muscle wasting and weakening from disuse.

THE LIVED EXPERIENCE

It is so discouraging to wake up feeling so stiff and sore every morning. Just getting out of bed seems like a real effort, but I usually feel better after I have moved around a bit. I was always so athletic, I can't understand how I have become so crippled up. And now I know that what my grandmother used to say about the weather affecting her rheumatism is really true. I can feel it when a storm is coming.

Mabel, age 80

I don't know how folks with arthritis can stand being uncomfortable so much of the time. I know Mabel takes medications, but she still seems to be in a lot of pain and has so much trouble moving about. I'll try to be as gentle as possible when I help her bathe.

Elva, student nurse

MUSCULOSKELETAL SYSTEM

The healthy musculoskeletal system not only allows us to be upright but also is necessary to allow us to comfortably carry out the most basic activities of daily living. For some, later life is an opportunity to explore the limits of their ability, taking their musculoskeletal system to the limits and becoming master athletes. For others, such as Mabel (above), late life is a time of significant compromise with disuse leading to sarcopenia, or slow wasting and weakening in the muscle itself. However, both the athletes and the nonathletes have to deal with the challenges presented by the normal aging changes in this important system.

The gerontological nurse attends to the musculoskeletal needs of older adults and works to promote healthy bones. In this chapter we discuss osteoporosis, the arthritis', and the implications for nursing intervention.

OSTEOPOROSIS

Osteoporosis means "porous bone." Primary osteoporosis is associated with the normal changes of aging. Secondary osteoporosis is caused by another disease state or by medications. Both are diseases that are characterized by low bone mass (or bone mineral density) and subsequent deterioration of the bone structure. It is a major medical, economic, and social health problem in the United States. Osteoporosis affects about 55% of persons over 50 in some way. Ten million people have osteoporosis, and another 34 million have a lesser (but perhaps a precursor) condition of bone loss called *osteopenia*. The primary site for fractures is the vertebra (700,000), hip (300,000), wrist (250,000), or other site (300,000) with a cost of $17 billion in 2001 (NIH, 2003).

Important to the nurse is the fact that osteoporosis itself is not necessarily a health problem and may be to some extent a naturally occurring condition. It is a silent condition, and a person may have no symptoms of any kind ever or for years. However, the most serious aspect of osteoporosis is the fall-related morbidity and mortality. One out of two women and one out of four men will eventually have a fracture. A striking 24% of persons who have an osteoporosis-related fracture will die within 1 year. One fourth of those who were ambulatory before a fracture will need long-term care afterwards; and many of them will need long-term care indefinitely. Six months after the fracture only 15% of persons will be able to walk unassisted (NIH, 2004).

In the normal process of growth the bones build up mass (formation) and strength while they are also losing both through resorption, known as bone turnover. Before about the age of 25 the formation is greater than the resorption; bone strength and density peak and then begin to decline. At first the loss of bone mineral density (BMD) is quite minimal, but then it speeds up. For women, the period of the fastest overall loss of BMD is in the 5 to 7 years immediately following menopause, with losses up to 20% (NIH, 2004).

Loss is seen in both the cortical bone (the outer shell of a bone and 80% of the skeleton) and the trabecular bone (the spongy meshwork inside the bone and 20% of the skeleton) in both men and women (Thorndyke, 2001). The DEXA scan (dual-energy x-ray absorptiometry) provides the most reliable measurement of bone integrity. The results are a calculated comparison "T-score," the density of the bone scanned compared with that of a 30-year-old healthy man or woman. If the bone loss is between −1 and −2.5 standard deviations from that of a healthy 30 year old, it is called osteopenia. If the bone loss is greater than −2.5 standard deviations, the person is diagnosed with osteoporosis.

The prevalence of osteoporosis varies with gender and race or ethnicity. Women are much more likely than men to develop the disease. In 2004 the NIH reported that 8 million women were affected compared with 2 million men. Only 5% of African American women had the disease compared with 10% of Hispanic women and 20% of Caucasian and Asian women. Thin white women of northern European descent are at the highest risk (NIH, 2004).

A number of other factors increase or decrease a person's risk for both osteopenia and osteoporosis. Some of these cannot be changed (e.g., gender, race or ethnicity), but others (e.g., calcium intake, exercise) are amenable to change (Box 19-1). At one time it was thought that weakened bones could not be strengthened, but current thought is that although old bones can never be young bones again, preventive and restorative measures can have some positive effect at any age.

Implications for Gerontological Nursing and Healthy Aging

Osteoporosis is diagnosed through a DEXA scan but can be presumed in most people who have nontraumatic fractures, especially of the hip, vertebra, or wrist. Other signs include a loss of height of more than 3 cm or kyphosis, the development of a C shape to the cervical vertebra (Figure 19-1). The nurse may be the one to identify the changes to the spine or realize that the person had a fracture or unexplained back pain but had not yet

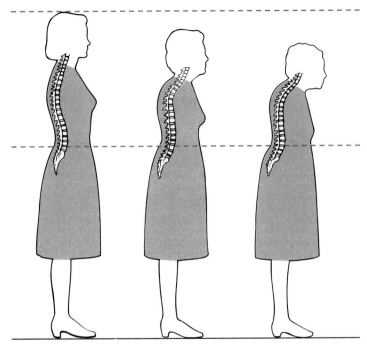

Figure 19-1   Osteoporosis spine alignment.

Box 19-1	Risk Factors for Osteoporosis

Nonmodifiable Factors
Female gender
Caucasian race
Northern European ancestry
Advanced age
Family history of osteoporosis

Modifiable Factors
Low body weight (underweight)
Low calcium intake
Estrogen deficiency
Low testosterone
Inadequate exercise or activity
Use of steroids or anticonvulsants
Excess coffee or alcohol intake
Current cigarette smoking

received a medical diagnosis. Without a diagnosis it is unlikely the person with have access to the full treatments that are available.

The nurse can also pay attention to the risk factors (see Box 19-1) and urge both formal screen-ing and lifestyle changes to minimize risk and enhance prevention. The U.S. Prevention Task Force recommends that all persons over the age of 65 and those with more than one risk factor have at least one screening DEXA scan, which is covered by Medicare (USPSTF, 2002). If the screen-ing is positive the nurse can advocate for the elder, regardless of residential setting, for treatment and initiation of more aggressive prevention approaches to both injury and exacerbation of the disease.

Reducing Risk and Injury
Measures to prevent injury and osteoporosis pro-gression include weight-bearing physical activity and exercise, nutrition, and lifestyle changes that reduce risk factors, including smoking cessation (Ali, Twibell, 1994). Education and fall prevention must be considered as well.

Weight-bearing physical activity and exercises help to maintain bone mass. Brisk walking and working with light weights provide mechanical force and spinal and long bone movement. Muscle-building exercises help to maintain skele-tal architecture by improving muscle strength and

Table 19-1 Calcium Content of Common Foods

Food Item	Serving Size	Calcium (mg)	% Daily Value
Plain yogurt, fat free	8 oz	450	45%
American cheese	2 oz	350	35%
Yogurt with fruit (low fat or fat free)	8 oz	315	31%
Milk	8 oz	300	30%
Cheese pizza	1 slice	220	22%
Ice cream, soft serve	4 oz	118	10%
Cooked dried white beans	1 oz	161	15%
Spinach	4 oz	122	10%
Turnip greens	4 oz	99	8%
Dried figs	10 figs	269	25%
Orange juice, calcium fortified	8 oz	300	30%

Source: National Institutes of Health: *Sources of calcium*, Washington, DC. Available at www.nichd.nih.gov/milk. Accessed 7/29/04.

flexibility. Participation in a variety of exercises that include all parts of the body is important to prevent boredom and promote continued interest in maintaining a program. The Asian art of Tai Chi has been used successfully for strengthening of both ambulatory and nonambulatory elders (Li et al, 2003). Tai Chi and exercise have the added advantage of improving balance and stamina, which may prevent falls or limit the damage if a fall should occur.

Nutrition, especially the adequate intake of calcium and vitamin D, is the cornerstone to all other treatments. Ideally optimal nutrition in late life has followed a lifetime of good eating habits. The diet during adolescence is probably a key to healthy bones later. A balanced diet that includes food sources of calcium is best (Table 19-1). Persons over 50 should take in 1200 mg of calcium per day, which can come from combined dietary and supplementary sources. If using supplements, the doses are best when spread over the course of the day (e.g., 400 mg of calcium in the morning, diet with 400 mg during the day, another 400 mg of calcium in the evening). Unless the person gets 15 minutes of sunshine each day, vitamin D supplementation is also necessary. Daily doses of 400 to 800 international units are sufficient and should not be exceeded (Jett, Lester, 2004). Patient teaching includes discussion of the factors that inhibit calcium absorption (e.g., excess alcohol, protein, or salt), excretion enhancers (e.g., caf-feine; excess fiber; phosphorus in meats, sodas, and preserved foods); and the influence of the body's response to stress (decreased calcium absorption, increased excretion of calcium in the urine).

Patient teaching also includes other key aspects of the prevention and treatment of osteoporosis. Knowledge about the sites most vulnerable to fracture through accidents, falls, back strain, and poor posture should be provided. Explanation should be given about changes in the upper spine that occur when vertebrae are weakened and about the pain that results from strain on the lower spine to compensate for balance and height changes attributable to alteration of the upper spine. Education also includes the appropriate way to take medications and how to handle their side effects.

Fall prevention is especially important to decrease the morbidity and mortality associated with osteoporosis. Shoes with good support should be worn. Handrails should be used, and walking in poorly lighted areas should be avoided. Basic body mechanics, such as not bending or lifting heavy objects, should be learned. Use of step stools or chairs for reaching things in high places should be discouraged. Home safety should include good lighting, railings, and other aids as needed. Walkways should be kept free of obstacles; loose rugs and electrical cords should be arranged so that they do not cause falls (see Chapter 22).

Pharmacological Interventions

Considerable progress has been made in the last decade in the development of pharmacological treatments for both the prevention and treatment of osteoporosis. The currently available medications include bisphosphonates, calcitonin, selective estrogen receptive modulators (SERMs), estrogen, and parathyroid hormone. Adequate intake of calcium and vitamin D are required for all of the prescribed treatments currently available.

Estrogen had been the primary treatment prescribed for many years. However, the Women's Health Initiative found that although estrogen is an excellent means to prevent bone loss, it also increased the rate of breast cancer, colon cancer, and heart disease (Bruckner, Youngkin, 2002). Because of these findings, estrogen is not usually prescribed for osteoporosis, and if it is, it is for a limited period of time. The SERM Raloxifene is a good substitute for estrogen and decreases the risk for breast cancer, but it can cause hot flashes and coagulation disorders so is contraindicated for someone with a history of a deep vein thrombosis (DVT) or someone who is taking warfarin (Coumadin).

The most common treatments that are seen in older adults are the bisphosphonates alendronate (Fosamax) and risedronate (Actonel). Alendronate must be used by the patient and administered by the nurse with caution. It must be taken on an empty stomach (when first awake), with a full glass of water, and the person must remain in an upright position for at least $\frac{1}{2}$ hour afterward. It has been associated with severe esophageal erosions. It should not be given to patients who are not able to follow these instructions exactly.

Another medication that is quite useful is calcitonin. Although the mechanism is not known, for some, it not only slows down bone resorption, but also reduces osteoporosis-related pain. It is given either subcutaneously or as a nasal spray.

The newest treatment for osteoporosis is daily injections of parathyroid hormone in the commercial form of teriparatide (Forteo). This has been found to have excellent results, but it can only be administered for 2 years (Jett, Lester, 2004). It is unknown what will happen to people after 2 years. The cost of this treatment can be over $1000 per month, which will not be possible for many people who do not have drug coverage.

One must be cautious, particularly with very old women, because long-range effects of these medications are unknown. Simple, effective, and risk-free treatment methods are not available at this time.

ARTHRITIS

Arthritis is the term used to refer to more than 100 diseases that affect 45 to 60 million individuals of all ages in the United States. Arthritis is the number one reason for activity limitations from middle age on (Callahan, Jonas, 2002). The three most common forms of the disease that the gerontological nurse will encounter are osteoarthritis (OA), rheumatoid arthritis (RA), and gout.

Osteoarthritis

Osteoarthritis (OA) is a degenerative joint disorder (DJD) that affects at least 20 million Americans. Risk factors include increased age, obesity, family history of the same, and repetitive use or trauma to the joint. Most persons over 65 will have x-ray evidence of OA even if they have no symptoms. Native Americans have the highest prevalence of OA and Asians and Pacific Islanders have the lowest. However, for all, arthritis causes joint stiffening and pain and impairs functioning.

The osteoarthritic joint is one in which the normal soft and resilient cartilaginous lining becomes thin and damaged. This causes the joint space to narrow and the bones of the joint to rub together causing destruction of the joint. Bone spurs (osteophytes) may develop in the spaces (Figure 19-2). It was previously thought to be a normal consequence of aging that had no cure (Kalunian, Brion, 2002). However, it is now known that OA results from a complex interplay of many factors, including genetic predisposition, local inflammation, joint integrity, mechanical forces, and cellular and biochemical processes.

In classic OA there is stiffness with inactivity relieved by activity and pain with activity relieved by rest (Concoff, 2002). The stiffness is greatest in the morning after the disuse of sleep but should resolve within 20 to 30 minutes. As the disease advances, there is pain at rest as well and more joints become involved. There may be joint instability, and crepitus may be felt or heard. This crepi-

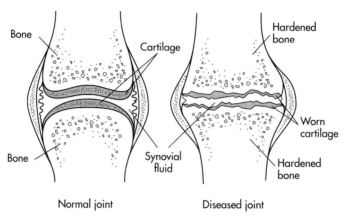

Figure 19-2 Normal joint and diseased joint.

tation is an indication of the deterioration of the synovial covering of the joint. The joint will enlarge, and range of motion will be reduced. The most common locations for OA are the knees, hips, neck (cervical spine), lower back (lumbar spine), fingers, and thumbs (Figure 19-3). Less frequently it is found in the shoulders.

OA is a condition that cannot be cured without a joint replacement. Many elders elect this procedure for hips and knees, and the nurse is involved in the perioperative period and active in the rehabilitation process when the person is learning to use the new joint.

Implications for Gerontological Nursing and Healthy Aging

Assessment. When assessing the musculoskeletal system, the nurse examines the joints for tenderness, swelling, warmth, redness, subluxation (partial dislocation of a joint), and crepitus (a crackling sound). The hands are examined for the presence or absence of osteophytes. If they appear in the distal joints of the fingers they are called Heberden's nodes, and they are called Bouchard's nodes in the proximal joints. If present these are often accompanied by deformities in the flexion of these joints.

Both passive range of motion and active range of motion are evaluated. How far can the person reach and bend all joints without assistance, and what are the reach, flexion, and extension with assistance? The testing of passive range of motion must go only to the point of discomfort and never to induce pain. Test the functional ability of the

What Areas Does Osteoarthritis Affect?

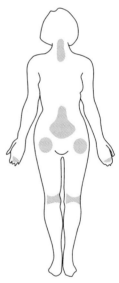

Figure 19-3 Common locations for osteoarthritis. (Source: National Institutes of Health: *Handout on health: osteoarthritis*, Washington, DC. Available at www.niams.nih.gov/hi/topics/arthritis/oahandout.htm. Accessed 7/29/04.)

arms by asking the person to touch the back of the head with both hands. Test the flexibility of the hands by surveying the movements as the individual uses eating utensils.

Interventions. The goals of intervention and management of OA are to control pain and minimize disability. The nurse is very involved with both of these in terms of pain assessment, medication administration, evaluation, and patient teaching.

Pain management and the minimization of disability are interconnected. To minimize disability the joint must be used, strengthened, and protected. Exercises will not be done if they cause pain. Too much pain medication will decrease the person's level of consciousness, and safe exercise will not be possible.

PHARMACOLOGICAL INTERVENTIONS. Acetaminophen (Tylenol) remains the drug of choice for the treatment of pain associated with mild arthritis (Jett, Lester, 2004). When this is not effective, the next choice is one of the nonsteroidal antiinflammatory drugs (NSAIDs), such as aspirin or ibuprofen; however, these are not without a significant risk for gastrointestinal problems, such as bleeding. To minimize this risk, the NSAID can be taken with a second, protecting agent, such as a proton pump inhibitor (e.g., omeprazole [Prilosec]) or in a combination drug, such as misoprostol (Arthrotec). Newer but more expensive alternatives to the traditional NSAIDs are the COX-2 inhibitors (celecoxib [Celebrex], valdecoxib [Bextra]), which have a much lower rate of gastric irritation and therefore bleeding (Chao, Vega, 2004), however their safety is now in question.

As the disease progresses or during exacerbations, stronger medications may be necessary to help control the pain, and the nurse may need to act as a patient advocate to make sure the pain is satisfactorily addressed. Tramadol is used for moderate to severe pain. Although it is not an opioid, the effect may be similar. It can cause nausea and vomiting and should be started in very low doses and increased very slowly to avoid side effects. Codeine and other opiates can be used for moderate to severe pain, with a bowel regimen. The goals of intervention and management of OA are to help the elder to prevent or control pain, to minimize disability, and to ensure optimal medical management. For older persons with chronic pain the nurse should be less concerned about the addictive quality of the medications and strive for pain relief adequate enough to allow the person to function at as high a level as possible.

For persistent and disabling pain in the knees, the patient may seek out joint injections. Either cortisone or the chemical hyaluronic acid (a derivative of hyaluronan) is used. In some cases these provide at least temporary and sometimes instantaneous relief. Repeated injections may be necessary (especially for hyaluronic acid), but there is a limit to how many injections can be done. The nurse should be aware that even after an injection the joint still will need protection and support.

Other pharmacological agents often used in OA management include topical capsaicin made from pepper plants and available over the counter in two strengths. It becomes effective after several days of use. Menthol and aspirin creams are also useful and are preferred by many elders.

SURGICAL INTERVENTIONS. For disabling pain in the knees and hips, surgical replacement of the joint (arthroplasty) may be highly successful and restore the person to his or her previous level of functioning. Surgical replacements are recommended for even the very old. The acute postsurgical nursing care is designed to restore the physiological functions: maintaining fluids, movement, and nutritional adequacy. Pain management is critical to ensure that the individual will move about as necessary and is essential to achievement of maximal recovery. It cannot be overstated that ongoing therapy from accredited physical therapists is essential for restoration of full movement. During the recovery period, weight loss (if the client is overweight) and muscle building are highly recommended. In many cases the increased ease and enhancement of the activities of daily living become highly motivating. Outcomes depend on the timing of surgery; the number of procedures that the surgeon and the hospital have to their credit; and the patient's medical status, perioperative and postoperative management, and rehabilitation (Hochberg et al, 1995). Nearly twice as many women as men have joint replacements, and more than 60% of all joint replacements are in individuals older than 65 years of age (U.S. Bureau of the Census, 1998).

NONPHARMACOLOGICAL NURSING INTERVENTIONS. To provide care to the whole person with OA the nurse works with a number of nonpharmacological approaches and teaches these to the person to enable and empower self-care. These approaches include the use of heat and cold, joint support and protection, exercise, and diet.

The use of heat and cold is well known for management of pain. Patient preference is important, but cold usually works best for an acute process, using cold packs that decrease muscle spasm, decrease swelling, and relieve inflammatory pain. Heat may be applied superficially or deep; either works well (Lozada, Altman, 2001). Ultrasound provides deep heat. Hot packs, hydrotherapy, and radiant heat provide superficial heat. Liquid paraffin baths can be purchased in most drug stores for the hands. Immersing the hand in the warmed paraffin easily provides deep heat and temporary relief. A recent device available for prolonged heat application is ThermaCare, which is a band applied to the affected area (e.g., neck, lower back, abdomen) that lasts for 8 to 12 hours. It is available without a prescription and can be worn under clothing throughout the day.

Devices and techniques are available that relieve some of the pressure to the joints and protect the joints from further stress and, in doing so, may decrease pain and improve balance. Canes, crutches, walkers, collars, shoe orthotics, and corsets are such devices. A cane can relieve hip pressure by 60%. A shoe lift can improve lumbar pain. A knee brace is useful for knees, especially if there is lateral instability (the knee "gives out"). If the hands are affected the person can resist carrying packages by the fingers or using larger rather than smaller grips of utensils and household equipment. Avoiding exposing the affected joints to cold temperatures may also help. The person is encouraged to wear leggings, gloves, or scarves as necessary while out-of-doors.

A careful exercise plan should be strongly encouraged. Working with a skilled physical therapist or rehabilitation nurse specialist may improve clinical outcomes. Regular exercise can improve flexibility and muscle strength, which in turn help to support the affected joints, reduce pain, improve function, and reduce falls (Brion, Concoff, 2002). Preventive occupational therapy has been shown to improve personal and social relationships in the Well Elderly Study (Agency for Healthcare Research and Quality, 2002).

Attention should also be given to diet. With the decreases in activity associated with pain, it is easy for the person to gain weight. Excess weight significantly increases the pressure and wear and tear of the joints, leading to less activity and more weight gain. Weight reduction should be considered for all persons who are overweight (body mass index [BMI] >25). The nurse can work with the person to identify weight and caloric goals and develop meal plans that are culturally acceptable but still balanced and healthy. The nurse can also refer the person to a registered dietitian and then lend support and encouragement.

COMPLEMENTARY AND ALTERNATIVE INTERVENTIONS. A number of complementary and alternative interventions show promise in contributing to pain relief for persons with arthritis. Among the most popular is the dietary supplement glucosamine. Available in most grocery stores and pharmacies it comes in tablets and capsules to be taken three times per day. Anecdotal reports are often positive, and whereas the research is promising, it is not yet conclusive (Blakeley, Ribeiro, 2004). McCaffrey and Freeman (2003) found a significant reduction in arthritic pain for persons who listen to music. Others have found the ancient techniques of acupuncture and acupressure also effective in some cases (Gaylord, Crotty, 2002; Roberts, 2003). Information about these and other techniques can be found at both the Arthritis Foundation and the National Institutes for Health websites (www.arthritis.org, www.niams.nih.gov).

These and other nursing interventions for OA are given in Box 19-2 as summarized by Kee and colleagues (1998).

Rheumatoid Arthritis

Rheumatoid arthritis (RA) is a chronic, systemic inflammatory joint disorder. It is considered an autoimmune disease in which an inflamed synovium (the lining of the joint) invades and destroys the cartilage and bone within the joint. The cause is unknown. RA affects more women then men (3:1). It most often starts in mid-life, with most cases seen between the ages of 40 and 60 (Anderson, 2004).

RA is characterized by pain and swelling in multiple joints and in a symmetrical pattern (e.g., if the left hand is affected, the right hand will be affected also). It generally affects the small joints of the wrist, knee, ankle, and hand, although it affects large joints as well. Whereas morning stiffness in OA lasts less than 30 minutes, in RA it is longer than 30 minutes, and the person may feel general fatigue and malaise. The joints are warm and tender (Gornisiewicz, Moreland, 2001). Weight loss is common. The natural course of RA is highly variable, with remissions and exacerbations; that is, there are good and bad periods. The

Box 19-2	Nursing Interventions in Osteoarthritis

Pain Management
Behavioral-cognitive pain control (imagery, relaxation, distraction)
Analgesic medications
Localized applications of heat

Exercise
Range of motion initially, progressing to aerobic exercise as tolerated or prescribed
Exercise alternated with rest
Avoiding prolonged rest periods

Diet
Weight loss if obese
Balanced, nutritious diet

Joint Protection
Avoiding high-impact activities in affected joints
Good body mechanics
Assistive devices: canes, commode extenders, Velcro-fastened clothing

Psychosocial Parameters
Assessment of coping strategies, self-efficacy beliefs, social support

Education
Nature of osteoarthritis disease process
Purpose of prescribed interventions

From Kee CC et al: Perspectives on the nursing management of osteoarthritis, *Geriatr Nurs* 19(1):19-26, 1998.

disease may be unremitting, with continuing progression, disability, and death, or it may be a remitting disease, but only rarely.

Early diagnosis is important because of the significant and irreversible destruction of affected joints within 1 to 2 years of onset (Paget, 1995). Nearly one half of those affected are disabled within 10 years (Luggen, 2003). Symptoms in late life tend to be acutely uncomfortable and spread throughout the joints of the body. Sometimes the disorder affects systems other than joints. An elevated rheumatoid arthritis factor (RF) combined with an elevated erythrocyte sedimentation rate (ESR) are most suggestive of RA.

In the past NSAIDs were the drugs of choice for early disease. It was thought that these would reduce the swelling and therefore the damage to the joints as well as address pain. However, it has been found that the disease is the most aggressive in the first 2 years and that prompt efforts must be made to halt or slow the damage as much as possible (Anderson, 2004). Persons diagnosed with RA are usually cared for by rheumatologists, and treatment involves the use of aggressive therapy using a class of drugs called disease-modifying antirheumatic drugs (DMARDs). All the DMARDS are potentially toxic and must be both prescribed (by a physician) and administered (by a registered nurse) with care.

Because of the unknown causes and unpredictable but persistent nature of RA, people often fall prey to worthless cure tactics. However, some may be effective because they act as placebos. Self-help and support groups are useful, but the individual often must simply learn to live with a certain degree of constant discomfort. It seems that feelings of self-efficacy, induced by increased knowledge and feelings of control, may have more positive outcomes even in the presence of increasing debilitation.

All the nonpharmacological nursing interventions discussed in the section on OA apply here. However, the use of dietary supplements cannot be recommended because of their potential and unknown interactions with the complex prescribed drug regimen. In helping the patient manage the associated pain and other symptoms, expert nursing care must be provided. See the discussion of pain management in Chapter 17 and the suggested interventions in Box 19-3.

Gout

Gout is another form of inflammatory arthritis that results from the accumulation of uric acid crystals in a joint. Gout may be a one-time acute illness, or it may become a chronic condition with acute attacks. The joint of the great toe is the most

Goals

Pain management and promotion of comfort
Exercise and rest interspersed
Psychological support
Reduction of swelling and inflammation
Prevention of deformity
Promotion of optimal lifestyle

Suggested Interventions

Provide realistic information.
Teach client self-care to promote comfort.
Assist client in modifying lifestyle appropriately.
Prescribe exercises for muscle maintenance.
Promote participation in weight reduction program if necessary.
Have client balance rest and activity.
Teach relaxation and stress reduction.
Teach client to avoid bending painful joints and to splint when joints are inflamed.
Teach client to maintain body alignment when standing, sitting, and lying down.

Data from Heckheimer EF: *Health promotion of the elderly in the community,* Philadelphia, 1989, WB Saunders.

typical site of an attack. Sometimes the ankle, knee, wrist, or elbow is involved.

Gout typically starts with an acute attack. The person complains of what is called exquisite pain in the affected joint, often starting in the middle of the night during sleep. The joint is bright red, hot, and too painful to touch. Gout may be exacerbated by drugs commonly taken by the elderly, particularly thiazide diuretics and salicylates (even in small dosages). A laboratory test finding of elevated uric acid is possible, but the uric acid level also may be normal.

The first goal of treatment during an attack is pain relief. This may include NSAIDs, colchicine, and sometimes injection of long-lasting steroids into the joint. The nurse ensures that the person takes in enough fluids to help flush the uric acid through the kidneys (2 L/day if not contraindicated).

After the acute attack the medical goal is to prevent another attack, systemic spread of the disease, and the development of chronic gout. This may be done with the avoidance of drugs or foods that are high in purine and alcohol both of which increase uric acid levels; with medications to either decrease uric acid production (e.g., allopurinol) or increase its excretion (e.g., probenecid). Weight reduction if the patient is overweight is also encouraged (Jett, Lester, 2004).

The nurse's roles include teaching the person how to decrease the likelihood of another attack by employing preventive measures. In administering gout-related medications the nurse pays close attention to renal function and notifies the physician or nurse practitioner of any impairment so that the dosages can be adjusted.

KEY CONCEPTS

- Most people over the age of 40 will have osteoarthritis at some point in their lives.
- Osteoporosis is a crippling problem for many elders, especially women. Although it cannot be completely prevented, it can be minimized by early interventions: exercise, weight bearing, and calcium intake.
- The most serious outcomes of osteoporosis are fractures, which are associated with a high mortality rate.
- Rheumatoid arthritis produces swelling, inflammation, intense pain, and distortion of the joints.
- Gout is both an acute and a chronic condition. One of the goals of treatment of gout is to minimize a future attack.
- Certain types of complementary and alternative interventions have been found to be very helpful to individuals with joint disorders and chronic discomfort; however, their exact usefulness or safety is unknown.

Activities and Discussion Questions

1. What are the most effective ways of preventing osteoporosis?
2. What lifestyle issues would you discuss with an individual with advanced osteoporosis?
3. What are the differences in appearance of osteoarthritis and rheumatoid arthritis?

NANDA and Wellness Diagnoses

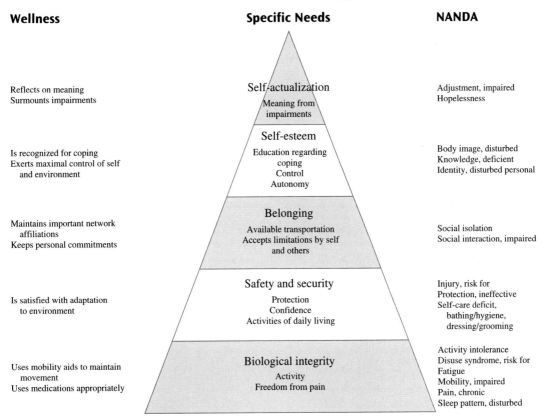

Wellness	Specific Needs	NANDA

Self-actualization
Meaning from impairments

Reflects on meaning
Surmounts impairments

Adjustment, impaired
Hopelessness

Self-esteem
Education regarding coping
Control
Autonomy

Is recognized for coping
Exerts maximal control of self and environment

Body image, disturbed
Knowledge, deficient
Identity, disturbed personal

Belonging
Available transportation
Accepts limitations by self and others

Maintains important network affiliations
Keeps personal commitments

Social isolation
Social interaction, impaired

Safety and security
Protection
Confidence
Activities of daily living

Is satisfied with adaptation to environment

Injury, risk for
Protection, ineffective
Self-care deficit, bathing/hygiene, dressing/grooming

Biological integrity
Activity
Freedom from pain

Uses mobility aids to maintain movement
Uses medications appropriately

Activity intolerance
Disuse syndrome, risk for
Fatigue
Mobility, impaired
Pain, chronic
Sleep pattern, disturbed

These are not all of the possible wellness or NANDA diagnoses that may be identified. The above are frequent examples of nursing diagnoses that should be considered when planning care for the older adult in whatever setting.

4. What advice would you give someone who is experiencing joint pain and mobility limitations?
5. Discuss your thoughts and experiences relating to alternative methods of dealing with chronic pain.
6. Which of your favorite activities would be difficult if you were afflicted with osteoarthritis?

RESOURCES

Websites

The Arthritis Foundation
www.arthritis.org

National Institute for Arthritis and Musculoskeletal Systems
www.niams.nih.gov

National Institute of Health
Office of Alternative Medicine
www.altmed.od.nih.gov

REFERENCES

Agency for Healthcare Research and Quality: AHRQ research has improved OA management, 2002. Available at www.ahrq.gov/research/osteoria/osteoria.htm.
Ali NS, Twibell KR: Barriers to osteoporosis prevention in perimenopausal and elderly women, *Geriatr Nurs* 15(4):201-205, 1994.

Anderson DL: TNF inhibitors: a new age in rheumatoid arthritis treatment, *Am J Nurs* 104(2):60-68, 2004.

Blakeley JA, Ribeiro VE: Glucosamine and osteoarthritis, *Am J Nurs* 104(2):54-59, 2004.

Brion PH, Concoff AL: Nonpharmacologic therapy of osteoarthritis, *UpToDate* 10(6), 2002. Available at www.uptodate.com.

Brucker MC, Youngkin EQ: What's a woman to do? Exploring HRT questions raised by the women's health initiative, *AWHONN Lifelines* 6(5):408-417, 2002.

Callahan LF, Jonas BL: Arthritis. In Ham RJ, Sloane PD, Warshaw GA, editors: *Primary care geriatrics: a case-based approach,* ed 4, St Louis, 2002, Mosby.

Chao S, Vega C: Alternative approaches to relieving the pain of osteoarthritis, *The Clinical Letter,* pp 21-26, Jan 2004.

Concoff AL: Clinical manifestations of osteoarthritis, *UpToDate* 10(1), 2002. Available at www.uptodate.com.

Gaylord S, Crotty N: Enhancing function with complementary therapies in geriatric rehabilitation, *Top Geriatric Rehab* 18(2):63-79, 2002.

Gornisiewicz M, Moreland LW: Rheumatoid arthritis. In Robbins L, editor: *Clinical care in the rheumatic diseases,* ed 2, Atlanta, 2001, Association of Rheumatology Health Professionals.

Hochberg MC et al: Guidelines for the medical management of osteoarthritis. I. Osteoarthritis of the hip, *Arthritis Rheum* 38(11):1535-1540, 1995.

Jett KF, Jester PB: Musculoskeletal disorders. In Youngkin EQ, Sawin K, Isreal D, editors: *Pharmcotherapeutics,* ed 2, Upper Saddle River, NJ, 2004, Prentice-Hall.

Kalunian KC, Brion PH: Classification and diagnosis of osteoarthritis, *UpToDate* 10(1), 2002. Available at www.uptodate.com.

Kee CC et al: Perspectives on the nursing management of osteoarthritis, *Geriatr Nurs* 19(1):19-26, 1998.

Li F et al: A simple 8-form easy Tai Chi for elderly adults, *J Aging Phys Act* 11(2):206-211, 2003.

Lozada CJ, Altman RD: Osteoarthritis. In Robbins L, editor: *Clinical care in the rheumatic diseases,* ed 2, Atlanta, 2001, Association of Rheumatology Health Professionals.

Luggen AS: Arthritis in older adults: current therapy with self-management as centerpiece, *Adv Nurs Pract* 11(3):26-35, 2003.

McCaffrey R, Freeman E: Effects of music on chronic osteoarthritis pain in older people, *J Adv Nurs* 44(5):517-524, 2003.

National Institutes of Health: *Osteoarthritis overview,* 2003. Available at www.nih.gov.

National Institutes of Health: *Fast facts on osteoporosis,* 2004. Available at www.osteo.org.

Paget S: Diagnostic guidelines. In The Institute for Medical Studies: *Diagnosis and treatment of rheumatoid arthritis: a special report for primary care physicians,* Laguna Niguel, Calif, 1995, HP Publishing.

Roberts D: Alternative therapies for arthritis treatment. 2, *Orthop Nurs* 22(6):412-420, 2003.

Thorndyke L: Osteoporosis. In Adelman AM, Daly MP, editors: *Twenty common problems in geriatrics,* New York, 2001, McGraw-Hill.

U.S. Bureau of the Census: *Statistical abstract of the United States: 1998,* ed 118, Washington, DC, 1998, U.S. Government Printing Office.

U.S. Prevention Services Task Force: *Screening for osteoporosis,* 2002. Available from www.acpr.gov.

Coping with Cardiac and Respiratory Disorders

Upon completion of this chapter, the reader will be able to:

- Identify the possible causes of heart failure.
- Discuss assessment of and intervention for the elder with heart failure (HF).
- State the most common respiratory disorders affecting the older adult.
- Discuss the interventions necessary to meet therapy goals for an older adult with chronic obstructive pulmonary disease (COPD).
- Explain the significance of pneumonia and tuberculosis in the older population and discuss means of prevention of each of these diseases.
- Develop a nursing care plan for the elder with congestive heart failure (CHF) and one for the elder with COPD.

GLOSSARY

Co-morbidity More than one disease or health condition existing at the same time.
Dyspnea The subjective report of shortness of breath
Morbidity Disability as the result of a health condition.

Mortality Death as a result of a condition.
Nosocomial Pertaining to the institutional setting as the source (as in nosocomial infection).

THE LIVED EXPERIENCE

When I first had that heart attack, I was so frightened it seemed I would die just from the fear. It was the first time I realized how comforting calm and efficient nurses could be. There was the one who came into the room a few days later and talked to me about the cardiac rehab program and that I could continue doing the things I had always done, except for changes in diet and more exercise. Even sex! I would never have asked that young thing, but she just told me it was OK.

Jerry, age 63

When Dad had that heart attack, it really scared us all, and I know we were afraid we would say or do something that would bring on another. I think he was also afraid of everything. I'm so grateful for the nurses at the hospital. They seem to give him lots of attention and information about the things he needs to know. He seems quite relaxed with himself now.

Ruth, Jerry's youngest daughter

Caring for older adults means caring for persons with cardiac problems, respiratory problems, or both. These two systems are interconnected. A problem in one is likely to precipitate or complicate a problem in the other. When the nurse is addressing a cardiovascular problem, such as heart failure, the respiratory system must also be seriously considered in the nursing plan of care. Conversely, in the elder with serious respiratory problems, such as pneumonia or emphysema, cardiac status must be a part of nursing assessment and care for the whole person. Nursing interventions frequently overlap. One carefully planned action can address several systems at the same time and achieve goals of homeostasis and energy conservation, therefore reducing morbidity and promoting as much health as possible.

CARDIAC DISORDERS

Heart disease is the number one cause of death for persons over 65 living in the United States and many other parts of the world, affecting both men and women in every ethnic group. The most common types of heart disease seen by nurses include coronary artery disease (CAD) and heart failure (HF), especially in long-term care settings. When the HF has advanced it is known as congestive heart failure (CHF) and when it advances to a life-threatening point, it is known as end-stage heart disease.

Coronary Artery Disease

The beating heart, like other muscles, needs oxygen and other nutrients to provide energy for its work. Despite all of the blood that passes through the heart, it cannot use the nutrients from the blood that passes through its chambers. The heart muscle, like all other muscles, receives its oxygen from arteries. Coronary artery disease (CAD) is blockage of the vessels that supply the heart with blood. This disease process is termed *arteriosclerosis*, commonly called "hardening of the arteries." In this process, cholesterol and other fats are deposited in the layers of the arteries, narrowing the channel for blood to flow and therefore limiting the amount of oxygen reaching the tissue (ischemia).

Ischemia may be experienced differently by younger and older adults. When ischemia occurs, a younger person may have chest pain (angina) and is said to be having a heart attack or a myocardial infarction (MI). Angina is described as a pressing or squeezing pain, usually in the chest under the breastbone, but sometimes in the shoulders, arms, neck, jaws, or back. It is often precipitated by exertion. Unfortunately, many elderly patients with heart attacks do not have this classical presentation and instead have what are called *silent MIs*. Their discomfort may be relatively mild and may be localized to the back, abdomen, shoulders, or either or both arms. Nausea and vomiting, or merely a feeling of heartburn, may be the only symptom. These less classical symptoms may not make patients think of a heart problem and may keep them from seeking medical help. In fact, up to 30% of heart attacks are diagnosed by taking a routine electrocardiogram (ECG) long after the fact.

Heart Failure

The damage to the heart from CAD may lead to heart failure (HF), the most frequent cause for hospitalization of an older adult and the second most common reason, after hypertension, for an office visit to a health care provider. Seventy-five percent of those with HF are over 65 (Ghosh, Gupta, 2002).

HF is a disease of the heart muscle in which the heart muscle malfunctions and can no longer pump enough blood to meet the needs of the body. The severity of malfunctioning depends on whether it is a mechanical or functional abnormality. Other causes of HF are hypertension, fever, hypoxia, anemia, metabolic disease (hyperthyroid or hypothyroid), and infection. Over time the heart is further damaged because of poor control of the underlying problem (e.g., hypertension or CAD) leading to more and more severe HF (Box 20-1). An unhealthy diet, smoking, and lack of exercise aggravate the development of heart disease and the extent of damage, especially for those who have a family history of heart disease and the genetic predisposition for heart disease. There is no cure for HF, only the management of symptoms and attempts to prevent worsening.

Clinical HF is categorized as left-sided, right-sided, or biventricular (both-sided) failure. It can

Box 20-1	Causes of Heart Failure

Impeded Forward Ejection
Systemic arterial hypertension or elevated systemic vascular resistance
Aortic valve stenosis
Coarctation of aorta
Subaortic stenosis
Obstructive hypertrophic cardiomyopathy
Pulmonary hypertension

Impaired Cardiac Filling
Ventricular hypertrophy
Prolonged myocardial relaxation time (diastolic dysfunction)
Pericardial constriction or tamponade
Restrictive endocarditis or myocardial heart disease
Ventricular aneurysm

Volume Overload
Valvular regurgitation
Increased intravascular volume
Metabolic demands: thyrotoxicosis, anemia
Arteriovenous shunts or fistulas

Myocardial Failure
Loss of muscle function (myocardial infarction; ischemia)
Cardiomyopathy
Myocarditis
Drug induced
Systemic disease (hypothyroid)
Chronic overload

Box 20-2	Classification of Heart Failure

Class I: Basically Asymptomatic
Cardiac disease without resulting limitations of physical activity

Class II: Mild Heart Failure
Slight limitation of physical activity
Comfortable at rest
An increase in activity may cause fatigue, palpitations, dyspnea, or anginal pain

Class III: Moderate Heart Failure
Marked limitation in physical activity
Comfortable at rest
Ordinary walking or climbing of stairs can quickly bring on symptoms of fatigue, palpitations, dyspnea, or anginal pain
Substantial periods of bed rest required

Class IV: Severe Heart Failure
Almost permanently confined to bed
Inability to carry out any physical activity without discomfort or severe symptoms
Some symptoms occur at rest
Chronic shortness of breath is common

also be described as either systolic or diastolic dysfunction (Marek et al, 1999). Left-sided and diastolic failure are the most common types found in the elderly. Long-standing left-sided HF eventually causes right-sided failure (Braunwald, 1992). The New York Heart Association provides us with a convenient way to classify the symptomatic experience of the HF, from symptom free to severely disabled (Box 20-2).

Common signs and symptoms of heart failure in the elderly include fatigue or shortness of breath (dyspnea) with exertion, inability to lie flat without getting short of breath (orthopnea), waking up at night gasping for air, weight gain, and swelling in the lower extremities. Dyspnea may be at rest, be only on exertion, or occur intermittently at night (paroxysmal nocturnal dyspnea). The dyspnea may be relieved by sitting up or sleeping on multiple pillows or with the head of the bed elevated. If a cough is present, it is worse at night.

In addition, the nurse should be alert for the atypical clinical presentation of exacerbations of HF in the elderly. The person may appear fatigued, confused, or delirious; begin falling; or complain of insomnia or urinary frequency at night (nocturia). He or she may complain of dizziness or may have syncope (fainting). Or more often, the nurse will notice that the person has the "droops," or malaise and a subtle decline in activity tolerance or in functional ability.

One of the major ways that cardiac conditions differ from other chronic problems is that when they become acute problems they can do so very rapidly and often require acute hospitalization and intensive treatment followed by rehabilitation. Many other chronic disorders are managed at home.

Peripheral Vascular Disease

The most common vascular disorders of the older adult are venous insufficiency and arterial insufficiency, which result in venous stasis ulcers or arterial complications, such as gangrene. A discussion of these can be found in Chapter 13.

Implications for Gerontological Nursing and Healthy Aging

Assessment

As with any assessment, obtaining a pertinent history of the events leading up to and including the presentation of HF is essential whether the history is from the elder patient or a caregiver. Monitoring of vital signs and laboratory results; assessment of the cardiac and respiratory systems by inspection, palpation, percussion, and auscultation; and obtaining a mental status level as well as kidney function (output) are essential. Determination of the person's ability to perform activities of daily living (ADLs) and instrumental activities of daily living (IADLs) is also part of the assessment of cardiac status. These and other assessment guidelines are listed in Box 20-3.

Box 20-3	Assessment for Heart Failure

Brief history of onset and course of condition
Vital signs
Cardiac and respiratory inspection and
    auscultation of heart and breath sounds
Mental status check
Activity capabilities
Lifestyle
Genitourinary: nocturia, oliguria
Weight change
Client's perception of condition, reaction to
    diagnosis, and treatment
General laboratory values: electrolytes,
    hemoglobin, hematocrit, coagulation

Data from Saunders SA: Atherosclerotic heart disease: heart failure. In Rogers-Seidl FF, editor: *Geriatric nursing care plans*, St Louis, 1991, Mosby; Havens LL, Weaver JW: Cardiovascular system. In Hogstel MO: *Clinical manual of gerontological nursing*, St Louis, 1992, Mosby.

Interventions

For the person with HF, the goals of therapy are to provide relief of symptoms, improve the quality of life, reduce mortality and morbidity, and slow or stop progression of dysfunction through the use of aggressive drug therapy (Gross, 1999). Concurrent and supportive therapies include diet modification by decreasing fat, cholesterol, and sodium intake; exercise such as walking 30 minutes each day or several times each week; education; and family and social supports (Schultz, 1998). The ultimate goal for elders with chronic HF is quality of life, not quantity of life (Kennedy-Malone et al, 2003).

Nursing interventions assist in the accomplishment of these goals. What specific interventions are used will depend on the severity of the HF. Nursing actions range from teaching the older adult about lifestyle changes in diet, activity, and rest to acute measures, such as the administration of oxygen and other emergent procedures in acute situations. In general, interventions about which the nurse should be knowledgeable include the following:

- Prescribed exercise
- Medication administration and the evaluation of medication effects
- Monitoring for signs and symptoms of CHF
- Monitoring fluid intake and output and diet
- Monitoring weight (either daily, biweekly, or weekly)
- Checking for jugular distention
- Auscultating heart and lung sounds
- Monitoring laboratory values
- Education related to all of the above

Vitally important for older adults, as well as for younger adults, is cardiac rehabilitation. Coronary problems are likely to produce a "cardiac cripple" when the individual believes that any exertion overtaxes the heart, and these problems may potentiate a return to CHF or a heart attack and death. In reality, few elders develop activity-induced ischemia. However, complicating illnesses, such as infections and bleeding episodes, may trigger acute decompensation. To prevent this, cardiac exercise rehabilitation programs must be encouraged for the physical, as well as mental, health of the individual. Exercise training of patients with heart disease has been found to increase work capacity and vagal tone and decrease resting heart rate, body weight, and the percentage of body fat (Stanley, 1999). Typical programs are prescribed by the physician or nurse practitioner and begin with light activity and progress to moderate activity under the supervision of a nurse or physical therapist. Women may need extra encouragement. Schuster et al (1995) found that women knew less about their heart disease and supportive treatment than men and were the poorest adherents to exercise regardless of whether the cardiac rehabilitation program was at home or in a rehabilitation center.

The nurse and the individual must be cautious about exercise. Postexercise orthostatic hypotension is more likely to occur with the older adult as a result of age-related decreased baroreceptor responsiveness, which controls the body's ability to respond to the need for changes in blood pressure. Because thermoregulation is impaired, exercise intensity must be reduced in hot, humid climates. Specific cardiac rehabilitation programs for elders emphasize activities that build endurance, increase fitness, reduce the risk of new cardiac problems, and promote self-reliance to facilitate self-care and improve the quality of life (Schultz, 1998). For more impaired elders, it is necessary to identify energy-conserving measures applicable to their daily tasks.

Risk reduction programs should be instituted with a clear understanding of the difficulties involved in attempts to alter harmful lifestyle practices such as smoking, overeating, habitual anger or irritation, and sedentary lifestyle. These practices may have been going on for a lifetime and are not easily changed by "education." The nurse's role in these instances is to discuss these practices in a nonjudgmental manner, providing acceptance, encouragement, resources, knowledge, and affirmation of both the difficulty of making lifestyle changes and the elder's right to choose.

RESPIRATORY DISORDERS

The normal physical changes with aging (see Chapter 7) result in a greater risk for respiratory problems, and when they occur, there is a higher mortality rate than seen in younger persons. Diseases of the respiratory system are identified as acute or chronic and as involving the upper or lower respiratory tract. They are further defined as

either *obstructive*—preventing airflow out as a result of obstruction or narrowing of the respiratory structures (e.g., COPD [emphysema]); or *restrictive*—causing a decrease in total lung capacity as a result of limited expansion (Lewis, Haggerty, 1999).

Chronic Obstructive Pulmonary Disease

Chronic obstructive pulmonary disease (COPD) is a nonspecific term used to "characterize persistent slowing of airflow during forceful expiration" (American Thoracic Society, 1995). It is the only major cause of death whose mortality rate is rising among adults, and it is now the fourth leading cause of death for both older men and women in most ethnic groups. The increase is largely driven by cumulative and residual effects of long-term cigarette smoking (80% to 90% of cases), occupational and community pollutants, exposure to secondhand smoke, and, to a lesser extent, familial and genetic factors. Damage to the lungs earlier in life may not be noticeable for 20 to 30 years, and usually about 50% of lung function has been irretrievably lost before symptoms appear suggestive of COPD (Stoller, 2002).

The most common symptoms of COPD are cough, dyspnea on exertion, and increased phlegm production (Estes, 2002). Chronic cough affects the majority of smokers or former smokers. Other common signs include wheezing, prolonged expiration with pursed-lip breathing, barrel chest, air trapping, hyperresonance, pale lips or nail beds, fingernail clubbing, and use of accessory breathing muscles (McCrory et al, 2001). In advanced cases, cyanosis, evidence of right-sided heart failure, and peripheral edema are present. A chest x-ray usually shows hyperinflation of the lungs and flattening of the diaphragm.

When respirations exceed 30/min the person with COPD may be having an exacerbation of his or her illness and intervention is necessary. An acute exacerbation of COPD represents an acute worsening of the baseline symptoms and signs of COPD, generally characterized by significantly worsened dyspnea and increased volume and purulence of sputum (McCrory et al, 2001). A number of factors, including viral or bacterial infections, air pollution or other environmental exposures, or changes in the weather, may trigger a change in the person's health.

Exacerbations are typical features of COPD in its moderate to severe stages, especially in patients with symptoms of chronic bronchitis. When the worsening of the condition occurs it frequently means that medications will need to be increased or changed or hospitalization may be necessary. The routine use of antibiotics is controversial because the exact cause of the worsening is often difficult to determine and may not be related to a bacterial infection. Antibiotics are generally indicated in patients with new pulmonary infiltrates on chest x-ray, fever, or purulent sputum. Although the acute phase of an exacerbation is usually over in 10 to 14 days, lung function may take 4 to 6 weeks to return to baseline.

As a category, COPD includes chronic bronchitis, asthma, and emphysema; and all worsen over time. The progressive nature of COPD can lead to malnutrition because energy is consumed by the tremendous effort expended for breathing. Eating requires further effort and is often neglected. Individuals and their families may be so concerned with the breathing difficulties that they are hardly aware of the diminished caloric intake. Anxiety and depression are associated with the disease because of the difficulty breathing and the progressive and debilitating aspects of the condition.

Implications for Gerontological Nursing and Healthy Aging

Assessment. The nursing assessment of the person with COPD usually focuses on the complaints of dyspnea and coughing. Dyspnea is a subjective report. Only persons experiencing it can really tell us what it is like for them. Visual analog scales and numeric rating scales, similar to those used to assess pain, may be helpful to use in the measurement (see Chapter 17). Persons can be asked how they would rate their breathing, from 1 (no dyspnea) to 10 (the worst dyspnea possible).

The assessment includes detailed information about the cough. When did it start? How long are the episodes of coughing? Is there any associated pain? What seems to make the cough better, and what makes it worse? Is the person using anything

to treat the cough? Is the person smoking (and how much) or exposed to smoke or other respiratory irritants? If the cough is productive, what are the color, texture, and odor of the mucus? Does the color change over the time of the day?

The remaining physical examination is the same as that used for persons with cardiac disease, since it is not always clear whether symptoms such as fatigue and shortness of breath are cardiac or respiratory in nature. Observation of airway clearance, breathing patterns, and mobility; the measurement of pulse oximetry; a mental status examination; and a functional assessment facilitate a clearer picture of the current status. Pulmonary function testing is most definitive in terms of lung capacity, and along with a chest x-ray examination, can show the extent of respiratory damage. Box 20-4 presents a model of respiratory assessment.

Box 20-4   COPD Assessment

History
Respiratory diseases
Smoking history
Symptoms

Physical Examination
Inspection*
Posture
Chest symmetry, shape, expansion
Respirations
Skin color
Capillary fill
Sputum (color, amount, consistency)
Palpation
Tenderness
Percussion
Areas of hyperinflation, consolidation
Auscultation*
Breath sounds

Functional Activity and Mobility
Levels of activity before dyspneic
Interferences from sensory impairments

Knowledge
Educational attainment
Understanding of disease processes in COPD

COPD, Chronic obstructive pulmonary disease.
*Most important of the four assessment techniques.

Interventions. As with heart failure, COPD cannot be cured. Nursing interventions are based on palliative goals, namely, stabilizing the disease, reducing the risk of exacerbations and hospitalizations, promoting maximal functional capacity, and preventing premature disability. Aspects that should be included are smoking cessation, secretion clearance techniques, identification and management of exacerbations, breathing retraining, education, rehabilitation, psychological support, management of depression and anxiety, nutritional support, the proper use and administration of medications, and supplemental oxygen therapy if and when it is necessary (Brown et al, 1999; Monahan, 1999).

Education should be considered in every aspect of pulmonary care. The older adult should be taught to recognize the signs and symptoms of respiratory infection, how to maintain adequate nutrition, how to use an inhaler or nebulizer, how to clean it, the use of oxygen and oxygen safety, the type of exercise that is beneficial, how to pace activities, coping strategies, and other issues, such as sexual function. Each of these areas requires teaching and has specific interventions that will be helpful to older adults and their families or other caregivers. The interventions that might lessen many of the problems encountered in COPD appear in Box 20-5.

Diet education should address the reason for monitoring weight and the signs of malnutrition. Weight loss can occur rapidly because of the energy expenditure needed to breathe. Dyspnea interferes with eating. In addition, satiation results from the intake of small amounts of food because of congestion in the abdomen caused by a flattened diaphragm. Anorexia or decreased appetite occurs as a result of sputum production and gastric irritation from the use of bronchodilators and steroids.

Activity and exercise tolerance should be assessed by the physician and respiratory therapist, and activities should be prescribed to increase endurance and improve respiratory status. Exercise may be done with or without oxygen as a supplement to control symptoms so that the older adult can spend enough time in exercise to benefit from it. The person should be informed that sex is still possible and should be provided with education and counseling information, either by the nurse or a professional counselor.

Medications are used to control dyspnea, cough, and sputum production. As with any medication teaching, the nurse can make sure that the older adult knows the purpose and correct dosing of any medication he or she is taking, its side effects, and what to do if side effects occur. Medications administered through inhalers or nebulizers have a more rapid onset, local efficiency of reaching the target organ, and fewer side effects. However, instruction on the use of the equipment is also very important, since fewer than 30% of patients use the inhaler correctly (Lewis, Haggerty, 1999). Return demonstrations are recommended. Inhalers may be troublesome for some older adults because of the coordination of inspiration with the inhaler or impaired manual dexterity, such as in patients with arthritis. Metered-dose or spacer devices may help elders use inhalers better and facilitate maximal drug delivery. There are also special adaptive devices for persons with limited hand strength. Figure 20-1 illustrates the use of the inhaler.

Rehabilitation is an important aspect of maximizing life with COPD. An older adult with COPD would be considered a candidate for pulmonary rehabilitation as long as he or she does not have severe COPD without pulmonary reserve or unstable heart disease. Rehabilitation programs for the older adult with COPD consist of drug therapy, reconditioning exercises, and counseling. A multidisciplinary team of health professionals works collectively to help the older adult achieve the following goals:

- Increase the level of independence
- Maintain individuality and autonomy
- Improve function in his or her environment
- Decrease the number of hospitalizations and need for hospitalization
- Increase exercise tolerance
- Increase self-esteem
- Improve the quality of life

The number of goals achieved depends on many factors, including extent of illness and of co-existing conditions.

Economic issues are always a concern for persons with chronic disease. A number of medications are used and are very expensive, especially when needed for an indefinite period of time. Regular Medicare does not cover prescriptions. The expense of oxygen therapy for elders with a limited income may also interfere with the ade-

| **Box 20-5** | **Interventions for Chronic Obstructive Pulmonary Disease** |

Nutrition

Eat small, frequent, nutrient-intense meals.

Eat foods with high protein and caloric content.

Serve meals on small plates (servings will not look overwhelming).

Select foods that do not require a lot of chewing.

Have food cut in bite-size pieces to conserve energy.

Establish a plan for fluid intake; drink 2 to 3 L of fluid daily (pineapple juice helps cut secretions; keep 1 L of water in the refrigerator or on the kitchen counter to be consumed each day in addition to other fluids).

Weigh at least twice each week.

Exercise

(Based on an established plan suggested by physician or rehabilitation team)

Walk daily all year round (in good weather, outdoors; in bad weather, go to the mall and walk indoors).

Walk up and down stairs in home (if present).

Use a stationary bicycle.

When buying shoes for activity and everyday wear, avoid shoes that require bending over to tie; instead, get a slip-on type and use a long-handled shoehorn to assist the heel into the shoe.

Activity Pacing

Avoid high levels of exertion in the early morning.

Arrange rest periods throughout the day.

Allow plenty of time to complete activities; do not hurry.

Schedule activities in advance to reduce pressure and anxiety.

Obtain and follow prescribed exercise program for maintenance of heart and lung capacity.

Activities of Daily Living (ADLs)

Allow ample time for bathing and dressing. Have a chair in the bathroom for bathing.

Arrange toiletries in easy reach.

Wear shoes that slip on or have Velcro closures, not ties.

Select clothing with elasticized waistbands; avoid constrictive clothing; use suspenders rather than belts.

Select and wear clothing that is easy to put on and remove.

Safety

Attempt to keep a dust-free environment.

Minimize or eliminate dander and use of aerosol sprays, fumes, contaminants.

Place plastic covers over mattresses; use hypoallergenic pillows and blankets.

Avoid carpet and rug floor coverings.

Emotional Support

Accept and encourage expression of emotions.

Be an active listener.

Be cognizant of conversational dyspnea; do not interrupt or cut off conversations.

Education

Teach breathing techniques:

   Pursed-lip breathing

   Diaphragmatic breathing

   Cascade coughing (series)

Teach postural drainage.

Teach medications:

   What, why, frequency, amount, side effects, and what to do if side effects occur

   Use and care of inhalers

Teach signs and symptoms of respiratory infection.

Teach about sexual activity:

   Sexual function improves with rest.

   Schedule sex around best-breathing time of day.

   Use prescribed bronchodilators 20 to 30 minutes before sex.

   Use a position that does not require pressure on the chest or support of the arms.

Avoid the use of alcohol or eating large quantities of food.

General Instructions

Listen to weather reports:

   Avoid going out in inclement weather.

   Wear a scarf over the nose and mouth in cold and windy weather; wear a hat.

   Avoid going out when air pollution is high.

Use an air conditioner to filter air and make it drier.

Avoid situations where you may encounter individuals with influenza or upper respiratory tract infections.

Obtain an annual flu shot if not allergic.

Obtain one-time multivalent pneumococcal immunization.

Notify health care provider of any temperature above 99° F (37.2° C).

Examine sputum; recognize and report changes to physician.

Do not use over-the-counter drugs unless provider approves.

1. Remove the cap, and hold the inhaler upright.
2. Shake the inhaler.
3. Tilt your head back slightly, and breathe out.
4. Use the inhaler in any one of these ways. (A and B are the best ways. B is recommended for young children, older adults, and those taking inhaled steroids. C is okay if you are having trouble with A or B.)
   A. Open mouth with inhaler 1 to 2 inches away.
   B. Use spacer (ask for the handout on spacers).
   C. Put inhaler in mouth, and seal lips around the mouthpiece.
5. Press down on the inhaler to release the medicine as you start to breathe in slowly.
6. Breathe in *slowly* for 3 to 5 seconds.
7. *Hold* your breath for 10 seconds to allow the medicine to reach deeply into your lungs.
8. Repeat puffs as prescribed. Waiting 1 minute between puffs may permit the second puff to go deeper into the lungs.

NOTE: Dry powder capsules are used differently. To use a dry powder inhaler, close your mouth tightly around the mouthpiece and inhale very fast.

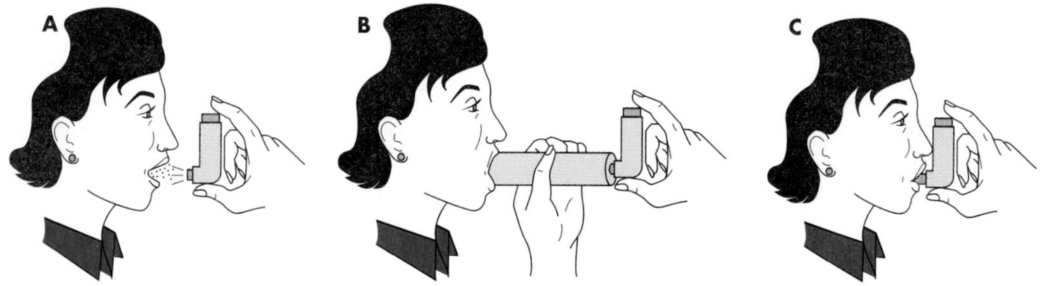

Figure 20-1   Using a metered-dose inhaler. (Redrawn from Nurses' Asthma Education Working Group: *Nurses: partners in asthma care*, NIH Pub No. 95-3308, 1995.)

quacy of therapy and create feelings of anxiety. Medicare coverage for oxygen is limited to those persons with a moderate to severe level of disease as determined by their oxygen saturation rates, and oxygen is never covered simply for comfort.

All efforts of professionals, family caregivers, and the older adult are directed toward creating a safe and comfortable environment that will maximize individual function and attainment of the highest level of function and wellness, with or without direct assistance.

Pneumonia

Pneumonia is a lower respiratory tract infection that causes inflammation of the lung tissue, generally by a bacterial agent. Pneumonia, combined with influenza, is the fifth leading cause of death of the elderly in the United States (CDC, 1999). Pneumonia-related mortality has not decreased appreciably since the 1950s (Karnath et al, 2003). The old-old (85 years and older) are five times more likely to die of pneumonia than young-old

or old adults. Particularly susceptible are elders with co-existing morbidity, such as alcoholism, asthma, COPD, or heart disease, or those who live in institutional settings (Koivula et al, 1994). Other factors that increase the risk of acquiring pneumonia relate to normal age changes of the respiratory system, such as a diminished cough reflex, increased residual volume, and decreased chest compliance (see Chapter 7).

Pneumonia is classified as either community acquired or nosocomial. The usual signs and symptoms of pneumonia manifested in younger persons are not commonly seen in the aged. Instead, falling, mental status changes or signs of confusion, general deterioration, weakness, anorexia, tachycardia, and tachypnea occur in the older adult. These atypical responses can easily lead to an incorrect diagnosis or a diagnosis made too late in the progression of the pneumonia (Kennedy-Malone et al, 2000).

Aspiration pneumonia is a high-risk condition for an obtunded client who is force fed or fed by a gastrostomy or PEG (percutaneous endoscopic gastrostomy) tube, a client with swallowing difficulties or esophageal disease, a client who regurgitates food, a client with an endotracheal tube or tracheostomy, and a client who is heavily sedated.

The most common pathogen causing a community-acquired infection is *Streptococcus pneumoniae* (15.3% of hospital admissions) (Karnath et al, 2003). Other less common bacterial pneumonias are caused by *Haemophilus influenzae, Staphylococcus, Pseudomonas,* or *Klebsiella,* but the cause for most is undetermined (Brown et al, 1999; Lewis, Haggerty, 1999).

Implications for Gerontological Nursing and Healthy Aging

The nurse has a role in reducing the mortality associated with pneumonia through prompt recognition of the potential signs of the problem and facilitating the prompt initiation of treatment. Especially for the frail elder, it is never appropriate to use a "wait and see" approach; elevations in temperature or in white blood count may not occur until the person is in a septic state, and chest x-rays in debilitated persons are often falsely negative at the beginning of the infection or with dehydration. More timely diagnosis requires sensitive clinical assessments by both the nurse and the other health care providers.

Where treatment is given is a critical issue. If the person is already in a skilled nursing facility, except in severe cases, treatment can occur there if oxygen therapy, parenteral fluids, and antibiotics can be administered by the nursing staff. If there is a person available to assume a caregiver role, care and treatment can occur in the elder's home with temporary home health service support. If the elder fails to improve or deteriorates in either setting, then hospitalization is often necessary, unless this is against the wishes of the patient. If the person is hospitalized, the sometimes prolonged rehabilitation for declined functioning is likely to occur in a long-term care setting.

The nurse's role is vital in caring for elders with pneumonia in acute and long-term care settings. Care will include a multitude of interventions. Medications will be administered for a specified period of time, depending on the responsible organism and extent of illness. Adequate rest is needed to preserve limited reserve capacity, and oxygen therapy is provided (if emphysema is present, then oxygen must be limited to 1 or 2 L). Optimizing pulmonary ventilation can be done by working with the person to breathe deeply, cough regularly, and frequently change position. Mouth care is very important, especially for the person receiving supplemental oxygen. Inadequate mouth care leads to the propagation of bacteria, which confounds an already serious situation. Sputum is considered infectious and requires appropriate handling.

Monitoring nutrition and obtaining nutrition consultation as necessary are the responsibility of the nurse in all settings. The nurse will also ensure that the person recovering from pneumonia is adequately nourished and hydrated while monitoring fluid volume to prevent overload in elders with cardiovascular disease and CHF. Mobilizing the older person and referring him or her for physical and occupational therapy to prevent or stop functional decline should occur as soon as the person's condition allows.

The nurse also has a role in the prevention of pneumonia. Adults older than 65 years of age and those with chronic conditions should be encouraged to receive the one-time pneumococcal vaccine (Pneumovax) unless they are at high risk. In that case, their health care providers may recommend a second immunization after about 5 years. Influenza-related pneumonias may be avoided or ameliorated with yearly (October to December) flu vaccinations. Finally, yearly dental cleanings and examinations should be encouraged, since dental caries and periodontal disease predispose one to develop pneumonia as a secondary infection (Karnath et al, 2003).

Tuberculosis

Tuberculosis (TB) is a communicable and infectious disease associated with one of several organisms, *Mycobacterium tuberculosis, Mycobacterium bovis,* and *Mycobacterium africanum.* The term *tuberculosis infection* refers to a positive TB skin test with no evidence of active disease. *Tuberculosis disease* refers to cases that have positive acid-fast smear or culture for *M. tuberculosis* or radiographical and clinical presentation of TB.

It is estimated that one third of the world's population is infected with *M. tuberculosis*

(Rajagopalan, Yoshikawa, 2000). *M. tuberculosis* was considered to be conquered in the 1950s with the development of the drug isoniazid (INH). Many of our present elders were treated following their acquisition of the disease during World War II. Many others contracted the disease in childhood. As they become immunocompromised as a result of chemotherapy, extreme old age, or human immunodeficiency virus (HIV) infection, the bacterium could be reactivated.

The number of cases of TB in the United States has steadily decreased from the 37,100 reported in 1970 to 15,075 in 2002 (CDC, 2003). In absolute numbers, the most cases of TB are seen in the over 65 population of black Americans; however, the percentage per population is only 12.6 per 100,000. Asians and Pacific Islanders have the highest rate by percentage at 27.8. In comparison, the rate is only 1.5 in white Americans (CDC, 2003).

Although these numbers are small, the vast majority of the cases of TB seen in persons over 65 occur in those who are living in nursing homes, with wide variation by area. In 2002 only three cases were documented in long-term care residents in Wyoming, but California, Texas, Florida, and New York City had 3169, 1550, 1086, and 1084 cases, respectively (CDC, 2003). Gerontological nurses working in these areas need to be particularly knowledgeable about this potentially life-threatening disease.

Although TB is not as contagious as once believed, the tubercle bacillus is becoming resistant to treatment. Therefore prevention is of high priority, especially among groups in close contact who have compromised immune systems; are malnourished; have co-morbidities such as diabetes mellitus, malignancies, and chronic renal failure; or have a body weight 10% below ideal, such as the very old in nursing homes (Brown et al, 1999; Kennedy-Malone et al, 2003). Symptoms include unexplained weight loss or fever and a cough lasting more than 3 weeks regardless of age group. Laboratory results in the elderly may show an increased sedimentation rate and lymphocytopenia.

Implications for Gerontological Nursing in Long-Term Care Settings

In promoting healthy aging the nurse must be proactive in the prevention of contagious disease and in the prompt treatment of those who become or are ill. This is especially important in the long-term care setting. There elders are at higher risk because of communal living situations and the high rate of medical frailty.

In 1990 the CDC recommended that every person entering a long-term care facility as a resident or an employee be tested for TB on an annual basis. Whereas some individual states have modified that recommendation, the CDC has not. The most accurate tuberculin skin test is the Mantoux test, in which 5 units of tuberculin purified protein derivative (PPD) are injected intradermally to detect delayed hypersensitivity to TB. The amount of induration is assessed after 48 to 72 hours, and the extent of induration (not erythema) should be measured across two diameters at right angles and the two measurements then averaged. An induration of ≥10 mm is considered positive. There are false negatives in about 30% of the persons with the disease (CDC, 1990); that is, in about 30% of the cases where there is actually an infection, the test will be negative. For those who test negative, the test is repeated in 7 to 10 days. Those with a positive PPD test should receive a chest x-ray and clinical evaluation for TB. A positive sputum culture is necessary to confirm a diagnosis of TB.

Successful completion of TB treatment regimens in the elderly patient is complicated by a high mortality rate of 22% during the first 3 months (Kaltenbach et al, 2001). Although a major concern with young adults is the use of directly observed therapy to ensure compliance, in the elderly biweekly liver function monitoring is of equal importance because of the frequency of drug-induced hepatitis (Janssens, Zellweger, 1999). The nurse's role in monitoring laboratory values (assessing for adverse drug reactions and monitoring drug compliance) is crucial to treatment effectiveness and the patient's well-being. Patients generally undergo pretreatment measurement of liver function, serum urea nitrogen, platelets, bilirubin, creatinine, and uric acid levels. Laboratory values should be monitored monthly during treatment and whenever symptoms suggesting adverse effects occur.

Sputum culture conversion among TB patients is the most important indicator of successful drug treatment in all patients. However, the elderly and non-Hispanic whites were the most unlikely to yield negative sputum culture results even after

NANDA and Wellness Diagnoses

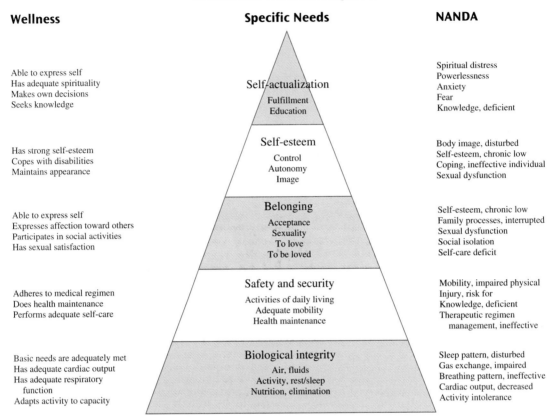

Wellness	Specific Needs	NANDA

Wellness

Able to express self
Has adequate spirituality
Makes own decisions
Seeks knowledge

Has strong self-esteem
Copes with disabilities
Maintains appearance

Able to express self
Expresses affection toward others
Participates in social activities
Has sexual satisfaction

Adheres to medical regimen
Does health maintenance
Performs adequate self-care

Basic needs are adequately met
Has adequate cardiac output
Has adequate respiratory
  function
Adapts activity to capacity

Specific Needs

Self-actualization
Fulfillment
Education

Self-esteem
Control
Autonomy
Image

Belonging
Acceptance
Sexuality
To love
To be loved

Safety and security
Activities of daily living
Adequate mobility
Health maintenance

Biological integrity
Air, fluids
Activity, rest/sleep
Nutrition, elimination

NANDA

Spiritual distress
Powerlessness
Anxiety
Fear
Knowledge, deficient

Body image, disturbed
Self-esteem, chronic low
Coping, ineffective individual
Sexual dysfunction

Self-esteem, chronic low
Family processes, interrupted
Sexual dysfunction
Social isolation
Self-care deficit

Mobility, impaired physical
Injury, risk for
Knowledge, deficient
Therapeutic regimen
  management, ineffective

Sleep pattern, disturbed
Gas exchange, impaired
Breathing pattern, ineffective
Cardiac output, decreased
Activity intolerance

These are not all of the possible wellness or NANDA diagnoses that may be identified. The above are frequent examples of nursing diagnoses that should be considered when planning care for the older adult in whatever setting.

treatment in a recent study (Liu et al, 1999). A positive finding on acid-fast smear or culture of the sputum after 5 months of treatment is considered a treatment failure. Failure can result from prescription of an inappropriate dosage or inadequate number of drugs, patient noncompliance, malabsorption, or organism resistance.

To ensure prompt identification of those persons with TB and limit its spread, especially in the long-term or extended care facility, nurses should develop and implement a surveillance plan (Box 20-6). If this is not already in place, the Centers for Disease Control and Prevention (CDC) and the state health departments are excellent sources of guidance and assistance.

KEY CONCEPTS

- Congestive heart failure is one of the most prevalent chronic problems of the aged. Any condition that stresses the heart may precipitate heart failure.
- The mortality associated with pneumonia in the elderly can be minimized through the use of pneumonia and influenza vaccinations.
- The goal of therapy for cardiac and respiratory disorders is to relieve symptoms, improve the quality of life, reduce mortality, stabilize and slow the progression of the disease, reduce the risk of exacerbation, and maximize functional capacity.

Box 20-6	Guidelines for Extended Care Monitoring for Tuberculosis

Screen all new residents on admission using two-step purified protein derivative (PPD).

Screen all residents every 2 years.

Perform chest x-ray examination of new residents on admission and of residents with documented positive reactions or in whom reactions turn positive or in whom suggestive symptoms are present.

Perform PPD testing on all previously negative residents immediately and again in 12 weeks if an active case of tuberculosis (TB) is documented in the facility.

Collect sputum for acid-fast bacillus (AFB) testing if a previously positive resident develops cough, bronchitis, pneumonia, or unexplained weight loss.

Notify local and state health departments as indicated.

- Careful attention to the early detection and prompt treatment of tuberculosis is necessary to continue in the attempts to eradicate this communicable disease.

Activities and Discussion Questions

1. What is congestive heart failure?
2. Discuss assessment and intervention for elders with a diagnosis of congestive heart failure, chronic obstructive pulmonary disease, and pneumonia.
3. Why is pneumonia so dangerous to the older adult?
4. What preventive measures can be instituted to prevent or lessen the severity of pneumonia and tuberculosis among the elder population?
5. Develop a nursing care plan for an elder with congestive heart failure or a respiratory condition using wellness and North American Nursing Diagnosis Association (NANDA) diagnoses.

RESOURCES

Websites

American Heart Association
www.americanheart.org

American Lung Association
www.lungusa.org

CDC Division of Tuberculosis Elimination (DTBE)
www.cdc.gov/nchstp/tb

Centers for Communicable Diseases
www.cdc.gov

REFERENCES

American Thoracic Society, Medical Section of the American Lung Association: Standards for the diagnosis and care of patients with chronic obstructive pulmonary disease (COPD) and asthma, *Am J Respir Crit Care Med* 152(5, pt 2):S77-S121, 1995.

Braunwald E: Pathophysiology of heart failure, *Heart Dis* 14:327, 1992.

Brown JB, Bedford NK, White SJ: *Gerontological protocols for nurse practitioners,* Philadelphia, 1999, Lippincott.

Centers for Disease Control and Prevention (CDC): Prevention and control of TB in facilities providing long term care to the elderly, *MMWR Morb Mortal Wkly Rep* 39(RR-10), 1990.

Centers for Disease Control and Prevention (CDC): *Health and aging: health status. National Center for Health Statistics, National Vital Statistics Systems,* 1999, Washington, DC.

Centers for Disease Control and Prevention (CDC): *Reported tuberculosis in the U.S.,* Atlanta, 2003, USDHHS, CDC.

Estes MEZ: *Health assessment and physical examination,* Albany, NY, 2002, Delmar.

Ghosh S, Gupta K: Congestive heart failure in the elderly populations: some common questions, *Ann Long Term Care* 10(12):29-39, 2002.

Gross SB: Heart failure: a review of current treatment strategies, *Adv Nurse Pract* 7(6):26-32, 1999.

Janssens JP, Zellweger JP: Clinical epidemiology and treatment of tuberculosis in elderly patients, *Schweiz Med Wochenschr* 129(3):80-89, 1999.

Kaltenbach G et al: Influence of age on presentation and prognosis of tuberculosis in internal medicine, *Presse Med* 30(29):1446-1449, 2001.

Karnath B, Agyeman A, Lai A: Pneumococcal pneumonia: update on therapy in the era of antibiotic resistance, *Consultant,* pp 321-326, March 2003.

Kennedy-Malone L, Fletcher KR, Plank LM: *Management guidelines for gerontological nurse practitioners,* Philadelphia, 2003, Davis.

Koivula I, Sten M, Makela PH: Risk factors for pneumonia in the elderly, *Am J Med* 96(4):313-320, 1994.

Lewis MFR, Haggerty MC: Topics in respiratory care. In Molony SL, Waszynski CM, Lyder CH, editors: *Gerontological nursing: an advanced practice approach,* Stamford, Conn, 1999, Appleton-Lange.

Liu Z, Shilkret KL, Ellis HM: Predictors of sputum culture conversion among patients with tuberculosis in the era of tuberculosis resurgence, *Arch Intern Med* 159(10):1110-1116, 1999.

Marek MA, Wilcox JA, Cocks AE: Topics in cardiovascular care. In Molony SL, Waszynski CM, Lyder CH, editors: *Gerontological nursing: an advanced practice approach,* Stamford, Conn, 1999, Appleton-Lange.

McCrory DC et al: Management of acute exacerbations of COPD: a summary and appraisal of the published evidence, *Chest* 119(4):1190-1209, 2001.

Monahan K: A joint effort to affect lives: the COPD Wellness Program, *Geriatr Nurs* 20(4):200-202, 1999.

Rajagopalan S, Yoshikawa TT: Tuberculosis in the elderly, *Gerontologie Geriatrics* 33(5):374, 2000.

Schultz S: Living with congestive heart failure, *Focus Geriatr Care Rehabil* 12(2):1, 1998.

Schuster PM, Wright C, Tomich P: Gender differences in the outcome of participants in home programs compared to those in structured cardiac rehabilitation programs, *Rehabil Nurs* 20(2):93-101, 1995.

Stanley M: Congestive heart failure in the elderly, *Geriatr Nurs* 20(4):180-185, 1999.

Stoller JK: Clinical practice: acute exacerbations of chronic obstructive pulmonary disease, *N Engl J Med* 346(13):988-994, 2002.

Cognitive Impairment and Older Persons

▶ **LEARNING OBJECTIVES**

Upon completion of this chapter, the reader will be able to:

- List several purposes of a cognitive assessment.
- Differentiate between dementia, delirium, and depression.
- Relate several ways in which cognitive impairment is measured.
- Explain the differences between hemorrhagic and ischemic stroke.
- Describe the effects of Parkinson's disease.
- Develop a nursing care plan for an individual with delirium.
- Develop a nursing care plan for an individual with dementia.

▶ **GLOSSARY**

Aberrant Abnormal or not following the expected course.

Ataxia An impaired ability to coordinate movement, especially a staggering gait.

Catastrophic An overwhelming behavioral response to a situation perceived as threatening.

Contracture An abnormal fixed position of a joint secondary to lack of movement, loss of elasticity, and shortening of muscle fibers.

Degenerative Gradual deterioration and changing to a less functional form.

Dysphagia Difficulty swallowing caused by obstruction or motor disorders of the esophagus.

Embolus A quantity of air, gas, or tissue that circulates and becomes lodged in a blood vessel.

Excess disability A reversible deficit that is more disabling than the primary disability. An example would be a patient with dementia who is kept in a wheelchair and therefore loses the ability to walk or a patient with a stroke who experiences a contracture or pressure ulcer on the affected side as a result of poor positioning or pressure relief.

Intracerebral Within the tissue of the brain.

Milieu The environment or setting.

Pseudodementia Affective disorder that mimics dementia, particularly severe depression.

Subarachnoid The space under the arachnoid membrane and above the pia mater, which may fill with blood during cerebral hemorrhage.

Thrombus A lump of platelets, fibrins, and cellular elements attached to the inner wall of an artery or vein, sometimes blocking the flow of blood.

Tomography An x-ray technique that produces a film representing a detailed cross section of tissue. Used primarily to diagnose space-occupying lesions.

Vascular dementia Deterioration of intellectual functioning caused by vascular disease that impairs circulation to the brain.

▶ **THE LIVED EXPERIENCE**

"The Alzheimer's patient asks nothing more than a hand to hold, a heart to care, and a mind to think for them when they cannot; someone to protect them as they travel through the dangerous twists and turns of the labyrinth. These thoughts must be put on paper now. Tomorrow they may be gone, as fleeting as the bloom of night jasmine beside my front door."

Diana Friel McGowin, who was diagnosed with Alzheimer's disease when she was 45 years old
From McGowin DF: Living in the labyrinth: a personal journey through the maze of Alzheimer's, New York, 1993, Dell Publishing, p viii.

COGNITIVE IMPAIRMENT AND OLDER PERSONS

Cognitive impairment is a term that describes a range of disturbances in cognitive functioning, including disturbances in memory, orientation, attention, concentration, judgment, learning ability, perception, problem solving, psychomotor ability, reaction time, and social ability (Warner, Butler, 2001). Common causes of cognitive impairment in the older adult are often related to degenerative processes of the central nervous system, such as those found in Alzheimer's disease (AD), Parkinson's disease (PD), or cerebrovascular accident.

Dementia, delirium, and depression have been called the three *D's* of cognitive impairment because they occur frequently in older adults and cause impairments in cognition. These conditions are not a normal consequence of aging, although the incidence increases as one grows older. Older people, particularly those with dementia and acute illnesses and stressors, are especially prone to delirium. Because cognitive and behavioral changes characterize all of the three *D's*, it can be difficult to diagnose delirium superimposed on dementia or depression. Inability to concentrate, with resulting memory impairment and other cognitive dysfunction, is common in late life depression. The term *pseudodementia* has been used to describe the cognitive impairment that may accompany depression in older adults (see Chapter 25). Knowledge about cognitive function in aging and appropriate assessment and evaluation are keys to differentiating these three syndromes. Table 21-1 presents the clinical features and the differences in cognitive and behavioral characteristics among delirium, dementia, and depression.

This chapter focuses on cognitive impairment, which includes delirium, AD and other dementias, brain attack (stroke), and PD. Cognitive assessment and nursing care for people experiencing dementia and delirium will be discussed.

DELIRIUM

Delirium is most often a complication of a medical illness, a drug or substance effect on the brain, or a surgical procedure involving general anesthesia. Environmental factors such as noise, relocation, and the use of invasive devices and restraints influence the development and escalation of delirium. The condition usually occurs as a result of complex interactions among multiple causes and is more common in older adults. Factors predisposing older adults to delirium include normal age-related changes in the brain and nervous system, diminished eyesight and hearing, greater use of medications, and diseases that injure the brain and predispose to delirium such as dementia. Delirium is given many labels: *acute confusional state*, *acute brain syndrome*, *confusion*, *metabolic encephalopathy*, and *toxic psychosis*.

The currently accepted definition of delirium from the American Psychiatric Association's *Diagnostic and Statistical Manual of Mental Disorders (DSM-IV)* (1994) is as follows:

> Delirium is a disturbance of consciousness with reduced ability to focus, sustain, or shift attention; a change in cognition; or the development of a perceptual disturbance that occurs over a short period of time and tends to fluctuate over the course of the day. Associated features of delirium may include sleep-wake cycle disturbances, altered psychomotor behavior (e.g., restlessness, agitation, inattention, somnolence), behavioral manifestations such as attempts to escape one's environment, disruptive vocalizations (e.g., screaming, calling out, cursing, moaning), removal of medical equipment, and aggressive behavior such as striking out (Rapp et al, 2001).

The exact pathophysiological mechanisms involved in the development and progression of delirium remain uncertain but are thought to be related to disturbances in the neurotransmitters in the brain that modulate the control of cognitive function, behavior, and mood. Poor cerebral blood flow is also a factor in the development of delirium (Flaherty, Morley, 2004). The causes of delirium are potentially reversible so accurate assessment and diagnosis are critical. Diseases and disorders that place older people at risk for delirium are presented in Box 21-1.

Table 21-1 Differentiating Delirium, Depression, and Dementia

Characteristic	Delirium	Depression	Dementia
Onset	Sudden, abrupt	Recent, may relate to life change	Insidious, slow, over years and often unrecognized until deficits obvious
Course over 24 hr	Fluctuating, often worse at night	Fairly stable, may be worse in the morning	Fairly stable, may see changes with stress
Consciousness	Reduced	Clear	Clear
Alertness	Increased, decreased, or variable	Normal	Generally normal
Psychomotor activity	Increased, decreased, or mixed Sometimes increased, other times decreased	Variable, agitation or retardation	Normal, may have apraxia or agnosia
Duration	Hours to weeks	Variable and may be chronic	Years
Attention	Disordered, fluctuates	Little impairment	Generally normal but may have trouble focusing
Orientation	Usually impaired, fluctuates	Usually normal, may answer "I don't know" to questions or may not try to answer	Often impaired, may make up answers or answer close to the right thing or may confabulate but tries to answer
Speech	Often incoherent, slow or rapid, may call out repeatedly or repeat the same phrase	May be slow	Difficulty finding word, perseveration
Affect	Variable but may look disturbed, frightened	Flat	Slowed response, may be labile

Adapted from Rapp CG, Mentes JC, Titler MG: Acute confusion/delirium protocol, *J Gerontol Nurs* 27(4):21-33, 2001.

Incidence

Delirium is a prevalent and serious disorder estimated to affect 14% to 80% of all older adults hospitalized for treatment of an acute physical illness; and it may develop in more than 8 out of 10 patients in the intensive care unit (ICU) (Ely et al, 2001; Foreman et al, 2001). As many as one quarter of all older adult patients in the hospital experience delirium, and the rates are even higher among those confined to an ICU or who have undergone surgery. Delirium is a common and serious problem in the acute care setting and one that is not often recognized by health care providers. Studies indicate that delirium is unrec-

ognized in 66% to 84% of patients (Inouye, 1994; Hustey, Meldon, 2002; Sanders, 2002). Sixty-five percent of physicians and 43% of nurses failed to recognize delirium in hospitalized older adults, and even when specifically asked to document cases of delirium, nurses identified fewer than 50% of those who were moderately to severely delirious (Foreman et al, 2001; Inouye et al, 2001).

Consequences

Delirium during hospitalization is highly predictive of future cognitive impairment, functional

Box 21-1	Diseases and Disorders Placing Older People at Risk for Delirium

Pharmacological agents, especially anticholinergics, hypnotics, anxiolytics, antipsychotics, nonsteroidal antiinflammatory drugs (NSAIDs), antidepressants

Hypoxemia and metabolic disturbances

Infection, especially respiratory and urinary tract

Dehydration, with and without electrolyte disturbances

Electrolyte imbalances

Withdrawal syndromes (alcohol and sedative-hypnotic agents)

Major medical and surgical treatments (especially hip fracture)

Nutritional deficiencies

Dementia

Circulatory disturbances (congestive heart failure [CHF], myocardial infarction [MI], cerebrovascular accident [CVA])

Anemia

Pain (either unrelieved or inadequately treated)

Sensory deficits

Social isolation, lack of family contact

Retention of urine and feces

Emergency admission or admission from a long-term care facility

Use of invasive equipment

Restraint use

Abrupt loss of significant person

Multiple losses in short span of time

Move to radically different environment (hospitalization, nursing home)

---

decline, and subsequent hospitalization (Flaherty, Morley, 2004). At the time of discharge from the hospital, approximately 30% to 90% of patients who experienced delirium continue to manifest symptoms. In a study of older patients admitted to a home care agency, 46% were delirious on admission. Of greater significance, 50% of that group lived alone. Several studies reported that patients with delirium continue to manifest symptoms up to 6 months after discharge, with persistent memory deficits of particular significance. Greater morbidity and mortality, loss of independence, cognitive decline, and hospital readmission have all been noted as consequences of delirium (Foreman et al, 2001).

Confusion: What Does it Really Mean?

Contributing to the problem of diagnosis of delirium is our lack of knowledge and understanding about cognition and behavioral changes that may occur in older adults. Cognitive changes in older people are often labeled confusion by nurses and physicians, are frequently accepted as part of normal aging, and are rarely questioned. In a landmark book entitled *Confusion: Prevention and Care*, Wolanin and Phillips (1981, p 2) were some of the first gerontological nurses to describe this phenomenon:

The term confusion is used to describe a constellation of behaviors that caregivers recognize as being deviant from those expected from the person in a certain place or at a certain time . . . . Confusion in the young is a temporary phenomenon. In the middle aged it is a reversible event that has a definite etiology. When the cause is removed, the confusional state clears. Historically, the confusional state of the elderly is linked to . . . hopeless and permanent dementia.

More recently, in a report on the occurrence of delirium in elderly patients with hip fracture, Milisen et al (2002, p 27) stated that "confusion is used as a descriptive term or symptom (e.g., dementia is characterized by severe confusion), or as a diagnosis (e.g., the patient is confused)." A variety of signs and symptoms are used by physicians and nurses when labeling a person confused. These include disorientation, inability to concentrate, memory loss, anxiety, restlessness, sleep disturbances, or psychotic symptoms such as delusions or hallucinations. There is a lack of clarity and agreement regarding the definition of confusion, and for many, confusion implies an irreversible, untreatable condition. Nurses may report clients' behavioral manifestations within their own framework, seldom exploring the meaning to the individual. It is essential to recognize and diagnose delirium rather than labeling all acute changes in mental status with the general term *confusion*. Confusion is not a consequence of normal aging, and any change in mental status of an older person needs thorough assessment. Failure to recognize delirium by assuming confusion to be normal contributes to the morbidity and mortality associated with this condition.

Clinical Subtypes of Delirium

Delirium is categorized according to the level of alertness and psychomotor activity. The clinical subtypes are hyperactive, hypoactive, and mixed. Box 21-2 presents the characteristics of each of these clinical subtypes. In non-ICU settings, approximately 30% of delirium is hyperactive, 24% is hypoactive, and 46% is mixed. Because of the increased severity of illness and use of psychoactive medications, hypoactive delirium may be more prevalent in the ICU. Whereas the negative consequences of hyperactive delirium are serious, the hypoactive subtype may be more

---

Box 21-2   Clinical Subtypes of Delirium

Hypoactive Delirium
"Quiet or pleasantly confused"
Reduced activity
Lack of facial expression
Passive demeanor
Lethargy
Inactivity
Withdrawn and sluggish state
Limited, slow, and wavering vocalizations

Hyperactive Delirium
Excessive alertness
Easy distractibility
Increased psychomotor activity
Hallucinations, delusions
Agitation and aggressive actions
Fast or loud speech
Wandering, nonpurposeful repetitive movement
Verbal behaviors (yelling, calling out)
Removing tubes
Attempting to get out of bed

Mixed
Unpredictable fluctuations between
    hypoactivity and hyperactivity

---

often missed and associated with a worse prognosis because of the development of complications, such as aspiration, pulmonary embolism, pressure ulcers, and pneumonia. Increased hospital stays, longer duration of delirium, and higher mortality have been associated with hypoactive delirium (Truman, Ely, 2003).

Risk Factors and Prevention

Identification of risk factors, prompt and appropriate assessment, and continued surveillance are the cornerstones of prevention of delirium. More than 35 potential risk factors have been identified for delirium. Acute illness, infections, metabolic disturbances, alcohol or drug abuse, sensory impairments, surgery, hip fracture, and cognitive impairment are common risk factors for delirium. Unrelieved or inadequately treated pain is a frequent cause of delirium. Medications account for 22% to 39% of all deliriums, and all medications, particularly those with anticholinergic effects and any new medications, should be suspect. Invasive equipment, such as nasogastric tubes, intravenous (IV) lines and catheters, and restraints, also contribute to delirium by interfering with normal feedback mechanisms of the body. The Acute Confusion/Delirium Protocol developed by Rapp et al (2001) provides a screening and surveillance form identifying risk factors that can be used on hospital admission and during the course of the hospital stay. A copy of the protocol and screening and surveillance forms can be obtained from http://www.nu.edu/library/N605.html.

Assessment

Several instruments can be used to assess the presence and severity of delirium. It is very important to determine the person's usual mental status in order to detect changes. If the person cannot tell you this, family or other caregivers who are with the patient can be asked to provide this information. If the patient is alone, a phone call to the responsible party or the institution transferring the patient should be made to gather this information. Do not assume the person's current mental status is representative of his or her usual state, and do not attribute altered mental status to age alone. All patients, regardless of their current cognitive function, should have formal mental status assessments to identify possible delirium, especially delirium superimposed on dementia. Strategies to assist in recognition of dementia in older hospitalized patients can be found at: http://hartfordign.org.

The Mini-Mental State Exam (MMSE) (Folstein et al, 1975) is considered a general test of cognitive status that helps in identifying mental status impairment. Although the MMSE alone is not accurate for assessing delirium, it represents a brief, standardized method to assess mental status and can provide a baseline from which to track changes. The MMSE is discussed in Chapter 14. Several delirium-specific assessment instruments are available: the Confusion Assessment Method (CAM) (Inouye et al, 1990) and the NEECHAM Confusion Scale (Neelon et al, 1996). The CAM-ICU is another instrument specifically designed to assess delirium in an intensive care population (Ely et al, 2001). The CAM and NEECHAM instruments are available on-line from the following websites: http://pccc.health.org/Tools/neecham_confusion_scale.htm and http://www.hartfordign.org/resources/education/tryThis.html.

Assessment using the MMSE, CAM, and NEECHAM should be conducted on admission to the hospital, throughout the hospitalization for all patients identified at risk for delirium, and for all patients who exhibit signs and symptoms of delirium or develop additional risk factors. Documenting specific objective indicators of alterations in mental status rather than using the global non-specific term *confusion* will lead to more appropriate prevention, detection, and management of delirium and its negative consequences.

Prevention

An awareness and identification of the risk factors for delirium and a formal assessment of mental status are the first-line intervention for prevention. Many nursing interventions, in addition to treatment of underlying physical causes, can assist in the prevention of delirium. A comprehensive program of delirium prevention in the acute care setting, the Elder Life Program (Inouye et al, 1999), focuses on managing six risk factors for delirium: cognitive impairment, sleep deprivation, immobility, visual impairments, hearing impairments, and dehydration. Patient outcomes with the use of this model include a 40% reduction in

the incidence of delirium and a decrease in the number of days and episodes of delirium. Most of the interventions can be considered quite simple and part of good nursing care. Examples include the following: offering herbal tea or warm milk instead of sleeping medications, keeping the ward quiet at night by using vibrating beepers instead of paging systems, silent pill crushers, removing catheters and other devices that hamper movement as soon as possible, encouraging mobilization, and correcting hearing and vision deficits. Fall prevention interventions such as bed and chair alarms, low beds, reclining chairs, volunteers to sit with restless patients, and keeping routines as normal as possible with consistent caregivers are other examples of interventions. Box 21-3 presents suggested interventions to prevent delirium.

Nursing Interventions

Outcomes of effective management of delirium are as follows: (1) episodes of delirium are resolved within 48 hours; (2) episodes of delirium are managed with the minimal use of physical and chemical restraints; and (3) the patient remains free from physical harm during episodes of delirium. Caring for patients with delirium can be a challenging experience. Patients with delirium can be difficult to communicate with, and disturbing behaviors such as pulling out IV lines or attempting to get out of bed disrupt medical treatment and compromise safety. Nonpharmacological interventions are aimed at improving orientation, decreasing sensory overload or deprivation, and providing reassurance and ensuring safety. Realize that behavior is an attempt to communicate something and express needs. The patient with delirium feels frightened and out of control. The more calm and reassuring the nurse is, the safer the patient will feel. Box 21-4 presents some communication strategies that might be helpful in caring for people with dementia.

Pharmacological interventions to treat the symptoms of delirium may be necessary but should not replace thoughtful and careful evaluation and management of the underlying causes of delirium. The atypical antipsychotics, short-acting benzodiazepines, and short-acting hypnotics for sleep may be used for agitation (Rapp et al, 2001). Chapter 15 discussed the appropriate use of these medications with older people.

Box 21-3   Suggested Interventions to Prevent Delirium

- Know baseline mental status, functional abilities, living conditions, medications taken, alcohol use.
- Assess mental status using Mini-Mental State Exam (MMSE), Confusion Assessment Method (CAM), or NEECHAM Confusion Scale, and document.
- Correct underlying physiological alterations.
- Compensate for sensory deficits (hearing aids, glasses, dentures).
- Encourage fluid intake (make sure fluids are accessible).
- Avoid long periods of giving nothing orally.
- Explain all actions with clear and consistent communication.
- Avoid multiple medications, and avoid problematic medications.
- Be vigilant for drug reactions or interactions; consider onset of new symptoms as an adverse reaction to medications.
- Avoid use of sleeping medications—use music, warm milk, noncaffeinated herbal tea to alleviate discomfort.
- Attempt to find out why behavior is occurring rather than simply medicating for it (e.g., need to toilet, pain, fear, hunger, thirst).
- Avoid excessive bed rest; institute early mobilization.
- Encourage participation in care for activities of daily living (ADLs).
- Minimize the use of catheters, restraints, or immobilizing devices.
- Use least restrictive devices (mitts instead of wrist restraints, reclining geri-chairs with tray instead of vest restraints).
- Hide tubes (stockinette over intravenous [IV] line), or use intermittent fluid administration.
- Activate bed and chair alarms.
- Place the patient near the nursing station for close observation.
- Assess and treat pain.
- Pay attention to environmental noise.
- Normalize the environment (provide familiar items, routines, clocks, calendars).
- Minimize the number of room changes and interfacility transfers.
- Do not place a delirious patient in the room with another delirious patient.
- Have family, volunteer, or paid caregiver stay with the patient.

Box 21-4   Communicating with a Person Experiencing Delirium

Know the person's past patterns.

Look at nonverbal signs, such as tone of voice, facial expressions, gestures.

Speak slowly.

Be calm and patient.

Face the person and keep eye contact—get to the level of the person rather than standing over him or her.

Explain all actions.

Smile.

Use simple, familiar words.

Allow adequate time for response.

Repeat if needed.

Tell the person what you want him or her to do rather than what you don't want him or her to do.

Give one-step directions; use gestures and demonstration to augment words.

Reassure of safety.

Keep caregivers consistent.

Assume that communication and behavior are meaningful and an attempt to tell us something or express needs.

Do not assume the person is unable to understand or is demented.

DEMENTIA

Dementia is considered a syndrome, not a diagnosis. There are more than 70 causes of dementia, and any person with symptoms of dementia should have a thorough workup to determine the etiology. Dementia is defined as "a clinical state in which a persistent change in cognitive function occurs, with memory loss, and at least one other type of cognitive deficit. These losses are severe enough to impair functioning and to be a clear change from a prior level of function, not occurring during the course of delirium" (Ham et al, 2002, p 253). Other clinical features of the syndrome of dementia include at least one of the following:

- Aphasia—loss of ability to speak with relevance and fluency
- Apraxia—inability to carry out purposeful movements although motor and sensory abilities are intact
- Agnosia—inability to recognize common objects or faces of familiar people despite intact sensory abilities
- Disturbances in executive functioning (planning, organizing, sequencing, abstracting)

Types of Dementia

Dementia can be categorized as primary or secondary. Primary dementias are progressive disorders caused by brain pathological conditions (e.g., AD); secondary dementias produce brain pathological conditions as a result of other conditions (e.g., dementia related to the effects of alcoholism). Many dementias in old age can be described as mixed dementias, produced by a combination of primary and secondary causes. For example, dementia can be caused by a combination of AD, vascular brain changes, and prior alcoholism (two primary causes and one secondary cause). Box 21-5 presents the primary dementias and common secondary dementias.

Although there are approximately 70 causes of dementia, dementia of the Alzheimer's type (AD) is the most common type of dementia. AD accounts for 50% to 60% of all dementias and affects approximately 7.5% of individuals older than 65 and 20% to 50% of people older than 80 (Ham et al, 2002). The prevalence of AD increases with age, doubling every 5 years after age 60. By

---

Box 21-5	Primary and Secondary Dementias

Primary, Progressive Dementias
Alzheimer's disease (dementia of the Alzheimer's type [DAT])
Diffuse Lewy body dementia
Vascular dementia (includes Binswanger's disease, multiinfarct dementia)
Frontotemporal dementia (includes Pick's disease)
Huntington's disease
Creutzfeldt-Jakob disease

Common Secondary Dementias
Alcohol-associated dementia
Parkinson's-associated dementia (subcortical)
Human immunodeficiency virus/acquired immunodeficiency syndrome–associated dementia
Postanoxic encephalopathy
Poststroke dementia
Progressive supranuclear palsy

---

the year 2050, the prevalence of AD is expected to more than triple. However, there are a number of other common causes of dementia. These include vascular dementia (VaD) (about 10% of dementias), diffuse Lewy body dementia (DLBD) (about 15% to 25% of dementias), and mixed dementias (usually DAT and vascular). Other less commonly occurring dementias are frontotemporal dementia (FTD), Creutzfeldt-Jakob disease (CJD) (subacute spongiform encephalopathy), and human immunodeficiency virus (HIV)–related dementia. Normal pressure hydrocephalus (NPH) causes a dementia characterized by ataxic gait, incontinence, and memory impairment. This disease is reversible and treated with a shunt that diverts cerebrospinal fluid away from the brain. Advances in technology and knowledge about dementia-type disorders have resulted in better diagnosis of the type of dementia. Accurate diagnosis is important since treatment and prognosis vary.

Assessment

An older person who presents with a change in cognitive function needs a thorough assessment to rule out reversible causes, as well as to accurately diagnose the type of dementia that may be present. A complete assessment, including laboratory workup, should be performed to rule out any medical causes of cognitive impairment. Screening for depression using instruments such as the Geriatric Depression Scale (GDS) should be conducted. Formal cognitive testing, neuropsychological examination, interview (family and patient), observation, and functional assessment are additional components of a comprehensive assessment. Computerized tomography (CT), magnetic resonance imaging (MRI), and an electroencephalogram (EEG) may be indicated in the diagnostic process. There are several evidence-based guidelines for assessment of changes in mental status and diagnosis of dementia, including assessing cognitive function (Foreman et al, 2003), altered mental status (AMDA, 1998), and diagnosis of dementia (Knopman et al, 2001). All these guidelines are available at http://www.guidlines.gov. Chapter 14 presents a discussion of assessment instruments that gerontological nurses may use to assess cognitive function.

Alzheimer's Disease

Alzheimer's disease (AD) was described by Dr. Alois Alzheimer in 1906 and is a cerebral degenerative disorder of unknown origin. AD destroys proteins of nerve cells of the cerebral cortex by diffuse infiltration with nonfunctional tissue called *neurofibrillary tangles* and *plaques*. The tangles and plaques represent the death of nerve cells throughout the brain. The brain shrinks to about one third of its normal weight. The tangles consist of a protein called *tau* that "clogs" the insides of brain cells and their connections. Deposits of beta amyloid accumulate abnormally in the brains of patients with AD. The disease is progressive and is accompanied by increasing memory loss, inability to concentrate, personality deterioration, and impaired judgment. The course of AD ranges from 1 to 15 years; typical life expectancy is 8 to 9 years after symptom onset, with death usually occurring as a result of pulmonary infections, urinary tract infections, pressure ulcers, or iatrogenic disorders. Risk factors include increasing age, family history and genetics, female gender, Down's syndrome, environ-

mental toxins, low formal education and occupational attainment, previous head trauma, and cerebrovascular disease.

Research continues related to the cause of AD, but the cause is still unknown. In addition to the genetic theories known and proposed, a number of other avenues are being pursued to find a cause for AD. Atherosclerosis, cerebrovascular disease, and AD have been linked. Much research is being conducted on plaques and tangles to determine whether they are the start of the disease process or the end product of the process. The beta-amyloid hypothesis suggests that plaques lead to neuronal cell death and neuronal synaptic loss with neurotransmitter effects, such as cholinergic deficits. The cholinergic theory is based on the understanding that acetylcholine, an important chemical neurotransmitter in the brain, is deficient. AD-affected areas of the brain have cholinergic activity that is reduced by 80% to 90%. Neurofibrillary tangles are being researched in terms of tau protein. A vaccine to prevent formation of amyloid is under investigation. Other research is investigating the role of inflammation, effects of cholesterol, estrogen, and homocysteine (Beier et al, 2004; Ham et al, 2002). The gerontological nurse needs to be knowledgeable about current research to be able to provide older adults and their families the most current information about causes and treatment of AD.

Diagnosis

Presently, the only accurate method of diagnosing AD is to perform a brain biopsy or autopsy. The clinical criteria for the diagnosis of probable, possible, and definite AD are quite complex, but nursing observations of behaviors and affect are important. AD is most thoroughly diagnosed based on the history from the family and testing ruling out other disorders that may mimic the disease. Probable AD can be clinically diagnosed if there is a typical insidious onset of dementia with progression and if there are no other systemic or brain diseases that could account for the progressive cognitive deficits. Symptoms are usually present several years before diagnosis is made. Box 21-6 presents the DSM-IV-TR criteria for dementia of the Alzheimer's type. There has been little research on the influence of culture and ethnicity on the recognition and interpretation of cognitive changes and the assessment, diagnosis, and treat-

Box 21-6	DSM-IV-TR Criteria for Dementia of the Alzheimer's Type

1. Multiple cognitive deficits manifested by the following:
   a. Memory impairment, and
   b. Aphasia, apraxia, or executive function disturbance
2. Significant impairment of social and work-related function caused by deficits in cognition in 1a and 1b and is a decline from previous functioning.
3. There is a gradual onset of deficits and progressive cognitive decline.
4. The cognitive deficits in 1a and 1b are not caused by the following:

a. Central nervous system disturbances that cause progressive memory deficits, such as Parkinson's disease, cerebrovascular disorders, subdural hematoma, brain tumor
b. Conditions known to cause dementia, such as hypothyroidism, pernicious anemia, folic acid deficiency, neurosyphilis, hyperparathyroid disease with hypercalcemia
c. Substances, drugs
5. The deficits are not caused by delirium.
6. The deficits are not accounted for by major depression or schizophrenia.

Adapted from American Psychiatric Association: *Diagnostic and statistical manual of mental disorders, DSM-IV-TR,* Washington, DC, 2000, The Association.

ment of AD and other dementias in minority populations. The Diversity Toolbox prepared by the Alzheimer's Association (http://www.alz.org) is an important resource for nurses and other health professionals working with culturally diverse older adults.

Drug Treatment

Drug therapy with cholinesterase inhibitors (CIs) has transformed the treatment of AD, offering hope for enhanced function and reduction of the speed of cognitive decline. CIs approved to treat AD include donepezil (Aricept), rivastigmine (Exelon), and galantamine (Reminyl). The most recently U.S. Food and Drug Administration (FDA)–approved drug, memantine (Namenda), is a new class of medication (*N*-methyl-D-aspartate [NMDA] antagonist) indicated for the treatment of moderate to severe DAT. Unlike the CIs, which increase the amount of acetylcholine in the brain, memantine blocks the effect of abnormal glutamate activity that may lead to neuronal cell death and cognitive dysfunction. Memantine may be used alone or in combination with the CIs. These medications may also positively affect the behavioral manifestations of AD.

Current treatment guidelines recommend CI therapy as first-line treatment in patients with mild to moderate AD. Duration of therapy should be long term, even if the patient shows a slight decline, provided that function is better than it would have been without treatment (Doody et al, 2001; Ham et al, 2002). Side effects are generally minor and include gastrointestinal disturbances, sleep disturbances, and sedation. Starting at a lower dose with slow titration is recommended to minimize side effects. Medication therapy is directed toward the symptoms of AD and does not affect the neuronal decline that will eventually produce severe disability. However, medications are likely to produce a plateau of brain function and functional abilities and delay the progression of AD. Positive effects on the behavioral manifestations of AD have also been shown with drug therapy.

STROKE AND ITS CONSEQUENCES

Epidemiology

Stroke is the leading cause of long-term disability among adults in the United States and the third leading cause of death, behind heart disease and cancer. Morbidity and mortality rates increase with age. Stroke occurs more often in men and in African Americans. Poorer outcomes (greater neurological impairment) are more common among minorities than whites. Higher rates of stroke-related impairments may be related to the incidence of type 1 diabetes and hypertension in minorities, but inadequate access to care and lack of preventive teaching and interventions may also contribute (Shen et al, 2004). Continued research on racial disparities in stroke outcomes as well as other diseases is essential.

The complications of stroke are devastating. There may be impairment of walking, seeing, feeling, remembering, speaking, and thinking. Strokes are cerebrovascular accidents that affect cerebral circulation through occlusive thrombi and emboli or, less often, hemorrhagic incidents occurring in the intracerebral or subarachnoid space. Symptoms of cerebral hemorrhage usually evolve over several hours and are often associated with headache. Hemorrhagic strokes are more life threatening but much less frequent than thrombotic strokes. Thrombotic strokes are most frequently a consequence of atrial fibrillation, which predisposes one to systemic emboli. It is important to differentiate between ischemic and hemorrhagic strokes because the treatment is different. A CT scan is the most useful means for making the determination (Ham et al, 2002). Figure 21-1 illustrates brain areas affected by stroke.

Risk factors for stroke include prior transient ischemic attack (TIA) or stroke, myocardial infarction, rheumatic heart disease, hypertension, diabetes, coronary artery disease, congestive heart failure, atrial fibrillation, hyperlipidemia, peripheral artery disease, smoking, lack of exercise, and obesity. A stroke risk sheet and other information useful for patients and providers are available from the National Institutes of Health, National Institute of Neurological Disorders and Stroke at: http://www.ninds.nih.gov/.

Vascular dementia (VaD) is more common in people who have had a history of hypertension, TIAs, and stroke. Box 21-7 lists conditions that may create cerebral anoxia or hypoxia leading to VaD. Whereas VaD often occurs in a mixed form of dementia with AD, criteria for differentiating VaD from AD include the following:
- Early gait disturbance
- History of unsteadiness or falls
- Early urinary symptoms
- Personality and mood changes
- History of stroke, hypertension, TIAs
- Sudden or step-wise deterioration

- Focal neurological signs (e.g., increased deep tendon reflexes, positive extensor plantar response, extremity weakness)
- Imaging evidence of cardiovascular disease, single infarct/diffuse and extensive white matter changes

Prevention

The best approach to stroke, despite new therapies and medications, is prevention. Identifying high-risk or stroke-prone older adults is important. Blood pressure reduction is essential, and reducing the blood pressure 5 mm Hg in a hypertensive person reduces risk of stroke 34%. With reduction of 10 mm Hg, it is reduced 56% (Sica, 2002). When a person has had a stroke, there is a high likelihood of another stroke. Attention needs to be given to preventing the next stroke through

---

Box 21-7   Vascular Brain Disease

Vascular brain disease may result from any of the following:
- Arteriosclerotic plaques blocking circulation to cerebral cells
- Blood dyscrasias interfering with platelet and clot formation
- Cardiac decompensation resulting in insufficient perfusion to the brain
- Cerebrovascular hemorrhage (strokes) of small or large magnitude
- Diabetic deterioration of blood vessels
- Primary hypertension causing deterioration of capillary walls because of sustained pressure (Cerebral cells dependent on the deteriorated capillaries no longer function. Over time, hypertensive persons show greater decrements in cognitive performance than persons with normal blood pressure.)
- Rupture of cerebrovascular or aortic aneurysms
- Sustained severe anemia
- Systemic emboli lodging in cerebrovascular pathway
- Transient ischemic attacks (TIAs) lasting up to 24 hours, resulting from spasms of blood vessels in certain segments of the brain, which produce temporary disturbances in sensation, cognition, and motor activity and are often a warning sign of impending stroke

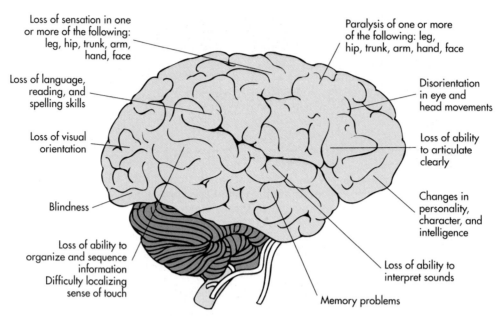

Loss of sensation in one or more of the following: leg, hip, trunk, arm, hand, face

Paralysis of one or more of the following: leg, hip, trunk, arm, hand, face

Loss of language, reading, and spelling skills

Disorientation in eye and head movements

Loss of visual orientation

Loss of ability to articulate clearly

Blindness

Changes in personality, character, and intelligence

Loss of ability to organize and sequence information Difficulty localizing sense of touch

Loss of ability to interpret sounds

Memory problems

Figure 21-1   Brain areas affected by strokes.

appropriate drug therapy and continued reduction of risk factors (Sica, 2002). See Chapter 15 for a discussion of medications.

Transient Ischemic Attacks

In addition to major brain attacks, there are transient ischemic attacks (TIAs) caused by impaired circulation from a temporary occlusion of a cerebral blood vessel. Most TIAs last less than 30 minutes, and symptoms resolve within 24 hours. TIAs signal the presence of significant atherosclerotic disease and are considered precursors to a stroke or myocardial infarction. Symptoms vary depending on the location of the circulatory impairment. In older people, TIAs can be precipitated by a sudden drop in blood pressure related to orthostatic hypotension, sudden changes in posture, or even overaggressive hypertension therapy. Symptoms of TIAs can include blurred vision, numbness of arms and legs, temporary amnesia or aphasia, confusion, unsteady gait, and difficulty with coordination of movement (Ham et al, 2002). One third of people who have a TIA will have a stroke. Most people who suffer an ischemic stroke do not reach the hospital in time for the currently available treatment (Fagan et al, 1998). It is

important to teach older adults the signs of TIAs and the effectiveness of immediate treatment.

The use of intravenous tissue plasminogen activator (rt-PA) can be an effective therapy for acute ischemic stroke. Immediate treatment, within 3 hours of the first symptoms, may prevent some of the brain cell death. Treatment begun within 90 minutes of the first symptoms doubles the chance of full recovery (Haney, 2002). An intracerebral hemorrhage is not amenable to this treatment. Anticoagulant therapy is advised for conditions in which thrombotic strokes may occur. Comprehensive guidelines for the management of acute stroke are available at www.strokeassociation.org/get with the guidelines.

Poststroke Care

Difficulties and handicaps following stroke often involve communication, continence, and functional impairments. The particular functional impairments will depend on the area of the brain attack. Some of the methods of testing functional disorders of the poststroke client can be seen in Box 21-8.

Preparation for rehabilitation must begin in the acute phase of stroke. Prevention of secondary

| Box 21-8 | Tests of Specific Disabilities That Commonly Follow Stroke |

Hemianopia (Loss of Part of Visual Field)

Sitting opposite the patient, hold up simultaneously two pens of different colors 30 cm in front of the patient and 30 cm apart; patients with hemianopia will be unable to see one of the pens or may turn the head toward the hemianopic side in an effort to see.

Proprioception (Awareness of Body in Space)

The wrist of the affected arm is held between the thumb and forefinger of the examiner; the patient's hand is raised and lowered, and the patient, with closed eyes, is asked the position of the hand; this exercise can also be done with fingers to determine even more specific loss of proprioception.

Sensation (Feeling Generated by Sensory Receptors)

With the patient's eyes closed, the examiner strokes the back of the unaffected hand and then the affected hand and in both cases asks the patient to describe the sensation. The affected side may have varying degrees of loss of sensation or total loss of feeling.

Balance (Body Poise)

The patient is asked to sit on the side of the bed with feet off the floor and maintain balance and sit unaided for 1 minute; it is usually readily apparent if the individual has a problem maintaining balance.

Arm Function (Range of Motion and Control)

The patient is asked to lift the affected arm to shoulder height and press against the examiner's upheld hand:

Complete paralysis = inability to move arm
Severe weakness = can move arm but not lift up or push
Moderate weakness = able to lift arm but unable to push
Slight weakness = able to do task requested but cannot push as hard as with unaffected arm
No weakness = no difference in abilities of either arm

Data from Anderson R: *The aftermath of stroke: the experience of patients and their families,* Cambridge, UK, 1992, Cambridge University Press.

complications and maintenance of functional abilities are important in the nursing care of patients with stroke. Complications such as pressure ulcers and contractures significantly add to the burden of disability and can be prevented. Dysphagia and aphasia are discussed in Chapters 3 and 10. Box 21-9 presents some of the secondary complications of stroke.

Rehabilitation involves timing and persistence. The expected functional improvement is based on the severity of disability 1 month after the stroke. Most clients with stroke disabilities regain the most function possible in terms of prestroke performance of activities of daily living (ADLs) within 9 months. At 18 months following the stroke there actually tends to be a small decline, which is thought to be a result of lowered motivation or discouragement with progress. Functional improvement is delayed in those of advanced age, social isolation, and emotional distress. Up to one third of stroke victims become profoundly depressed in the year following stroke. The American Heart Association and the American Stroke Association websites (listed in Resources at the end of the chapter) all provide excellent information for patients and professionals as well as comprehensive guidelines for the prevention and treatment of stroke. A comprehensive guideline for the early management of patients with ischemic stroke (Adams et al, 2003) can be found at http://stroke.ahajournals.org/cgi/content/full/34/4/1056.

Assessment of Needs

To maximize the benefits of interventions, a multidisciplinary team must activate a comprehensive rehabilitation plan as soon as the individual is physiologically stabilized. The assessment of needs following stroke is extremely complex and requires evaluation by neurologists, physiatrists, speech therapists, ophthalmologists, physical therapists, psychologists, and environmental planners. A multidisciplinary team is essential in

Box 21-9	High-Risk Physical and Psychosocial Complications of Stroke

Physical

Joint contractures of affected side

Shoulder separation of the affected side

Pulmonary embolus/deep vein thrombosis (DVT)

Aspiration pneumonia

Constipation

Urinary incontinence

Trauma to areas with decreased sensation (pressure ulcers, skin tears, bruising)

Edema in flaccid extremities that are allowed to dangle for long periods of time in dependent positions

Sensory deprivation (in terms of the sensations available in the environment—if aphasic, people may not talk to you)

Whole areas of the body fail to sense stimuli from the environment

Fatigue and major amounts of time to accomplish routine activities of daily living (ADLs)

Psychosocial

Body image greatly affected when major portions of the body lack sensation or cease to function

Social isolation at high risk, especially with communication deficits; may see self as a tremendous burden to others, or others may communicate that he or she is an unwanted burden

Depression, hopelessness of any improvement in one's status, sadness at one's state in life

Anxiety over risk of using up one's resources as the disability drags on

Fear of another stroke

Shifting from independence to dependence can be catastrophic for individuals who highly value their independence

the evaluation of the needs of an elder following stroke. Caretakers of the client, as well as the elder, must be included at every stage of planning to the extent possible. The nursing role involves coordinating team efforts in recognition of the client's energy levels and capacities. This involves clearly documenting all of the functional capacities that are retained and those that are impaired. Reassessment must be completed routinely to adjust care plans to the client's progress.

Stroke Support Groups

Nurses are becoming much more aware of the devastation a stroke produces as they study the reported experiences of elders recovering from stroke. Easton (1999) analyzed several reports and identified six stages common to stroke survivors: agonizing, fantasizing, realizing, blending, framing, and finally owning. The important idea is that the individual stroke survivor goes through many stages toward acceptance. Nurses must respect the process and realize that some survivors never accept the assault to their sense of self. Small-group support is an ideal way for victims of stroke to become aware of the various stages they experience. The group ideally provides an environment for problem solving and feedback,

support, acceptance, and encouragement to relearn and understand from others with similar limitations and struggles. When members have great difficulty verbalizing, it may be useful and relieve some tension to have part of each group designed toward nonverbal, nondominant brain expressions, such as art, music, or psychomotor activities. The success of a stroke group largely depends on the skill of the group facilitator. Experience with neurosurgical disorders and a background in gerontology and rehabilitation are desirable.

PARKINSON'S DISEASE

Etiology and Symptoms

Parkinson's disease (PD) results from the progressive loss of dopaminergic cells from the substantia nigra in the brainstem (Moore, Clarke, 2001). Although the etiology of primary parkinsonism is unknown, the death of the substantia nigra cells within the basal ganglia results in a marked reduction in dopamine and is the cause of symptoms of tremor, muscular rigidity, akinesia, and loss of postural reflexes. There is an 80% to 90% loss of the dopamine-producing cells by the time a person becomes overtly symptomatic (Burke, Laramie, 2000). The mean age at onset is 65 with both men and women affected equally. First-degree relatives have twice the risk of developing PD (Moore, Clarke, 2001). Risk factors are not clear, but preliminary investigation suggests that environmental toxins may be a factor. Diagnosis is often one of exclusion; however, the diagnosis requires two of four cardinal symptoms: resting tremor, bradykinesia, cogwheel rigidity, and postural instability (Boss, 2002). The most common early symptom is tremor of one hand and the pill-rolling motion of the fingers. Depression may be an early symptom and may occur in 80% of individuals with PD. Secondary Parkinson's is caused by several medications, with antipsychotics being the most common. Older people are especially prone to the development of Parkinson's-like symptoms in response to antipsychotic medications, and any older adult receiving these medications should be routinely screened for extrapyramidal symptoms (EPS) (see Chapter 15).

Essential Tremor

Essential tremor (sometimes called *familial tremor*) is somewhat similar in appearance to PD and is said to be the most prevalent movement disorder, peaking in the fifties. It primarily affects the hands and the head and may significantly impair communication and activities requiring fine motor control, as well as impact psychosocial adjustment. The disorder may become apparent in young adulthood and will grow progressively worse as one ages. Etiology and management are poorly understood. Beta blockers are the most effective treatment and usually improve the tremor so that it does not interfere with normal activities. In some people, the tremor disappears completely. Other medications used include primidone (Mysoline), lorazepam (Ativan), and alprazolam (Xanax). Many people find that drinking small amounts of alcohol temporarily relieves tremor, but heavy drinking should be avoided.

Management

Typically, individuals with PD are given a combination of carbidopa and levodopa (Sinemet), which often loses effectiveness as the amino acid

levodopa competes with other amino acids for absorption at both the intestinal wall and the blood-brain barrier. Several other medications are available for treatment of Parkinson's (see Chapter 15). Restricting dietary protein is sometimes effective. In many clients with PD the medication regimen may create illusions or hallucinations. Medications and individualized treatment plans are critical to the care of the person with PD. The challenge to client, family, and nurse is to maintain the highest possible level of hope. At times the deterioration is rapid, but most clients remain functional for many years.

Because of the slow progression of the disease and the disability that accompanies it, individuals experience a change in roles, activities, and social participation. Tremors may produce embarrassing moments. The expressionless face, slowed movement, and soft, monotone speech may give the impression of apathy, depression, and disinterest. Others, observing these symptoms, may react with disinterest. A sensitive nurse is aware that the visible symptoms produce an undesired facade that may hide an alert and responsive individual who wishes to interact and generate interest. Persons with PD experience great functional problems in mobility, communication, and home management. Safety is a major care concern related to gait disturbances. The following suggestions may be of benefit in coping with some of the symptoms that disturb the client with PD:

1. Movement of the limbs decreases the tremors; when walking, one should swing the arms. A regular exercise program should be implemented (see Resources at end of chapter for a video on exercise and PD).
2. Holding an object helps control the tremors; individuals should hold something in their hands when sitting quietly.
3. Contractures and deformities are avoided if the individual walks as much as possible and avoids remaining still for long periods; range of motion and balancing exercises need to be prescribed by a physical therapist and practiced faithfully.
4. Skin must be kept dry and clean, and oil-free lotion should be applied every few hours to avoid seborrhea and skin breakdown; air mattresses and sheepskins are advisable for beds.
5. Constipation may be avoided by high fluid intake and a high-residue diet.

6. Speaking and reading aloud should be encouraged to enhance communication; sometimes speech therapy is warranted. A discussion of the dysarthria that may accompany PD can be found in Chapter 3.

7. Depression and low self-esteem may be partially countered by direct discussion of feelings about changes in self-image, sexuality, and functional ability. Selective serotonin reuptake inhibitors (SSRIs) are useful in treating depression in patients with PD.

8. Support system encouragement and information about the disease are essential if the family and the person are to cope with the losses associated with PD. Whitney (2004), in an analysis of the stories of older adults with PD, suggested that learning what gives the person purpose and meaning in life and helping these persons understand what is happening to their bodies can assist in coping with the loss of prior abilities.

9. Self-help groups are often useful because the members solve their problems collectively. The American Parkinson Disease Foundation is an excellent resource for patients and their families and professionals.

Dementia and Parkinson's Disease

About 30% of people with PD develop dementia, and dementia is most common in those older than 70 or who have had PD a long time (Boss, 2002). It remains controversial whether the dementia that occurs in clients with PD is related to the pathological findings of the disease or whether it is a disorder quite distinct from PD without dementia. Diffuse Lewy body dementia (DLBD) is a common type of dementia that shares similarities with AD and PD. DLBD accounts for about 15% to 20% of dementias and is more common than VaD. The relationship between DLBD and PD is an area of considerable controversy. Crystal (2004) notes that "when motor features of PD appear first and predominate over cognitive symptoms, the diagnosis is believed to be PD. When cognitive impairment and behavioral disturbances are prominent symptoms, DLBD is believed to be the diagnosis" (accessed 8/30/02 from http://www.emedicine.com/neuro/topic91.htm).

Symptoms of DLBD differ from those of AD, and the typical clinical picture includes Alzheimer's-like dementia, parkinsonian symptoms, prominent psychotic symptoms, and extreme sensitivity to antipsychotic medications (Stewart, 2003). Symptoms generally vary more from day to day than symptoms of AD, deterioration is more abrupt than in AD, and the presence of hallucinations and psychotic symptoms is high, occurring early in the disease. Treatment includes the use of levodopa and carbidopa, dopamine agonists, and CIs. Orthostatic hypotension is common and predisposes the patient to falls. Environmental safety is very important, and medications that cause orthostasis should be avoided. Most important, patients with DLBD should not be treated with antipsychotic agents since severe akinesia, dystonias, and neuroleptic malignant syndrome are common reactions to even low doses of the older typical antipsychotic medications. These medications also contribute to the cognitive decline. Patients may tolerate low doses of atypical antipsychotic medications such as quetiapine (Seroquel) or olanzapine (Zyprexa) if hallucinations and psychotic symptoms interfere with function and cannot be managed with environmental adaptation. Risperidone (Risperdal) is not well tolerated.

CARING FOR THE PERSON WITH DEMENTIA

There is no cure for AD, and although new medications offer hope for improved function, the most important treatment for the disease is competent and compassionate person-centered care—the kind of care that fosters abilities, supports limitations, ensures safety, enhances quality of life, prevents excess disability, and offers hope. Gerontological nurses know that the person, not the disease, is always the focus of care, and they practice from the belief that the person with dementia is still a whole person, someone who can think, feel, learn, grow, and be in a relationship (Touhy, 2004). Sifton (2001, p iv) states: "Since Alzheimer's affects mind and personality, as well as physical function, there is a great danger that the person can become obscured by the disease, defined by symptoms rather than by her or his unique spirit and continuing sense of self."

The current view of Alzheimer's in the popular and professional press is negative, hopeless, and frightening. We hear people with Alzheimer's described as victims, empty shells (Moore, Hollett, 2003), ex-people (Pulsford, 1997), and bodies from which the personhood has been removed (Keane, 1994). Nursing students used the terms *afraid, frustrated, sad,* and *nervous* to describe their feelings when caring for a person with dementia (Beck, 1996). We read about the actions of people with dementia described as aggressive, agitated, catastrophic, inappropriate, and burdensome (Fazio, 2001; Talerico, Evans, 2000). The emphasis on the decline associated with the disease, the catastrophic behaviors, and the loss of humanness promotes despair, hopelessness, and fear for professional caregivers, patients, and families (Touhy, 2004).

Care for persons with Alzheimer's is more than keeping their bodies alive, safe, and clean; performing tasks; and managing behavior—the care must also nourish their souls (Touhy, 2004). Care that nourishes souls is care that establishes connections and a sense of security; respects and appreciates the person; and supports the person's need to love and be loved, to be known and accepted, to give and to share, to be productive and successful, to still become, and to have hope (Bell, Troxel, 2001). Research conducted by nurses and other gerontological professionals has made significant contributions to understanding and caring for people with dementia.

Nursing Models of Care for Persons with Dementia

Gerontological nurses often provide direct care for people with dementia in the community, hospitals, and long-term care facilities. They also work with families and staff, teaching best approaches to care and providing education and support. Much of the care of people with dementia takes place in the home and is provided by a spouse or other family member or in a nursing home where it is provided by nursing assistants. Gerontological nurses will be most effective when they assist the caregivers in whatever setting to understand the nature of dementia and the interventions likely to be most effective. Overall, interventions must match expectancies with capacities, incorporate earlier life skills and interests, and provide a calm, caring, and structured environment.

Several nursing models of care are useful in guiding practice and assisting families and staff in providing care to people with dementia.

The progressively lowered stress threshold (PLST) model (Hall, Buckwalter, 1987; 1994) was one of the first models used to plan and evaluate care for people with dementia in every setting. The PLST model categorizes symptoms of dementia into four groups: (1) cognitive or intellectual losses, (2) affective or personality changes, (3) conative or planning losses that cause a decline in functional abilities, and (4) loss of the stress threshold causing behaviors such as agitation or catastrophic reactions. Symptoms such as agitation are a result of a progressive loss of the person's ability to cope with demands and stimuli when the person's stress threshold is exceeded. Five common stressors that may trigger these symptoms are fatigue; change of environment, routine, or caregiver; misleading stimuli or inappropriate stimulus levels; internal or external demands to perform beyond abilities; and physical stressors such as pain, discomfort, acute illness, and depression.

Using this model, care is structured to decrease the stressors and provide a safe and predictable environment. Outcomes reported when the model was used on an Alzheimer's special care unit included increased hours of sleep, decreased nighttime awakening, decreased sedative and tranquilizer use, increased food intake and weight, increased socialization, decreased episodes of anxious, agitated, combative behaviors, increased caregiver satisfaction with care, and increased functional level (Hall, Buckwalter, 1987). Hall (1994) offers many suggestions for both institutional caregivers and families caring for a person with dementia at home. Using principles of the PLST model, DeYoung et al (2003) designed a behavior management unit in a long-term care facility. Reported outcomes included a decrease in aggressive, agitated, and disruptive behaviors. Staff training was an important part of this program and included an emphasis on knowing the patient well and modifying the environment. Box 21-10 presents the principles of care derived from the PLST model.

The need-driven, dementia-compromised behavior (NDB) model (Algase et al, 2003; Kolanowski, 1999; Richards et al, 2000) is a framework for the study and understanding of

| Box 21-10 | Principles of Care Derived from PLST Model |

1. Maximize functional abilities by supporting all losses in a prosthetic manner.
2. Establish caring relationship, and provide person with unconditional positive regard.
3. Use behaviors indicating anxiety and avoidance to determine appropriate limits of activity and stimuli.
4. Teach caregivers to try to find out causes of behavior and to observe and evaluate verbal and nonverbal responses.
5. Identify triggers related to discomfort or stress reactions (factors in the environment, caregiver communication).
6. Modify the environment to support losses and promote safe function.
7. Evaluate care routines and responses on a 24-hour basis, and adjust plan of care accordingly.
8. Provide as much control as possible— encourage self-care, offer choices, explain all actions, do not push or force the person to do something.
9. Keep environment stable and predictable.
10. Provide ongoing education, support, care, and problem solving for caregivers.

Adapted from Hall GR, Buckwalter KC: Progressively lowered stress threshold: a conceptual model of care of adults with Alzheimer's disease, *Arch Psychiatr Nurs* 1(6):399-406, 1987.

behavioral symptoms of dementia. The NDB model proposes that the behavior of persons with dementia carries a message of need that can be addressed appropriately if the individual's past history and habits, physiological status, and physical and social environment are carefully evaluated (Kolanowski, 1999). Rather than viewing behavior as disruptive, it is viewed as having meaning and expressing needs. Behavior reflects the interaction of background factors (cognitive changes as a result of dementia, gender, race, education, personality, responses to stress) and proximal factors (physiological needs [e.g., hunger, pain], mood, physical environment [light, noise]) with social environment (staff stability and mix, presence of others) (Richards et al, 2000). Optimal care is provided by manipulating the proximal factors that precipitate behavior and by maximizing strengths and minimizing the weaknesses of the background factors. For instance, sleep disruptions are common in people with dementia. If the person is not getting adequate sleep at night, agitated or aggressive behavior may signal a need for rest. Interventions to modify proximal factors interfering with sleep, such as noise, frequent awakenings during the night, and daytime boredom, can contribute to meeting the need for rest and sleep and decrease agitation or aggression.

Cohen-Mansfield's Treatment Routes for Exploring Agitation (TREA) model (2000) is another useful framework for detecting the needs of the person with dementia, and the decision-making algorithms for understanding and responding to behaviors such as verbal agitation and physical aggression based on the model are helpful in designing interventions. Table 21-2 presents some reasons for unmet needs in people with dementia using Maslow's framework.

Other authors have discussed the importance of viewing all behavior as meaningful rather than disruptive or problematical and encourage nurses to avoid labeling the behavior of persons with dementia as aggressive (Cohen-Mansfield, 2000; Mahoney et al, 2000; Talerico, Evans, 2000; Volicer, Mahoney, 2002). Talerico and Evans (2000) suggest that terms such as *disruptive, problematic,* and *aggressive* focus on the caregiver's negative response (disturbed, disrupted) rather than on the perspective of the person with dementia (fearful, protective). Using labels such as *disruptive* or *catastrophic* when describing behaviors often leads to attempts to control the behavior through the use of psychoactive medications or restraints and does not help caregivers focus on understanding the reasons behind the behavior from the perspective of the person with dementia. Behavioral symptoms more often occur during personal care activities and are associated with higher levels of disability and communication deficits. Fear, pain, discomfort, illness, fatigue,

Table 21-2 Reason for Unmet Needs in Persons with Dementia

Maslow's Hierarchical Needs	Internal and External Conditions Affecting Need Fulfillment
Physiological—rest, fluids and nutrition, elimination, pain and comfort	Unable to communicate needs, unaware of needs of self, lack of availability of caregiver, caregiver unresponsiveness or inability to understand and respond to needs
Safety, protection from injury, feeling secure	Unaware of needs, safety risks, limitations; unable to use prior coping mechanisms
Love and belonging, acceptance, need for social contacts	Unable to obtain the means for meeting needs, unable to communicate easily, environment not supportive of establishing connections, limited interaction and stimulation
Self-esteem, respect, control	Does not receive positive feedback, environment does not provide support, often viewed as "nonperson"
Self-actualization, finds meaning in life and death	No meaningful activities offered, communication limited, no opportunities to meet spiritual needs, may be seen as "empty shell" with no higher-level needs

Adapted from Cohen-Mansfield J: Nonpharmacological management of behavioral problems in persons with dementia: the TREA model, *Alzheimer Care Q* 1(4):23, 2000.

depression, delusions and hallucinations, need for autonomy and control, caregiver approach, and environmental stressors are frequent precipitants of behavioral symptoms (Cohen-Mansfield, 2000; Richards et al, 2000). Box 21-11 presents some conditions that may precipitate behavioral symptoms.

The overuse of psychoactive medications to treat behavioral responses is of concern in light of the side effects of such medications. Research indicates that only 20% of patients respond favorably to these drugs (Richards et al, 2000). Although use of psychoactive medications may be indicated for hallucinations and other psychotic-type behaviors that cause distress and decrease functional abilities, a careful understanding of behavior and adaptation of responses and the environment is often a more therapeutic response. Chapters 15 and 25 discuss the appropriate use and monitoring of psychoactive medications. Nonpharmacological interventions and nursing responses derived from use of the frameworks described above place the focus of care on understanding the person with the disease. Gerontological nurses with this focus create environments and relationships that value and respect older adults with dementia rather than ones that punish or control.

Common Care Concerns

Communication, nutrition, ADLs, maintenance of health and function, safety, and caregiver needs and support are the major care concerns for patients, families, and staff who care for people with dementia. Special considerations for gerontological nursing interventions to enhance nutrition, sleep, rest, activity, safety, fluids and continence, emotional health, and communication for people with dementia are covered in Chapters 3, 10, 11, 12, 22, and 25. Caregiving concerns of families are discussed in Chapter 23, and therapeutic group work is discussed in Chapter 5. Additional helpful resources for older adults with dementia and their families are listed under Resources at the end of this chapter.

Mary Opal Wolanin, a gerontological nursing pioneer, suggested that nurses are not as interested in the neurofibrillary tangles in the brain as they are in trying to smooth out the environmental and relational tangles. The overriding goals in caring for older adults with dementia are to maintain function and prevent excess disability, structure the environment and relationships to maintain stability, compensate for the losses associated with the disease, and create a therapeutic milieu that nurtures the personhood of the individual and maintains quality of life.

Box 21-11	Conditions Precipitating Behavioral Symptoms in Persons with Dementia

- Communication deficits
- Pain or discomfort
- Acute medical problems
- Sleep disturbances
- Perceptual deficits
- Depression
- Need for social contact
- Hunger, thirst, need to toilet
- Loss of control
- Misinterpretation of the situation or environment
- Crowded conditions
- Changes in environment or people
- Noise, disruption
- Being forced to do something
- Fear
- Loneliness
- Psychotic symptoms
- Fatigue
- Environmental overstimulation or understimulation
- Depersonalized, rushed care
- Restraints
- Psychoactive drugs

Adapted from Talerico K, Evans L: Making sense of aggressive/protective behaviors in persons with dementia, *Alzheimer Care Q* 1(2):78, 2000.

Box 21-12	Needs of the Person with Dementia

Persons with dementia need the following:
- A safe environment but not one that restricts their freedom
- To understand and be understood, but not talked down to or shouted at
- To be kept physically fit
- To feel needed
- Nurses who understand their complex needs and respond appropriately
- They DO NOT need nurses who restrain, overmedicate, feed into their delusions, or try to reason with them
- Nurses who can assess the underlying cause of their behavior, such as pain and fear
- Nurses who understand who they are as a person and do not mistake lifelong patterns or peculiarities as confusion
- Nurses who make their environments as familiar and comfortable as possible
- Nurses who can assess the needs of their families, direct them toward the necessary resources, and support them when it comes time to make really tough choices

Source: Donna Ihle, Senior BSN student, 1993. Florida Atlantic University.

Box 21-12 presents the needs of the person with dementia from the perspective of a senior nursing student.

The remainder of this chapter will focus on two common care concerns that gerontological nurses and family caregivers may encounter when caring for people with dementia: bathing and wandering. Environmental modifications in homes and nursing homes that have been found to be effective in assisting people with dementia to remain as functional as possible will also be discussed.

Providing Care for Activities of Daily Living

The losses associated with dementia interfere with the person's normal communication patterns and ability to understand and express thoughts and feelings. Perceptual disturbances and misinterpre-tations of reality contribute to fear and mis-understanding. People with dementia struggle to understand the world and make their needs known. Often, bathing and the provision of other care for ADLs, such as dressing, grooming, and toi-leting, are the cause of a great deal of distress for both the person with dementia and the caregiver. Bathing and care for ADLs, particularly in nursing homes, can be perceived as an attack by persons with dementia, who may respond by screaming or hitting. A rigid focus on tasks or institutional care routines, such as a shower three mornings each week, can contribute to the distress and distress-ing behaviors. Being touched or bathed against one's will violates the trust in caregiving relation-ships and is a major affront (Rader, 2000). The behaviors that may be exhibited by the person with dementia are not deliberate attacks on care-givers by a violent person. The message is, in the words of Rader and Barrick (2000, p 49), "Please find another way to keep me clean, because the

| Box 21-13 | Framework for Asking Questions About the Meaning of Behavior |

What?

What is being sought? What is happening? Does the behavior have a physical or emotional component or both? What are the person's responses? What would be done if the person was 20 years old instead of 80? What is the behavior saying? What is the emotion being expressed?

Where?

Where is the behavior occurring? Environmental triggers?

When?

When does the behavior most frequently occur? After what (e.g., activities of daily living [ADLs], family visits, mealtimes)?

Who?

Who is involved? Other residents, caregivers, family?

Why?

What happened before? Poor communication? Tasks too complicated? Physical or medical problem? Person being rushed or forced to do something? Has this happened before and why?

What Now?

Approaches and interventions (physical, psychosocial)?
Changes needed and by whom?
Who else might know something about the person or the behavior or approaches?
Communicate to all and include in plan of care.

Adapted from Hellen C: *Alzheimer's disease: activity focused care*, Boston, 1998, Butterworth-Heinemann; Ortigara A: Understanding the language of behaviors, *Alzheimer Care Q* 1(4):91, 2000.

way you are doing it now is intolerable." To care effectively for older adults with dementia, nurses and other caregivers need to try to put themselves in the place of the person with dementia and try to see the world from his or her eyes. The following paragraph will illustrate:

> You are asleep in the chair at home when suddenly you are woken up by a person you have never seen before trying to undress you. Then they put you naked into a hard, cold chair and wheel you down a hallway. Suddenly cold water hits you in the face and the person is touching your private areas. You don't understand why they are trying to do this to you. You are embarrassed, frightened, cold, angry. You hit and scream at this person and try to get away.

It is very important to remember that behavior is an expression of needs, and as such, the focus needs to be on understanding what the person is trying to communicate through behavior. Family members and nurses caring for people with dementia must understand that they are the ones who must change their reactions, behaviors, and approaches because the person with dementia

cannot do this. Modification of communication techniques, expectations of care and care routines, and the environment is the foundation for responding appropriately. Box 21-13 presents a framework for asking questions about the possible meanings and messages behind observed behavior.

In research in nursing homes, Rader, Barrick (2000) have provided comprehensive guidelines for bathing people with dementia in ways that are pleasurable and decrease distress. Asking the question "What is the easiest, most comfortable, least frightening way for me to clean the person right now?" guides the choice of interventions (Rader, Barrick, 2000, p 42). Knowing the person's lifetime bathing routines and preferences; providing care only when the person is receptive; respecting refusals to participate in care; explaining all actions; realizing that a bath is not an essential intervention; encouraging self-care to the extent possible; making bathrooms and shower areas warm, comfortable, and safe; being attentive to pain and discomfort; and using alternative bathing methods, such as a towel bath or sponge bath, are some suggested responses. Box 21-14

Box 21-14 Guidelines for Bathing Persons with Dementia

- Speak calmly, slowly, facing the person, and using his or her name.
- Tell the person what you are doing at all times, and avoid surprises.
- Praise and reassure.
- Bathe the person before he or she is dressed for the day.
- Wash the most sensitive area (as defined by the person being bathed) last.
- Keep covered and warm.
- Minimize the number of moves during the bath or shower.
- Pat dry rather than rub to decrease discomfort.
- Medicate for pain before bathing if indicated.
- Keep room and water temperatures comfortable. Install an extra heater in the tub room so the air and water temperatures are not as disparate.
- Avoid background noises and conversations. Hang beach towels in the bathing room if there is a lot of "echo" from sounds.
- Wash hair last, be sure patient is well covered and warm, wet head with washcloths, use small amount of baby shampoo, and rinse using small amounts of water from a small pitcher or bowl, deflecting water from face and ears.
- Give the person a tub bath, shower, bed bath, sponge bath at sink, or towel bath, depending on preference of the resident. Assess the best time of day for the person's bath—usually when the resident is the most calm and does not have other activities or appointments challenging his or her stress threshold. Follow accustomed patterns for bathing (method, frequency, time of day).
- If the person is very resistive, postpone the bath, return when more receptive. Do not push or force. Bathing is rarely an emergency situation.
- Transfer residents with sufficient staff, proper techniques, and proper equipment. Do not use a shower chair to transfer the person to the bathing room. Replace tubs with hydraulic chair lifts with ones that use an easy-access side panel.
- Undress the person in the bathing room. As the person is undressed, cover each unclothed area with a bath blanket. If comforting, put the person in the tub with bath blankets or towels that cover the person and are raised only in the area needed to allow a hand and washcloth to do the washing.
- Run the water into the tub before the person enters the bathing room. Running water before bringing the person to the tub room not only keeps the tub room warm, but also controls

unwanted noise and distraction. It also allows the caregiver and person to engage in conversation. Some people can tolerate 1 inch of water, and some are not bothered by 5 inches. Keep this and other likes and dislikes in the care plan.
- Have all equipment, linens, and clothing ready and organized before the person enters the bathing room to facilitate an organized and consistent bathing process.
- Allow the resident to feel the water before getting into the tub. Use reassuring phrases such as "This is nice" or "This feels good."
- Try some aromatherapy. Give the resident a choice between two. For example, allow the resident to smell the bath oils and ask, "Do you like the rose or herb scent?"
- Use a calm, unhurried approach. Have one consistent caregiver give the bath, explaining what will be done and asking the person if he or she is comfortable. Use reassuring words, especially when the person seems confused or fearful.
- Keep stimulation as singular and focused as possible. For example, two people should not bathe different parts of the body. If water is running, decrease or stop tactile stimulation.
- Encourage the resident to participate in the bath when possible. If the person has difficulty, try putting your hand over the person's hand while washing.
- Give the person a washcloth or shampoo bottle to hold during the bath, and encourage self-care to the extent possible.
- Placing a sock or pillowcase over the shower head decreases the force of the spray. Use only a hand-held shower to provide focused and controlled spraying.
- Use music to redirect and relax. Songs with which the caregiver and person can sing along can be helpful in giving the person control of the bath.
- Decorate the tub room in a homelike fashion. The tub room should look like a bathroom, not a laboratory. Encourage the staff to bring their personalities into the bathing routine. Pictures of children, pets, and familiar landscapes and objects are helpful for supporting engaging behaviors.
- "Seize the moment." If an accidental food spill soils the clothes, it may be the perfect time to change clothes in the tub room and suggest a bath. "As long as we're changing your clothes let's freshen up, wash your face and hands, and soak your feet a while."

From Kovach CR, Meyer-Arnold EA: Preventing agitated behaviors during bath time, *Geriatr Nurs* 18(3):107-111, 1997; Rader J: Ways that work: bathing without a battle, *Alzheimer Care Q* 1(4):35-49, 2000.

Box 21-15	Recommendations to Avoid People with Dementia Getting Lost

Do not leave the person with dementia alone in the home.

Secure the environment so that the person cannot leave by himself or herself while the caregiver is asleep or busy.

If the person lives in a nursing facility, keep in supervised area; do frequent checks; use bed, chair and door alarms and Wanderguard bracelets; identify potential wanderers by special arm bands; and disguise doorways.

Place locks out of reach, hide keys, and lock windows.

Consider motion detectors or home security systems that alert when doors are opened.

Register the person in the Safe Return program of the Alzheimer's Association, and ensure that the person wears the Safe Return jewelry or clothing tags at all times.

Let neighbors know that a person with dementia lives in the neighborhood.

Prepare a search and rescue plan in case the person becomes lost.

Keep copies of up-to-date photos ready for distribution to searchers, police, hospital, and the media.

Conduct a search immediately if the person becomes lost.

Call the local law enforcement agency and the Safe Return program to report the missing person.

If the person is not found within 6 to 12 hours (or sooner depending on weather conditions), search any wooded areas or fields near where the person was last seen. People with dementia may not seek help or respond to calls and may try to hide from searchers; search in an organized manner with as many searchers as possible.

Adapted from Rowe M: People with dementia who become lost, *Am J Nurs* 103(7):32-39, 2003.

presents a summary of some of these guidelines that both nurses and family caregivers may find helpful.

Wandering

Wandering is one of the most difficult management problems encountered in home and institutional settings. Wandering has been defined as purposeless walking that involves random movement and frequent changes in direction, pacing, or doing laps (Rowe, 2003). Wandering can lead to falls, elopement (leaving the home or facility), disturbances in care routines such as eating, and interference with the privacy of others (Algase et al, 2003). Wandering behavior may also result in people with dementia going outside and getting lost, a phenomenon studied by Rowe (2003). The Alzheimer's Association estimates that 60% of people with dementia will wander and become lost in the community at some point. Conclusions from Rowe's (2003) research, a retrospective review of records of Safe Return (a nationwide, federally funded identification program of the Alzheimer's Association), advised that all people

with dementia should be considered capable of becoming lost. Caregivers need to prevent people with dementia from leaving homes or care facilities unaccompanied, register the person with dementia in the Safe Return program, and have a plan of action in case the person does become lost. Rowe also suggests that police must respond rapidly to requests for searches and the general public should be informed how to recognize and assist people with dementia who may be lost (Rowe, 2003). Box 21-15 presents specific recommendations from this study.

An understanding of wandering behavior is important so that approaches can be individualized. The stimulus for wandering arises from many internal and external sources. Agenda behaviors were identified and studied by Rader et al (1985) and are defined as "the verbal and nonverbal planning actions that cognitively impaired persons use in an effort to fulfill their felt social, emotional, and physical needs" (p 196). Rader and colleagues proposed three factors that may contribute to wandering: fear caused by separation from people and environments with which the person was

Box 21-16	Interventions for Wandering or Exiting Behaviors

Face the person, and make direct eye contact (unless this is interpreted as threatening).

Gently touch the person's arm, shoulders, back, or waist if he or she does not move away.

Call the person by his or her formal name (e.g., Mr. Jones).

Listen to what the person is communicating verbally and nonverbally; listen to the feelings being expressed.

Identify the agenda, plan of action, and the emotional needs the agenda is expressing.

Respond to the feelings expressed, staying calm.

Repeat specific words or phrases, or state the need or emotion (e.g., "You need to go home, you're worried about your husband.").

If such repetition fails to distract the person, accompany him or her and continue talking calmly, repeating phrases and the emotion you identify.

Provide orienting information only if it calms the person. If it increases distress, stop talking about the present situations. Do not "correct" the person or belittle his or her agenda.

At intervals, redirect the person toward the facility or the home by suggesting, "Let's walk this way now" or "I'm so tired, let's turn around."

If orientation and redirection fail, continue to walk, allowing the person control but ensuring safety.

Make sure you have a backup person, but he or she should stay out of eyesight of the person.

Have someone call for help if you are unable to redirect. Usually the behavior is time limited because of the person's attention span and the security and trust between you and the person.

Adapted from Rader J, Doan J, Schwab M: How to decrease wandering: a form of agenda behavior, *Geriatr Nurs* 6(4):196-199, 1985.

previously most connected and comfortable; frustration that develops when the agenda is thwarted by caregivers with a different agenda; and the need to be needed.

Algase et al (2003) described how the NDB model can be used to research, understand, and design interventions related to wandering. With this framework, predisposing background factors (level of cognitive impairment, perceptual disturbances, language skills, previous work roles and activity levels, lifelong patterns of coping with stress) and proximal factors (type of environment, caregiver communication, noise) all play a role in wandering behavior. Wandering behaviors can be predictable through careful observation and knowing the person's patterns. For example, if the person with dementia starts wandering or trying to leave the home around dinner time everyday, meaningful activities such as music, exercise, and refreshments can be provided at this time. Research suggests that wandering may be less likely to occur when the person is involved in social interaction. Environmental interventions such as camouflaging doorways, providing enclosed outdoor gardens and paths for walking, electronic bracelets that activate alarms at exits, exercise, ambulation, and meaningful activity programs are some examples. Box 21-16 presents suggestions for additional interventions. A guideline for approaches to prevent and manage wandering in hospitalized older adults can be found at http://www.hartfordign.org.

Listening, really listening, to the person with dementia and reading books, articles, and poetry written by people with dementia can teach us a lot about what the person is feeling and experiencing. Several of these are listed in the Resources at the end of the chapter. The following excerpts about wandering from an article by Laurenhue (2001) provide a great deal of insight into this concern:

Wandering and restlessness is one of the by-products of Alzheimer's disease . . . When the darkness and emptiness fill my mind, it is totally terrifying . . . Thoughts increasingly haunt me. The only way I can break the cycle is to move (Davis, 1989, p 96).

Very often I wander around looking for something which I know is very pertinent, but then after a while I forget all about what it was I was looking for. When I'm wandering around, I'm trying to touch base with—anything, actually. If anything appeared I'd probably enjoy it, or look at it or examine it and wonder how it got there. I feel very foolish when I'm wandering around not knowing what I'm doing and I'm not always quite sure how to do any better. It's not easy to figure out what the heck I'm looking for (Henderson, 1998, p 24).

Clearly, wandering is a complex behavior that calls for observation, investigation, and a variety of individualized approaches. Peatfield et al (2002), in a report of an integrative review of the research literature on wandering, discuss many of the interventions proposed and call for intervention studies to develop evidence-based guidelines for the management of this concern. The safety and comfort of the person are essential so that wandering and getting lost do not result in injury or death.

Environmental Alterations

Both home and institutional settings can be modified to be more supportive for people with dementia. Many nursing homes resemble little hospitals and can be cold, impersonal, and confusing places for people with dementia. The present trend is to have special care units (SCUs) designed for the needs of people with cognitive impairment. In nursing homes, space can be designed to be a more homelike environment with smaller areas more like rooms in a real house. Family rooms, small-group dining rooms, kitchens on the unit where residents can participate in meal preparation and eat together, private spaces, natural light, elimination of noise such as overhead paging, spalike bathrooms, and outdoor walking and sitting areas are some examples. There are many other ideas and descriptions of more appropriate designs for institutions (Eastman, 2001; Lindstrom, 2004). Examining safety in the home from the perspectives of the physical environment and caregiver competence, Hurley et al (2004) developed a home safety/injury model that may be helpful in teaching caregivers how to create safer homes. Resources to assist caregivers in both institutional and home settings in making environmental modifications to maintain function and ensure safety are listed under Resources at the end of this chapter as well as Chapter 22.

IMPLICATIONS FOR GERONTOLOGICAL NURSING AND HEALTHY AGING

Many of the interventions to prevent delirium and to care for people with cognitive impairment are achieved by applying the principles of good gerontological nursing care. An understanding of these principles and how to adapt responses and the environment to people with cognitive impairment will ensure the meeting of basic needs and enhance quality of care and quality of life. Some may seem like simple basic nursing, but they are often not practiced, leading to a great deal of iatrogenesis, distress, and excess disability. Often these consequences are more problematic than the illnesses themselves. Our care, however well intentioned, must not increase disability. It must be based on knowledge and research to be considered best practice. We also have a responsibility to teach others about these best practices.

The four roles of a successful caregiver for someone with dementia presented by Rader and Tornquist (1995) provide a framework for competent and compassionate gerontological nursing care and healthy aging for older adults with cognitive impairment:

- Magician role: To understand what the person is trying to communicate both verbally and nonverbally, we must be a magician who can use our magical abilities to see the world through the eyes, ears, and feelings of the person. We know how to use our tricks to turn an individual's behavior around or prevent it from occurring and causing distress.
- Detective role: The detective looks for clues and cues about what might be causing distress and how it might be changed. We have to investigate and know as much about the person as possible to be a good detective.
- Carpenter role: By having a wide variety of tools and selecting the right tools for the job, we build individualized plans of care for each person.
- Jester role: Many people with dementia retain their sense of humor and respond well to the appropriate use of humor. This does not mean making fun of but rather sharing laughter and fun. "Those who love their work and do it well employ good doses of humor as part of the care of others as well as for self-care" (Rader, Barrick, 2000, p 42). The jester spreads joy, is creative,

NANDA and Wellness Diagnoses

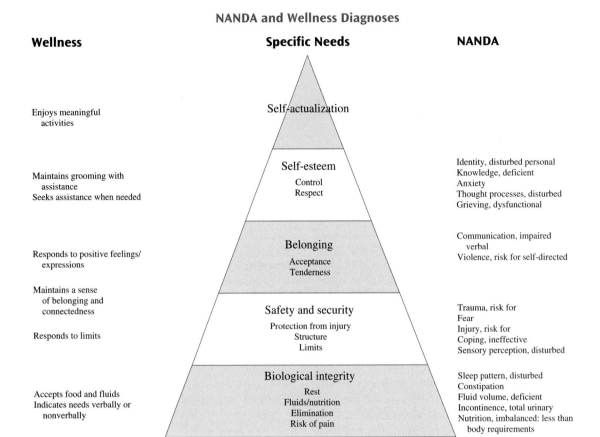

Wellness	Specific Needs	NANDA

Wellness

Enjoys meaningful
    activities

Maintains grooming with
    assistance
Seeks assistance when needed

Responds to positive feelings/
    expressions

Maintains a sense
    of belonging and
    connectedness

Responds to limits

Accepts food and fluids
Indicates needs verbally or
    nonverbally

Specific Needs

Self-actualization

Self-esteem
Control
Respect

Belonging
Acceptance
Tenderness

Safety and security
Protection from injury
Structure
Limits

Biological integrity
Rest
Fluids/nutrition
Elimination
Risk of pain

NANDA

Identity, disturbed personal
Knowledge, deficient
Anxiety
Thought processes, disturbed
Grieving, dysfunctional

Communication, impaired
    verbal
Violence, risk for self-directed

Trauma, risk for
Fear
Injury, risk for
Coping, ineffective
Sensory perception, disturbed

Sleep pattern, disturbed
Constipation
Fluid volume, deficient
Incontinence, total urinary
Nutrition, imbalanced: less than
    body requirements

These are not all of the possible wellness or NANDA diagnoses that may be identified. The above are frequent examples of nursing diagnoses that should be considered when planning care for the older adult in whatever setting.

energizes, and lightens the burdens (Laurenhue, 2000; Rader, Barrick, 2003).

APPLICATION OF MASLOW'S HIERARCHY

Consistent with the philosophy of this book, the nursing care of older adults with dementia presented in this chapter is focused not only on meeting basic needs, but also on creating environments and relationships that promote growth, self-actualization, and quality of life. Despite their inability to express their thoughts and feelings in ways that we are accustomed to, people with cognitive impairment still have higher-order needs, such as those for belonging, self-esteem, and a meaningful life. The care relationships and the environment need to support the meeting of all their needs. Surely we would want the same for ourselves. "The relationship between the caregiver and care recipient is the central determinant of quality of life and quality of care" (Rader, Barrick, 2000, p 36).

▶ **KEY CONCEPTS**

- Cognitive impairment that is significant is a disease process and must be regarded as such. Some of the dementias are treatable, and some are not. Nurses need to advocate for thorough assessment of any elder who appears to be experiencing genuine cognitive decline and inability to function in important aspects of life.

- Delirium is a result of physiological imbalances and may be caused by a variety of biological disturbances and other stressors. Delirium is characterized by fluctuating levels of consciousness, sometimes in a diurnal pattern, and frequent misperceptions and illusions. It is often unrecognized and attributed to age or dementia. Knowledge of risk factors, preventive measures, and treatment of underlying medical problems is essential to prevent serious consequences.
- Medications and pain are frequently the cause of delirious states in the older adult.
- Irreversible dementias follow a pattern of inevitable decline accompanied by decreased intellectual function, personality changes, and impaired judgment. The most common of these is Alzheimer's disease.
- Alzheimer's disease has been the subject of enormous amounts of research in attempts to understand the causes. Genes, latent viruses, enzyme and neurotransmitter deficiencies, environmental toxins, and psychosocial stressors have all been implicated to some degree. Research is continuing in attempts to discover ways to protect against or halt the progression of the disease. At this time there is no known cure, although some medications being developed seem to slow the progression of the dementia for a time.
- Vascular brain disorders (brain attacks) are caused by interruption of the blood supply to the brain because of clots, hemorrhages, and vascular spasm or occlusion. Identification of risk factors and prevention are important. Many of these situations can be remedied and serious brain damage prevented if treatment is immediate.
- Assessment of cognitive impairment is complex. Nurses may perform preliminary assessments with any number of brief mental status examinations and need to request more thorough assessment when there is an indication of dementia.
- Individuals with cognitive impairment respond best to calmness and patience, adaptations of communication techniques, and

environments and relationships that enhance function, support limitations, ensure safety, and provide opportunities for a meaningful quality of life. Since they may be unable to express their feelings or needs, the gerontological nurse must always try to understand the world from their perspective.

Activities and Discussion Questions

1. What are the differences among delirium, dementia, and depression?
2. What are some of the risk factors for development of delirium?
3. Discuss the most useful way to provide information for a person experiencing delirium.
4. Why is it important to ensure that the person experiencing any change in mental status receives a thorough assessment and evaluation?
5. What would you say to a person who reports to you that he or she has had symptoms of a transient ischemic attack (TIA)?
6. How do the symptoms of Parkinson's disease affect functional abilities? What nursing interventions would be important when caring for a person with Parkinson's disease?
7. Brainstorm with fellow students how it would feel to be bathed by a total stranger.
8. Describe how you would design a special care unit for individuals with dementia.
9. A family caregiver tells you that his or her loved one keeps trying to leave the house to find the children. What are some strategies you might share with the caregiver to deal with this situation?
10. The nursing assistants in a nursing home complain to you that Mr. G. hit them when they were trying to give him his required twice weekly shower. How might you assist them in meeting Mr. G's need for bathing?

RESOURCES

Books and Publications

Hellen C: *Alzheimer's disease: activity focused care,* Boston, 1998, Butterworth-Heinemann.

Loveday B, Kitwood T, Bowe B: *Improving dementia care: a resource for training and professional development,* Philadelphia, 1998, Hawker Publications.

Mahoney E, Volicer L, Hurley A: *Management of challenging behaviors in dementia*, Baltimore, 2000, Health Professions Press.

Reade H: *Speaking from experience: nursing assistants share their knowledge of dementia care*, Brooklyn, NY, 2002, Cobble Hill Health Center.

Santo Pietro M, Ostuni E: *Successful communication with Alzheimer's disease patients: an in-service manual*, Boston, 1997, Butterworth-Heinemann.

Santo Pietro MJ, Boczko F: *The breakfast club*, Vero Beach, Fla, 1997, The Speech Bin.

Snyder L: *Speaking our minds: personal reflections from individuals with Alzheimer's*, New York, 1999, WH Freeman and Co.

Warner M: *The complete guide to Alzheimer's proofing your home*, Lafayette, Ind, 2000, Purdue University Press.

Organizations

Alzheimer's Association
225 N. Michigan Avenue, Floor 17
Chicago, IL 60601
(800) 272-3900
website: http://www.alz.org

Alzheimer's Disease Education and Referral Center
PO Box 8250
Silver Spring, MD 20907
(800) 438-4380
website: http://www.alzheimers.org

Alzheimer's Solutions
3122 Knorr Street
Philadelphia, PA 19149
(212) 624-2098
website: http://www.caregiving-solutions.com

American Heart Association
7272 Greenville Avenue
Dallas, TX 75231
www.americanheart.org

American Stroke Association
7272 Greenville Avenue
Dallas, TX 75231
www.strokeassociation.org

American Parkinson Disease Association
1250 Hylan Boulevard, Suite 4B
Staten Island, NY 10305
(800) 223 -2732
website: http://www.apdaparkinson.org

National Alliance for Caregiving
4720 Montgomery Lane, 5th floor
Bethesda, MD 20814
website: http://www.caregiving.org

National Parkinson Foundation, Inc.
1501 NW 9th Avenue/Bob Hope Road
Miami, FL 33136
(800) 327-4545
website: http://www.parkinson.org

The Parkinson's Disease Foundation, Inc.
710 W. 168th Street
New York, NY 10032
(800) 457-6676
website: http://www.pdf.org

Perspectives—a quarterly newsletter for individuals diagnosed with Alzheimer's disease
Available from:
Lisa Snyder, Alzheimer's Disease Research Center
9500 Gilman Drive—0948
La Jolla, CA 92093
(858) 622-5800

Website

Alzheimer's Caregiver Support Online
http://www.alzonline.net

Video

Motivating Moves for People with Parkinson's: a video/DVD on exercise
Available from www.motivatingmoves.com or The Parkinson's Disease Foundation (www.pdf.org)

REFERENCES

Adams HP Jr et al: Guidelines for the management of patients with ischemic stroke, *Stroke* 34(4):1056-1083, 2003.

Algase D, Beel-Bates C, Beattie E: Wandering in long-term care, *Ann Long-Term Care* 11(1):33-39, 2003.

American Medical Directors Association (AMDA): *Altered mental status*, Columbia, Md, 1998, American Medical Directors Association.

American Psychiatric Association: *Diagnostic and statistical manual of mental disorders (DSM-IV)*, ed 4, Washington, DC, 1994, The Association.

Beck CT: Nursing students' experiences caring for cognitively impaired elderly people, *J Adv Nurs* 23(5):992-998, 1996.

Beier M, Peskind E, Sey M: Optimizing care management plans across the spectrum of Alzheimer's disease, *Suppl Ann Long Term Care Clin Geriatr*, pp 1-9, March 2004.

Bell V, Troxel D: Spirituality and the person with dementia: a view from the field, *Alzheimer Care Q* 2(2):31-45, 2001.

Boss B: Alterations of neurological function. In McCance K, Huether S, editors: *Pathophysiology: the biologic basis for disease in adults and children*, ed 4, St Louis, 2002, Mosby.

Burke MM, Laramie JA: *Primary care of the older adult: A multidisciplinary approach*, St Louis, 2000, Mosby.

Cohen-Mansfield J: Nonpharmacological management of behavioral problems in persons with dementia: the TREA model, *Alzheimer Care Q* 1(4):22-34, 2000.

Crystal H: Dementia with Lewy bodies. Accessed 8/25/04 from http://emedicine.com/neuro/topic91.htm.

Davis R: *My journey into Alzheimer's disease*, Wheaton, Ill, 1989, Tyndale House Publishers, Inc.

DeYoung S, Just G, Harrison R: Decreasing aggressive, agitated, or disruptive behavior: participation in a behavior management unit, *J Gerontol Nurs* 28(6):22-31, 2003.

Doody RS et al: Practice parameter: management of dementia (an evidence-based review): report of the Quality Standards Subcommittee of the American Academy of Neurology, *Neurology* 56(9):1154-1166, 2001.

Eastman P: Environmental therapy aids for Alzheimer's patients, *Caring for the Ages* 2(9):1, 18, 2001.

Easton KL: The poststroke journey: from agonizing to owning, *Geriatr Nurs* 20(2):70-75, 1999.

Ely EW et al: Evaluation of delirium in critically ill patients: validation of the Confusion Assessment Method for the Intensive Care Unit (CAM-ICU), *Crit Care Med* 29(7):1370-1379, 2001.

Fagen SC, Morgenstern LB, Petitta A et al: Cost-effectiveness of tissue pasminogen activator for acute ischemic stroke, NINDA V1-PA Stroke Study Group, *Neurology* 50(4):883-890, 1998.

Fazio S: Person-centered language is an essential part of person-centered care, *Alzheimer Care Q* 2(2):87-90, 2001.

Flaherty JH et al: A model for managing delirious older inpatients, *J Am Geriatr Soc* 51(7):1031-1035, 2003.

Flaherty J, Morley J: Delirium: A call to improve current standards of care, *J Gerontology* 59A(4):341-343, 2004.

Folstein MF, Folstein SE, McHugh PR: "Mini-mental state": a practical method for grading the cognitive state of patients for the clinician, *J Psychiatr Res* 12(3):189-198, 1975.

Foreman M, Fletcher K, Mion L, Trygstad L: Assessing cognitive function. In Mezey M et al, editors: *Geriatric nursing protocols for best practice*, New York, 2003, Springer Publishing Company.

Foreman MD et al: Delirium in elderly patients: an overview of the state of the science, *J Gerontol Nurs* 27(4):12-20, 2001.

Hall GR: Caring for people with Alzheimer's disease using the conceptual model of progressively lowered stress threshold in the clinical setting, *Nurs Clin North Am* 29(1):129-141, 1994.

Hall GR, Buckwalter KC: Progressively lowered stress threshold: a conceptual model for care of adults with Alzheimer's disease, *Arch Psychiatr Nurs* 1(6):399-406, 1987.

Ham R, Sloane P, Warshaw G: *Primary care geriatrics*, St Louis, 2002, Mosby.

Haney DQ, Faster ER: Care team treats stroke better, Associated Press, Sunday, Feb. 10, 2002.

Henderson C: *Partial view: an Alzheimer's journal*, Dallas, 1998, Southern Methodist University Press.

Hurley A, Gauthier M, Horvath K et al: Promoting safer home environments for persons with Alzheimer's disease, *J Gerontol Nurs* 30(6):43-51, 2004.

Hustey F, Meldon S: The prevalence and documentation of impaired mental status in elderly emergency department patients, *Ann Intern Med* 39:248-253, 2002.

Inouye SK: The dilemma of delirium: clinical and research controversies regarding diagnosis and evaluation of delirium in hospitalized elderly medical patients, *Am J Med* 97(3):278-288, 1994.

Inouye SK et al: Clarifying confusion: the confusion assessment method: a new method for detection of delirium, *Ann Intern Med* 113(12):941-948, 1990.

Inouye SK et al: A multicomponent intervention to prevent delirium in hospitalized older patients, *N Engl J Med* 340(9):669-676, 1999.

Inouye SK et al: Nurses' recognition of delirium and its symptoms: comparison of nurse and researcher ratings, *Arch Intern Med* 161(20):2467-2473, 2001.

Keane WL: The patient's perspective: the Alzheimer's association, *Alzheimer Dis Assoc Disord* 8(suppl 3):151-155, 1994.

Knopman DS et al: Practice parameter: diagnosis of dementia (an evidence-based review): report of the Quality Standards Subcommittee of the American Academy of Neurology, *Neurology* 56(9):1143-1153, 2001.

Kolanowski AM: An overview of the Need-Driven Dementia-Compromised Behavior Model, *J Gerontol Nurs* 25(9):7-9, 1999.

Kovach CR, Meyer-Arnold EA: Preventing agitated behaviors during bath time, *Geriatr Nurs* 18(3):107-111, 1997.

Laurenhue K: Each person's journey is unique, *Alzheimer Care Q* 2(2):79-83, 2001.

Laurenhue K: Learning to increase comfort, *Alzheimer's Care Quarterly* 1(4): 93-97, 2000.

Lindstrom A: Designer's challenge, *Caring for the Ages* 5(4):1, 16, 18, 27, 2004.

McGowin DF: *Living in the labyrinth: a personal journey through the maze of Alzheimer's*, New York, 1993, Dell Publishing, p viii.

Milisen K, Foreman M, Wouters B, et al: Documentation of delirium in elderly patients with hip fracture, *J Gerontol Nurs* 28(11):23-29, 2002.

Moore A, Clarke C: PD, *BMJ Clinical Evidence*, issue 6, Dec 2001.

Moore T, Hollett J: Giving voice to persons living with dementia: the researcher's opportunities and challenges, *Nurs Sci Q* 16:164-167, 2003.

Neelon VJ et al: The NEECHAM confusion scale: construction, validation, and clinical testing, *Nurs Res* 45(6):324-330, 1996.

Ortigara A: Understanding the language of behaviors, *Alzheimer Care Q* 1(4):89-92, 2000.

Peatfield J, Futrell M, Cox C: Wandering: an integrative literature review, *J Gerontol Nurs* 28(4):44-50, 2002.

Pulsford D: Therapeutic activities for people with dementia—what, why . . . and why not? *J Adv Nurs* 26(4):704-709, 1997.

Rader J, Barrick A: Ways that work: bathing without a battle, *Alzheimer Care Q* 1(4):35-49, 2000.

Rader J, Doan J, Schwab M: How to decrease wandering, a form of agenda behavior, *Geriatr Nurs* 6(4):196-199, 1985.

Rader J, Tornquist E: *Individualized dementia care*, New York, 1995, Springer Publishing Co.

Rapp CG, Mentes JC, Titler MG: Acute confusion/ delirium protocol, *J Gerontol Nurs* 27(4):21-33, 2001.

Richards K, Lambert C, Beck C: Deriving interventions for challenging behaviors from the need-driven, dementia-compromised behavior model, *Alzheimer Care Q* 1(4):62-76, 2000.

Rowe MA: People with dementia who become lost, *Am J Nurs* 103(7):32-39, 2003.

Sanders AB: Missed delirium in older emergency department patients: a quality-of-care problem, *Ann Emerg Med* 39(3):338-341, 2002.

Shen JJ, Washington EL, Aponte-Soto L: Racial disparities in the pathogenesis and outcomes for patients with ischemic stroke, *Manage Care Interface* 17(3):28-34, 2004.

Sica D: ACE inhibitors and stroke: new considerations, *J Clin Hypertens* 4(2):126, 2002.

Sifton C: Life is what happens while we are making other plans, *Alzheimer Care Q* 2(2):iv-vii, 2001.

Stewart JT: Defining diffuse Lewy body disease: tetrad of symptoms distinguishes illness from other dementias, *Postgrad Med* 113(5):71-75, 2003.

Talerico K, Evans L: Making sense of aggressive/protective behaviors in persons with dementia, *Alzheimer Care Q* 1(4):77-88, 2000.

Touhy TA: Dementia, personhood, and nursing: learning from a nursing situation, *Nurs Sci Q* 17(1):43-49, 2004.

Truman B, Ely EW: Monitoring delirium in critically-ill patients: using the confusion assessment method for the intensive care unit, *Crit Care Nurse* 23(2):25-36, 2003.

Warner J, Butler R: *Alzheimer's disease: clinical evidence number 6*, London, 2001, BMJ Publishers.

Whitney CM: Maintaining the square: how older adults with Parkinson's disease sustain quality in their lives, *J Gerontol Nurs* 30(1):28-35, 2004.

Wolanin MO, Phillips LR: *Confusion: prevention and care*, St Louis, 1981, Mosby.

Maintaining Mobility and Environmental Safety

LEARNING OBJECTIVES

Upon completion of this chapter, the reader will be able to:

- Specify risk factors for impaired mobility.
- Discuss the effects of impaired mobility on general function and quality of life.
- Be familiar with factors that increase vulnerability to falls.
- Identify older adults at risk for falls and list several measures to prevent falls.
- Describe assessment measures to determine gait and walking stability.
- Name several assistive devices that facilitate mobility for elders.
- Develop a nursing care plan appropriate for an elder at risk of falling.
- Understand the effects of restraints and alternate safety interventions.
- Recognize hazards in the home and environment that threaten the safety of elders.
- Identify numerous factors in the environment that contribute to the safety and security of the aged.
- Relate strategies for protecting the older person from injury and accidents in the home and in the community.

GLOSSARY

Extrapyramidal Pertaining to structures outside the pyramidal tracts of the brain that are associated with body movement.

Hypoxia Inadequate oxygen for cellular metabolism. Ischemia Decreased supply of oxygenated blood to a body part or organ.

Paresthesia Subjective sensation experienced as numbness, tingling, or "pins and needles."

Postural hypertension A drop in blood pressure when a person assumes an upright position after being in a supine position.

Proprioception Sensations from within the body regarding spatial position and muscular activity.

Syncope Brief lapse in consciousness caused by transient cerebral hypoxia.

Vertebrobasilar Pertaining to the vertebral and basilar artery junction at the base of the skull.

Vestibular In this chapter it is associated with the sense of equilibrium.

THE LIVED EXPERIENCE

After that fall last year when I slipped on the urine in the bathroom, I feel so insecure. I find myself taking small, shuffling steps to avoid falling again, but it makes me feel awkward and clumsy. When I was younger, I never worried about falling, but now I'm so afraid I will break a bone or something.

Betty, age 75

MOBILITY, SAFETY, AND SATISFACTION

Mobility is the capacity one has for movement within the personally available environment. In infancy, moving about is the major mode of learning and interacting with the environment. In old age, one moves more slowly and purposefully, sometimes with more forethought and caution. Throughout life, movement remains a significant means of personal contact, sensation, exploration, pleasure, and control.

This chapter focuses on maintaining maximal mobility in health and in the presence of various disorders, the assessment of gait and mobility status, the effects of restraints and immobility, risk factors related to falls and preventive actions that nurses may take to reduce the risks, and aids and interventions that are useful when mobility is impaired. Specific information will be provided to promote a safe environment. Also included are transportation and driving as essential aspects of environmental safety.

Mobility and Agility

Mobility and comparative degrees of agility are based on muscle strength, flexibility, postural stability, vibratory sensation, cognition, and perceptions of stability. Aging produces changes in muscles and joints, particularly of the back and legs. Strength and flexibility of muscles decrease markedly; endurance decreases to a somewhat lesser extent, especially if there is a decrease in activity as one ages. Movements and range of motion become more limited. Normal wear and tear reduce the smooth cartilage of joints. Movement is less fluid as one ages, and joints change as regeneration of tissue slows and muscle wasting occurs. Some normal gait changes in late life include a narrower standing base, wider swaying when walking, slowed responses, a greater reliance on proprioception, diminished arm swing, and increased care in gait. These changes are less pronounced in those who remain active and at a desirable weight. Exercise and strength training, even for frail elders, improves mobility and function.

Various degrees of immobility are often temporary or permanent consequences of illness. On a broader scale, elders frequently have limited environmental mobility because of lack of transporta-

tion or loss of a driver's license. In summary, many normal and abnormal changes affect the fluidity and comfort of movement and the capacity for involvement with surroundings. Impairment of mobility is highly associated with poor outcomes in older people (Morley et al, 2003).

Disorders Affecting Mobility

Common conditions that accompany the normal changes of aging, as well as disorders that occur more frequently in older adults, merit special attention. Osteoporosis, gait disorders, Parkinson's disease, strokes, and arthritic conditions markedly affect movement and functional capacities. Mobility may also be limited by paresthesias; amputations; neuromotor disturbances; fractures; foot, knee, and hip problems; and illnesses that deplete one's energy. In long-term care facilities, comprehensive rehabilitation and restorative programs can assist in maintenance of mobility and prevent wheelchair dependence. Many elders in later years have some of these afflictions, with women significantly outnumbering men in this respect. Bone and joint problems affecting mobility are discussed in Chapter 19.

FALLS: CAUSES AND CONSEQUENCES

Falls are one of the most important gerontological syndromes and the leading cause of morbidity and mortality for peoples over the age of 65 (Cesari et al, 2002). Injury as a result of falls is the leading cause of death in older adults. The fall-related mortality rate increases with advanced age. Of those who fall and require hospitalization, 50% will die within 1 year. One third of people over the age of 65 fall at least one time each year, and about half of those fall repeatedly. Falls account for 40% of nursing home admissions annually. Up to 20% of hospitalized patients and 45% of those in long-term care facilities will fall. In hospitals and nursing homes, falls are the largest category of adverse incident reports. The acute care cost of treating injurious falls has been estimated in the billions of dollars (Perell et al, 2001).

Falls are a symptom of a problem, although they become the focus of a problem when they occur. Falls may indicate neurological, sensory,

Table 22-1 Fall Factors

Psychogenic	Physiological	Environmental
Poor evaluation of ability and environment	Neurological	Slippery floor: urine or fluid on the floor, loose throw rugs
Depression	Dementias	
Disinterest in surroundings, no concern for safety, subliminal suicide	Somnolence	Uneven and obstructed walking surfaces: electrical cords, furniture, pets, children, uneven door steps or stair risers, loose boards, cracked sidewalks
Fear or anxiety	Normal pressure hydrocephalus	
Distraction, scattered perceptions	Neurosensory and visual deficits: loss of proprioception; peripheral neuropathy; vestibular dysfunction; dizziness; vertigo; syncope; seizures, brain tumors or lesions; Parkinson's disease; cervical spondylosis	Inadequate visual supports: glaring; low-wattage bulbs; lack of night-lights for bathroom, stairs, and halls; poor marking of steps and other hazards
	Cardiovascular disorders	Inadequate construction: absence of railing, lack of grab bars on shower or tub, poorly designed stairs and walkways
	Cerebrovascular insufficiency, strokes and transient ischemic attacks (TIAs), carotid sinus syncope, vertebral artery insufficiency	
	Arrhythmias: Stokes-Adams	
	Valvulopathies	
	Congestive heart failure	
	Hypotension: postural hypotension, postprandial drop in blood pressure, medication induced, male micturition when urethral obstruction present, hypovolemia (dehydration, hemorrhage), impaired venous return (venous pooling, Valsalva's maneuver), impaired vasoconstriction (autonomic disorders, vasovagal)	
	Metabolic disorders: anemia, hypoxia, hypoglycemia, hyperventilation	
	Debilitating disease: cancer, pulmonary disease, immunosuppressant disorder	

cognitive, medication, musculoskeletal problems or impending physical illness (Table 22-1). Falls are rarely benign in older people. Incomplete diagnosis of reasons for a fall can result in repeated incidents. It is essential that nurses evaluate each older adult's risk for falls. Postfall assessments are also important to identify circumstances of the fall and determine fall prevention interventions. Intrinsic changes in the capacities of older adults, disease processes, medications, foot and gait abnormalities, psychological factors, and extrinsic factors all contribute to falls in an interactive manner. A fall is usually an interaction between an environmental factor, such as a wet floor, and an intrinsic factor, such as limited vision, cognitive impairment, or gait problems. In institutional settings, iatrogenic factors such as limited staffing, lack of toileting programs, and restraints and side rails also interact to increase fall risk.

Factors Contributing to Falls

Falls are generally classified as extrinsic (related to environmental factors), intrinsic (related to host

Box 22-1   Fall Risk Factors for Elders

Conditions

Female or single (incidence increases with age)
Maternal history of hip fracture
Sedative and alcohol use, psychoactive
   medications
Previous falls, unsteadiness, dizziness
Acute and recent illness
Pathological conditions, drop attacks
Cognitive impairment, disorientation
Weakness of lower extremities
Abnormalities of balance and gait
Foot problems
Depression, anxiety
Decreased vision or hearing
Fear of falling
Postural hypotension
Postprandial drop in blood pressure
Terminal drop (dies in following 1 to 2 years)
Skeletal and neuromuscular changes
   that predispose to weakness and postural
   imbalance
Acute and severe chronic illness, debilitation
Functional limitations in self-care activities
Multiple disorders and medications
Wheelchair bound
Sensory deficits
Decreased weight
Inability to rise from a chair without using the
   arms
Slow walking speed
Predisposing physiological and psychological
   conditions

Preoccupation with stressors
Anxiety related to previous falls

Situations

Urinary urgency, particularly nocturia
Environmental hazards
Recent relocation, unfamiliarity with new
   environment
Inadequate response to transfer and toileting needs
Assistive devices needed for walking
Inadequate or missing safety rails, particularly in
   bathroom
Poorly designed or unstable furniture
Low stools
High chairs and beds
Uneven floor surfaces
Glossy, highly waxed floors
Wet, greasy, icy surfaces
Inadequate lighting
General clutter
Pets that inadvertently trip an individual
Electrical cords
Loose or uneven stair treads
Reaching for a high shelf
Changing positions (sitting to standing, or
   transferring to or from a bed or wheelchair)
Inability to reach personal items, lack of access to
   call bell or inability to use
Side rails, restraints
Lack of access to bathrooms
Lack of staff training in fall prevention
   techniques

Data from Tinetti ME, Speechley J, Ginter SF: Risk factors for falls among elderly persons living in the community, *N Engl J Med* 319(26):1701-1707, 1988; Rubinstein T, Alexander N, Hausdoff J: Evaluating fall risk in older adults: steps and missteps, *Clin Geriatr* 11(1):52-61, 2003.

factors), or iatrogenic (related to treatment factors). After age 65 individuals fall most frequently because of external reasons; however, with increasing age, internal and locomotor reasons become increasingly prevalent. Fall risk factors that increase proportionally as one ages are disturbances in visual acuity, postural hypotension, cardiac arrhythmias, lower extremity weakness, and gait disturbances. Abnormal gait affects 20% to 50% of people over age 65 and increases susceptibility to falls. Arthritis

of the hip, knee, and foot deformities are common causes of gait disturbances and instability (Rubenstein, Trueblood, 2004). Declines in depth perception, proprioception, vibratory sense, and normotensive response to postural changes are important factors, although the majority of falls occur in individuals with multiple medical problems. Those who fall more often are women, more functionally impaired, and taking more medications. Box 22-1 presents fall risk factors.

Special Considerations Related to Falls

Fear of Falling

Even if a fall does not result in injury, falls contribute to a loss of confidence that leads to reduced physical activity, increased dependency, and social withdrawal (Cesari et al, 2002; Rubinstein et al, 2003). Fear of falling (fallophobia) may restrict an individual's life space (area in which an individual carries on activities). Fear of falling is an important predictor of general functional decline and a risk factor for future falls. Frequent falls contribute significantly to the downward spiral in frail older people (Morley, 2002). Resnick (2002) suggests that nursing staff may also contribute to fear of falling in their patients by telling them not to get up by themselves or using restrictive devices to keep them from independently moving about. More appropriate nursing responses would be to assess fall risk and design individual prevention interventions and safety plans that enhance mobility and independence and decrease fall risk.

A falls efficacy scale, an instrument to measure fear of falling based on self-perceived ability to avoid falls during nonhazardous activities of daily living (ADLs), will be useful in predicting functional decline based on limitations induced by fear (Tinetti et al, 1990, 1994). In research with this instrument, elderly individuals named activities they most avoided because of fear of falling as follows: reaching into cabinets or closets, taking a bath or shower, walking around the house, and getting in and out of bed. When performing a functional or home assessment, these activities should be assessed and suggestions provided for ways the person can alter the activities and feel more secure.

The Problem of Restraints

Restraints have been used historically for the "protection" of the client and for the security of the client and staff. Physical restraints were originally used to control the behavior of individuals with mental illness considered to be dangerous to themselves or others (Evans, Strumpf, 1989). Some common reasons for restraining patients today include prevention of falls, altered mental status, prevention of harming self or others, wandering, agitation, and prevention of interference with treatment. Stilwell's (1988) definition of physical

restraints was developed as part of her investigations as an expert witness and remains the clearest and most inclusive. Physical restraints are devices, materials, and equipment that (1) are attached to or are adjacent to the patient's body; (2) prevent free body movement to a position of choice (standing, walking, lying, turning, sitting); and (3) cannot be controlled or easily removed by the patient. Temporary immobilization of a part of the body for the purpose of treatment, such as casts, splints, and arm boards, is not included in this definition.

The problems of restraint usage were first brought to the forefront of nursing attention by a request from Doris Schwartz, one of the pioneer gerontological nurses, for information from practicing nurses regarding their observations and concerns about restraint usage. In the intervening time, and largely through the efforts of Schwartz, her colleagues, and substantial nursing research, the use of restraints has been drastically reduced (Evans, Strumpf, 1989).

Mechanical restraints are associated with serious injuries, including higher mortality rates, injurious falls, nosocomial infections, incontinence, immobility, contractures, and pressure ulcers. Prevention of falls and injury is most frequently cited as the primary reason for using restraints; however, restraints do not prevent serious injury and may increase the risk of injury and even death. For example, vest restraints, which have been found to be the cause of strangulation deaths, are still commonly used in hospitals. Other common reasons offered for the use of restraints include inadequate staffing, patient interference with medical treatment, agitation or aggression, patients who wander or appear confused, and fear of legal liability. The American judicial system has upheld the idea that restraint use is undesirable and impairs quality of life. There appears to be no change in rate of serious injury related to falls before and after restraint-removal programs, and in fact, several studies have found fall rates for previously restrained long-term care residents to be almost equal to those who have never been restrained. The use of restraints is a source of great physical and psychological distress to older adults and may intensify agitation and contribute to depression. The following quotes from a qualitative study on restraints by Strump et al (1992, p 126) illustrate:

I felt like a dog and cried all night. It hurt me to have to be tied up. I felt like I was nobody, that I was dirt. It makes me cry to talk about it. The hospital is worse than a jail.

I don't remember misbehaving, but I may have been deranged from all the pills they gave me. Normally, I am spirited, but I am also good and obedient. Nevertheless, the nurse tied me down, like Jesus on the cross, by bandaging both wrists and ankles. . . . It felt awful, I hurt and I worried. Callers, including men friends, saw me like that and I lost something. I lost a little personal prestige. I was embarrassed, like a child placed in a corner for being bad. I had been important . . . and to be tied down in bed took a big toll . . . I haven't forgotten the pain and the indignity of being tied.

Restrictions on restraint usage dictated by the Omnibus Budget Reconciliation Act (OBRA) provide specific guidelines for restraint use in long-term care facilities. All long-term care facilities must comply with statements from the *Federal Register* (1991) that relate to restraints and abuse in order to receive Medicare licensure (Box 22-2). Since the advent of OBRA, long-term care facilities have markedly reduced or eliminated restraint use and have developed effective fall prevention and safety programs that are a resource for other institutions. The Joint Commission on Accreditation

of Health Care Organizations also provides specific requirements related to restraint use in acute care settings.

With the move toward freedom from restraints and the promotion of the least restrictive environment, the establishment of safety plans is essential. Removing restraints without careful attention to safety promotion and effective alternatives can jeopardize safety. Many of the suggestions on safety and fall prevention provided in this chapter can be used to promote a safe and restraint-free environment. Delirium, dementia, and associated behaviors that contribute to safety concerns are discussed in Chapter 21. The methods are limited only by the creativity of the nurse. Tying people down is neither effective nor part of best practice nursing. Gerontological nurses must take the lead in education about restraint and restraint alternatives. For suggestions on how to maintain safety without restraints, see the Hartford Geriatric Nursing Institute Try This best practice guidelines, which can be found at http://www.hartfordign.org/resources/education/tryThis.html. The *RN+ Safe-T-Net* online newsletter provides helpful information about fall safety and restraint reduction (http://www.rnplus.com).

The use of side rails is also coming under scrutiny through nursing research. Historically, side rails have been used to prevent falling from the bed, but this practice is being replaced by careful evaluation of the need and benefits of side rails. Side rails are no longer viewed as simply attachments to a patient's bed but may be considered restraints with all of the accompanying concerns discussed above. When side rails impede the person's desired movement or activity, they meet the definition of restraint. Evaluation of the appropriate use of side rails is required in long-term care. A gerontological nurse researcher, Elizabeth Capezuti, has extensively studied the use of side rails and bed-related fall outcomes, as well as individualized interventions (Capezuti et al, 2002). Some alternatives to restraint and side rail use are enumerated in Box 22-3.

Fall Assessment

A comprehensive assessment, including attention to the conditions and situations noted above, and nursing observations of function are essential in assessing fall risk. The nurse is most likely to have

---

Box 22-2	**Statements on Use of Restraints and Abuse**

The resident has the right to be free from any physical or chemical restraints imposed for purposes of discipline or convenience, and not required to treat the resident's medical symptoms. The resident has the right to be free from verbal, sexual, physical, and mental abuse, corporal punishment, and involuntary seclusion.

The facility must develop and implement written policies and procedures that prohibit mistreatment, neglect, and abuse of residents.

The facility must ensure that the resident's environment remains as free of accidental hazards as possible, and that each resident receives adequate supervision and assistance devices to prevent accidents.

From *Federal Register* (V56187), Step 26, p 48825, 1991.

Box 22-3   Residential Problems and Interventions

Problems with Mobility

Inability to move in bed without assistance
- Install trapeze.
- Place unilateral or bilateral transfer enabler, such as bed handle, bed grab bar, transfer pole, quarter or half side rail.
- Refer to occupational therapist for upper extremity strengthening exercises.
- Install easily accessible call bell or bulb (pressure sensitive).

Inability to transfer safely without assistance
- Refer to physical or occupational therapist for transfer training, balance and strengthening, and gait training.
- Encourage recreational activities to complement rehabilitation therapies (e.g., dancing, Tai Chi).
- Place unilateral or bilateral transfer enabler, such as bed handle, bed grab bar, transfer pole with handrail that rotates 360 degrees, quarter or half side rail.
- Place folding bed board under mattress.
- Lock or remove wheels of bed.
- Adjust bed height specific to resident's lower leg length: low beds or very low adjustable-height beds.
- Use nonskid, rubber-backed rugs at bedside.
- Use nonslip bath mats or wet floor safety matting.
- Install easily accessible call bell or bulb (pressure sensitive).
- Use nursery or baby monitor.
- Identify high–fall risk residents. Use colored tags or dots (falling leaves or stars) on patient records, outside room doors, and above beds.
- Use weight-change sensor alarms for bed and chair.
- Install movement sensor alarm (usually placed on thigh).

Inability to safely transfer as a result of dizziness and/or postural hypotension
- Refer to physician or nurse practitioner for evaluation, including medication review.
- Teach resident to rise slowly from lying and sitting positions.
- Refer to physical or occupational therapist for transfer training: lying to sitting to standing, standing to commode, sitting on toilet or commode to standing.
- Teach correct method of sitting on toilet: do not sit until legs are against the seat, then

place hands on handrails, finally sit down slowly.
- Teach prevention of Valsalva's maneuver related to excessive straining when defecating or straining to urinate in residents with BPH.

Inability to safely ambulate as a result of specific lower extremity problems: pain, weakness, limited ROM, or contractures
- Refer to physician or nurse practitioner for evaluation, including medication review and prescription of scheduled analgesic agents.
- Refer to physical or occupational therapist for evaluation, including need for specific rehabilitation therapies.
- Use hot packs.
- Consider joint mobilization.
- Incorporate conditioning, strengthening, and ROM exercises.
- Obtain assistive ambulatory devices, such as a walker "sled."
- Explore gait training.
- Encourage slow, prolonged stretching preceded by heat or ultrasound.
- Use leg length discrepancy pads.
- Use extra-wide walker.
- Use hemi-ambulator walker.
- Use slide walker or walker "sled" plus walker skis.
- Install hand grips for walker.
- Provide unit-based ROM and walking program.
- Use bicycle helmets, knee and elbow pads to protect from injury.
- Provide comfortable and well-fitted seating.

Inability to navigate well because of foot problems
- Place antiskid acrylic wax on floors.
- Use nonskid, rubber-backed rugs at bedside.
- Apply skid-proof strips near bed.
- Teach resident the importance of wearing footwear when walking to bathroom.
- Refer to podiatrist for evaluation.
- Obtain podiatry prescription for appropriate shoe gear and orthotics (e.g., shoes to correct leg length discrepancy and fit over deformities).

Inability to negotiate environment in low light
- Install night-lights with bulb wattage specific to resident's need.
- Keep light in bathroom on at night.
- Install pull cord for light within resident's reach in bed.
- Use motion sensor light.

Continued.

Box 22-3	Residential Problems and Interventions—cont'd

- Place cordless press-on light at bedside.
- Use low buff on waxed floors.
- Install bulb (pressure sensitive) call bell.
- Ensure eyeglasses are easily accessible from bed.

Inability to negotiate path between bed and bathroom
- Rearrange furniture and objects to provide an obstacle-free path and compensate for specific problems (e.g., macular degeneration).
- Use side rail on one side (resident's weaker side) to encourage one path to bathroom.
- Outline path to bathroom with fluorescent tape in contrasting color to floor or wall, such as red or orange.
- Rearrange bed closer to bathroom or provide a rest stop (e.g., chair placed midway between bed and bathroom).
- Use bedside commode (without wheels) placed on resident's stronger side, specific to resident's size.
- Provide illustration of toilet on bathroom door.
- Avoid slippery floor surface.
- Attach stop sign or material or vinyl strip across doorways not to enter.
- Use knob locks, such as "knob knots."

Difficulty transferring on and off toilet
- Refer to occupational therapist to evaluate need for toilet to be fitted with a secured raised seat and grab rails on each side, adjustable toilet seat, or adjustable toilet seat and rails.
- Apply skid-proof strips near toilet.
- Use accessible, glare-free light.
- Place cordless press-on light near commode.
- Refer to physical or occupational therapist for transfer training: standing to toilet or commode, sitting on toilet or commode to standing.
- Teach transferring techniques, including sitting on a commode: wait until legs are against the seat, then place hands on handrails, finally sit down slowly.
- Teach prevention of Valsalva's maneuver related to excessive straining when defecating or straining to urinate in residents with BPH.
- Refer to physical or occupational therapist to teach exercises to increase strength of hip extensor-abductor and ankle plantar-flexor muscles.
- Use easily removable night clothing.
- Place alarm cord near toilet in bathroom.

Potential for Injury

Potential for fall-related injury from bed
- Use full body pillows or long immobilization bags.
- Use bed bolsters or pillows or rolled blanket under mattress edges.
- Use very low bed or very low adjustable-height bed.
- Adjust bed height specific to resident's lower leg length: low or very low adjustable-height beds.
- Place bed mattress on floor.
- Use raised-edge mattress.
- Place nonskid, rubber-backed rugs at bedside.
- Place egg-crate mattress on floor near bed if unable to walk.
- Use mat (4×6 to 8 feet) with nonslip surface.
- Apply hip protector pads.
- Use weight-change sensor alarm for bed.
- Use movement sensor alarm (usually placed on thigh).
- Apply call bell cord to clothing (alarm when disconnected) or alarm attached to clothing.
- Place motion sensor light close to bed.
- Use nursery or baby monitor.
- Install video monitor.
- Place signs at strategic locations to alert staff of fall risk.
- Place residents at risk for falling near the nursing station for close observation.

Potential for injury (skin tears) related to involuntary movements during sleep
- Position resident in center of bed (on back and both sides).
- Use body-length pillows bilaterally.
- Use full body–molded foam cushion.
- Use bed bolsters.
- Apply pillows or cushions for positioning of joints.
- Apply leg separator pads.
- Use very low beds: 5-, 8-, 11-inch deck heights or very low adjustable-height beds.
- Place bumper wedge on side rail.
- Attach sheepskin side rail pad.
- Attach side rail pad/bumper; bumper with see-through window.
- Use side rail pads for small-stature residents or sheepskin side rail pad.

| Box 22-3 | Residential Problems and Interventions—*cont'd* |

Nocturia and Incontinence

Nocturia
- Conduct elimination rounds (individual-specific frequency).
- Place urinal or bedpan near bedside.
- Place bedside commode (without wheels) on resident's strongest side, specific to resident's size; use drop arm commode.
- Use nonskid, rubber-backed rugs at bedside that can absorb urine.
- Apply nonskid, raised-tread socks.
- Place nonslip bath mats or wet floor safety matting near bed and bathroom.
- Refer to physician or nurse practitioner for evaluation of urination frequency changes.

Incontinence
- Refer to continence specialist, physician, nurse practitioner for evaluation.
- Conduct elimination rounds (individual-specific frequency).
- Use extra-absorbent incontinence pads.
- Use bed pads.
- Apply incontinence covers for cushions.
- Install incontinence sensor with alarm.
- Apply raised-tread socks.

Sleep

Lack of comfort or inability to relax
- Refer for evaluation by physician or nurse practitioner for anxiety, depression, restless leg syndrome, paroxysmal nocturnal dyspnea, and sleep apnea.
- Refer for medication review by physician or nurse practitioner.
- Evaluate sleep hygiene: excessive daytime napping, lack of regular exercise, and exposure to daylight and overuse of caffeine.
- Install noise conditioner or "white noise."
- Turn radio and television on or off; play soothing music based on previous lifestyle preferences.
- Use body-length pillow.
- Install firm mattress or folding bed board under mattress.
- Use egg-crate mattress.
- Use air mattress.
- Apply sheepskin mattress pads.
- Use specific position (i.e., elevated, bent knees for back pain).
- Use pillows or cushions for positioning.
- Apply leg separator pads.
- Apply heel pads, bed cradle, and foot support.
- Install foot board.

Modified from Capezuti E et al: Individualized assessment and intervention in bilateral siderail use, *Geriatr Nurs* 19(6):322-330, 1998.

BPH, Benign prostatic hypertrophy; *ROM*, range of motion.

had extended opportunities to observe the elder's function whether in the community or in an institution. Families' observations also provide important data. Older people may be reluctant to share information about falls because of fear of losing independence so the gerontological nurse must use judgment and empathy in eliciting information about falls, assuring the person that there are many modifiable factors to increase safety and help maintain independence.

Assessment should include evaluation of fall risk, history of falls, evaluation of previous falls, and physical examination including evaluation of cognition, balance, gait, strength, chronic illnesses, mobility, nutrition, and medications (Perell et al, 2001). A history of falls is an important predictor of future falls, and fall histories should be taken at least once per year for all older adults over the age of 65. The Minimum Data Set (MDS) requires information about a history of falls and hip fractures in the last 180 days, and the fall resident assessment protocol (RAP) provides an excellent overview of fall risk and fall assessment. Box 22-4 presents fall RAP triggers identified on the MDS 2.0. See Chapter 14 for discussion of MDS. Assessment of home safety and environmental factors should also be included in a comprehensive fall assessment of community-dwelling elders. A comprehensive assessment of safety for homebound older adults was presented by Tanner (2003). The tool incorporates risk for falls, history of falls, and risk for injury, fire and disasters, and

Box 22-4	**Fall Resident Assessment Protocol Triggers Identified on the MDS 2.0**

Alzheimer's disease or other dementia
Arthritis
Cane, walker, crutch
Cardiac dysrhythmia
Cardiovascular, psychotropic, diuretic
    medications
Decline in cognition
Decline in functional status
Delirium
Device or restraint
Dizziness, vertigo, syncope
Fracture of hip, history of falls
Incontinence
Hemiplegia or hemiparesis

Hypotension
Impaired hearing or vision
Joint pain
Loss or arm or leg movement
Manic depression
Missing limb
Osteoporosis
Pacemaker
Parkinson's disease
Seizures
Unstable chronic or acute condition
Unsteady gait
Wandering

Adapted from Buckwalter K, Katz I, Martin H: Guide to the prevention and management of falls in the elderly, II, *CNS Long-Term Care* 3(2):31, Spring 2004.

crime. Table 22-2 presents a home safety assessment. Physical examination should include evaluation for acute illness such as infection, dehydration, and anemia; evaluation of hearing and visual acuity; and a complete assessment of the cardiovascular, musculoskeletal, and neurological systems. Key elements include assessment of heart rate and rhythm, blood pressure and pulse supine and standing, evaluation of lower extremity joint function, foot deformities, pain or limitations in range of motion, coordination, gait, balance, and mental status.

Use of quick, reliable, and valid fall risk assessment to identify older adults at high risk for falls is an essential part of assessment, particularly for community-dwelling older people. However, most physicians do not use any type of formal screening test (Rubinstein et al, 2003). A variety of risk assessment instruments are available. A nursing fall risk assessment that has been successfully used in both the acute care and the long-term care settings is the Morse et al (1989) Fall Scale (available at http://www.patientsafety.gov/FallPres/Morse.html). Risk factors in the Morse Scale include history of falls, secondary diagnosis, ambulatory aid, gait/transferring impairment, and mental status. Perrell et al (2001) suggest that in the nursing home setting where the majority of patients will score as high risk, implementation of an overall fall prevention program may be

more appropriate than relying on individual risk assessments. The presence of dementia contributes to fall risk and may call for specific risk assessment and fall prevention interventions. A dementia-specific fall risk assessment and fall safety program are available from http://www.geriatric-resources.com.

Balance and walking assessment also need to be included in assessment. The get-up-and-go test is a practical assessment tool for older adults and can be conducted in any setting (Mathias et al, 1986; Resnick et al, 2001). In this test, the older person is asked to rise from a straight-backed chair, stand briefly, walk forward about 10 feet, turn, walk back to the chair, turn around, and sit down. Performance is graded on a 5-point scale from 1 (normal) to 5 (severely abnormal). The quality of movement is assessed for impaired balance. A score of 3 or higher suggests a high risk for falling. A copy of the get-up-and-go test is available at http://www.americangeriatrics.org/education/falls.shtml. Gait speed and agility have been found to correlate well with functional level. A more quantitative version, the timed up-and-go test is also available (Podsiadlo, Richardson, 1991, Rubenstein, Trueblood, 2004). The Tinetti Performance-Oriented Mobility Assessment (POMA) scale is also widely used and is a good predictor of fall likelihood (Tinetti, 1986). Functional assessments of ADLs and instrumental activities of daily

Table 22-2   Assessment and Intervention of the Home Environment for Older Persons

Area or Activity	Problem	Intervention
BATHROOM	Getting on and off toilet	Raised seat; side bars; grab bars
	Getting in and out of tub	Bath bench; transfer bench; hand-held shower nozzle; rubber mat; hydraulic lift bath seat
	Slippery or wet floors	Nonskid rugs or mats
	Hot water burns	Check water temperature before bath; set hot water thermostat to 120° F or less
		Use bath thermometer
	Doorway too narrow	Remove door and use curtain; leave wheelchair at door and use walker
BEDROOM	Rolling beds	Remove wheels; block against wall
	Bed too low	Leg extensions; blocks; second mattress; adjustable-height hospital bed
	Lighting	Bedside light; night-light; flashlight attached to walker or cane
	Sliding rugs	Remove; tack down; rubber back; two-sided tape
	Slippery floor	Nonskid wax; no wax; rubber-sole footwear; indoor-outdoor carpet
	Thick rug edge/doorsill	Metal strip at edge; remove doorsill; tack tape down edge
	Nighttime calls	Bedside phone; cordless phone; intercom; buzzer; lifeline
KITCHEN	Open flames and burners	Substitute microwave; electrical toaster oven
	Access items	Place commonly used items in easy-to-reach areas; adjustable-height counters, cupboards, and drawers
	Hard-to-open refrigerator	Foot lever
	Difficulty seeing	Adequate lighting; utensils with brightly colored handles
LIVING ROOM	Soft, low chair	Board under cushion; pillow or folded blanket to raise seat; blocks or platform under legs; good armrests to push up on; back and seat cushions
	Swivel and rocking chairs	Block motion
	Obstructing furniture	Relocate or remove to clear paths
	Extension cords	Run along walls; eliminate unnecessary cords; place under sturdy furniture; use power strips with breakers
TELEPHONE	Difficult to reach	Cordless phone; inform friends to let phone ring 10 times; clear path; answering machine and call back
	Difficult to hear ring	Headset; speaker phone; adapted handles
	Difficult to dial numbers	Preset numbers; large button and numbers; voice-activated dialing
STEPS	Cannot handle	Stair glide; lift; elevator; ramp (permanent, portable, or removable)
	No handrails	Install at least on one side
	Loose rugs	Remove or nail down to wooden steps
	Difficult to see	Adequate lighting; mark edge of steps with bright-colored tape
	Unable to use walker on stairs	Keep second walker or wheelchair at top or bottom of stairs

Continued.

Table 22-2 Assessment and Intervention of the Home Environment for Older Persons—*cont'd*

Area or Activity	Problem	Intervention
HOME MANAGEMENT	Laundry	Easy to access; sit on stool to access clothes in dryer; good lighting; fold laundry sitting at table; carry laundry in bag on stairs; use cart; use laundry service
	Mail	Easy-to-access mailbox; mail basket on door
	Housekeeping	Assess safety and manageability; no-bend dust pan; lightweight all-surface sweeper; provide with resources for assistance if needed
	Controlling thermostat	Mount in accessible location; large-print numbers; remote-controlled thermostat
SAFETY	Difficulty locking doors	Remote-controlled door lock; door wedge; hook and chain locks
	Difficulty opening door and knowing who is there	Automatic door openers; level doorknob handles; intercom at door
	Opening and closing windows	Lever and crank handles
	Cannot hear alarms	Blinking lights; vibrating surfaces
	Lighting	Illumination 1-2 feet from object being viewed; change bulbs when dim; adequate lighting in stairways and hallways; night-lights
LEISURE	Cannot hear television	Personal listening device with amplifier; closed captioning
	Complicated remote	Simple remote with large buttons; universal remote control; voice control–activated remote control; clapper
	Cannot read small print	Magnifying glass; large-print books
	Book too heavy	Read at table; sit with book resting on lap pillow
	Glare when reading	Place light source to right or left; avoid glossy paper for reading material; black ink instead of blue ink or pencil
	Computers keys too small	Replace keyboard with one with larger keys

Modified from Rehabilitation Engineering Research Center on Aging (RERC-Aging), Center for Assistive Technology, University at Buffalo.

living (IADLs) should also be included in fall assessments. The MDS also includes a balance assessment and functional assessment for older adults residing in long-term care facilities.

Interventions and Prevention of Falls

Because of the multifactorial nature of falls, fall prevention interventions need to be multifactorial as well, combining medical, rehabilitative, and environmental strategies in an interdisciplinary approach. Components of a fall prevention program include gait training; exercise programs with balance training, appropriate use of assistive devices, medication reviews and modification of medication usage, particularly psychotropics, treatment of postural hypotension, and modification of environmental hazards (Rubinstein et al, 2003). Prevention programs are most effective when tailored to individual risk factors. Prevention of falls also requires education of the individual (and informal and formal caregivers) in all aspects of environmental hazards and the awareness that falling may be an indication of other

Box 22-5   Postfall Assessment

History
Obtain a description of the fall from the resident or witness
Obtain the resident's opinion of the cause of the fall
Circumstances of the fall (trip or slip)
Person's activity at the time of the fall
Presence of co-morbid conditions, such as a previous stroke, Parkinson's disease, osteoporosis, seizure disorder, sensory deficit, joint abnormalities, depression, cardiac disease
Medication review
Associated symptoms, such as chest pain, palpitations, light-headedness, vertigo, fainting, weakness, confusion, incontinence, or dyspnea
Time of day and location of the fall
Presence of acute illness

Physical Examination
Vital signs: postural blood pressure changes, fever, or hypothermia
Head and neck: visual impairment, hearing impairment, nystagmus, bruit
Heart: arrhythmia or valvular dysfunction
Neurological signs: altered mental status, focal deficits, peripheral neuropathy, muscle weakness, rigidity or tremor, impaired balance
Musculoskeletal signs: arthritic changes, range of motion (ROM), podiatric deformities or

problems, swelling, redness or bruises, abrasions, pain on movement, shortening and external rotation of lower extremities

Functional Assessment
Observe and inquire about the following:
  Functional gait and balance: observe resident rising from chair, walking, turning, and sitting down
  Balance test, mobility, use of assistive devices or personal assistance, extent of ambulation, restraint use, prosthetic equipment
  Activities of daily living: bathing, dressing, transferring, continence

Environmental Assessment
Staffing patterns, unsafe practice in transferring, delay in response to call light
Faulty equipment
Use of bed, chair alarm
Call light within reach
Wheelchair, bed locked
Adequate supervision
Clutter, walking paths not clear
Dim lighting
Glare
Uneven flooring
Wet, slippery floors
Poor-fitting seating devices
Inappropriate footwear
Inappropriate eye wear

---

underlying problems. Acute and long-term care facilities need a well-developed prevention protocol tailored to their patients, staff, and environment. The American Geriatrics Society provides excellent resources for professionals and patients on falls in older adults, including the *Guideline for the Prevention of Falls in Older Persons* and *A Patient's Guide to Preventing Falls* (http://www.americangeriatrics.org). The American Medical Directors Association also provides a practice guideline of falls and fall risk in long-term care (http://www.amda.com).

Postfall Assessment

When a fall occurs, immediate assessment involves identifying and treating any injury. A

comprehensive postfall assessment should also be conducted to identify the circumstances associated with the fall so that appropriate interventions and prevention plans can be instituted to prevent future falls. A fall history should also be conducted when an older person reports a past fall. Factors to be evaluated include when, where, and how the fall occurred (including associated movements or activities that may have contributed to the fall); environmental hazards involved; presence of associated symptoms (palpitations, dizziness) at the time of the fall; injuries that occurred; and whether the person was able to get up right away (Rubinstein et al, 2003). In the institutional setting, plans of care should be reevaluated and modified after a fall. Box 22-5 presents a postfall assessment.

MOBILITY AIDS

Assistive Devices

Assistive devices have been used throughout history to assist in mobility and often to indicate status or fashion trends. In ancient times the cane or staff was a symbol of authority, and in Victorian times, a walking stick was essential to a gentleman's attire. Even now, many older persons carry elaborate walking sticks even though canes and walkers are primarily designed to augment security and independence.

Arthritic hips and knees may cause considerable pain. To relieve the pressure, the use of a cane on the uninvolved side is helpful. When both sides are involved, a walker may relieve the pressure equilaterally. Many devices are available that are designed for very specific benefits. Proper evaluation of the type of assistive device, as well as training on its use, is important. Occupational and physical therapists can provide expert assistance in proper selection, fit, and use. An assistive device used improperly can be a risk factor for falls. Medicare may cover up to 80% of the cost of assistive devices with a written prescription. Assistive technologies are devices or services that enhance an individual's functional abilities. A wide range of assistive technologies are available for assistance with personal safety, mobility, and making the home safer and more comfortable. A comprehensive website can be found at http://www.nau.edu, and additional resources are listed at the end of the chapter. Many of these devices are inexpensive and easy to obtain, but many older people are unaware of them.

When the correct mobility device is obtained, the client will need assistance in learning to use it. This, again, should be taught by specialists in physical therapy. In general, the following principles should be observed:

- Move the assistive device first, then the weaker leg, and finally the stronger leg.
- Always wear low-heeled, nonskid shoes.
- When using a cane on stairs, step up with the stronger leg and down with the weaker leg. Use the cane as support when lifting the weaker leg. Bring the cane up to the step just reached before climbing another step. When descending, place the cane on the next step down and move the disabled leg down, followed by the good leg.
- When using a walker, stand upright and lift the walker with both hands.
- Place all of the walker's legs down at a comfortable distance. Step toward it with the weaker leg, and then bring the stronger leg forward. Do not climb stairs with a walker.
- Every assistive device must be adjusted to individual height; the top of the cane should align with the crease of the wrist.
- Choose a size and shape of cane handle that fits comfortably in the palm; like a tight shoe, it will be a constant irritant if it is not properly fitted.
- Cane tips are most secure when they are flat at the bottom and have a series of rings. Replace tips frequently, because a worn tip is not reliable.

Wheelchairs

Wheelchairs are a necessary adjunct at some level of immobility. Medicare coverage assists in the payment for these devices with a prescription. Ideally, a physical therapist or medical supply specialist will assist in the selection of a wheelchair that is appropriate to the size of the individual and is comfortable; proper fit of the wheelchair is important. There are various types of motorized chairs that can be handled with ease. These are more expensive than hand-propelled chairs but are sometimes available secondhand through advertisements, senior center bulletin boards, or congregate care settings. For those dependent on wheelchairs, wheelchair mobility can be taught. Often, physical and occupational therapists can assist in wheelchair mobility programs. At one Veterans Affairs Medical Center, the physical therapy department routinely offered driving and safety classes for wheelchair users. This is particularly important for motorized wheelchairs and scooters.

ENVIRONMENTAL SAFETY

A safe environment is one in which one is capable, with reasonable caution, of carrying out the ADLs and the IADLs, as well as the activities that enrich one's life, without fear of attack, accident, or imposed interference. It is the job of nurses and other health team members to ensure, to the greatest extent possible, a safe environment for individuals within their care in the institution or in the home.

Accidents and Injury

Older adults make up approximately 11% of the population, but they suffer 23% of all accidental deaths. When accidents happen to older adults, they are more likely to have a severe injury and tend to heal more slowly. Individuals over age 75 are particularly subject to falls and motor vehicle accidents. Falls create the most accidental fatalities, and the majority of these occur in the home. The second highest cause of accidental deaths of individuals over 80 years of age is motor vehicle accidents.

Environmental Hazards

Older adults are more susceptible than younger people to the impact of environmental variations, including pollutants, pesticides, impure water supplies, toxic substances, and climatic and altitudinal environmental extremes.

High Altitude

When elders briefly visit areas of high altitude, they may become hypotensive or develop cardiac symptoms. Older persons may experience dizziness, shortness of breath, and headache at high altitudes. They should be advised to rise to a standing position slowly and to reduce their activity level to a point of comfort. They may need additional rest periods. High altitudes and air travel may precipitate aural discomfort or disequilibrium as a result of changes in atmospheric pressure. It is helpful to let people know that any major environmental change is likely to be physically stressful, but specific discomforts should not be ignored. When an older person experiences a specific, intermittent uncomfortable reaction or one sustained over several hours, he or she should seek medical attention. Too often, a real problem is dismissed as just a symptom of old age.

Hyperthermia

When body temperature rises above normal ranges because of environmental or metabolic heat loads, a clinical condition called heat illness, or hyperthermia, occurs. Hyperthermia is a temperature-related illness and is classified as a medical emergency. There are numerous deaths among elders annually from temperature extremes, and these could be almost entirely prevented with education and caution. Although most of these problems occur in the home among individuals who do not have air conditioning or sufficient heat during temperature extremes, older adults with multiple physical problems residing in institutions may be especially vulnerable to temperature changes. Elders with cardiovascular disease, diabetes, or peripheral vascular disease and those taking certain medications (anticholinergics, antihistamines, diuretics, beta blockers, antidepressants, antiparkinsonian drugs) are at risk. Interventions to prevent hyperthermia when ambient temperature exceeds 90° F (32° C) include the following:

- Drink 2 to 3 L of cool fluid daily.
- Minimize exertion, especially during the heat of the day.
- Stay in air-conditioned places, or use fans when possible.
- Wear hats and loose clothing of natural fibers when outside; remove most clothing when indoors.
- Take tepid tub baths or showers.
- Apply cold wet towel compresses, or immerse the hands and feet in cool water.
- Avoid heavy, hot foods.
- Evaluate medications for risk of hyperthermia.
- Avoid alcohol.

Hypothermia

Hypothermia and the prevalence of deaths from exposure and cold have paralleled the increase in energy costs, indicating that many older persons may not be able to afford sufficient heat in their homes. Unfortunately, a dulling of awareness accompanies hypothermia, and persons experiencing it rarely recognize the problem or seek assistance. For the very old and frail, environmental temperatures below 65° F (18° C) may cause a serious drop in core body temperature to 95° F (35° C) or less. The median oral temperature of elderly persons is 96.8° F (36° C). Factors that increase the risk of hypothermia are numerous, as shown in Box 22-6.

Under normal temperature conditions, heat is produced in sufficient quantities by cellular metabolism of food, friction produced by contracting muscles, and the flow of blood. Paralyzed

Box 22-6   Factors That Increase the Risk of Hypothermia in the Elderly

Thermoregulatory Impairment
Failure to vasoconstrict promptly or strongly on
    exposure to cold
Failure to sense cold
Failure to respond behaviorally to protect oneself
    against cold
Diminished or absent shivering to generate heat
Failure of metabolic rate to rise in response to
    cold

Conditions That Decrease Heat Production
Hypothyroidism, hypopituitarism, hypoglycemia,
    anemia, malnutrition, starvation
Immobility or decreased activity (e.g., stroke,
    paralysis, parkinsonism, dementia, arthritis,
    fractured hip, coma)
Diabetic ketoacidosis

Conditions That Increase Heat Loss
Open wounds, generalized inflammatory skin
    conditions, burns

**Conditions That Impair Central or Peripheral
Control of Thermoregulation**
Stroke, brain tumor, Wernicke's encephalopathy,
    subarachnoid hemorrhage
Uremia, neuropathy (e.g., diabetes, alcoholism)
Acute illnesses (e.g., pneumonia, sepsis,
    myocardial infarction, congestive heart failure,
    pulmonary embolism, pancreatitis)

Drugs That Interfere with Thermoregulation
Tranquilizers (e.g., phenothiazines)
Sedative-hypnotics (e.g., barbiturates,
    benzodiazepines)
Antidepressants (e.g., tricyclics)
Vasoactive drugs (e.g., vasodilators)
Alcohol (causes superficial vasodilation; may
    interfere with carbohydrate metabolism and
    judgment)
Others: methyldopa, lithium, morphine

From Worfolk JB: Keep frail elders warm! *Geriatr Nurs* 18(1):7-11, 1997.

or immobile persons lack the ability to generate significant muscle heat by muscle activity and become cold even in normal room temperatures. It is important to closely monitor body temperature in older people and pay particular attention to lower than normal readings. Older people with some degree of thermoregulatory impairment, when exposed to cold temperatures, are at high risk for hypothermia if they undergo surgery, are injured in a fall or accident, or are lost or left unattended in a cool place. Persons who are emaciated and with poor nutrition lack insulation, as well as fuel for metabolic heat-generating processes, so they may be chronically mildly hypothermic. Box 22-7 lists factors that may induce low basal body temperature in elders.

Recognition of clinical signs and severity of hypothermia is an important nursing responsibility. Confusion and disorientation may be the first overt sign. Nurses are responsible for keeping frail elders warm for comfort and prevention of problems. For older people living at home, frequent contact during cold weather is crucial. Assessment of the available warmth in the environment,

teaching related to preventing heat loss, and providing information about energy assistance available in most communities for those on limited incomes are important. Specific interventions to prevent hypothermic reactions are shown in Box 22-8.

Transportation

Even though one is physically able to move about, there may be many hindrances to full use of public space. Available transportation is a critical link in the ability of the elderly to remain independent and functional. The lack of accessible transportation may contribute to other problems, such as social withdrawal, poor nutrition, or neglect of health care. Even when a municipal transportation service is available, elders may not use it. Urban buses and subways not only are physically hazardous, but also are often dangerous. A "crisis in mobility" exists for many older people because of the lack of an automobile, an inability to drive, limited access to public transportation, health factors, geographical location, or economic considerations.

Box 22-7   Factors Associated with Low Body Temperature in the Elderly

Aging
Increases risk of thermoregulatory dysfunction
Increases risk of acute and chronic conditions
  that predispose to hypothermia

Low Environmental Temperature
Risk of hypothermia increased below 65° F

Thinness and Malnutrition
Very thin people have less thermal insulation,
  higher surface area/volume ratios
Prolonged malnutrition can decrease the
  metabolic rate by 20% to 30%

Poverty
Increases risk of thinness and malnutrition,
  inadequate clothing, low environmental

temperature secondary to poor housing
  conditions and inadequate heat

Living Alone
Associated with poverty, delayed detection of
  hypothermia, delayed rescue if person falls

Nocturia/Night Rising
Associated with falls; if rescue delayed and person
  lies immobilized for a long time, hypothermia
  may develop as heat is conducted away from
  the body to the cold floor.

Orthostatic Hypotension
An indicator of autonomic nervous system
  impairment; dizziness and postural instability
  are associated with falls

From Worfolk JB: Keep frail elders warm! *Geriatr Nurs* 18(1):7-11, 1997.

Box 22-8   Nursing Interventions to Prevent Cold Discomfort and the Development of Accidental Hypothermia in Frail Elders

Desired outcomes: hands and limbs warm; body
  relaxed, not curled; body temperature >97° F;
  no shivering; no complaints of cold.

Interventions
Maintain a comfortably warm ambient temperature
  no lower than 65° F. Many frail elders will
  require much higher temperatures.
Provide generous quantities of clothing and
  bedcovers. Layer clothing and bedcovers for best
  insulation. Be careful *not* to judge your
  patient's needs by how *you* feel working in a
  warm environment.
Limit time patients sit by cold windows to short
  periods in which they are warmly dressed.
Provide a head covering whenever possible—in bed,
  out of bed, and particularly out-of-doors.
Cover patients well during bathing. The standard—a
  light bath blanket over a naked body—is not
  enough protection for frail elders.

Cover naked patients with heavy blankets for
  transfer to and from showers; dry quickly
  and thoroughly before leaving shower room;
  cover head with a dry towel or hood while
  wet.
Dry wet hair quickly with warm air from an
  electric dryer. *Never* allow the hair of frail elders
  to air dry.
Use absorbent pads for incontinent patients
  rather than allow urine to wet large areas of
  clothing, sheets, and bedcovers. Avoid skin
  problems by changing pads frequently,
  washing the skin well, and applying a
  protective cream.
Provide as much exercise as possible to generate
  heat from muscle activity.
Provide hot, high-protein meals and bedtime snacks
  to add heat and sustain heat production
  throughout the day and as far into the night as
  possible.

From Worfolk JB: Keep frail elders warm! *Geriatr Nurs* 18(1):7-11, 1997.

Older persons may desire increased contact with friends and relatives; however, even more crucial is the need to reach medical services, shopping areas, and service agencies. The emphasis on a "barrier-free" (structurally revised) transportation system and reduced fares has been helpful to many older people, but some cannot avail themselves of public transportation because of physical disability or residence in a high-crime area. County, state, or federally subsidized transportation is being provided in certain areas to assist older people in reaching social services, nutrition sites, health services, emergency care, medical care, recreational centers, mental health services, day care programs, physical and vocational rehabilitation, continuing education, and library services.

Some effective local transportation programs include the following services:
- Reduced fares
- Informal, volunteer drivers
- Demand-response transit vehicles
- Specially constructed vehicles for the handicapped
- Door-to-door minibuses requiring advance reservations
- Use of subsidized taxicab services
- Radio-equipped response vehicles
- Dial-a-ride
- Charter bus trips to special events

The greatest problems in transportation exist among the rural aged, who may be unable to drive and have limited, if any, public transportation.

Driving

As a group, older drivers are some of the United States' safest drivers. Older drivers drive fewer overall miles than younger drivers and tend to drive less at night, during adverse weather conditions, or in congested areas. Fewer speed or drive after drinking alcohol than drivers of other ages. However, compared with younger age groups, people over the age of 70 are more likely to be involved in a crash and more likely to die in that crash (accessed 8/15/04 from http://www.niapublications.org/engagepages/drivers.asp). Older adults are also more likely to be involved in accidents involving multiple vehicles (McGregor, 2002). The increased crash rate has been attributed to age-related changes in driving skills in addition

to various medical illnesses and functional impairments.

Many older people depend on driving in order to maintain their basic needs, and the inability to drive can cause depression and isolation. For many, alternate transportation is not readily available, and consequently, they may continue driving beyond the time when it is safe. The issues of driving in the older adult population are the subject of a great deal of public discussion. Many older drivers and their families struggle with issues related to continued safety in driving and when and how to tell older people they are no longer safe to drive. It is the responsibility of health care providers, including gerontological nurses, to identify impairments that affect safe driving, correct them when possible, and offer alternatives for transportation. Vehicle adaptations, sensory aids, elder driver training, and driving assessment programs are helpful in promoting safe driving. A mnemonic, SAFE DRIVE, addresses key components to screen for in older drivers. The components include the following: *s*afety record, *a*ttention skills, *f*amily report, *e*thanol (alcohol), *d*rugs, *r*eaction time, *i*ntellectual impairment, *v*ision or visuospatial function, and *e*xecutive functions (McGregor, 2002). The American Medical Association in partnership with the National Highway Traffic Safety Administration provides the *Physician's Guide to Assessing and Counseling Older Drivers* with step-by-step plans for assessing older driver safety (www.amaassn.org/ama/pub/category/8925.html). Other resources are listed at the end of the chapter.

IMPLICATIONS FOR GERONTOLOGICAL NURSING AND HEALTHY AGING

The capacity to move about on two legs, horses, and wheeled vehicles has been portrayed from the earliest recorded time. The gerontological nurse can be significant in facilitating this most fundamental human need and can assist older people in moving as far as their reach extends and as far as our imagination will allow. Gerontological nurses play an important role in the maintenance of mobility and safety for older adults. Health promotion interventions to maintain fitness and mobility, as well as teaching older adults, their caregivers, and staff about fall risk factors, fall prevention interventions, and restraint-appropriate care, are important in all settings. For older adults with mobility limitations, nurses need to be knowledgeable about assistive devices and technology, environmental modifications, and resources to aid in maintaining independence and functional abilities. Gerontological nurses often work as members of interdisciplinary rehabilitation teams and bring expert knowledge of patient activities, abilities, and needs from a 24 hr/day, 7 days/wk perspective to help the team implement the most appropriate interventions. For community-dwelling older adults, nurses need to have knowledge of home, community, and environmental safety factors and modifications to ensure safety and comfort. Maintenance of mobility and safety for older adults is one of the most important components of gerontological nursing, and all nurses working with older adults need to be competent in these areas. Accidents and injuries among older adults in all settings are significant in terms of morbidity and mortality. Utilizing evidence-based practice can ensure improvement of many modifiable and preventable injuries as well as mobility limitations and functional decline.

APPLICATION OF MASLOW'S HIERARCHY

Movement is integral to the attainment of all levels of need as conceived by Maslow. Needs met by maintaining mobility include basic biological function, activity, security, social contacts, pride, and dignity. Thus maintaining mobility is an exceedingly important issue. Restrictions of mobility affect older people's ability to meet basic needs, their independence, and their ability to enjoy a sense of belonging and maintain desired activities.

▶ KEY CONCEPTS

- Mobility provides opportunities for exercise, exploration, and pleasure and is the crux of maintaining independence.

- Ease of mobility is thought to be the most visible measure of one's overall health and survival capacity.
- Changes in bones, muscles, and ligaments with aging affect one's balance and gait and increase instability.
- Gait disorders are often an obvious index of systemic problems and should be investigated thoroughly.
- A thorough nursing assessment must include assessment of fall risk, balance, and gait assessment, as well as intrinsic, extrinsic, and iatrogenic factors.
- Prevention of falls is one of the most important proactive considerations to preserve health and function for the elderly.
- Fear of falling (fallophobia) and extreme caution actually increase falling propensity in the elderly. A history of falls is the most significant factor in prediction of future falls.
- Physical restraints are not appropriate for "safety" and, in fact, increase injuries related to falls. Restraint-appropriate care, fall prevention interventions, and a safe environment are essential to best practice care for elders.
- Transportation for the elderly is critical to their physical, psychological, and social health.

▶ Activities and Discussion Questions

1. Put your shoes on the wrong feet, and then ask another student to analyze your gait.
2. Borrow a pair of bifocals from someone, and then attempt to go up and down stairs.
3. Evaluate the safety of your living quarters using Box 22-3 as a guide.
4. Discuss your activities that increase your fall vulnerability.
5. Discuss falls you have had and their consequences. Consider how it might have been different if you were 75 years old.
6. Obtain a wheelchair, and sit in it for 20 minutes with a restraining belt around your waist. Discuss your feelings with a partner. Reverse the process with your partner.
7. Discuss the various reasons why you might need to ensure safety for a hospitalized elder, and identify several alternatives that might be appropriate.

NANDA and Wellness Diagnoses

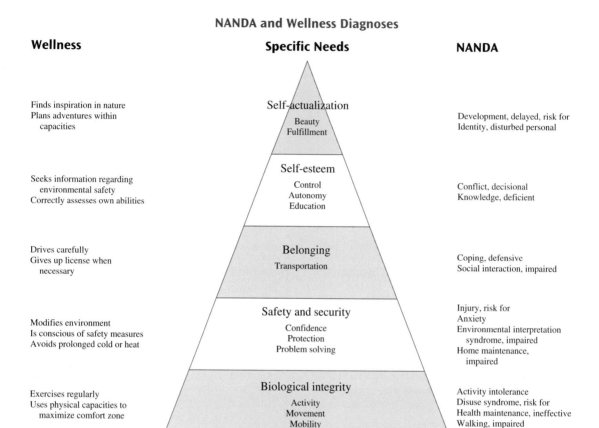

Wellness

Finds inspiration in nature
Plans adventures within
    capacities

Seeks information regarding
    environmental safety
Correctly assesses own abilities

Drives carefully
Gives up license when
    necessary

Modifies environment
Is conscious of safety measures
Avoids prolonged cold or heat

Exercises regularly
Uses physical capacities to
    maximize comfort zone

Specific Needs

Self-actualization
Beauty
Fulfillment

Self-esteem
Control
Autonomy
Education

Belonging
Transportation

Safety and security
Confidence
Protection
Problem solving

Biological integrity
Activity
Movement
Mobility

NANDA

Development, delayed, risk for
Identity, disturbed personal

Conflict, decisional
Knowledge, deficient

Coping, defensive
Social interaction, impaired

Injury, risk for
Anxiety
Environmental interpretation
    syndrome, impaired
Home maintenance,
    impaired

Activity intolerance
Disuse syndrome, risk for
Health maintenance, ineffective
Walking, impaired

These are not all of the possible wellness or NANDA diagnoses that may be identified. The above are frequent examples of nursing diagnoses that should be considered when planning care for the older adult in whatever setting.

RESOURCES

Organizations

American Geriatrics Society (tool kit on falls and
    practice guidelines for prevention of falls in older
    persons)
The Empire State Building
350 Fifth Avenue, Suite 801
New York, NY 10118
(212) 308-1414
website: http://www.americangeriatrics.org/
    education/falls.shtml

Arizona Technology Access Program (comprehensive
    list of resources for older adults with disabilities)
Jill Sherman, Project Director, AzTAP
Institute for Human Development
Northern Arizona University

4105 N. 20th Street, Suite 260
Phoenix, AZ 85016
(800) 477-9921
website: http://www.nau.edu/ihd/aztap

National Center for Patient Safety
Department of Veterans Affairs
PO Box 486
Ann Arbor, MI 48106-0486
(734) 930-5890
website: http://www.patientsafety.gov

The National Resource Center on Supportive
    Housing and Home Modification
USC Andrus Gerontology Center
3715 McClintock Avenue
Los Angeles, CA 90089
(213) 740-1364
website: http://www.usc.edu/dept/gero/nrcshhm

Untie the Elderly (educational and training program for providers of long-term care on the use of physical and chemical restraints in nursing facilities)
The Kendal Corporation
PO Box 100
Kennett Square, PA 19348-0100
(610) 388-5580
website:http://www.kendal.org

Websites

American Academy of Family Physicians
Decision-making tool kit for older drivers and their families
(800) 944-0000 or on-line at http://www.aafp.org

Dependable Acceptable Technology Solutions
Information on adaptive environments, assistive technology, home modification, safety and risk assessments
website: http://www.gdewsbury.ukideas.com

The National Institute on Aging
Age Page Health Information: Preventing Falls and Fractures, Crime and Older People, Hyperthermia, Hypothermia, Older Drivers
website: http://www.niapublications.org

"The Fire Risk Series: Fire Risks for Older Adults"
Available from http://www.cornellaging.com/gem/injury_fire_risk.html

"Home Safety Checklist"
Available from http://www.cornellaging.org/gem/injury_falls_checklist.html

RN+ Safe-T-Net (newsletter: patient safety, restraint alternatives, article reviews on safety by Dr. Rein Tideiksaar)
Website: http://rnplus.com

"Side Rail Decision Making Guide"
Available at http://www.ec-online.net/Knowledge/Articles/siderails.html

REFERENCES

American Geriatrics Society, British Geriatrics Society, and American Academy of Orthopaedic Surgeons Panel on Falls Prevention: Guideline for the prevention of falls in older persons, *J Am Geriatr Soc* 49(5):664-672, 2001.

Capezuti E et al: Individualized assessment and intervention in bilateral siderail use, *Geriatr Nurs* 19(6):322-330, 1998.

Capezuti E et al: Side rail use and bed-related fall outcomes among nursing home residents, *J Am Geriatr Soc* 50(1):90-96, 2002.

Cesari M et al: Prevalence and risk factors for falls in an older community-dwelling population, *J Gerontol A Biol Sci Med Sci* 57(11):M722-M726, 2002.

Evans LK, Strumpf NE: Tying down the elderly: a review of the literature on physical restraint, *J Am Geriatr Soc* 37(1):65-74, 1989.

Federal Register (VG6187), p 48825, Sept. 26, 1991.

Mathias S, Nayak US, Isaacs B: Balance in elderly patients: the "get up and go" test, *Arch Phys Med Rehabil* 67(6):387-389, 1986.

McGregor D: Driving over 65: proceed with caution, *J Gerontol Nurs* 28(8):22-26, 2002.

Morley J: A fall is a major event in the life of an older person, *J Gerontol A Biol Sci Med Sci* 57(8):M492-M495, 2002.

Morley JE, Flaherty JH, Thomas DR: Geriatricians, continuous quality improvement, and improved care for older persons, *J Gerontol A Biol Sci Med Sci* 58(9):M809-M812, 2003.

Morse J, Morse R, Tylko S: Development of a scale to identify the fall-prone patient, *Can J Aging* 8:366-377, 1989.

Perell KL et al: Fall risk assessment measures: an analytic review, *J Gerontol A Biol Sci Med Sci* 56(12):M761-M766, 2001.

Podsiadlo D, Richardson S: The timed "Up & Go": a test of basic functional mobility for frail elderly persons, *J Am Geriatr Soc* 39(2):142-128, 1991.

Resnick B: In Henkel G: Beyond the MDS: team approach to falls assessment, prevention and management, *Caring for the Ages* 3(4):15-20, 2002.

Resnick B, Corcoran M, Spellbring A: Gait and balance disorders. In Adelman AM, Daly MP, editors: *Twenty common problems in geriatrics*, New York, 2001, McGraw-Hill.

Rubenstein L, Trueblood P: Gait and balance assessment in older person, *Ann Long-Term Care* 12(2):39-46, 2004.

Rubinstein T, Alexander N, Hausdoff J: Evaluating fall risk in older adults: steps and missteps, *Clin Geriatr* 11(1):52-61, 2003. Available at www.mmhc.com.

Stilwell EM: Use of physical restraint on older adults, *J Gerontol Nurs* 14(6):42-43, 1988.

Strumpf N et al: *Reducing restraints: individualized approaches to behavior*, Huntington Valley, Pa, 1992, The Whitman Group.

Tanner EK: Assessing home safety in homebound older adults, *Geriatr Nurs* 24(4):250-256, 2003.

Tinetti ME: Performance oriented assessment of mobility problems in elderly patients, *J Am Geriatr Soc* 34(2):119-126, 1986.

Tinetti ME, Richman D, Powell L: Falls efficacy as a measure of fear of falling, *J Gerontol* 45(6):P239-P243, 1990.

Tinetti ME et al: Fear of falling and fall-related efficacy in relationship to functioning among community-living elders, *J Gerontol* 49(3):M140-M147, 1994.

Older Adults and Their Families

Upon completion of this chapter, the reader will be able to:

- Identify the variations of relationships that people identify as "family."
- Relate several functions of grandparenting and the contributions elders make to family life.
- Identify the range of caregiving situations and the potential challenges and opportunities of each.
- Describe the nursing role in supportive networks serving elders.
- Identify ways in which the nurse can support the family in its caregiving role.
- Identify the elder at risk for abuse.
- Identify the signs and symptoms of potential abuse.
- Discuss the nurse's responsibility in regard to assessing, intervening, and reporting in cases of suspected elder abuse.

▼ GLOSSARY

Caregiving The act of providing assistance to those who are unable to care entirely for themselves. Caregivers may be informal (family, friends and others who volunteer this service) or formal (those persons hired to provide the care).

Competent The status that one is able to make some decisions alone. There is a wide range of levels of competence from minimal to complex.

Ombudsman An advocate.

Respite A relief in caregiving, providing benefit to both the caregiver and the care recipient.

Surrogate kin Those persons with bonds of affection toward one another who function as family members but are not related by blood or marriage.

Undue influence When a person uses his or her power over another person in a negative way.

▼ THE LIVED EXPERIENCE

It is so irritating when Madge tries to help me do things. After all, I have lived 85 years and have done very well. I think she wants to put me away somewhere. I wish she would just leave me alone. I'm sure I could manage if she just wouldn't interfere.

John, the father

I just can't stand watching as my father becomes weaker and is unable to do the things he always did so naturally and well. Yesterday he got lost on his way to the market. He was always my guide and protector. I knew I could count on him no matter what. It makes me feel sort of alone in the world.

Madge, the daughter

FAMILIES

The idea of family evokes strong impressions of whatever an individual believes the typical family should be. Because everyone comes from a family, these impressions have powerful symbolic meaning. However, in today's world, the definition of a family is in a state of flux. As recently as 100 or so years ago the norm was the extended family made up of parents, their grown children, and the children's children, often living together and sharing resources, strengths, and challenges. As cities grew and adult children moved to them in pursuit of work, parents did not always come along, and the nuclear family evolved. The norm in the United States became two parents and their two children, or at least this was the norm in what has been considered mainstream America. This pattern was not as common, nor is it yet, in many families of color, especially living in what are called "ethnic neighborhoods," where the extended family is still the norm.

Other variations on the idea of family have developed. Approximately 42% of today's families are married couples without children. The high divorce and remarriage rate results in households of blended families of children from previous marriages and the new marriage. Single-parent families, blended families, childless families, and fewer families altogether are common. Four- and five-generation families are also becoming common (Kutza, 2001).

Still other families are composed of same-gender couples, which may or may not include children. Others without biological families either by choice or circumstance have created their own "families" through communal living with siblings, friends, or others. Indeed, it is not unusual for childless persons residing in long-term care facilities to refer to the staff as their new "family."

Family members, however they are defined, form the nucleus of relationships for the majority of the older adults and the support system if they become dependent. Most older adults possess a large intergenerational web of significant people, including sons, daughters, stepchildren, in-laws, ex-in-laws, nieces, nephews, grandchildren, and great-grandchildren, as well as partners and former partners of their offspring. All these people may play an important part in maintaining satisfaction in later life.

In coming to know the older adult, the gerontological nurse comes to know the family as well, learning of their special gifts and their life challenges. The nurse works with the elder within the unique culture of his or her family of origin, present family, and support networks, including friends.

This chapter deals with the nature of family and relationships, the range of caregiving, the mistreatment of frail elders, and legal issues particularly relevant for older adults.

Roles and Relationships

As families change, the roles of the members or expectations of one another may change as well. Grandparents may assume parental roles for their grandchildren if their children are unable to care for them; or grandparents and older aunts and uncles may assume temporary caregiving roles while the children, nieces, and nephews work. Adult children of any age may provide limited or extensive caregiving to their own parents or aging relatives who become ill or impaired. A spouse or sometimes a sibling may become a caregiver as well when needed. This caregiving may be temporary or long term.

Close-knit families are more aware of the needs of their members and work to resolve problems and find ways to meet the needs of members, even if they are not always successful. Emotionally distant families are less available in times of need and have greater potential for conflict. If the family has never been close and supportive, it will not magically become so when members have unmet needs. Resentments long buried may crop up and produce friction or psychological pain. Long-submerged conflicts and feelings may return if the needs of any one family member exceed those of the others.

Traditional Couples

The traditional couple in the United States is husband and wife or, for the purposes of discussion, the long-standing unmarried heterosexual couple (formerly called "common-law"). Although this relationship is often the most binding if it extends into late life, the chance of a couple going through old age together is exceedingly slim. Approximately 40% of men and 80% of women over age 75 have no spouse (U.S. Administration on Aging, 2000). Men who survive their spouse into old age ordinarily have multiple opportunities to remarry if they wish. A woman is less likely to have an opportunity for remarriage in late life.

Couple relationships are becoming more diverse, involving varying degrees of habit, culture, intimacy, shared backgrounds, and instrumental and emotional support. In late marriages or remarriage, developing an intimate, sharing relationship between individuals who have had 75 or 80 years of separate experiences and who often bring conflicting ideologies into the new relationship is an enormous challenge.

Couples in late life have needs, tasks, and expectations that differ from those in their earlier years. Some couples have been married more than 60 or 70 years. These years together may have been filled with love and companionship, or abuse and resentment or anything in between. For all couples, the normal physical and sociological circumstances in late life present challenges. Some of the issues that strain many of these relationships include: (1) the deteriorating health of one or both partners, (2) limitations in income, (3) conflicts with children or other relatives, (4) incompatible sexual needs, and (5) mismatched needs for activity and social activities.

Elders and their Adult Children

By and large elders and their children have relationships that are reciprocal in nature. These relationships are both the most important and potentially the most conflicted. Family resources are shared from birth and usually in some way until and after death. These resources may be tangible, such as money, belongings, and housing. Intangible resources may include advice, support, guidance, and day-to-day assistance with life. Elders provide a family history perspective, models for growing old, assistance with grandchildren, a sense of continuity, and a philosophy of aging. The older family members often serve as kin-keepers. *Kin-keeper* is a term used to denote a family member who arranges get-togethers, develops the family history and rituals, and in other ways promotes solidarity and unity among the kin (Rosenthal, 1985).

Consider the example of Grandma Daisy, who always merited a special visit from any of the kin in her vast northwestern network. A pioneer settler in her small community, she knew the names, ages, and whereabouts of the children and spouses and the grandchildren and spouses of all of her eight children. They seldom saw one another but always felt a connecting link through Grandma Daisy. When she died at age 94, a great portion of the family history and sense of solidarity died with her. She was a true kin-keeper.

There are no accurate estimates of the value of family exchanges. It is not known how much tangible support flows from the older generation to the younger ones, but a considerable amount is given to educate and launch the younger generations. In many situations there are additional transfers at the time of death of the elder when goods, assets, and properties are bequeathed. The younger generation may provide a sense of meaning and purpose to the elders. If either the child or the parent is functionally or physically impaired, personal assistance may be exchanged as well. Children provide the majority of the assistance required when an elder is unable to meet his or her own needs.

Siblings

Late-life sibling relationships are poorly understood and have been neglected by researchers. There are many possible sibling relationships in old age: intimate, congenial, loyal, apathetic, distant, friendly, hostile, advisory, competitive, and envious. For some elders, the significance of siblings grows with age. Siblings share a unique history—a similar biological and cultural heritage—albeit with numerous variable personal interpretations. These relationships may become increasingly important because they have a long history of memories and are of the same generation, similar backgrounds, and often ambivalent early relationships (Bedford, Avioli, 2001). They become particularly important when they are part of the support system, especially among single or widowed elders living alone. The strongest of sibling bonds is thought to be the relationship between sisters. When blessed with survival, these relationships remain important into late old age (Scott, 1996). Freedman (1996) found that having even one sibling significantly reduced the likelihood of institutionalization. Widowed, divorced, and never-married siblings may share a home and travel together.

The loss of siblings has a profound effect in terms of awareness of one's own mortality, particularly when those of the same gender die. When an elder reaches the age of the sibling who died, the reaction can be quite disruptive. Not only is grieving activated, but rehearsal for one's own death may occur. In cases where an elder sibling survives younger ones, there may be not only a deep grief but also some pangs of guilt: "Why them and not me?"

Other Relatives
The family with older members often includes collateral kin (cousins, aunts, uncles, nieces, nephews). The quality of the relationships varies but is still a potential source of joy, support, assistance, or conflict. Maternal kin (related through female bloodlines) may be emotionally closer than those in one's paternal line (related through male bloodlines) (Jett, 2002). These relatives may provide a reservoir of kin from which to find replacements for missing or lost intimate relationships for persons who are childless or estranged from their own offspring. Attachments with other relatives may be strong both ways and should be respected as such.

Friends
Friends are often a significant source of support in late life. Lifelong friendships are often sustaining in the face of overwhelming circumstances. They provide the critical elements of satisfactory living that family may not, providing commitment and affection without judgment. Personality characteristics between friends are compatible because the relationships are chosen and caring is shared without obligation. Friends may share a lifelong perspective or may bring a totally new intergenerational viewpoint into one's life. Late-life friendships often develop out of changing situations, such as shared tenancies, widowhood, moves, and involvements in volunteer pursuits (O'Connor, 1993). As desires and pursuits change, some friendships evolve that the persons never would have considered in their youth.

Friends function in many ways: (1) act as surrogate kin, (2) to ease the loneliness of widowhood or widowerhood, and (3) to validate one's generational viewpoint. Considering the obvious importance of friendship, it seems to be a neglected area of exploration and a seldom-considered resource by professionals assisting the aged.

Nontraditional Couples
As the variation in families grows, so do the types of coupled relationships. Among the types of couples we see today are same-gender couples. Although these couples are less often seen in the older population, they are still there but may not be obvious because of long-standing discrimination and fear. As society becomes more willing to accept persons in these relationships, they may be more willing to share with us who they are.

Although the issue of same-gender couples marrying is before the courts, it is still not legal in all states. In some cases the couples enter into marriage-type commitments and, where possible, legally register as "domestic partners." Lesbian women and gay men in long-term committed relationships often share homes, resources, and professional interests. Their families may include children (biological and adoptive), parents, siblings, and friends. However, in many cases the couples are estranged from families of origin and come to late life with a network of close friends who make up their "family." These nonrelatives become surrogate family and take on the instrumental and affection attributes of family. Because these family members are not relatives in the traditional sense they may not be recognized by the health care system, leading to considerable added stress to all involved. When the relationship was unknown to the public, the grief surrounding the loss of the partner becomes difficult because the loss may be unrecognized by others and may pass without ritual or social sanctions. This type of grief has been defined as "disenfranchised grief," which can be particularly difficult to resolve (Doka, 2002).

CAREGIVING
Gerontological nurses are most likely to encounter elders with their family and friends in situations relating to caregiving of some kind. The face of informal caregiving has changed and may include family, friends, and paid and unpaid workers, as well as volunteers in the home. Some middle-aged adults may also be involved in caring for the elderly parents of previous mates. Even though generally considered a women's issue, in more and more cases, male caregivers, including those other than spouses (e.g., brothers, nephews, sons), are

assuming the full range of caregiving roles (Houde, 2001).

While caregiving is a means to "give back" to a loved one and can be a source of joy in the giving, it is also stressful and can be physically and emotionally demanding. Caregivers are considered to be "the hidden patient" in that their own needs are set aside to meet the needs of the care recipient (Schulz, Beach, 1999, p 2216). Caregivers frequently experience depression and physical and emotional exhaustion (Yates et al, 1999). Whereas not all caregivers experience consequential stress, the circumstances that are more likely to cause problems with caregiving include competing role responsibilities (e.g., work and home), advanced age of the caregiver, high-intensity caregiving needs, insufficient resources, dementia of the care recipient, and prior relational conflicts between the caregiver and care recipient (Whitlack, Noelker, 1996; Zarit, Zarit, 1998; Navaie-Waliser et al, 2002).

The majority of this caregiving takes place at home. In 2004 a study by the National Alliance for Caregiving estimated that there were 44.4 million caregivers in 22.9 million homes. Caregiving may take place in the elder's home or that of the caregiver. At any one time only 4.5% of the nation's elders over 65 reside in nursing homes. However, the number of elders in nursing homes varies with age, from only 1.1% of those 65 to 74, to 18.2% of those over 85 (AOA, 2002). If the person in need of care moves from home to a long-term care facility, the informal caregiver (e.g., spouse) then often works alongside the formal caregiver, such as the nurse and aide.

As the population shifts toward increasing numbers of frail elders with multiple problems, the number in need of care will increase markedly. The nurse is a key person in both assessing the needs of elders and their families and working with them in finding ways to meet these needs.

Variations in Caregiving

Caregiving situations range from grandparents caring for grandchildren or other minor relatives to elders caring for their spouses or even their own, more elderly, parents. However, we know the most about caregiving from a parent–adult child perspective.

Caring for Parents

Adult children are sometimes said to reverse roles with parents when the parents become old and dependent. This scenario has a demeaning connotation, as if the elder becomes a child again. Regardless of the state of illness or disability of the parent, he or she is still the parent, and the child would like the parent to remain in this role if it were possible. These dynamics often make the child as caregiver role very complex and potentially difficult.

Filial obligation is associated with a sense of duty toward one's parents that is inherent in the relationship. In some cultures and in many ethnic groups this sense of duty is strong (Sokolovsky, 1997). As result, it is expected that children will set aside their own needs in order to meet those of the parent. Should the children have active lives and demanding careers or face multiple needs of their own children, conflicts with the needs of the parents are fairly certain. Many children find ways to overcome the conflicts and provide a substantial amount of elder care as noted above. The major concerns arise when the child caregiver is not available or willing to assume these responsibilities if he or she is needed.

Caring for Persons with Dementia

Each year more and more people are diagnosed with Alzheimer's or other dementing disorders. These disorders leave the person with progressively deteriorating cognitive function. Because of the progressive nature of these diseases, all persons with dementia will eventually need caregiving and the needs of the person will increase over time until at some point assistance is required 24 hours per day, usually provided by a spouse. In addition to the intensity of needs, the personality changes and impairments in communication make caregiving in this situation a special challenge. Spousal caregivers express a significant sadness in the loss of the companionship in the relationship, and child caregivers mourn the loss of the parent well before the physical death of the person with dementia.

One man said, "Caring for my wife is difficult now because she no longer recognizes me as her husband. I have become a stranger to her and she treats me as such. Because I am no longer viewed as her husband, she will not let me touch her or share the same bed. And, I have been told more than once to 'get out of the house because it's not your home'" (American Society on Aging, 2002, p 6).

Caregivers, be they spouses, family members, or professionals, need to learn new skills and to be given a significant amount of support. A daughter caring for her elderly mother with Alzheimer's disease said she had previously thought it was important to focus on reality. On one occasion, after trying unsuccessfully to convince her mother that the month was May and not April, she went to get a calendar to show her. By the time she returned, her mother had forgotten all about it. "It was then I realized that reality doesn't matter. That was the biggest breakthrough. If she thought it was April, what did it matter? I found that when I stopped correcting her and went along with her, it saved us both a lot of heartache. The content of the conversation did not matter as much as the feeling" (Hoffman, 1996).

Caring for Disabled Adults
Although we tend to think of caregivers as middle-age adults caring for elders, an unknown number of elders are caring for their middle-age children who are physically and mentally disabled. Earlier in the last century these developmentally disabled children usually died before reaching adulthood; now, with improved care they are surviving. Often this has been a burden carried by parents for their entire adult life and will end only with the death of the parent or the adult child. In a study of 115 older mothers (ages 58 to 96 years) caring for mentally retarded offspring, religion and prayer emerged as critical aspects of their coping, although they often questioned why God was letting them suffer so (Tobin et al, 1994). At present, little is being done about this situation, but the Society of Friends is giving serious attention to it as an issue of aging that has been neglected (Schwartz, Kelly, 1996).

A well elder can also become physically disabled at any time especially because of cerebral vascular accidents (strokes). Elderly spouses caring for disabled partners have special needs. The spouse may have significant health problems that are neglected in deference to the greater needs of the incapacitated partner. The disabled partner may need physical care that is beyond the capabilities of the spouse/caregiver, such as in small women caring for large men. It is most difficult when the partner is aphasic or incontinent. Availability of children, relatives, and friends is significant in easing the load and increasing the satisfaction of caregiving.

Long-Distance Caregiving
Because of the increasing mobility of today's society there are more and more situations in which children move away from home for education or employment and do not return home. When the parent needs help it must be provided "long distance." In 2004 the national Alliance for Caregivers estimated that more than 7 million caregivers lived more than 1 hour away from the care recipient. Seventy percent of these caregivers were employed full time, and most lost work hours regularly because of their added responsibilities (NCOA, 2004). This is perhaps one of the most difficult situations and presents unique challenges. The usual impulse is to move the elder to an accessible location for the family, but this may not be best for an elder who has lived a long time in one community and has many supports there. Plans and alternatives should be discussed before emergency events and may prevent the need for hasty decisions. Conferring with a case manager in advance of any evidence of problems may forestall the need to move the parent into the adult child's home. Issues that need to be considered include identifying a local person who will be available quickly in emergency situations; identifying reliable individuals or services that will provide daily monitoring if necessary; identifying acceptable facilities for assisted living if that becomes necessary; determining which family member is most likely to be free to travel to the elder if needed; and being sure that legalities regarding advance directives, a will, and powers of attorney (for health care and financial) have been established (Box 23-1).

A profession and industry have emerged to assist the geographically distant family member to ensure that an elderly relative will be taken care of; this profession is made up of geriatric care managers, only some of whom are nurses or social workers. A care manager can be hired to do everything a family member would do if able to do so, from being available in an emergency to helping with estate planning to making arrangements for the move to a nursing home. Often care managers know of resources that can allow the elder to

---

| Box 23-1 | Planning to Add an Aged Member to the Household |

Questions You Need to Ask
- What are the needs of the new member and of the family?
- Where will space be allotted for the new member?
- How will this new member be included in existing family patterns?
- How will responsibilities be shared?
- What resources in the community will assist in the adjustment phase?
- Is the environment safe for this new member?
- How will family life change with the added member, and how does the family feel about it?
- What are the differences in socialization and sleeping patterns?
- What are the aged person's strong needs and expectations?
- What are the aged person's skills and talents?

Modifications You Need to Make
- Arrange semiprivate living quarters if possible.
- Regularly schedule visits to other relatives to give each family times of respite and privacy.
- Arrange day care and senior activities for the older person to help keep contact with members of his or her own generation.

Discuss Potential Areas of Conflict
- *Space:* especially if someone has given up his or her space to the aged relative.
- *Possessions:* old person may want to move possessions into house; others may not find them attractive or may insist on replacing them with new things.

- *Entertaining:* times when old and young feel the need or desire to exclude the other from social events.
- *Responsibilities and chores:* old may feel useless if he or she does nothing and in the way if he or she does something; young may feel that his or her position is usurped or may be angry if he or she must wait on parent.
- *Expenses:* increased cost of home maintenance, food, clothing, and recreation may not be shared appropriately.
- *Vacations:* whether to go together or alone; the young may feel uneasy not taking older person but resentful if they must.
- *Child rearing:* disagreement over child-rearing policies.
- *Child care:* grandparental babysitting may be welcomed by family and resented by older person, or if not allowed, older person may feel lack of trust in capability.

Decrease Areas of Conflict
- Respect privacy.
- Discuss space allocations.
- Discuss elderly person's furnishings before move.
- Make it clear ahead of time when social events include everyone or exclude someone.
- Clear decisions about household tasks—all should have responsibility geared to ability.
- Pay a share of expenses and maintain a separate phone to reduce strain and increase feelings of independence.

---

remain independent and yet assure the family that safety and other needs are being met. Case management services can be particularly useful to families who are geographically remote. At present these services are primarily available to those who are able to pay for them since they are not covered by private insurance or public agencies of any kind. Although these services are expensive, they are far less expensive than alternative living arrangements or institutional placement.

Similar but simpler services may be available for persons with very low incomes by contacting the local Area Agency on Aging and asking about the local "Community Care for the Elderly" programs. In some states there are also programs called nursing home diversions to provide home support to those who would otherwise qualify for Medicaid coverage for a nursing home stay. For persons with incomes too high to qualify for Medicaid and too low to pay for private care managers, they and their families have no other options than doing the best they can. Long-distance care then depends on the goodness of neighbors, local friends, and apartment managers and frequent trips by the long-distance caregiver to the elder.

Formal (Nonfamily) Caregivers

Close relationships often develop between older adults and their formal, nonfamily caregivers. More than 50% of family caregivers use nurses, homemakers, and other personal care providers to assist in the care of their elder dependents (Piercy, 2001). These providers may include friends and hired or volunteer caregivers from a church or agency. Piercy found that only 40% of the care recipients using formal caregivers actually had living relatives. The caregivers not only provide substantial physical care, but also are often involved with the elder, when possible, in social activities such as dining, concerts, and church events. Conditions that foster closeness include continuity of caregiver, social isolation of the elder, homogeneity of the client and caregiver, and the caregiver performing extra tasks and small personal attentions. The client will sometimes describe a paid caregiver as "my family."

Grandparenting

About 72% of elders over age 65 have three or more grandchildren. Only about 13% of adults over age 65 have no grandchildren (NCOA, 2002). Somewhere between 400,000 and 600,000 of these grandparents have assumed parental roles for their grandchildren (NAC, 2004).

Traditionally grandparents provide gifts, money, and other forms of intermittent support to younger family members when possible. They also provide a sense of continuity, knowledge of family heritage, rituals, news, and folklore. Grandparents often provide respite for parents by temporarily watching the minor children.

In recent years more grandparents have become, by default, the primary caregivers of grandchildren because the parents are incapable of providing the care needed as a result of child abuse, imprisonment, joblessness, drug and alcohol addictions, illness, and social problems of the children's parents (Kelly, 1993). Estimates suggest that grandparents or other relatives are raising more than 2 million children with no parents present. This number has increased by more than 50% since 1990 and continues to grow. Approximately one third of these children are within the formal foster care system. Another 2.5 million children are living with grandparents or other relatives, but one or both parents reside with them. Twenty percent of these grandparents were over 65 years of age, and 50% of the children were under 6 years of age (Troope, 2000).

Too often both the children and their grandparent are in need of help. As expected many of these children are deeply disturbed, have multiple loss and grief issues, and need mental health services (Brown-Standridge, Floyd, 2000). Ghuman and colleagues (1999) found that 51 youths among a group of 233 youths being treated at a community mental health center were living with grandparents. Grandparents frequently experience problems with legal issues, housing, and the educational system. They also report financial and health problems related to the additional burden of caring for grandchildren. In spite of all that, grandmothers tend to report that the grandchildren provide purpose that keeps them going, and in some cases children raised solely by grandparents fare better than those in single-parent families (Roe, Minkler, 1998-1999).

The U.S. government has recognized that increasing number of older adults are raising grandchildren, great-grandchildren, and other younger relatives. Some of the funds distributed to each state through the Older Americans Act have been earmarked to find ways to reach out and support this needy group. Nurses can refer the grandparents to their local Area Agency on Aging to see what might be available to them.

Implications for Gerontological Nursing and Healthy Aging

Nurses are often the primary care providers and case managers for elders and their families both in the home and the institutional setting. The nurse monitors progress and manages chronic disorders of the elder within the context of the family.

Assessment

A comprehensive assessment of the elder includes assessment of the family: who are the members, what are their usual roles and their strengths, contributions, and deterrents to the function of the family unit. Assessing the family's needs, strengths, and stresses, as well as its sources of stress, particular methods of coping, meaning of caregiving, support system, and family dynamics, will assist the nurse in gaining a holistic picture of

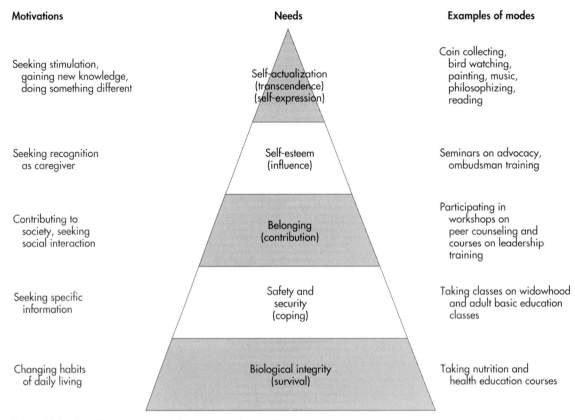

Figure 23-1   Family support problems and interventions.

the interventions that may strengthen the family unit. Maslow's Hierarchy of Needs provides a useful framework for both the assessment of the family and interventions (Figure 23-1). Ideally the assessment is conducted by a team of professionals, including the nurse, social worker, mental health counselor, and occupational therapist. In the skilled nursing facility, the MDS (Minimum Data Set) (see Chapter 4) is such a comprehensive assessment. If the assessment includes an informal caregiver, the Caregiver Strain Index developed by Robinson (1983) is recommended. This source is available through the John A. Hartford Foundation Institute for Geriatric Nursing, which has blanket permission to use it professionally (Sullivan, 2002).

A mutually constructed, written assessment of a family's needs and coping capacities can be both comprehensive and specific and becomes a docu-

ment of the family's strengths in times of stress. Including the family in the discussion of the outcome of the assessment is recommended for all settings, especially long-term care facilities.

Interventions

As the needs of the care recipient increase, so often do the number of informal and formal services. Coordinating the services, continuing to assess needs, and providing for the health needs of the family unit are important activities of the registered nurses and advanced-practice nurses working with caregivers. A major expectation of nurses is that they will teach, demonstrate, and evaluate the ability of caregivers to provide necessary interventions with elders in their care. The nurse also works to maintain health and wellness of the entire family structure. The New York University Spouse Caregiver Intervention Study

Table 23-1 Positive Outcomes Reported by Clients and Caregivers as a Result of Counseling and Support

Outcomes	Caregivers' Comments	Clients' Comments
Social enjoyment	—	It was an outing. An excuse to go out and talk to people!
Increased knowledge	I am more aware now. I know what things to look for.	I enjoyed the assessment. I learned from it.
Reduced stress	The support was very good. There was a tremendous amount of guilt going on. . . . Assessment helped us to deal with these things.	I was reassured that this was part of an illness. I had an explanation why this was happening.
Enhanced skills and feelings of competence	It proved very useful for our learning process in terms of her management (referring to client) and my own coping.	I learned how to cope better with my disability. I'm more positive as a result of it.
Better family communication and collaboration	They helped with communication with family. Our children now better understand how to support me.	—
Improved decision making	I don't know what we would have done without the geriatric services . . . It helped us to make decisions.	—
Greater access to services	Everything came out of that assessment: the diagnosis, home services, day program.	—
Positive health outcomes	If it wasn't for the assessment she wouldn't be here today. She may have died in her apartment.	—

From Aminzadeh F et al: Comprehensive geriatric assessment: exploring clients' and caregivers' perceptions of the assessment process and outcomes, *J Gerontol Nurs* 28(6):6-13, 2002.

reported by Mittleman (2002) found the most useful of the interventions studied included a few sessions of counseling to the caregiver and other involved family members and a support group for primary caregivers, as well as ongoing telephone support. These interventions, when available, can potentially alleviate much of the stress of caregiving. Some of the positive outcomes for families that can result from nursing assessment and intervention are listed in Table 23-1.

Interventions with caregivers must always take into account the great variability in family structures, resources, traditions, and history. The range of adaptations is enormous, and the goal is always to restore the balance of the system to the great-est extent possible and support caregivers in their caring. The family can be visualized as a mobile with many parts, and when one is touched, each part shifts to regain the balance. The intrusion of professionals into a family system will temporarily unbalance the system and may provide an opportunity to restore the balance in a healthier manner, sometimes by adding an element or increasing the weight of one or decreasing the weight of another. When working with a family who is from a different culture and who may have rituals and routines unfamiliar to the nurse, he or she needs to be particularly careful to respect these differences. The nurse can work with the family to make the best use of their strengths, whatever they may be. Each family member can be valued for what he or she brings to the situation.

If an elder is beginning to need help, the following suggestions to family members may be useful:

1. Involve the parent in all decisions that affect care.
2. Assist the elderly parent in remaining as independent as possible, and provide assistance only for those things that are needed.
3. Seek resources that provide options between independent living and a nursing home.

Respite.   Respite is the provision of temporary relief to the caregiver and is perhaps the most significant intervention with families. Respite may be in many forms, including the temporary stay of the elder in a care facility, a few hours' visit to a day care setting, or in-home relief by a relief informal or formal caregiver. Stephens (1996) found that day care respite can be effective for some caregivers if it allows sufficient relief, creates no additional stress, is at least partially subsidized, and provides information about other resources that may be helpful. Transportation of the elder is frequently a problem, since programs do not necessarily fit their hours to a working family's needs.

There are also audiotapes and videotapes that have been designed to provide mild stimulation or entertainment for elders with limited cognitive abilities. These show promise of effectively providing temporary distraction and, in doing so, providing respite for caregivers of persons with high levels of need (Camberg et al, 1996).

Institutionalization.   When the care needs exceed those available in the community, care within an institutional setting may be the solution. Institutional care takes place in group homes, assisted living facilities, nursing homes, and skilled nursing facilities. This is considered formal care, where care is exchanged for a fee. The fee is most often paid by the individual or family. When the elder has a low income and limited assets the fee may be paid through state funds, such as Medicaid. It is important to note that care of the person's personal needs is never covered by Medicare. Persons who do not qualify for state assistance programs but cannot afford the private charges are left in a precarious position of which we know very little.

Some families are either not willing or not able to provide care to their needy members. Family

relations that have never been warm or supportive will likely be less so with the dependencies of aging. There are also some elders who do not wish to be cared for by family. The elder may be fiercely independent and fear becoming what he or she considers a burden. It is the nurse's responsibility to accept and support the decisions of elders and their family members in this regard and to work with all in promoting as healthy and satisfying a solution as possible.

When a move to an institutional setting is necessary, family caregivers may feel defeated or guilty. The efforts they have expended are rewarded with decline. It is imperative that nurses reinforce the family's adequacy and importance to the older member. Family support groups may be helpful in dealing with the ambivalence and distress of institutionalizing an elder. Goals of these groups can be seen in Box 23-2.

Caregiving issues are likely to remain in the forefront of discussions of public policy and concerns about family life. There is a continuing need for investigations that identify potentially modifiable features of caregivers' situations and that contribute to the development and evaluation of interventions to assist families (Zarit, 1991).

Box 23-2   Goals of Family Support Groups

Learn to accept the elder as he or she is now; let go of the past.
Learn the balance between protectiveness and smothering.
Recognize one's own needs as fundamental to caring for others.
Learn to share and cope with disappointment.
Discuss resurgence of feelings of loss during holidays and anniversaries.
Share knowledge of how to deal with family and community.
Develop a caring and sharing network within the group.
Deal with feelings of guilt, helplessness, and hopelessness.
Identify realistic ways to assist in the care of the elder.

Modified from Richards M: Family support groups, *Generations* 10(4):68, 1986.

ELDER ABUSE AND NEGLECT

Unfortunately, a person in need of the assistance of others is at risk for harm and injury at the hands of a frustrated, angry, fraudulent, careless, or disturbed caregiver. Mistreatment of older frail and vulnerable adults is found in all socioeconomic, racial, and ethnic groups in the United States. It can be seen in any configuration of family and in every setting. Mistreatment includes several types of abuse and neglect; however, the definitions of exactly what constitutes any of these vary somewhat by state. The most common types of abuse are physical, psychological, sexual, and financial (see Appendix 23-A). Medical abuse is also seen, wherein the person is subjected to unwanted treatments or procedures, or medical neglect is seen when desired treatment is withheld. Neglect implies that the caregiver has not met his or her obligation. Self-neglect is recognized when a person is not caring for herself or himself in the manner in which most peers would do so. In all cases the vulnerable person is harmed.

There are undoubtedly numerous cultural differences in the identification and definition of abuse. Given our diverse society, this must be taken into consideration. Moon and Williams (1993) obtained responses from African American, Caucasian, and Korean-American elderly women regarding their perceptions of abusive situations. The Korean-Americans were much less likely than the others to perceive a given situation as abusive.

Although up to 2 million cases of abuse are thought to occur each year, it is believed that only one in five cases is recognized (Harrell et al, 2002). The majority of abuse occurs in the home setting, where the majority of caregiving occurs. The incidence of elder abuse is expected to increase with the increase of numbers of persons in need of care, the increased conflicting demands on the caregiver's time, and the increased pressure to report suspicions of abuse.

Elder abuse requires an abuser, an elder, and the context of caregiving (Burke, Laramie, 2004). The abuse tends to be episodic and recurrent rather than isolated. There are multiple risk factors for one to be or become an abuser or abused (Box 23-3). Persons who are abusing alcohol or other substances, have emotional or mental illnesses, or have a history of abusing or being abused are more likely to be abusers, as are caregivers who are

---

Box 23-3	Profiles of Abused and Abusers

Abused Elders
Woman age 80 or older
Lives alone or with abuser
Mental or physical disability
Dependency on abuser

Abusers
Middle-age male sibling or offspring
Mental health and substance abuse problems
Financially dependent on abused
History of abuse and being abused

Adapted from Utley R: Screening and intervention in elder abuse, *Home Care Provid* 4(5):198, 1999.

---

exhausted and frustrated. The abuser is usually the caregiver but may also be the care recipient. Caregivers, be they informal (e.g., spouses) or formal (e.g., nursing assistants), may be subjected to verbal and physical abuse by the person they are caring for. This may be a lifelong pattern that intensifies in the current situation.

Whereas any older person who is impaired and therefore vulnerable can be abused, women are at particular risk. This risk is intensified if they have been abused in the past or if their behavior is aggressive, combative, or provocative; that is, they are viewed as overly demanding or unappreciative (Harrell et al, 2002). The level of dependency is also a factor; the more dependent the elder, the more vulnerable he or she is to being abused. Men or women who had abused the caregiver earlier in life may be at risk for retaliation.

Since both the majority of caregiving and the majority of abuse occur within the family, this is the context. Caregiver/care recipient relationships that were conflicted earlier in life will continue to be so. Abuse and exploitation can also occur in the situation of a hired caregiver. When there are a number of providers, monitoring becomes especially difficult. Situations of potential formal caregiver abuse include those in which there is inadequate supervision of patient care, poor coordination of services, inadequate staff training, theft and fraud, drug and alcohol abuse by staff, tardiness and absenteeism, unprofessional and criminal conduct, and inadequate record keeping.

More frequently than we know, undue influence is exerted on the elder, and a companion or home care provider will manage to convince the elder to transfer assets and even the deed to the home. These situations are being examined more carefully in the courts, and some states are activating legal protections against undue influence (Quinn, 1999; Quinn, Tomita, 1997). The nurse should pay particular attention to the caregiver who is alone, with no support from others and no opportunities for respite.

Most often victims are unwilling or afraid to report the problem because of shame, embarrassment, intimidation, or fear of retaliation. The abuser may be the only caregiver available to the elder, and reporting or complaining could leave him or her without care at all. The abuse may be a lifelong pattern in which the victim has always felt somewhat at fault and will remain in the situation.

IMPLICATIONS FOR GERONTOLOGICAL NURSING AND HEALTHY AGING

Nurses must be vigilant in their sensitivity to the potential for abuse, observing for signs and symptoms in all their interactions with vulnerable elders. In addition to the physical signs (see Appendix 23-A), the nurse looks for more subtle signals. Is there an unusual delay between the beginning of a health problem and when help is sought? Are appointments often missed without reasonable explanations? Are there inconsistencies between the history given by the elder and that of the caregiver?

There also may be behavioral indications suggestive of an abusive situation. Does the caregiver do all of the talking in a situation, even though the elder is capable? Does the caregiver appear angry, frustrated, or indifferent while the elder appears hesitant or frightened? Is the caregiver or the care recipient aggressive toward one another or the nurse?

If abuse is suspected, a full assessment should be done, including a determination of the safety of the victim and the desires of the victim if competent. Assessment of mistreatment involves several components. Terry Fulmer at the Hartford Foundation presents a detailed assessment that is considered one of the best practice protocols. Her tool can be found in Appendix 23-B.

Intervention

The goals of intervention are to stop exploitation of elders, protect the victim and society from inappropriate and illegal acts, hold perpetrators of mistreatment accountable, rehabilitate the offender, and order restitution of property and payment for expenses incurred as a result of the perpetrator's conduct. However, most of these are beyond the nurse's usual scope of practice. The most important information for nurses to know are the requirements for mandatory reporting in their states and to participate in prevention in the promotion of healthy aging.

Mandatory Reporting

In most states and U.S. jurisdictions licensed nurses are required to report suspicions of abuse to the state, usually to a group called adult protective services. Most often these reports are anonymous. Allegations of abuse should not be made on casual suspicions but on solid evidence. If the nurse believes the elder to be in immediate danger, the police should be notified. How the nurse accomplishes this varies with the work setting. In hospitals and nursing homes this is often reported first internally to the facility social worker. In the home care setting, the report is made to the nursing supervisor. It would be very unusual for the nurse not to go through his or her employer. However, the nurse who is a neighbor, friend, or privately paid caregiver may be under obligation to make the report. In the nursing home or licensed assisted living facility the nurse has the additional resource of calling the state long-term care ombudsman for help. In each state, ombudsmen are either volunteers or paid staff members who are responsible for acting as advocates for vulnerable elders in institutions. All reports, either to the state ombudsman or to adult protective services, will be investigated. A unique aspect of elder abuse compared with child abuse is that the physically frail but mentally competent adult can refuse assessment and intervention and often does. Abused but competent elders cannot be removed from harmful situations without their permission, much to the frustration of the nurse and other health care providers.

Prevention of Abuse

In the ideal situation, gerontological nurses are alert to potential mistreatment of vulnerable elders and take steps to prevent the occurrence of abuse or neglect. In some situations the abuse may be preventable, and in others, it is less likely to be preventable. If the abuse is the result of psychopathological conditions, especially if the situation is long-standing, the nurse is unlikely to be able to prevent the abuse. However, nurses can make sure that the potential victims know how to get help if it is needed and the resources that are available to them, and nurses can provide support and encouragement that it is possible to leave the situation. The nurse can also work with the elder, caregiver, and community supports to increase the exposure of the elders to others.

If the abusive behavior is learned or a response to stress, the situation may be subject to change. Learned abuse, theoretically, can be unlearned and may respond to a close working relationship with a mentoring professional who can demonstrate positive problem solving and new ways of managing difficult situations.

If the abuse is based in the stress of the caregiving situation, nurses can be very proactive and help all involved do things to lessen the stress. This may include finding respite services, changing the situation entirely (giving permission to the caregiver to give up the role), referring to support groups for ventilation of frustrations and peer support, teaching people how to use crisis hotlines, professional consultation, victim support groups, victim volunteer companions, and, above all, thoughtful and compassionate care for the victim and the perpetrator (Wolf, Pillemer, 1994; Reis, Nahmiash, 1995; Quinn, Tomita, 1997).

Patwell (1988) provides a nice summary of community actions that may either prevent abuse or lead to quick intervention. These actions include the following:
- Make professionals aware of potentially abusive situations.
- Educate the public about normal aging processes.
- Help families develop and nurture informal support systems.
- Link families with support groups.
- Teach families stress management techniques.
- Arrange comprehensive care resources.
- Provide counseling for troubled families.
- Encourage the use of respite care and day care.
- Obtain necessary home health care services.
- Inform families of resources for meals and transportation.

- Encourage caregivers to pursue their individual interests.

Finally, for elders who become mentally incompetent, legal protection may be necessary. Gerontological nurses can become familiar with the laws that specifically affect older adults in their state. This can be done by speaking with an attorney or selecting continuing education programs to update knowledge in the field of client legal protections. Once informed of the laws affecting frail elders, nurses are in a position to assist elders and family members in seeking legal representation when necessary and in selecting the approach that will solve the problems in the least restrictive manner possible. Whereas initiating these interventions is usually the responsibility of the social worker and enacted by lawyers and judges, the nurse should understand the basic concepts and the types of legal protection for elders and other incapacitated persons.

Legal Protection

Situations occur in the care of older adults when the elder is either not strong enough or competent enough to exert measures to protect his or her own interests. When this occurs there are several means that can be used to protect the person. These include conservatorship, guardianship, and powers of attorney.

Conservatorships

A conservatorship (also called guardianship) is a legally restrictive process in which the court appoints a person to make decisions for someone who can no longer make or can no longer communicate safe or sound decisions for himself or herself; for someone who is unable to properly provide for his or her personal needs for physical health, food, clothing, or shelter; or for someone who appears to be highly susceptible to fraud or undue influence. A court hearing is held, and someone demonstrates the incapacity of the elder. Often the elder is not present. If the courts agree, then a conservator is appointed. The conservator may be responsible for the person's finances, his or her person (meaning what happens to his or her body), or both. The elder is then considered a ward, and all decision-making rights are lost. All decision making is the legal right and responsibility of the conservator or guardian.

In some states limits are set according to the degree of protection needed. *Total dependency* means the person cannot meet basic needs for survival and is unable to manage the environment in any self-sustaining way. *Some dependency* means the person may be able to manage certain challenges of life; health or judgment may interfere with management of other needs.

Whereas a conservator is the person appointed to control the finances of the ward, the person appointed to be responsible for the person is usually called the guardian. The conservator or guardian continues in that role until the court rescinds the order and in no other way. Each state is slightly different in how this is handled. In many, the ward, as a person without any legal standing, is unable to petition the courts to have his or her rights restored.

There are considerable pros and cons in the use of conservatorships and guardianships, including high risk for exploitation by the conservator. These should only be considered in extreme cases. Nurses working with older adults and their families can encourage the use of advanced planning, including the appointments of health care surrogates and powers of attorney as alternatives that are less restrictive, noting that the definitions and rules vary from state to state.

Power of Attorney

A power of attorney is a legal device in which a person designates another person to act on his or her behalf. The person appointed in a power of attorney becomes known as the attorney-in-fact. The person who is acting on behalf of another based on a standard durable power of attorney usually has the right to make financial decisions, pay bills, and so forth.

If decisions are related to health care, the power of attorney must so designate and is usually called a durable power of attorney for health care. The appointed person is also known as the health care surrogate. A health care surrogate is expected to use "substituted judgment" in making decisions; that is, the decision is expected to be that which the person would have made for herself or himself if able to do so and not what the surrogate would make for herself or himself in the same situation. Whether or not the health care surrogate is able to make end-of-life decisions is determined by state statutes.

Powers of attorney are only in effect at the specific request of the elder or in the event that he or she is unable to act on his or her own behalf. As soon as the person regains abilities, the power of attorney is no longer in force. The elder retains all of the rights and responsibilities afforded by usual law. An important aspect of the power of attorney is that persons who are given decision-making rights are those who are have been chosen by the elder rather than a court.

Advocacy

Because so many older frail people cannot speak for themselves, nurses often find themselves in the position of having to do the "talking"—being an advocate. An advocate is one who maintains or promotes a cause; defends, pleads, or acts on behalf of a cause for another; fights for someone who cannot fight; and often gets involved in getting someone to do something he or she would not otherwise do.

Topics for advocacy can include protection of specific rights, such as promoting the least restrictive alternative for a client, finding the best nursing home, or telling court personnel one's opinion of a proposed conservator. Other areas include the rights of medical patients, the right to have in-home supportive services, and maintenance of government benefits, such as veterans' benefits, Medicare, social security (SS) and supplemental security income (SSI), and food stamps.

Advocates function in various arenas: with their own and other disciplines within their own agencies, with other agencies, with physicians, with families, with neighbors and community representatives, with legislators, and with courts.

Strengthening Families

In this era of diverse lifestyles and family patterns, it is becoming increasingly important to preserve the integrity of the primary support systems. There is a prevalent feeling in the United States that too little is being done to help families care for their elders. Most older adults, or indeed anyone, when in need of assistance, must rely on the good will and intentions of those closest to them, whether nuclear or extended family, alternative family systems, friends, or neighbors. Support networks, families, and others are made up of ordinary people with needs, frailties, and frustrations. Each participant sometimes functions

NANDA and Wellness Diagnoses

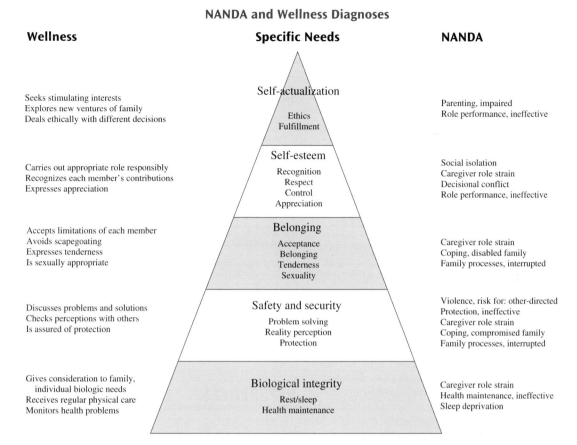

Wellness	Specific Needs	NANDA

Wellness (left side):

Seeks stimulating interests
Explores new ventures of family
Deals ethically with different decisions

Carries out appropriate role responsibly
Recognizes each member's contributions
Expresses appreciation

Accepts limitations of each member
Avoids scapegoating
Expresses tenderness
Is sexually appropriate

Discusses problems and solutions
Checks perceptions with others
Is assured of protection

Gives consideration to family,
   individual biologic needs
Receives regular physical care
Monitors health problems

Specific Needs (pyramid):

Self-actualization
Ethics
Fulfillment

Self-esteem
Recognition
Respect
Control
Appreciation

Belonging
Acceptance
Belonging
Tenderness
Sexuality

Safety and security
Problem solving
Reality perception
Protection

Biological integrity
Rest/sleep
Health maintenance

NANDA (right side):

Parenting, impaired
Role performance, ineffective

Social isolation
Caregiver role strain
Decisional conflict
Role performance, ineffective

Caregiver role strain
Coping, disabled family
Family processes, interrupted

Violence, risk for: other-directed
Protection, ineffective
Caregiver role strain
Coping, compromised family
Family processes, interrupted

Caregiver role strain
Health maintenance, ineffective
Sleep deprivation

These are not all of the possible wellness or NANDA diagnoses that may be identified. The above are frequent examples of nursing diagnoses that should be considered when planning care for the older adult in whatever setting.

---

well and sometimes barely. At times it becomes necessary to bring legal action into situations that have become destructive or dysfunctional. Considerable effort is needed to preserve the integrity of elders and their families. Making resources available that decrease stress and increase effectiveness may restore the balance of the family. A particularly important nursing function is to make individuals fully aware of the bonds that connect them and the special qualities each person appreciates of the other.

▶ **KEY CONCEPTS**

- Elders and their family members carry a long history. Current family dynamics must be understood within the context of family history.
- Sibling relationships may increase in importance during old age as individuals cope with various losses.
- Grandparenting is a significant role among elders. Grandparents are the primary provider for young children and function as parents in an increasing number of families.
- Caregiving of impaired elders is one of the major social issues of our times. Most spouses will spend some time caring for one another, and most adult children will spend some time caring for aged parents. Many of the children travel long distances to provide care.
- Frail elders are generally considered to be those who are in tenuous physiological, mental, or

emotional balance and who maintain their integrity within a small margin.

- Vulnerable elders may be placed under the legal protections of another who may or may not advocate or make decisions to their best advantage.
- Vulnerable elders are also those who live in situations that are potentially neglectful or outright abusive.
- Abuse may be financial, physical, sexual, financial, psychological, or extreme neglect, and either committed intentionally or unintentionally.
- Adult Protective Services is the usual state agency whose responsibility it is to respond to concerns of elder abuse and neglect.
- Nursing responsibilities are to be alert to signs of abuse and neglect of an elder and to report known cases to the appropriate state agency, as required by law.
- Abusive situations can emerge from overburdened caregivers who have little assistance, great frustration, and little respite.
- Elders rarely report family members who abuse them because they are uncertain whether an alternative situation would be an improvement.
- Nursing responsibilities include assisting caregivers in finding resources to alleviate or partially relieve a stressful situation.

▶ ### Activities and Discussion Questions

1. Discuss your position in the family and how that has affected your relationship with siblings and parents.
2. What do you suppose your role will be when your parent or parents need help?
3. Write a brief essay discussing the ways in which your grandparents have affected your life.
4. What would you find most difficult in regard to assisting your aged parent?
5. In what ways are nurses involved in protection of the rights of elders?
6. Discuss with a group the situations you have encountered in which you felt an elder was vulnerable or had been mistreated. What were the factors that influenced your feelings about this situation?

RESOURCES

Organizations

AARP Grandparent Information Center
American Association of Retired Persons
601 E Street NW
Washington, DC 20049
www.aarp.org

National Alliance for Caregiving
4720 Montgomery Lane, Suite 642
Bethesda, MD 20814
(301) 718-8444; (301) 652-7711 (fax)
www.caregiving.org

Websites

National Association of Professional Care Managers
www.caremanager.org

National Council on Aging
www.ncoa.org

National Family Caregivers Foundation
www.caregivingfoundation.org

National Guardianship Association
www.guardianship.org

REFERENCES

Administration on Aging (AOA): *A profile of older Americans 2003*, Washington, DC, 2003, U.S. Government Printing Office. Available at www.aoa.gov.

American Society on Aging: *CARE Pro-Module 3*, June 2002. Available at www.asaging.org.

Bedford VH, Avioli PS: Variations on sibling intimacy in old age, *Generations* 25(2):34, 2001.

Brown-Standridge MD, Floyd CW: Healing bittersweet legacies: revisiting contextual family therapy for grandparents raising grandchildren in crisis, *J Marital Fam Ther* 26(2):185-197, 2000.

Burke MM, Laramie JA: *Primary care of the older adult: a multidisciplinary approach*, ed 2, St Louis, 2004, Mosby.

Camberg L et al: Methods to evaluate an audiotape intervention for Alzheimer's patients. Paper presented at the meeting of the Gerontological Society of America, Washington, DC, Nov 19, 1996.

Doka KJ: Disenfranchised grief: lessons for those serving older clients, *Aging Today* 23(4):13, 2002.

Freedman VA: Family structure and the risk of nursing home admission, *J Gerontol B Psychol Soc Sci Soc* 51(2):S61-S69, 1996.

Fulmer T: Our elderly—harmed, exploited, abandoned. In *Reflections*, third quarter, Indianapolis, 1999, Sigma Theta Tau.

Fulmer T: Elder abuse and neglect assessment. Try this: best practices in nursing care to older adults, *Hartford Institute for Geriatric Nursing,* no. 15, May 2002.

Ghuman HS, Weist MD, Shafer ME: Demographic and clinical characteristics of emotionally disturbed children being raised by grandparents, *Psychiatr Serv* 50(11):1496-1498, 1999.

Harrell R et al: How geriatricians identify elder abuse and neglect, *Am J Med Sci* 323(1) 34, 2002.

Hoffman D: Complaints of a dutiful daughter, *Alzheimer's Caregiver* 9(1):1, 1996.

Houde SC: Men providing care to older adults in the home, *J Gerontol Nurs* 27(8):13-19, 2001.

Jett KF: Making the connection: seeking and receiving help by elderly African-Americans, *J Qualitative Health Res* 12(3):373-387, 2002.

Kelly SJ: Caregiver stress in grandparents raising grandchildren, *Image J Nurs Sch* 25(4):331-337, 1993.

Kutza EA: Living longer, living better: policy presumptions and new family structures, *Pub Pol Aging Rep* 11(3):12, 2001.

Mittleman MS: Family caregiving for people with Alzheimer's disease: results of the NYU spouse caregiver intervention study, *Generations* 26(1):104, 2002.

Moon A, Williams O: Perceptions of elder abuse and help-seeking patterns among African-American, Caucasian-American, and Korean-American elderly women, *Gerontologist* 33(3):386, 1993.

National Alliance for Caregiving (NAC): *Miles away: the Metlife study of long distance caregiving,* Bethesda, Md, 2004. Available at www.cargiving.org.

National Council on the Aging (NCOA): *American perceptions of aging in the 21st century,* Washington, DC, 2002, NCOA. Available at www.ncoa.org.

Navaie-Waliser M et al: When the caregiver needs care: the plight of vulnerable caregivers, *Am J Public Health* 92(3):409-413, 2002.

O'Connor P: Same-gender and cross-gender friendships among the frail elderly, *Gerontologist* 33(1):24-30, 1993.

Patwell T: Familial abuse of the elderly: a look at caregiver potential and prevention, *Home Healthc Nurse* 4(2):10, 1988.

Piercy KW: We couldn't do without them: the value of close relationships between older adults and their nonfamily caregivers, *Generations* 25(2):41, 2001.

Pratt C et al: Burden and coping strategies of caregivers to Alzheimer's patients, *Fam Relations* 34(1):27, 1985.

Quinn M, Director, San Francisco City and County Probate Court: Personal communication, June, 1999.

Quinn MJ, Heisler CJ: The legal system: civil and criminal responses to elder abuse and neglect, *Public Policy and Aging Report, Policy Institute of GSA* 12(2):8, 2002.

Quinn M, Tomita S: *Elder abuse and neglect: causes, diagnosis, and intervention strategies,* ed 2, New York, 1997, Springer.

Reis M, Nahmiash D: When seniors are abused: an intervention model, *Gerontologist* 35(5):666, 1995.

Robinson BC: Validation of a caregiver strain index, *J Gerontol* 38(3):344-348, 1983.

Roe KM, Minkler M: Grandparents raising grandchildren: challenges and responses, *Generations* 22(4):25, 1998-1999.

Rosenthal CJ: Kinkeeping in the familial division of labor, *J Marriage Fam* 47:965, 1985.

Schulz R, Beach SR: Caregiving as a risk factor for mortality: the Caregiver Health Effects Study, *JAMA* 282(23):2215-2219, 1999

Schwartz D, Kelly C: Personal communication, Sept 16, 1996, Gwynedd, Pa.

Scott JP: Sisters in later life: changes in contact and availability. In Roberto K, editor: *Relationships between women in later life,* New York, 1996, Haworth Press.

Sokolovsky J: *The cultural context of aging: a worldwide perspective,* Westport, Conn, 1997, Bergin & Garvey.

Stephens MAP: Day care and family strain: testing the effects of interventions. Paper presented at the meeting of the Gerontological Society of America, Washington, DC, Nov 19, 1996.

Sullivan MT: *Caregiver strain index, from Robinson,* New York, 2002, John A Hartford Foundation Institute for Geriatric Nursing.

Tobin S, Fulimer E, Smith GC: Coping with a developmentally disabled offspring. In Thomas E, Eisenhandler S, editors: *Aging and the religious dimension,* Westport, Conn, 1994, Auburn House.

Troope M: *Grandparents and other relatives raising children,* Washington, DC, 2000, Generations United.

U.S. Administration on Aging: Facts about older Americans, 2000. Available at www.aoa.gov.

Utley R: Screening and intervention in elder abuse, *Home Care Provid* 4(5):198, 1999.

Whitlack CJ, Noelker LS: Caregiving and caring. In Birren JE, editor: *Encyclopedia of gerontology: age, aging and the aged,* San Diego, 1996, Academic Press.

Wolf RS, Pillemer K: What's new in elder abuse programming? Four bright ideas, *Gerontologist* 34(1):126, 1994.

Yates ME, Tennstedt S, Chang BH: Contributors to and mediators of psychological well-being for informal caregivers, *J Gerontol B Psychol Sci Soc Sci* 54(1):P12-P22, 1999.

Zarit SH: Methodological considerations in caregiver intervention and outcome research. In Lebowitz BD, Light E, Niederche G, editors: *Alzheimer's disease and family stress,* Rockville, Md, 1991, National Institute of Mental Health.

Zarit SH, Zarit JM: *Mental disorders in older adults,* New York, 1998, Guilford Press.

Appendix 23-A *The National Elder Abuse Incidence Study*

DEFINITIONS OF DOMESTIC ELDER ABUSE, EXPLOITATION, AND NEGLECT

The following definitions of domestic elder abuse, exploitation, and neglect pertain to elders living in domestic settings. The perpetrator of this abuse may or may not be the caregiver of an elderly person or a member of the elderly person's family. Furthermore, some signs and symptoms are characteristic of several kinds of maltreatment and should be regarded as indicators of possible maltreatment. The most important of these are:

- an elder's frequent unexplained crying; and
- an elder's unexplained fear of or suspicion of a particular person(s) in the home.

Physical abuse is defined as the use of physical force that *may* result in bodily injury, physical pain, or impairment. Physical abuse may include but is not limited to such acts of violence as striking (with or without an object), hitting, beating, pushing, shoving, shaking, slapping, kicking, pinching, and burning. In addition, the inappropriate use of drugs and physical restraints, force-feeding, and physical punishment of any kind also are examples of physical abuse.

Signs and symptoms of physical abuse include but are not limited to:

- bruises, black eyes, welts, lacerations, and rope marks;
- bone fractures, broken bones, and skull fractures;
- open wounds, cuts, punctures, untreated injuries, and injuries in various stages of healing;
- sprains, dislocations, and internal injuries/ bleeding;
- broken eyeglasses/frames, physical signs of being subjected to punishment, and signs of being restrained;
- laboratory findings of medication overdose or underutilization of prescribed drugs;
- an elder's report of being hit, slapped, kicked, or mistreated;
- an elder's sudden change in behavior; and
- the caregiver's refusal to allow visitors to see an elder alone.

Sexual abuse is defined as nonconsensual sexual contact of any kind with an elderly person. Sexual contact with any person incapable of giving consent also is considered sexual abuse. It includes but is not limited to unwanted touching, all types of sexual assault or battery such as rape, sodomy, coerced nudity, and sexually explicit photographing.

Signs and symptoms of sexual abuse include but are not limited to:

- bruises around the breasts or genital area;
- unexplained venereal disease or genital infections;
- unexplained vaginal or anal bleeding;
- torn, stained, or bloody underclothing; and
- an elder's report of being sexually assaulted or raped.

Emotional or psychological abuse is defined as the infliction of anguish, pain, or distress through verbal or nonverbal acts. Emotional/psychological abuse includes but is not limited to verbal assaults, insults, threats, intimidation, humiliation, and harassment. In addition, treating an older person like an infant; isolating an elderly person from his/her family, friends, or regular activities; giving an older person a "silent treatment"; and enforced social isolation also are examples of emotional/psychological abuse.

Signs and symptoms of emotional/psychological abuse may manifest themselves in such behaviors of an elderly person as:

From National Center on Elder Abuse: *Elder abuse informational series no. 3,* Washington, DC, 1996, National Center on Elder Abuse.

- being emotionally upset or agitated;
- being extremely withdrawn and noncommunicative or nonresponsive;
- unusual behavior usually attributed to dementia (e.g., sucking, biting, rocking); and
- an elder's report of being verbally or emotionally mistreated.

Neglect is defined as the refusal or failure to fulfill any part of a person's obligations or duties to an elder. Neglect may also include a person who has fiduciary responsibilities to provide care for an elder (e.g., pay for necessary home care services, or the failure on the part of an in-home service provider to provide necessary care). Neglect typically means the refusal or failure to provide an elderly person with such life necessities as food, water, clothing, shelter, personal hygiene, medicine, comfort, personal safety, and other essentials included in the responsibility or agreement to an elder.

Signs and symptoms of neglect include but are not limited to:
- dehydration, malnutrition, untreated bedsores, and poor personal hygiene;
- unattended or untreated health problems;
- hazardous or unsafe living conditions/arrangements (e.g., improper wiring, no heat, or no running water);
- unsanitary and unclean living conditions (e.g., dirt, fleas, lice on person, soiled bedding, fecal/urine smell, inadequate clothing); and
- an elder's report of being mistreated.

Abandonment is defined as the desertion of an elderly person by an individual who has assumed responsibility for providing care for an elder, or by a person with physical custody of an elder.

Signs and symptoms of abandonment include but are not limited to:
- the desertion of an elder at a hospital, a nursing facility, or other similar institution;
- the desertion of an elder at a shopping center or other public location; and
- an elder's own report of being abandoned.

Financial or material exploitation is defined as the illegal or improper use of an elder's funds, property, or assets. Examples would include but are not limited to: cashing an elderly person's checks without authorization/permission; forging an older person's signature; misusing or stealing an older person's money or possessions; coercing or deceiving an older person into signing any document (e.g., contracts, a will); and the improper use of conservatorship, guardianship, or power of attorney.

Signs and symptoms of financial or material exploitation include but are not limited to:
- sudden changes in bank account or banking practice, including an unexplained withdrawal of large sums of money by a person accompanying the elder;
- the inclusion of additional names on an elder's bank signature card;
- unauthorized withdrawal of the elder's funds using the elder's ATM card;
- abrupt changes in a will or other financial documents;
- unexplained disappearance of funds or valuable possessions;
- substandard care being provided or bills unpaid despite the availability of adequate financial resources;
- discovery of an elder's signature being forged for financial transactions and for the titles of his/her possessions;
- sudden appearance of previously uninvolved relatives claiming their rights to an elder's affairs and possessions;
- unexplained sudden transfer of assets to a family member or someone outside the family;
- the provision of services that are not necessary; and
- an elder's report of financial exploitation.

Self-neglect is characterized as the behaviors of an elderly person that threaten his/her own health or safety. Self-neglect generally manifests itself in an older person's refusal or failure to provide himself/herself with adequate food, water, clothing, shelter, personal hygiene, medication (when indicated), and safety precautions. The definition of self-neglect *excludes* a situation in which a cognitive/mentally competent older person (who understands the consequences of his/her decisions) makes a conscious and voluntary decision to engage in acts that threaten his/her health or safety as a matter of personal preference.

Signs and symptoms of self-neglect include but are not limited to:
- dehydration, malnutrition, untreated or improperly attended medical conditions, and poor personal hygiene;

Continued.

Appendix 23-A *The National Elder Abuse Incidence Study—cont'd*

- hazardous or unsafe living conditions/arrangements (e.g., improper wiring, no indoor plumbing, no heat or no running water);
- unsanitary or unclean living quarters (e.g., animal/insect infestation, no functioning toilet, fecal/urine smell);
- inappropriate and/or inadequate clothing, lack of the necessary medical aids (e.g., eyeglasses, hearing aid, dentures); and
- grossly inadequate housing or homelessness.

NATIONAL CENTER ON ELDER ABUSE (NCEA)

Consortium Organizations

American Public Welfare Association (APWA)
810 First Street NE
Suite 500
Washington, DC 20002-4267

National Association of State Units on Aging (NASUA)
1225 I Street NW
Suite 725
Washington, DC 20005

University of Delaware
College of Human Resources
Department of Textiles, Design, and Consumer Economics
Newark, DE 19716

National Committee for the Prevention of Elder Abuse (NCPEA)
c/o Institute on Aging
The Medical Center of Central Massachusetts
119 Belmont Street
Worcester, MA 01605

Appendix 23-B   *Abuse and Neglect Assessment*

1. General Assessment	Very Good	Good	Poor	Very Poor	Unable to Assess
a. Clothing					
b. Hygiene					
c. Nutrition					
d. Skin integrity					
Additional Comments:					

2. Possible Abuse Indicators	No Evidence	Possible Evidence	Probable Evidence	Definite Evidence	Unable to Assess
a. Bruising					
b. Lacerations					
c. Fractures					
d. Various stages of healing of any bruises or fractures					
e. Evidence of sexual abuse					
f. Statement by elder re: abuse					
Additional Comments:					

3. Possible Neglect Indicators	No Evidence	Possible Evidence	Probable Evidence	Definite Evidence	Unable to Assess
a. Contractures					
b. Decubiti					
c. Dehydration					
d. Diarrhea					
e. Depression					
f. Impaction					
g. Malnutrition					
h. Urine burns					
i. Poor hygiene					
j. Failure to respond to warning of obvious disease					
k. Inappropriate medications (under/over)					
l. Repetitive hospital admissions due to probable failure of health care surveillance					
m. Statement by elder re: neglect					
Additional Comments:					

From Fulmer T: Elder abuse and neglect assessment. Try this: best practices in nursing care to older adults, *Hartford Institute for Geriatric Nursing,* no. 15, May 2002.

Continued.

Appendix 23-B *Abuse and Neglect Assessment—cont'd*

4. Possible Exploitation Indicators	No Evidence	Possible Evidence	Probable Evidence	Definite Evidence	Unable to Assess
a. Misuse of money					
b. Evidence					
c. Reports of demands for goods in exchange for services					
d. Inability to account for money/property					
e. Statement by elder re: exploitation					
Additional Comments:					

5. Possible Abandonment Indicators	No Evidence	Possible Evidence	Probable Evidence	Definite Evidence	Unable to Assess
a. Evidence that a caretaker has withdrawn care precipitously without alternate arrangements					
b. Evidence that elder is left alone in an unsafe environment for extended periods without adequate support					
c. Statement by elder re: abandonment					
Additional Comments:					

6. Summary	No Evidence	Possible Evidence	Probable Evidence	Definite Evidence	Unable to Assess
a. Evidence of abuse					
b. Evidence of neglect					
c. Evidence of exploitation					
d. Evidence of abandonment					
Additional Comments:					

24

Financing Health Care for Older Adults

LEARNING OBJECTIVES

Upon completion of this chapter, the reader will be able to:

- Describe the major methods of financing health care for older adults.
- Compare the costs to the consumer between Medicare and Medicaid.
- Explain the fundamentals of Medicare, Medicaid, and TRICARE sufficiently to assist elders in accessing the services needed.
- Discuss the potential impact of health care financing in long-term care and home health.
- Describe the roles of the nurse as case and care managers.

▶ **GLOSSARY**

CMS The Centers for Medicare and Medicaid Services (formerly Health Care Financing Administration [HCFA]), the federal agency under the U.S. Department of Health and Human Services responsible for the administration of Medicare and Medicaid.

Custodial care The provision of personal assistance related to one's inability to perform the activities needed in daily living. This care may be provided informally by family and friends or formally by nursing assistants.

Prospective payment system (PPS) A system in which the payment of a health service is calculated in advance and based on a number of factors, including diagnosis and age of the patient rather than the actual costs and length of the care needed.

Skilled care The provision of a level of care that requires professional expertise and training, such as that provided by licensed nurses, physical therapists, or occupational therapists.

The Social Security Act The legislation passed in 1935 that provides regular income for older persons.

Title XVIII of the Social Security Act The federal legislation providing for Medicare to all eligible persons over age 65 and the disabled.

Title XIX of the Social Security Act The federal legislation providing for Medicaid to individuals over age 65 or the disabled with very low incomes.

Title XX of the Social Security Act The federal legislation providing for the establishment of senior centers throughout the United States.

▶ **THE LIVED EXPERIENCE**

When I was growing up life was hard. We were so poor we couldn't do much but to hold on tight. When I was lucky I could get work plowing a field and make $1.00 an acre. You work hard, and you make do. There were not such things as going to a doctor or a hospital, you just did the best you could do and pray you don't get sick. Then when I turned 65 I got a little check from the government and a red, white, and blue insurance [Medicare] card. The check isn't much, only about $564 a month, but you know I just consider myself blessed and better off than ever before. And now I don't worry about my health, I will be taken care of.

Aida, age 74

*P*eople growing up in the United States represent all levels of education, experience, and income. However, all have in common the potential need for health care. It is rare to meet an older adult who does not have experience in some way with both the past and present health care system in the United States. It is a system in a state of flux and stress as it finds a way to care for the ever increasing number of older adults in the face of skyrocketing costs. In order for gerontological nurses to provide the best care to older adults, it is helpful to have a basic understanding of the financing associated with the care they provide.

SOCIAL SECURITY

The health care system of today and its financing began in 1935. Not only were there more elders in numbers, but also they were living longer than they ever had. There had been an exodus from the country and farms and into the city and the factories in the early 1900s, changing the financial basis of the family. In the country, an elder worked in some way until death, but this was not possible in the exceedingly difficult work of the factories. For the first time people were retiring by choice or by reason of disability. The word *retiring,* which had meant "to withdraw from public" in the 1800s, now meant "no longer qualified," with dramatically different implications (Achenbaum, 1978).

The family, no longer able to provide all the care to their elders, looked to the federal government for help. In 1935 the Social Security Act was passed. The Social Security program, established at the time of the Great Depression, was considered by many to be one of the most successful federal programs. Its primary function was to provide monetary benefits to American citizens and legal residents over the age of 65 to prevent destitution and dependency in older age and for younger people who were significantly disabled (Weinberger, 1996). The amount of the benefit was calculated in part by the person's average salary during his or her working years. This has been most beneficial to white men, who have worked consistently and historically earned the highest salaries, and less beneficial to others.

The program has been managed on what is called a pay-as-you-go system. Payroll taxes collected from employees and employers are immediately distributed to beneficiaries (retirees, the disabled). As long as the amount of contributions from the workers exceeds those paid to the beneficiaries, the program, as designed, can exist. At the time of its inception the system was constructed to transfer funds from those believed to be relatively well off (workers) to those believed to be relatively poor (retirees).

Later amendments were made to the Social Security Act authorizing funding of Medicare and Medicaid and of a program called Supplementary Security Income (SSI). SSI was established to make sure that all persons who are at least 65 or blind or disabled receive a minimum income regardless of their earning power in their working years. In 2003 this rate was set to make sure that all single persons have incomes of at least $564 per month and all couples receive at least $846 per month. If one's regular Social Security income is below the threshold, then the income is supplemented with SSI funds (SSA, 2003).

In recent years there has been a great concern that the balance between the contributions made to the program and the payments made out is shifting and that the Social Security trust fund will "run out" of money in the early 2000s. In an attempt to forestall the loss of the Social Security program the age of retirement is rising. While all eligible persons can receive partial retirement benefits at the age of 62, the age when one may receive full benefits is rising. At this time full benefits are available at 65 only for those persons born before 1937. For each year of birth after 1937 the age of retirement increases, reaching 66 for those born between 1943-54 and 67 for those born in 1960 or later (USDHHS, n.d.).

The Social Security program is intimately tied to the financing of the majority of health care provided to persons over 65 in the United States. Indeed, the federal government is the primary (no. 1) payer for health care through Medicare, Medicaid (shared with states), and the Veterans Administration.

Medicare and Medicaid

History

In 1934 President Franklin D. Roosevelt tried to organize a plan to provide universal health insurance in the United States. This was met with unbeatable opposition from groups such as the American Medical Association (Goodman, 1980) and, by poll, the majority of the American public (Cantril, 1951). Except for a few successful insurance plans for working people, health care was on a fee-for-service, out-of-pocket basis. This meant that each health care service could be purchased for a fee from one's own funds, or "pocket." When costs were reasonable, older adults could continue to pay for their care, especially since they had a guaranteed income of some kind through Social Security. However, as the number of elders grew greater, lived longer, had more health problems, and charges rose, paying for the costs of health care out-of-pocket grew harder.

In 1965 through the efforts of President Lyndon B. Johnson, legislation (Title XVIII of the Social Security Act) was passed creating an insurance plan (Medicare A) covering the costs of hospitalization for all persons eligible for Social Security, SSI, or railroad retirement benefits. A second policy (Medicare B) could be purchased as a medical supplement to cover the costs of seeing health care providers. The costs of outpatient medications have never been covered by Medicare. While recent changes have made discount coupons for some medications available to Medicare recipients, true coverage has yet to be provided.

Medicare was meant to provide insurance coverage of medical care to the elderly and disabled regardless of their financial situation. Another amendment (Title XIX) to the Social Security Act created a second form of insurance for the elderly, the disabled, and children with low incomes, known as Medicaid. Medicaid was designed to defray expenses for those who did not qualify or could not afford to purchase the supplemental policy (Medicare B) or to pay the co-payments required. All persons eligible for SSI are automatically eligible for Medicaid. Medicaid, however, is left to the individual state's discretion; therefore it varies in coverage nationwide. Most aged persons today receive Medicare; some receive Medicaid benefits instead of or in addition to Medicare.

Medicare

More than 40 million adults in the United States have health insurance coverage through Medicare (CMS, 2003). To be eligible for Medicare, the adult must have worked legally at least 5 years in the United States and be at least 65 years old or be under 65 with severe disabilities or end-stage renal disease (ESRD). Medicare only covers select services and requires that these services be considered medically necessary (Box 24-1). This means that the services must be needed for the diagnosis or treatment of a medical condition, meet the standards of good medical practice, and are not for the convenience of the health care provider (CMS, 2004b). Box 24-2 provides definitions for various terms related to health care payments and benefits.

Medicare A.   A person automatically receives a Medicare card (red, white, and blue) indicating Medicare A coverage when he or she turns 65. If a person has not worked before the age of 65 he or she may be eligible to purchases Part A coverage for a monthly fee. Medicare A is a hospital insurance plan covering acute care and acute and short-term rehabilitative care and some costs associated with hospice care and home health care under certain circumstances. Rehabilitative care, usually provided in skilled nursing facilities, is only paid for if it occurs within 3 days of a hospital discharge and as long as the patient requires what is called skilled care, or only that which is provided by a licensed nurse or physical or occupational therapist. Medicare A will pay 100% of the first 20 days of a nursing home stay, with a co-pay of up to $150 per day for days 21 to 100 and no coverage after that (USHHS, 2003). At any time the person no longer needs skilled care, Medicare coverage stops. Medicare does not cover additional charges that may be incurred during a long-term care stay, such as incontinence supplies and laundry.

When only assistance with personal care or medication supervision is required, it is not covered by Medicare at all. Similarly, for home health care, for the costs to be paid by Medicare the care must be provided at the written direction and supervision of a physician (only), through a certified agency, and for the purposes of active rehabilitation as seen in the nursing home setting. There are no co-payments for home health or hospice care.

Medicare Part A is supported through a dedicated payroll tax on current workers and by the co-payments of the beneficiaries. When acute care is needed, the co-payments can be quite high, including on-time co-pay of $912 (as of 2005) for

Box 24-1	Fundamentals of Medicare*

Medicare Part A

Medicare Part A is designed primarily to partially cover the costs of inpatient hospital care and other specialized care as listed below:

- Acute hospitalization coverage, through a prospective payment system, includes costs of semiprivate rooms, meals, nursing services, operating and recovery room, intensive care, drugs, laboratory and radiology fees, blood products, and other necessary medical services and supplies. There is a deductible for days 1-60. This is repeated anytime the person is rehospitalized after 60 days. After 60 days there is a daily co-pay that increases over time. No coverage after 150 days. Deductibles and co-pays increase every year. The deductibles and co-pays are either paid out-of-pocket or by Medicaid or Medigap policies.
- Nursing home care is covered by Medicare only if the person had been in an acute care setting for 3 days before the admission and only as long as a skilled service is needed and for a maximum of 100 days. While the facility is paid on a prospective payment system similar to the acute care setting, for the patients, the first 20 days are covered at 100%, and for days 21-100 a substantial daily co-pay is required. There is no coverage if skilled care is not continuously needed.
- Home health care may be covered by Medicare (also prospective payment) on an intermittent and/or part-time basis for skilled nursing care, physical therapy, and rehabilitative services. The person must be ill enough to be

considered homebound. Custodial care is not covered. Medicare pays 80% of the approved amount for durable medical equipment and supplies.

- Hospice care is provided for terminally ill persons expected to live less than 6 months who elect to forgo traditional medical treatment for the terminal illness. Medicare pays for all but limited costs for outpatient drugs and inpatient respite care. Hospice Medicare replaces Medicare A and B for all costs associated with the terminal condition.
- Inpatient psychiatric care is limited number of days in a lifetime; partial payment and other limitations apply.

Medicare Part B

Medicare Part B is designed to cover some of the costs associated with outpatient or ambulatory services. Deductibles and co-pays are required in most cases:

- Physician and nurse practitioner services, including some prescribed supplies and diagnostic tests
- Physical, occupational, and speech therapy for the purpose of rehabilitation
- Limited durable medical equipment
- Clinical laboratory services fully covered if deemed medically necessary
- Outpatient hospital treatment, blood, and ambulatory surgical services
- Limited preventive services
- Diabetic supplies (excluding insulin and other medications)

*See www.cms.gov for the latest information about covered services and associated costs. These are all subject to change.

days 1 to 60 and then an increasing daily co-pay for days 61 to 150. After 150 days in an acute care setting there is no coverage.

Medicare B. In the 7 months surrounding the 65th birthday (from 3 months before), a person who is eligible for Part A must apply for Part B through the local Social Security Administration offices (www.socialsecurity.gov). At that time the person will be asked to choose one of the Medicare B plans that are available in his or her area. The possible plans include the Original Medicare Plan or one of the Medicare Advantage

Plans (formerly called Medicare + Choice). Medicare B covers the costs associated with the services provided by physicians; nurse practitioners; outpatient services (e.g., lab); qualified physical, speech, and occupational therapy; and some home health care.

The *Original Medicare Plan* is based on a traditional fee-for-service arrangement; the patient receives services from a provider for a medical problem, a bill for the costs of the care is sent to Medicare (through a carrier) or to the patient, who can submit the claims, and the provider or the

Box 24-2   Terms

Managed care organization (MCO): A for-profit or not-for-profit company that manages a system of health care delivery in which patients agree to use health care providers from a panel of physicians, nurse practitioners, therapists, hospitals, pharmacies, and home care agencies among others designated by the MCO. The MCO monitors the cost of care provided to patients in order to control the cost of care.

Integrated delivery systems: A group of individual entities, such as a hospital and physicians that join together into a single entity to provide integrated health care services to contracted clients or patients.

Payers: In the health care context, payers are the entities who pay for health care on behalf of persons who have paid premiums or fees to the payer or, in the case of some government programs, on behalf of persons who are unable to pay themselves.

Providers: One who provides something; a generic term referring to all persons and agencies that provide health care.

Insurer: An individual or organization that underwrites an insurance risk and that agrees to pay compensation or benefits to the insured according to a contract. The insured is the person covered by the insurance contract; with a health insurance contract, the insured is the patient.

Beneficiary: A person who derives a benefit from something; in health care, the person who is a subscriber to an MCO or HMO or who is receiving benefits through Medicare is said to be a beneficiary of those organizations since the person receives medical benefits from his or her association with the organizations.

Preferred provider organization (PPO): A health care delivery system through which providers contract to offer medical services to benefit plan enrollees on a fee-for-service basis at various reimbursement levels in return for more patients and/or timely payment. Enrollees may use any provider in the PPO or outside the PPO, but they have a financial incentive (e.g., lower co-insurance payments) to use providers within the PPO.

Health maintenance organization (HMO): A health insurance company to which subscribers (patients) pay a predetermined premium or fee in return for a range of medical services from physicians and other health care providers who are approved by the organization. Premiums or fees may also be paid by employers and other organizations on behalf of their employees or members.

---

patient is reimbursed. Charges incurred are paid by Medicare at a rate of 80% of what Medicare considers an "allowable charge" (mental health is limited to 50%). The patient is responsible for the remaining 20% (or 50%) of the charge. In addition, the patient is responsible for an annual deductible of $110 and a monthly premium ($78.20/mo in 2005). The premium is usually deducted directly from the monthly Social Security check. Any co-payments must come from whatever other financial resources the elder may have. The premiums usually increase on a yearly basis along with raises in Social Security (CMS, 2004b).

The advantages of the Original Medicare Plan include choice and access. The person can seek the services of any provider of his or her choice, without a referral. If the provider accepts the Medicare rate, the provider is obligated to bill Medicare for the 80% and can only bill the patient the uncovered 20% of the allowable charge rather than the provider's usual charge. There are providers all over the United States who accept Medicare, and a person can change providers as often as desired. Many people with the Original Medicare Plan purchase what are called Medigap policies to cover the deductibles and co-pays.

The *Medicare Advantage Plans*, depending on location, may include a private fee-for-service plan, a preferred provider organization plan, and/or any number of managed care plans. Not all plans are offered at all locations. Although these plans may provide extra benefits (e.g., limited drug coverage), they may have small co-pays, they all have special rules that must be followed, and they may charge extra premiums for the added services.

Under the private-fee-for-service plan Medicare pays a portion of the premium of a private insurance plan and the consumer pays the rest. Whereas all the traditional services covered by both Medicare A and B must be provided, additional services, co-pays, and deductibles are determined by the insurance company.

The preferred provider organization (PPO) plan works like the Original Medicare except that only specific providers can be used (those in the network), and in most cases a referral from a selected or assigned primary care provider is required to see a specialist. The additional services and fees or co-pays vary by plan. A patient may choose to be seen by a provider outside the PPO network for an additional charge.

In managed care plans (MCPs; also known as health maintenance organizations [HMOs]) the consumer is also restricted to certain providers and hospitals. There are fewer out-of-pocket costs unless an individual decides to see a provider or seek a service without a referral or outside the system to which he or she has subscribed, which are not usually covered at all. Medicare contracts with MCPs to provide comprehensive services for the elderly, financed by Medicare premiums. The best of these are complete health care systems with highly trained physicians, nurse practitioners, and nurses working out of single or regional, completely equipped medical center. MCPs differ from other medical services in that they emphasize preventive medicine, comprehensive care, periodic physical examinations, and immunizations, and they cover more services than are ordinarily covered under the Original Medicare Plan or the PPO plans. There may be a minimum monthly charge to the participant or the participant's former employer and a service fee for each visit and for each prescription.

Capitation is imposed on managed care plans by Medicare; this means that the plan is paid a certain fixed amount each day for each enrollee regardless of the amount of care given, and from this amount all care needed must be provided. This has created abuses and horror stories in which elders were denied needed treatments to save money for the corporate providers. Now patient protection laws are in place that allow consumers to lodge complaints and initiate legal action against these abuses. The Center for Patient Advocacy supported a much-needed bill that

became law in October 1999, which allows appeals when an MCP denies care, guarantees access to specialists when needed, ensures that health-related decisions are made by health care providers rather than bureaucrats, and holds MCPs legally accountable for medical decisions that cause harm. See Resources at the end of this chapter for further information regarding complaints.

HMOs that have been granted Medicare per capita waivers cannot refuse applicants based on preexisting health conditions, and the supplemental services offered may save the participant a considerable amount in the costs of medications, assistive devices, and professional consultation charges. The negative aspects of HMOs and managed care are the access barriers to specialists and high-tech procedures and treatments. Some HMOs provide extensive health education services, support groups, and telephone support services to the homebound.

Medicare is administered by the Centers for Medicare and Medicaid Services (CMS), formerly the Health Care Financing Administration, and is a part of the U.S. Department of Health and Human Services, a special entity created to improve the administration of programs.

Medicaid

For elders with low incomes (including all persons receiving SSI), Medicaid may be available to offset the high Medicare co-pays and deductibles, as well as to provide additional health benefits.

In 2000 Medicaid provided health care insurance to 4.1 million persons 65 or older (10% of all Medicaid beneficiaries) at a cost of about $11,345 per person, and for 7.5 million disabled persons at $10,040 per person. State Medicaid programs paid for 41% of all of the U.S. nursing home and home health care. This included $34.5 billion ($20,220 per beneficiary) for 1.7 million of the people in nursing homes and $3.1 billion ($3135 per person) for 995,000 at home (CMS, 2004a).

Within the broad guidelines established by the federal government each state establishes its own eligibility criteria, determines the types and extent of services to be covered, sets the payment rates to providers, and administers its own programs (CMS, 2003). In most cases Medicaid covers more services than Medicare, including custodial care in nursing homes and preventive care with no co-pays or deductibles; however, this is highly variable by state and by the year and depends on the state's fiscal health and political priorities.

More states are turning to Medicaid managed care plans (MCPs) and waiver programs in an attempt to control costs. Sometimes the MCP is optional for the beneficiary, and sometimes enrollment is mandatory. Waiver programs are designed to allow the states to design and implement innovative delivery models to keep Medicaid-eligible elders out of nursing homes. Medicaid does not help the near-poor, who cannot qualify for aid but cannot afford basic health care, even with the partial aid of Medicare.

The premise of Medicare and Medicaid managed care is that better outcomes will result from systems of care that integrate professionals in responsive teams, maximize the use of subacute care, and provide incentives to reduce the reliance on institutional acute care (Rosenfeld, 1996). Managed care systems are most effective for individuals enrolled over a long period who use ongoing primary care and preventive strategies to maintain health and avoid high-cost emergency services and intensive treatment (Twentieth Century Fund, 1995).

The American Association of Managed Care Nurses was established in 1994 in response to an identified need to educate nurses regarding managed health care (see Resources).

CARE FOR VETERANS

Nearly 7 million World War II veterans and 3 million Korean War veterans are now over 65 years old. Medical program expenses for the veterans of our wars have become a major fiscal responsibility, totaling $16.9 billion in 1997. The Veterans Health Administration (VA) system has long held a leadership position in gerontological research, medical care, and extended care. In fact, a great deal of the research that has guided gerontologists in earlier years was generated through the VA system, as were innovations in care. In addition, the vast majority of gerontological fellowships have been provided through the Department of Veterans Affairs (VA) hospitals. The VA system has been a forerunner of the various continua of care providers in place at present. Early on, this system provided VA-run nursing homes, home care and community-based programs, respite care, blindness rehabilitation, mental health, and numerous other services in addition to acute medical/surgical provisions.

Persons and their dependents who have been part of the uniformed services may be eligible for health care services through veterans hospital networks or through TRICARE. At one time veterans hospitals and services were available on an as-needed basis for anyone who had served at any time. It was not necessary for individuals to use their Medicare benefits. However, this system is undergoing a process of significant change. One of the first changes that veterans noted was restrictions placed on the use of Veterans Hospitals and services. Instead of coverage of any health problems, priorities were set for those problems that were in some way deemed "service connected"; in other words, the health care problem had to be linked to the time the person was on active duty. Veterans older than 65 are now expected to obtain and use Medicare for their non–service-connected health problems, with the responsibilities for co-pays and deductibles the same as for other beneficiaries. There was an outcry among veterans and veteran groups that resulted in the development of a free Medigap policy known as TRICARE for Life (TFL).

TRICARE for Life

TRICARE is the health care insurance program provided by the Department of Defense for eligible beneficiaries. The TRICARE for Life plan (TFL) is for Medicare-eligible beneficiaries age 65 and older and their dependents or widows or widowers older than 65. This plan requires that the person enroll in both Medicare A and B and pay the premiums for Part B. As a Medigap policy, TFL covers those expenses not covered by Medicare, such as co-pays and prescription medicines. Dependent parents or parents-in-law may be eligible for pharmacy benefits if they turned age 65 on or after April 1, 2001 and are enrolled in Medicare B. For more information about this see www.tricare.osd.mil.

LONG-TERM CARE INSURANCE

Some persons are electing to purchase additional insurance (long-term care insurance [LTCI]) for their potential long-term care needs. Ideally these policies would cover the expenses related to co-pays for long-term care and coverage for what is called custodial care or help with day-to-day needs (as opposed to skilled care). Traditionally these policies were limited to care in long-term care facilities and provided a flat-rate reimbursement to residents for their costs. However, these policies are becoming more creative and innovative and may cover home care costs instead or in addition to under some circumstances. Many plans are being marketed at present. Even the American Nurses Association (ANA) has a plan available to ANA members that is underwritten by American Express.

LTCI plans are not for everyone. Since they do not receive any governmental funding support, the costs can be prohibitive. The purchaser must be cautioned to read the policy carefully and understand all the details, limitations, and exclusions. There are particular concerns related to Alzheimer's disease because many policies exclude these individuals from home benefits and include very limited institutional benefits. The best LTCI packages that have been negotiated by a large employer or state organization or association. It is also advisable to have the elder or family member check consumer reports of the particular insurance company and its reliability before applying for a policy.

IMPLICATIONS FOR GERONTOLOGICAL NURSING AND HEALTHY AGING

Nurses are increasingly at the frontlines as primary care providers, case and care managers, and members or leaders of interdisciplinary care teams, all charged with working within the above described funding plans to make sure that the elder not only gets the best care possible, but also is able to achieve the highest level of wellness possible.

Case and Care Management

The nurse is probably most able to influence the quality of care elders receive in the current system through the roles of care manager and case manager. As a care manager the nurse makes sure

that the care an elder receives is the best it can be. In the role of the case manager, the nurse ensures that the care provided is done in the most efficient and effective manner possible. In the strictest sense, a case manager works within a system with the primary intent of efficiency—of both time and money, whereas a care manager is working for the client to provide the best service at the least cost.

Although the terms *case manager* and *care manager* have slightly different connotations, in real practice the roles are seldom that clear and there is much overlap. Both these roles include advocate, broker, leader, manager, counselor, negotiator, administrator, and communicator. Ideally the care or case manager follows the person through the entire continuum of care. Care or case managers must be experts regarding community resources and understand how these can best be used to meet the client's needs. They are expected to make appropriate referrals with consideration of the client's expectations and the system's limits and to monitor the quality of any arranged services. The care or case manager is a resource person whom the client can seek for advice and counsel and for brokering (negotiating, arranging) the flow of services. As a gatekeeper, the case or care manager controls the entrances and exits to services to make sure that the elder gets what is needed while avoiding resource waste (Box 24-3).

Community-based case or care management as a method of controlling costs and avoiding premature institutionalization has increased immensely in the last 15 years. Care managers are usually paid privately, less often by Medicare or Medicaid managed care plans and rarely through public funding from agencies such as Area Agencies on Aging (see Chapter 23). Care that is well managed is believed to be a solution to both the spiraling cost and the fragmentation of care experienced by elders with multiple needs. The case or care manager works to optimize the resources and outcome for the client and the agency or community in which the person resides.

In response to the emergence of case management, the Case Management Society of America (CMSA), an international, nonprofit organization, was founded in 1990 (see Resources at the end of this chapter). The CMSA developed the Standards of Practice for Case Management and the Standards of Practice and Ethics Statement. Education,

Box 24-3	Ten Commandments of Case Management During Hospitalization

1. Be visible in the acute care setting; the case manager must follow the client through any level of care.
2. Communicate routinely with the hospital discharge planner (HDP); when the client is hospitalized, immediately call the HDP to alert him or her to your involvement.
3. Provide support for the hospitalized client. Ideally, visit daily and keep the client informed of discharge plans.
4. Provide for necessary monitoring of the home while the client is absent, such as pet care.
5. Monitor the client's hospital progress and make staff aware of previous functional needs and abilities.
6. Recommend appropriate levels of discharge to the HDP; when meeting resistance,

negotiate for a trial period in the least restrictive level of care.
7. Maximize benefits of hospitalization by initiating assessment and care of conditions that the client may have been neglecting before hospitalization.
8. Encourage early discharge; hospitalization is dangerous to elders.
9. Begin discharge planning on the day of hospital admission. Discuss with the HDP a package of potential services needed on discharge.
10. Make placement recommendations based on experience with the quality of care or special facilities in specific institutions; seek the least restrictive alternative. At times you must educate the physician or acute care staff regarding the differences in levels of long-term institutional care.

Modified from Peters B: The ten commandments of case management during hospitalization: a practice perspective. In Pelham AO, Clark WF, editors: *Managing home care for the elderly: lessons from community based agencies,* New York, 1986, Springer.

research, and networking to create professionalism and accountability are top priorities of the organization.

Multidisciplinary Care Team Planning

The nurse also influences health outcomes and promotes healthy aging through participation in and leading of multidisciplinary care team meetings as a part of the responsibility of the care or case manager, as a representative of an insurer, or as a health care provider (e.g., nurse in a nursing home). The basic case management team for the care of an individual and family involves a physician and/or nurse practitioner, licensed nurse, rehabilitation specialist, and social worker. It also may include chaplains, dietitians, and certified nursing assistants.

As the health care system becomes more complex, the need for collaboration among these interested parties becomes more important. The special knowledge and skills of a dozen or more professionals may be required in working with a single elder and his or her family. A functioning multidisciplinary team will reduce care redun-

dancy, fragmentation, and waste by making use of the resources available in a coordinated and cost-effective manner.

Ensuring Quality of Care

Nurses are also influential in and responsible for ensuring continuous quality improvement and quality management in all health care settings regardless of the financial arrangements. Funders, licensing agencies, accrediting bodies, and patients all depend on the nurse to make sure that the care provided is the care that is actually needed and that the care is effective and efficient. Funding sources, especially the federal government through Medicare, have taken steps to ensure that their standards are met and that their monies are not wasted through audits and through the required documentation of care (see Chapter 6).

Recently there has been a strong move toward outcome assessments involving efficacy, effectiveness, and efficiency. *Efficacy* is based on the expected value of an intervention in ideal circumstances; *effectiveness* is the result obtained under usual circumstances; and *efficiency* considers the benefit of the service in relation to the cost. In 1994 the outcome-based quality improvement (OBQI) system was established to measure all aspects of quality, including providers, discharge and ongoing planning, and efficacy of supports. The broad case management approach to quality care emphasizes consumer rights, client involvement, and satisfaction. Many of these elements are subjective, and clients' perspectives may be shaped by the events of the day on which they are assessed rather than by their ongoing quality of life. However, the general move toward more assessment of clients' perspectives rather than structural adequacy seems to be an important consideration.

THE NURSE AND COMMUNITY-BASED CARE

An array of public and privately financed services has developed across the United States to support the desire of impaired elders to remain at home. Community-based services may be funded through a combination of Medicare and Medicaid (Titles XVIII and XIX of the Social Security Act), the Social Services Amendment (Title XX of the Social Security Act), Title III of the Older Americans Act, the Department of Veterans Affairs, and out-of-pocket—either the elder's pocket or that of their friends and family members. Medicaid waiver programs are available in many communities. If the person is eligible for a nursing home stay covered by Medicaid, the state may instead offer services directed by a case manager that would enable the person to remain at home. The type of services provided is determined by both the needs of the person and the resources available. The majority of the services needed at home are provided by family members (see Chapter 23). Most of this service is care that is uncompensated, although some states have experimented with providing low-income family caregivers a small monthly stipend.

Just about any services can be purchased for a fee (see Chapter 23), but persons may be unaware of what is needed or where it can be obtained. In these situations, case managers may help individuals identify specific needs and find the appropriate services (see above). Case managers may be found through city and county referral services or private agencies that provide case management on a fee-for-service basis.

Those who cannot afford the out-of-pocket expenses of purchased services must rely on those available through community agencies funded by the states and by the federal government via the Area Agencies on Aging. As with Medicaid services, the resources available depend on the economics and politics of the state and the power of elder advocates. Some frail and needy elders desire to remain in their homes even when few services and minimal assistance are available to them. This situation is often distressing to the nurse, but as competent adults, elders have a right to make their own life choices, and staying home with less may be selected over going to a nursing home with more. However, nurses can continue to advocate for and support the elder in any way possible and acceptable to them.

It has become clear as we face the burgeoning population of very old survivors and the entry of the baby boomers into the ranks of older persons that many aspects of the health care system must be modified. Because nurses are pivotal players within the system and occupy diverse roles, there are abundant opportunities for professional growth and gratification in working with the aged in our ever-shifting health care system. Nurses are case managers and primary care coordinators in the home. We expect that nurses will continue to occupy a pivotal role in home care as client advocates and to carefully evaluate care plans, quality outcomes, and costs.

▶ KEY CONCEPTS

- A combination of Social Security and Supplementary Security Income payments provide persons with a regular income after the age of 65 or earlier if disabled. The total amount varies greatly and is dependent on qualified earned income during the working years.

- Medicare, Medicaid, and TRICARE are insurance plans for specific groups of people. Almost all of the older adults in the United States have some kind of coverage for expenses related to health care needs.

- Medicaid pays for a large portion of the cost associated with long-term home and nursing home care.

NANDA and Wellness Diagnoses

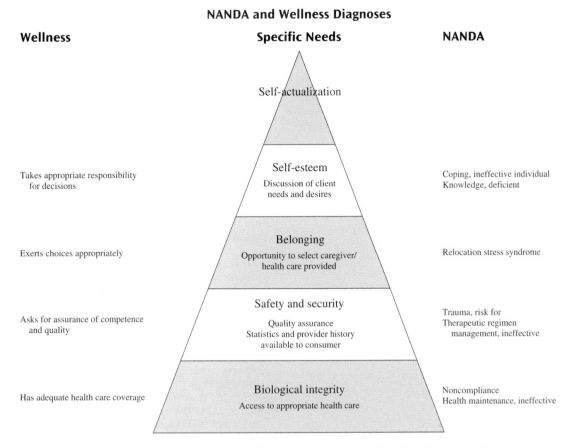

Wellness

Takes appropriate responsibility
for decisions

Exerts choices appropriately

Asks for assurance of competence
and quality

Has adequate health care coverage

Specific Needs

Self-actualization

Self-esteem
Discussion of client
needs and desires

Belonging
Opportunity to select caregiver/
health care provided

Safety and security
Quality assurance
Statistics and provider history
available to consumer

Biological integrity
Access to appropriate health care

NANDA

Coping, ineffective individual
Knowledge, deficient

Relocation stress syndrome

Trauma, risk for
Therapeutic regimen
management, ineffective

Noncompliance
Health maintenance, ineffective

These are not all of the possible wellness or NANDA diagnoses that may be identified. The above are frequent examples of nursing diagnoses that should be considered when planning care for the older adult in whatever setting.

- There may be substantial out-of-pocket costs associated with the receipt of health care today.
- In order for Medicare to pay for the expenses related to long-term care or home health care, strict criteria of medical necessity must be met.
- Good case management is a mode of care management that considers cost, quality, and coordination of services for the benefit of the client.
- Nurses have key roles in the assurance of quality care to older adults.

▶ **Activities and Discussion Questions**

1. Interview a nurse case manager, and ask about the components of the position that are gratifying and those that are the most difficult.

2. Discuss your thoughts about specific activities that are different for case managers and care managers.
3. Describe the role of the nurse-advocate in relation to health and consumer protections.
4. Explain the fundamentals of Medicare and Medicaid sufficiently to assist elders in obtaining more specific information.
5. Interview an elder in a rehabilitation center, and ask about his or her experiences with acute hospitalization, long-term care, and Medicare.
6. Discuss with this elder his or her thoughts about Medicare and how it does or does not meet his or her needs. Write a brief summary, and present it to the class.

RESOURCES

Books and Publications

Consumers' Guide to Health Plans. Publication that has rated health care maintenance organizations (HMOs) across the nation as excellent, very good, good, fair, or poor. This guide also gives information on keeping costs down and getting the best care when enrolled in a plan. Contact Health Plan Guide, 733 15th Street NW, Suite 821, Washington, DC 20005.

Consumers' Guide to Health Plans. Similar publication; available from the Center for the Study of Services; call (202) 347-7283, (510) 397-8305, or (800) 475-7283. See also the CMS website: www.cms.gov.

Self-Help for Public Benefits. Brochure prepared by the Legal Counsel for the Elderly/AARP, PO Box 96474, Washington, DC 20090-6474; www.aarp.org.

Social Security Retirement and Survivors Benefits. Booklet available from all Social Security offices listed in the telephone book or by calling (800) 772-1213; www.ssa.gov.

Organizations

American Association of Managed Care Nurses
4435 Waterfront Drive, Suite 101
PO Box 4975
Glen Allen, VA 23058
(804) 747-9698
www.aamcn.org

Case Management Society of America
1101 17th Street NW, Suite 1200
Washington, DC 20036
www.cmsa.org

Websites

Information about supplementary security income
www.ssa.gov

Medicaid at a Glance, 2003
Available at www.ssa.gov

Medicare and Medicaid information for professionals and for consumers
www.cms.gov

Medicare information
www.medicare.gov

Social Security Administration
www.ssa.gov

TRICARE
www.tricare.osd.mil

REFERENCES

Achenbaum WA: *Old age in a new land,* Baltimore, 1978, Johns Hopkins Press.

CalPERS: Making your health plan decision, *Perspective,* p 1, Fall 1996 (California Public Employees' Retirement System newsletter).

Cantril H: *Public opinion 1935-1946,* Princeton, NJ, 1951, Princeton University Press.

Center for Medicare and Medicaid Services (CMS): *What is Medicare,* 2003. Available at www.cms.gov.

Center for Medicare and Medicaid Services (CMS): *Medicaid: a brief summary,* 2004a. Available at www.cms.gov.

Center for Medicare and Medicaid Services (CMS): *Your Medicare benefits. Pub no. CMS-10116,* July 2004b. Avaialble at www.medicare.gov.

Department of Health and Human Services (USDHHS): Medicare coverage of skilled nursing facility care, August 2003, U.S. Printing Office, Baltimore.

Goodman JC: The regulation of medical care: is the price too high? *Cato Public Policy Research Monograph,* no. 3, San Francisco, 1980, Cato Institute.

Rosenfeld A: Managed care for the elderly: what's the problem, where's the problem? *Public Policy Aging Rep* 7(2):1, 1996.

Social Security Administration (SSA): *SSI fact sheet,* 2003. Available at www.ssa.gov.

Social Security Administration (SSA): Finding your retirement age, Available at www.socialsecurity.gov/retirementchartred.htm

Twentieth Century Fund: *Medicaid reform: a Twentieth Century Fund guide to the issues,* New York, 1995, Twentieth Century Fund Press.

Weinberger M: *Social Security: facing the facts,* Washington, DC, 1996, Cato Project on Social Security Privatization. Available at www.socialsecurity.org/pubs/ssps/ssp3.html.

25

Emotional Health in Late Life

Upon completion of this chapter, the reader will be able to:

- Identify emotional needs of elders.
- Describe crises and stressors that are likely to occur in the lives of the elderly in the community; list those that are likely for the institutionalized elder.
- Discuss the concept of anxiety, and explain several reactions that may be used to reduce the discomfort.
- Name the three most common mental health problems of elders.
- List symptoms of late-life depression, and discuss assessment, treatment, and nursing interventions.
- Recognize elders at risk of suicide, and utilize appropriate techniques for suicide assessment.
- Specify several indications of the possibility of substance abuse.
- Evaluate interventions aimed at promoting emotional health in older adults.

Compulsion An insistent and repetitive urge to perform an act contrary to the person's ordinary desires. It is a mechanism to control anxiety, and if it is interfered with, the individual will become very anxious. The classical compulsion is repetitious hand washing.

Delusion A false belief not in keeping with the individual's experience that is not subject to logic.

Denial An unconscious defense mechanism to protect against realities that the individual is not able to cope with.

Dysthymia At least 2 years of depressed mood for more days than not, accompanied by additional depressive symptoms, but symptoms do not meet the criteria for a major depressive episode.

Hallucination A false sensory perception in the absence of a real stimulus (e.g., hearing voices that no one else can hear).

Illusion Misinterpretation of a real experience (e.g., thinking a curled rope is a snake).

Major depression Five or more of the following symptoms are present for 2 weeks or more: (1) depressed mood, (2) diminished interest or pleasure, (3) loss or gain of more than 5% of body weight

within 1 month, (4) insomnia or excessive sleeping, (5) movement agitation or retardation, (6) excessive fatigue, (7) feelings of worthlessness or inappropriate guilt, (8) inability to concentrate or make decisions, (9) recurrent thoughts of death or suicide. Detailed discussion can be found in the *Diagnostic and Statistical Manual of Mental Disorders (DSM-IV)* (APA, 1994, p 327).

Minor depression The presence of at least two but fewer than five depressive symptoms, including depressed mood or loss of interest in normal activities, during the same 2-week period with no history of major depressive episode or dysthymic disorder but with clinically significant impairment or distress.

Obsession A persistent unwanted thought that cannot be eliminated by logic or reasoning; a common and benign obsession is the repetitious intrusion of a particular song into one's thoughts.

Paranoia The development of an unrealistic belief system that interprets events as persecutory. The individual may be convinced of his or her superiority or unique abilities.

Posttraumatic stress disorder Characteristic symptoms of intense psychological distress recurring, often for years, following exposure to extremely traumatic events that have incurred horror, helplessness, and paralyzing fear.

Projection An unconscious defense mechanism in which emotions unacceptable to self are attributed to others (e.g., believing your husband is unfaithful when unconsciously you would like to have an affair).

Psychoneuroimmunology The investigation of how the psyche and neurological system interact to weaken or strengthen the immune system.

Somatic displacement Physical symptoms that are caused by emotional factors and that are focused on a single organ system; commonly, back problems with no identifiable physiological explanation.

THE LIVED EXPERIENCE

An elderly man wrote his philosophy succinctly:
"I have no ideas about what would constitute happiness for anyone else, considering the differences in taste and preferences, and no spate of ideas about improving the lot of the aged. But I am sure that among other things, a calm acceptance of the facts of life is a great help. I consider serenity and peace of mind two of the greatest gifts I have, although I cannot tell you where they come from or how to get them."

From Burnside IM: Listen to the aged, Am J Nurs 75(10):1800-1803, 1975.

EMOTIONAL HEALTH IN LATE LIFE

Emotional health of the elderly is difficult to define because a lifetime of living results in many variations in personality, coping, and life patterns. One can generally say what 5 year olds or 15 year olds are like, but the same is not true for older people. Each individual becomes more uniquely himself or herself the older he or she becomes. Well-being in late life can be predicted by cognitive and affective functioning earlier in life (Qualls, 2002). The accumulation of life experience, as well as particular situations, emphasizes certain aspects of personality and appearance and diminishes others. Some apparently negative personality characteristics, such as being crusty, disagreeable, grouchy, or grumpy, may be adaptive. Thus an old man coping with a severe illness and stoically protecting others from awareness of his pain might be mentally healthy although extremely cantankerous.

Emotional health can be simply defined as a satisfactory adjustment to one's life stage and situation. An emotionally healthy person is "one who accepts the aging self as an active being, engaging available strengths to compensate for weaknesses in order to create personal meaning, maintain maximum autonomy by mastering the environment, and sustain positive relationships with

others" (Qualls, 2002, p 12). Put quite simply, "We all try to do the best with what we have" (Kivnick, 1993, p 24). Emotional health is not different in late life, but the level of challenge may be greater. What it means to be emotionally healthy is subject to many interpretations and familial and cultural influences. Emotional health, as with general health, can be thought of as being on a fluctuating continuum from wellness to illness. The absence of emotional illness does not mean one is emotionally healthy, nor does the presence of psychological symptoms mean one is emotionally or mentally ill. Individuals move back and forth on the continuum as stressors, supports, health, and resources are ample or scarce.

This chapter presents concepts of mental and emotional health and disturbances common in later life and provides specific nursing strategies to maintain and promote emotional health, self-esteem, and satisfaction of older individuals. Nurses caring for older people need to consider clients' basic human needs when attempting to assess emotional health and adaptation. Anyone who has survived the past 80 or so years has been exposed to many stressors and crises and has developed tremendous resistance. It is our task to discover the strengths and adaptive mechanisms that will assist older people to cope with stress and anxiety and to avert crises. As part of a research study on hope, spirituality, and connectedness with others among institutionalized elders, one of the authors (TT) was interviewing a 100-year-old woman who was very frail, wheelchair bound, and blind. As part of the interview, I asked her to rate her current level of hope on a scale of 0 to 10. I prepared myself to hear her say "0," and after much thought on her part, she said instead, "Oh, I think maybe an 8 or 9." Maintaining hope in the midst of losses requires a deep inner strength that many older people possess. We can learn much from older people about coping with life and thriving, not merely surviving. Gerontological nurses must create relationships and environments of hope to promote emotional health for older people.

Demographics and Services

Currently, nearly 20% of people over the age of 55 experience emotional disorders that are not a part of normal aging, and these figures are expected to significantly increase in the next 25 years. The most prevalent disorders are anxiety, severe cognitive impairment, and mood disorders. These mental disorders are underreported. The rate of suicide is higher in older adults than in any other age group, with those age 85 and over having the highest suicide rate—twice the national average. Stigma about having a mental or emotional disorder (being "crazy"), particularly for older people, discourages many from seeking treatment. Less than one half of elders who acknowledge mental health problems receive any treatment from any provider. The rate of utilization of mental health services is less than that of any other age group.

Moorehead and Brighton (2001) report several studies suggesting that a substantial number of elders are suffering anxiety, substance abuse, and somatoform disorders that were unrecognized and untreated. Medical patients with chronic illnesses present with psychiatric disorders in 25% to 33% of cases, although they are unrecognized by primary health practitioners much of the time. Lack of knowledge on the part of health care providers about emotional health in late life presents another barrier to appropriate diagnosis and treatment. Older people underutilize mental health services when they are available; only one half of those who acknowledge their mental disorder receive treatment. Less than 3% see mental health professionals for treatment (APA Fact Sheet on Mental Health and Aging; accessed 8/8/04 from http://www.apa.org). Compounding the problem of inadequate services is the limited coverage for mental health care under Medicare and Medicaid. Several gaps exist in the delivery of mental health services to the elderly both in the community and in long-term care settings.

Prevalence of mental illness among nursing home residents is high with estimates that two thirds of residents have diagnosable mental disorders and one fourth have depression (Frampton, 2004). Staff members in nursing homes are often ill prepared to provide mental health care (Beck et al, 2002). A recent report of the Surgeon General in 2000 spoke of the mental health needs of the elderly population and verified the need for therapy services in long-term care. Whereas some services are available and reimbursed, the mainstay of treatment is medication with little attention to individual counseling or group work. (Chapter 5 discusses reminiscence and life review techniques that can be effective for depression.) The various revisions of the Omnibus Budget Reconciliation Act (OBRA) and the implementation of the Minimum Data Set (MDS) have resulted in reduction of chemical and physical restraints in nursing homes, but more attention must be paid to the mental health of older people in these settings.

Gerontological nurses must be advocates for better and more appropriate treatment of mental health needs for older people and should closely monitor proposals for federal and state revisions and budget cuts in this area. Geropsychiatric nursing is the specialty care that nurses provide to elders with mental health disorders. Few educational programs focus on this specialty, but all gerontological nurses should be knowledgeable about geropsychiatric nursing care.

EMOTIONAL NEEDS IN LATE LIFE

There is much that we do not yet understand about the connection between emotions and health and illness, although we know that some emotions for some people result in illness. Stress theorists are interested in understanding the process by which demands exceed the adaptive capacity of the organism and result in psychological and biological changes that place the person at risk of disease. Many studies in psychoneuroimmunology (PNI) are being conducted to more clearly determine the connection between mind and body.

According to Maslow (1970), the author of the model we have found most useful in caring for older people, certain human needs must be fulfilled to ensure maximal function and satisfaction. In later life, when the basic physiological systems are gradually losing efficacy over time, the needs for safety and security, a sense of belonging, and intimacy become supremely important.

Safety and Security

The external issues of safety and security are considered in Chapter 22. These are relatively simple to address if there is a real desire to do so. A deep, internal sense of insecurity develops as elders discover that the body they have taken for granted most of their lives begins to betray them; organ systems work less effectively, and automatic actions and reactions require concentration. This then becomes the source of much anxiety and erodes one's security. Compensation for impairments and sensory deficits and the opportunity to continue personal rituals that provide daily structure and security will help ensure feelings of safety and reduce anxiety. Specific manifestations of anxiety and interventions are considered later in this chapter. Appropriate living situations significantly affect one's sense of security and safety. These are discussed in Chapter 27.

Belonging

As individuals in the support system become less readily available and the society moves forward without the elder's input or major contributions, the sense of belonging is diminished and the opportunity to be an active participant with others is steadily decreased. The family and its elder members are considered in Chapter 23. Elders without involved family or partners and geriatric orphans, especially those who are institutionalized, will need to develop surrogate family or caring groups and affiliations that meet their need for belonging. Gerontological nurses in long-term care settings often fill these needs in what has been referred to as "like family."

Intimacy and Sexuality

The need for closeness and intimacy remains throughout life regardless of opportunity. Many older individuals say that they enjoy simply being cuddled and held, but others seek sexual satisfaction through intercourse. The opportunity for intimacy and for sexual expression as a component of intimacy may be virtually unattainable for very old persons whose lifelong partner has died or for elders who are institutionalized. Although professionals give lip service to this need, some are surprised when actually confronted with it. Many elders consider physical intimacy an important aspect of their lives.

In assessing the need for sexual activity, one must be wary of reticence and of inflicting one's own values. A 95-year-old man was found to be actively involved with prostitutes who would come to his low-rent high-rise apartment when he requested it. His housekeeper was upset when she discovered this, as were the nursing students involved in his health care. The housekeeper feared that the prostitutes would steal from him, and the students feared that he might contract a sexually transmitted disease (STD). These are legitimate concerns, but the first and most important issue is the confrontation of health care providers' attitudes toward elders and sexual activities. Suggestions for discussing sexuality with elders are presented in Box 25-1 and may be helpful guidelines for nurses not sure how to approach this discussion.

The normal sexual changes of aging are considered in Chapter 7. Erectile dysfunction (impotence) is a common problem among older men and one that may be personally devastating. Erectile dysfunction in old age is frequently related to disease entities, such as diabetes, medications, alcohol, depression, and long periods of abstinence. There are several medical strategies for erectile dysfunction, but with the advent of sildenafil citrate (Viagra) and vardenafil hydrochloride (Levitra), these may be less often necessary. Some men have had penile implants and find them satisfactory. The method of maintaining an erection must be effective and acceptable to the man and his partner. Nurses are responsible for identifying and addressing health-related issues that interfere with life satisfaction, and therefore it is appropriate for nurses to ask, "Are your needs for intimacy being met?" The nurse may assist the elderly in obtaining information and referrals.

Box 25-1	Guidelines for Health Care Providers in Talking to Older Adults About Sexual Health

Health Care Providers Should Spend Time with Older Adults
- Be available to discuss the subject.
- Give us your full attention.
- Allow time to ask questions.
- Take time to answer questions.

Health Care Providers Should Use Clear and Easy-to-Understand Words
- Use plain, everyday language.
- Explain medical terms in plain English.
- Give explanations or answers to questions in simple terms.

Health Care Providers Should Help Older Adults Feel Comfortable Talking About Sex
- Help us to break the ice.
- Make us feel comfortable in asking questions.
- Offer permission to express feelings and needs.
- Do not be afraid or embarrassed to discuss sexuality problems.

Health Care Providers Should Be Open Minded and Talk Openly
- Do not assume there are no concerns.
- Be open.
- Ask direct questions about sexual activity and attitudes.
- Discuss sexual concerns freely.
- Answer questions honestly.
- Just talk about it.
- Do not evade sexual concerns.
- Be willing to discuss sexual problems.
- Probe sexual concerns if elder wishes.

Health Care Providers Should Listen
- Be prepared to listen.
- Listen so we feel you are interested in our problems.
- Let us talk.

Health Care Providers Should Treat Older Adults with a Respectful and Nonjudgmental Attitude
- See us as individuals with sexual needs.
- Accept us for what we are: gay, straight, bisexual.
- Be nonjudgmental.
- Show genuine concern and respect.

Health Care Providers Should Encourage Discussion
- Make opportunities for one-to-one discussion.
- Provide privacy.
- Promote candid discussion.
- Provide discussion groups to ask questions.
- Develop support groups.

Health Care Providers Can Give Advice or Suggestions
- Provide information.
- Offer to find solutions and alternatives to given situations.
- Provide explicit pamphlets; explain sexual positions, lubrication.
- Discuss old taboos.
- Give suggestions of ways to help solve sexual problems.

Health Care Providers Need to Understand That Sex Is Not Just for the Young
- Try to eliminate the idea that sex and love are just for younger people.
- Acknowledge that sexual impulses are healthy and do not disappear as individuals age.
- Treat older adults as normal sexual beings and not as asexual elderly people.
- Recognize that sex can improve—can become even better when one is older.

From Johnson B: Older adults' suggestions for health care providers regarding discussions of sex, *Geriatr Nurs* 18(2):65-66, 1997.

Unmet Needs

Unmet needs may be submerged and appear in the form of various defense mechanisms or behavioral distortions. Deprivations result in reactions that may or may not be health enhancing. The nurse's task is to provide appropriate resources for resolving the issue to the extent possible and to listen, knowing that we all are connected and will be that individual with the same need at some point. To be truly heard provides the feelings of security, belonging, and intimacy that are so necessary but often unavailable in our economically and mechanistically oriented society. When the needs are not addressed or even recognized, various manifestations will occur.

Psychological Assessment of Elders

General issues in the psychological assessment of older adults involve distinguishing among normal, idiosyncratic, and diverse characteristics of aging and pathological conditions. Using standardized tools and functional assessment is valuable, but the data must be placed in the context of the person's early life and hopes and expectations for the future. Distinguishing normal from pathological aging in a particular individual depends on these factors. Although some age-appropriate assessment instruments are available, many of the tools available were developed for younger people. Further research is needed in developing appropriate tools, especially for people with dementia.

Assessment of mental health includes examination for cognitive function or impairment and the specific conditions of anxiety and adjustment reactions, depression, paranoia, substance abuse, and suicidal risk. Assessment of mental health must also focus on social intactness and affectual responses appropriate to the situation. Attention span, concentration, intelligence, judgment, learning ability, memory, orientation, perception, problem solving, psychomotor ability, and reaction time are assessed in relation to cognitive intactness and must be considered when making a psychological assessment (see Chapter 14 for assessment tools). Cognitive function is considered in Chapters 8 and 21.

Obtaining assessment data from elders is best done during short sessions after some rapport has been established. Performing repeated assessments at various times of day and in different situations will give a more complete psychological profile. It is important to be sensitive to a client's anxiety, special needs, and disabilities and vigilant in protecting the person's privacy. The interview should be focused so that attention is given to strengths and skills as well as deficits. It is also useful to take a psychological inventory of the older adult client (Box 25-2).

STRESS AND STRESSORS IN LATE LIFE

The experience of stress is an internal state accompanying threats to self. Healthy stress levels motivate one toward growth, whereas stress overload diminishes one's ability to cope effectively. Ongoing stressors may create moderate anxiety and be accompanied by unconscious alterations in behavior, such as repetitive actions, that discharge the anxious feelings in specific and observable symptoms. Many changes and losses compounded may result in anxiety that has no specific trigger that the elder can identify. Among the older adults, stress is likely to appear as cognitive impairment.

During the course of the later years many situations and conditions occur that erode confidence in one's self and stir negative feelings. Restoration of a sense of control is basic to moving beyond the helplessness experienced during crises, stress, and illness. No generation has faced so many changes or had its mettle so tested. This provides a beginning focus of discussion with elders feeling uncertain and incapable of making the changes necessary in their situation. It is sometimes necessary to remind elders of all the major events that they have survived (see Chapter 1 for discussion of these) and help them call on the coping strategies used that may be helpful in dealing with current crises. Our task is to restore faith in one's adaptive capacity and self-directed action. Older people who are resilient (getting back up when circumstances get them down) deal with problems and losses better. These skills can be learned or strengthened in late life and certainly benefit younger people as well. Resilient persons cope with changing circumstances and deal with the problems of daily life by doing the following:

- Talking to people who can do something to fix the problem
- Sharing their feelings and making a plan of action
- Finding ways to compensate for their losses
- Relying on and trusting their faith or spirituality
- Using their sense of humor to reduce tension
- Using their life experiences to solve problems
- Keeping an overall positive outlook

Stressors in the present, whether acute or chronic, require action and inner resources to

| **Box 25-2** | **Inventory of Psychogeriatric Client: Function and Care Plan** |

1. List client's strengths:
- Ability to take initiative in caring for self, finances, work project
- Ability to express feelings
- Ability to stand up for his or her rights
- Ability to make decisions
- Ability to care for self; for example, dressing, going to meals
- Ability to share with others or show concern for others
- Enjoyment of music and arts
- Active participation in organizations
- Interest in sports
- Enjoyment of reading
- Imagination and creativity
- Special aptitudes; for example, mechanical ability, gardening

2. Identify predominant defensive coping styles:
- Denial
- Projection
- Displacement
- Passive aggression
- Positive identification

3. Identify highly adaptive coping styles:
- Affiliation
- Altruism
- Humor
- Self-assertion
- Sublimation

4. Identify defensive breakdown patterns:
- Delusional projection
- Psychotic suspiciousness
- Psychotic denial
- Immobilizing fears
- Psychotic distortions
- Apathetic withdrawal

5. Determine client needs and problems based on the following:
- Reason for seeking assistance by patient, family, and others

- Medical history and findings (physical, mental, neurological, and psychological examinations and tests)
- Drug use profile (use of prescribed and nonprescribed drugs)
- Laboratory and diagnostic tests
- Psychiatric history
- Social history
- Mental status
- Other background information provided by patient, family, and each staff person who has interviewed the patient

6. Develop a nursing care plan considering the following:
- Patient's problems, needs, and strengths
- Mutually identified short-term goals
- Mutually identified long-term goals

7. State expected outcome of care in terms that can be measured. The following are examples of goals stated in measurable terms:
- Socializes more
- Dresses appropriately—puts on coat or jacket when going outside in cold weather
- Improves personal hygiene—brushes teeth daily without being reminded
- Shows improvement in problem areas
- Improves attitude—discusses problems or concerns instead of hitting or resisting
- Increases functional independence
- Reduces hostility—responds when spoken to in a friendly manner
- Improves self-esteem—goes 1 day without self-criticism
- Reduces depression—expresses interest in one outside activity
- States increased enjoyment of activities
- Reduces suspiciousness—eats a meal without expressing fear of poisoning

8. Review progress periodically, and revise goals as necessary and appropriate.

---

avert crises. Some that are common to older adults include the following:
- Caregiving of a spouse with dementia
- Illness or health care system concerns
- Relocation and dispersal of significant belongings
- Loss of children, cohorts, siblings, or friends
- Incompetency proceedings
- Inheritance conflicts

- Abandonment: fear of dying alone, not being found, or painful death
- Hospitalization or institutionalization, costs, and loss of independence
- Separation from the elder's personal physician
- Sensory changes (vision and hearing)
- Housing and home maintenance
- Lack of protection when frail and vulnerable

- Limited mobility and lack of transportation
- Unnamed concerns about the future
- Fear of dementia
- Social losses or loss of the elder's driver's license
- Acute and chronic pain
- Medications
- Abuse and neglect
- Loss of pet
- Uncertainties about financial resources
- Designing interventions for stress management

The following are suggestions to consider in designing interventions for stress management:

- Change is stressful; therefore interventions should impose as few changes as possible.
- Older people may be reluctant to seek help because of pride of independence, stoic acceptance of difficulty, unawareness of resources, and fear of being "put away."
- Older people who are resilient (getting back up when circumstances get them down) deal with problems and losses better. These skills can be learned or strengthened.
- Continuity of personnel and having as few persons as possible to administer services leave the client more energy to deal with the problem at hand.
- Timing is important. Individuals have personal time clocks that order their peak efficiency daily, monthly, and developmentally; use the best times to introduce change.
- Another aspect of timing to consider is the timing of stresses. More energy will be needed to integrate events that have occurred within the previous 6 weeks, 6 months, or 1 year than those occurring in the remote past.
- Older people often experience multiple, simultaneous stresses, and reduction of anxiety is necessary before options for intervention can be considered.
- Some older people are in a chronic state of grief because losses are never fully resolved before another one occurs; stress then becomes a constant state of being. Further discussion of grief can be found in Chapter 26.
- The individual needs to understand that resolution may be slower than expected if he or she has recently been bombarded with change.
- Exercise, yoga, and relaxation strategies may be helpful to include in a stress management program.

Posttraumatic Stress Disorder

Posttraumatic stress disorder (PTSD) has become part of our national vocabulary and reminds us of the deep and lasting toll that national disasters take. PTSD was originally recognized as an outcome of overwhelmingly stressful experiences of individuals in the war in Vietnam. Only recently realized is that many World War II veterans have lived the majority of their lives under the shadow of PTSD without it being recognized. Seniors now under our care have also experienced the Great Depression, the holocaust, racism, and the Korea conflict (Kennedy, 2001). Rape, child abuse, physical violence, assault, mugging, natural or man-made disasters, and life-threatening illnesses with all of the attendant medical treatments and torments are traumatic events that may leave permanent psychological scars.

PTSD is a syndrome characterized by the development of symptoms following an extremely traumatic event, which involves experiencing, witnessing, or unexpectedly hearing about an actual or threatened death or serious injury to oneself or another closely affiliated person. It can also result from prolonged exposure to lowered level, but still significant, emotional trauma. Individuals often re-experience the traumatic event in episodes of fear and experience symptoms such as helplessness, flashbacks, intrusive thoughts, memories, images, emotional numbing, loss of interest, avoidance of any place that reminds of the traumatic event, startle reactions, poor concentration, irritability, jumpiness, and hypervigilance. These episodes may occur periodically for years, although they frequently remain submerged until activated by the losses of aging. An instrument to assess post-traumatic stress can be found at www.hartfordign.org.

A person who becomes cognitively impaired may no longer be able to control thoughts, flashbacks, or images. This can be the cause of great distress that may be attributed to aggressive or hostile behavior. An example of this occurred in a Veterans Administration (VA) nursing home with an 80-year-old WWII veteran resident who became very agitated and attempted to hit others around him when he was placed in the large day room with other residents. The staff recognized this as a PTSD reaction from his years as a prisoner of war and always placed him in a smaller day room near the nursing station away from the other residents. The aggression stopped without the need for medications. Bludau (2002) described the concept of second institutionalization that occurs in nursing home residents who are Holocaust survivors.

PTSD prevention and treatment are only now getting the research attention that other illnesses have received over the years (Culpepper, 2000). The care of the individual with PTSD involves awareness that certain events may trigger inappropriate reactions, and the pattern of these reactions should be identified when possible. Cognitive-behavioral therapy with pharmacological therapy is of benefit. Sertraline and paroxetine have U.S. Food and Drug Administration (FDA) approval for treatment of PTSD. Nursing supports include humor, distraction, teaching relaxation techniques, back massage, support groups with guided imagery, therapeutic touch, and information provided to family members (Moorehead, Brighton, 2001). Effective coping with extremely traumatic events that created intense fear and helplessness seems to be associated with secure and supportive relationships; the ability to freely express or fully suppress the experience; favorable circumstances immediately following the trauma; productive and active lifestyles; strong faith, religion, and hope; a sense of humor; and biological integrity.

Crises

Crises and stressful situations occur throughout life but are thought to occur less frequently in the later years, although with more devastating effects, when one may have less reserve adaptive capacity and fewer available supports. *Stress* and *crisis* are not the same. Crisis events always create stress, but stressful situations do not necessarily precipitate crises. Any stressors that occur in the lives of older adults may actually be experienced as a crisis if the event occurs abruptly, is unanticipated, requires skills or resources the elder does not possess, or results in personality disorganization or psychological immobility.

Psychological homeostasis, comparable with and intertwined with physiological homeostasis, fluctuates in the elderly within a reduced range of normal. The daily habits and rituals provide points of security and bolster stress immunity. When crises and cumulative stresses stretch the limits of coping capacity beyond one's individu-

---

Box 25-3	Crises Common to Older Adults

- Abrupt internal and external body changes and illnesses
- Other-oriented concerns: children, grandchildren, spouse
- Loss of significant people
- Acute discomfort and pain
- Breach in significant relationships
- Fires, thefts
- Injuries, falls
- Translocation
- Aphasia, abrupt loss following stroke
- Abrupt loss of mobility or source of transportation
- Major unexpected drain on economic resources (e.g., house repair, illness)
- Abrupt changes in housing, especially without warning, to a new location, home, apartment, room, or institution
- Death of roommates in institutions

---

ally established range, adaptive behavior temporarily deteriorates. Helplessness, lack of control, and dependency may emerge, as well as personality aberrations. It is important to remember that these are temporary conditions and will generally subside as some degree of personal power is restored. Crises common to the older adults include those listed in Box 25-3.

Some individuals have developed, through a lifetime of coping with stress, a tremendous stress tolerance, whereas others will be thrown into crisis by changes in their life with which they feel unable to cope. The critical factor is personal perception of an event. The degree of personal disorganization is reflective of one's self-esteem and sense of capability more than the magnitude of the event. Reactions to a perceived crisis include (1) anxiety, fear, a sense of unreality, and detachment; (2) restlessness, inability to sit still, searching for something to do, disorganized behavior, and repetitiously performing behaviors that are no longer effective; (3) detachment and watchful waiting; (4) ruminating thoughts of guilt, incompetence, helplessness, questioning, confusion, and paranoia; and (5) physical reactions of exhaustion, anorexia, and other symptoms of grief as explained in Chapter 26.

Recognizing characteristics of and reactions to crises will alert nurses to organize crisis intervention strategies. We have most frequently observed detachment, apathy, inability to make decisions, and disorganized behavior in elders experiencing a crisis. Crises and stressful situations may produce emotions that erode the health of the frail older person. When the events exceed a critical, but individually variable, level of demand on the already-vulnerable physical homeostasis, illness is likely. The numerous unexpected natural disasters that occur each year leave many elderly displaced or homeless. Tornadoes, hurricanes, cyclones, floods, tropical storms, firestorms, and earthquakes are examples of such events. In addition, there are terrorist acts, bombings, killings, and accidents that occur suddenly and without preparation. All these are likely to generate crises and difficulty coping. They may or may not resolve quickly, depending on the person, as well as the quality and immediacy of interventions. These events may trigger PTSD, as discussed earlier. Events that evoke personal body threat and terror are most difficult to integrate.

Crisis Intervention Strategies

Crisis intervention is designed to resolve the immediate problem and to restore the person to the level of function that existed before the crisis occurred. The immediate interventions must be geared to alleviating some of the anxiety and the problem that most disturbs the elder. Immediate actions must decrease discomfort sufficiently to gain the elder's attention and cooperation.

Dealing with older persons in crisis differs from dealing with younger persons. Increased chronic medical problems, decreased ability to manage without assistance, and living alone combine to produce a situation requiring supportive therapy. Crisis management may involve many referrals and ongoing case management. Some specific suggestions for crisis intervention with older adults include the following:

1. Maintain routine and usual habits as much as possible.
2. Clarify cognitive perception of the disruptive event.
3. Learn the person's characteristic behavior.
4. Encourage reminiscing to learn about self-esteem, affect, character, past coping patterns, and uniqueness and to restore a sense of control and capability.
5. Encourage expression of feelings toward tension discharge and mastery.
6. Listen to complaints; do not dismiss any as unimportant; help resolve predominant complaints.
7. Develop a readily available support system; identify and use existing systems when they are supportive; and build up external supports.
8. Give adequate information to the client, but avoid overload; sometimes the information will need to be written and/or repeated.
9. Attend to physical comfort measures.
10. Use touch as appropriate.

Crisis as Growth

Growth occurs through crisis if the process is recognized and coping efforts are supported and augmented as needed. Many symptoms of emotional disorders are evidence of an ineffective search for resolution of an earlier problem. Recognizing these symptoms may assist nurses in reassuring clients of their potential strength. Rather than attempting to ameliorate or ignore symptoms of crisis states, we might encourage recognition and acceptance. Nurses may wish to pose alternative solutions long before the client has reached a state of readiness. This is not helpful. Timing is critical. Recognize stages, and validate verbally (e.g., "It seems as if your thoughts are going in circles. That is a necessary step before you can move on to resolution of the problem.").

The next section of the chapter discusses psychiatric conditions as well as symptoms that may be seen in older people that do not meet the criteria for diagnosable psychiatric illness or psychotic disorders. Some symptoms and presentations may be considered coping strategies or temporary states in response to stress and crisis. The incidence of late-life onset of psychotic disorders is low among older people, but psychosis can occur as a secondary syndrome in a variety of disorders, the most common being Alzheimer's disease. Psychotic symptoms in Alzheimer's disease require different assessment and treatment than long-standing psychotic disorders (see Chapter 21). Depression (the most common emotional health problem in late life), suicide, and alcohol and drug dependence are also discussed.

ANXIETY REACTIONS

A general definition for anxiety is unpleasant and unwarranted feelings of apprehension, which may be accompanied by physical symptoms. Anxiety itself is a normal human reaction and part of a fear response; it is rational, within reason. Anxiety becomes problematic when it is prolonged, is exaggerated, and interferes with function. Anxiety meeting the criteria for a diagnosable disorder ranges from 3.5% to 10% of older people. In women over 65 years of age 10% to 15% find anxiety symptoms sufficiently distressing to visit a physician (Hegel et al, 2002). Risk factors for anxiety disorders in older people include the following: female; urban living; history of worrying or rumination; poor physical health; low socioeconomic status; high stress life events; and depression and alcoholism. Generalized anxiety disorder (GAD) is the most common anxiety disorder in the elderly, although it is underdiagnosed and undertreated. GAD is commonly related to life events, such as illness, bereavement, social and financial status changes, and cognitive impairment. Worry is the primary feature of GAD, and anxiety symptoms frequently co-exist with depression (Frampton, 2004). Other anxiety disorders that occur in older people include phobic disorder, obsessive-compulsive disorder, and panic disorders.

The general and pervasive nature of anxiety may make diagnosis difficult in older adults. In addition, older people tend to deny psychological symptoms, attribute anxiety-related symptoms to physical illness, and have co-existent medical conditions that mimic symptoms of generalized anxiety. Some of the medical disorders that cause anxiety responses include cardiac dysrhythmias, delirium, depression, dementia (probably the most common cause of anxiety), congestive heart failure, hyperthyroidism, hypoglycemia, postural hypotension, pulmonary edema, and pulmonary emboli. Drugs that cause anxiety reactions are anticholinergics, caffeine, digitalis, theophylline, antihypertensives (clonidine), beta blockers, beta-adrenergic stimulators (albuterol), corticosteroids, and over-the-counter drugs such as appetite suppressants, nicotine, and cough and cold preparations containing ephedrine. Withdrawal from alcohol, sedatives, and hypnotics will cause symptoms of anxiety. Some strategies used by older

Box 25-4	Defense Mechanisms Used to Reduce Anxiety

- *Denial* may be intrinsic to aging and necessary to maintain one's equilibrium in the face of major losses and impending demise of self.
- *Projection* is often used to give vent to inexpressible wishes and feelings; it signals high levels of internal stress.
- *Regression* may be temporarily necessary to mobilize energy and resources to cope with external stressors.
- *Displacement* may help the elder to submerge feelings of anxiety and fasten on something more concrete and controllable.
- *Somatization* is a common means of dealing with psychosocial problems and is very hard to circumvent, since it brings secondary gains if not overused.
- *Selective* memory tends to focus one on the memories that exemplify and corroborate present feelings, whatever they may be.
- *Compulsivity* allows one to keep control in a comforting way of certain aspects of life when the larger issues are overwhelming.

adults that might appear as maladaptive personality traits if predominant in other situations are effective in reducing anxiety in elders and should be respected (Box 25-4).

It is important to assess the older adult for anxiety symptoms as well as investigate other possible causes, such as medical conditions and depression. Clinical signs that suggest an anxiety reaction include restlessness, edginess, fatigue, difficulty concentrating, irritability, tension, and sleep disturbances. When co-morbid conditions are present, they need to be treated. A review of medications is in order, eliminating those that cause anxiety. When dealing with anxiety reactions, look for daily disturbances, such as staff or caregiver changes, room changes, or events over which the individual feels a lack of control or influence. By themselves, these circumstances seldom provoke an anxiety reaction, but they may be "the straw that breaks the camel's back," particularly in frail elders.

Medications that have been found to be especially useful are paroxetine and venlafaxine, particularly when depression is present (Reuben et al, 2002). Benzodiazepines (lorazepam, oxazepam) may be recommended for short-term therapy. All these medications can have problematic side effects, such as sedation, falls, altered mental status, and dependence (see Chapter 15). Although useful, they are often prescribed without adequate assessment of the multitude of factors contributing to anxiety symptoms. Nonbenzodiazepine anxiolytic agents (buspirone) may also be used. Buspirone has fewer side effects but requires a longer dosing time for effectiveness. Other interventions such as cognitive-behavioral therapy, relaxation training, exercise, anxiety management, supportive interventions, and interpersonal psychotherapy, often in combination with medication, have been shown to be of benefit and need further study in this population (Hegel et al, 2002). Anxiety disorders and their treatment have not been well studied, particularly in older people.

Obsessive-Compulsive Disorder

Obsessive-compulsive disorder (OCD) is characterized by recurrent and persistent thoughts, impulses, or images (obsessions) that are repetitive, purposeful, and intentional urge or ritualistic behaviors (compulsions) that improve comfort level but are recognized as excessive and unreasonable. OCD is an anxiety disorder that significantly interferes with function and consumes more than 1 hour each day (APA, 1994). OCD symptoms are common among elderly people, seem to have a genetic component, and occur mainly in women. These disorders are exaggerated manifestations of a need for control and order and a way of warding off anxiety. Often in elderly people, symptoms are not sufficient to be considered a disorder but rather a coping strategy. If symptoms progress to the point where they disrupt the lifestyle, they will need clinical attention.

In older adults, these disorders are often displayed as obsessions about body functions, particularly elimination and sleep. The compulsive rituals that accompany these thoughts are an effort to ward off anxiety and discharge tension. Carrying out these tension-relief behaviors must be respected if they do not interfere with important aspects of life. As with other anxiety disor-

ders, exercise and cognitive-behavioral therapy have been shown to be effective in management of OCD, in combination with pharmacological therapy if indicated. Medication therapy with sertraline, paroxetine, fluoxetine, and fluvoxamine is recommended (Reuben et al, 2002).

Excessive Suspicion and Paranoia

Paranoia is characterized by suspiciousness and insecurity. Many older people with no previous history of mental disturbance develop a suspicious or paranoid viewpoint. Various estimates of the prevalence of paranoia range from 5% to 10% of the older adult population. These reactions are sometimes induced by alcoholism or medications, and hearing impairment may accentuate these feelings. Fear and a lack of trust originating from a reality base may become magnified, especially when one is isolated from others and does not receive reality feedback. The majority of reactions, however, originate in attempts to exert control in an unsatisfactory situation or to feel capable. Inability to correctly evaluate the social milieu because of isolation or cognitive disturbance is a significant factor.

Paranoia is an early symptom of Alzheimer's disease, appearing approximately 20 months before diagnosis. In his description of a woman with a peculiar disease of the cerebral cortex, Dr. Alois Alzheimer described the first noticeable symptoms of the illness as suspiciousness of her husband and believing that people were out to murder her. Memory loss and forgetfulness may result in an elder being convinced that items are being stolen. The dynamics seem to be loss of control and inability to evaluate the social milieu appropriately, with the feeling of external forces controlling one's life, which in many instances is true.

In addition to these dynamics, an unknown number of elders have a paranoid personality disorder that has simply grown old and more pronounced. These individuals have had a pervasive distrust and suspiciousness of others' motives all of their adult life, assuming that others will harm, exploit, or even deceive them, although they have no basis to support these beliefs (APA, 1994). It is sometimes difficult to determine the reality of an apparent paranoid reaction. Many cases have been encountered in which plots against an older person were real.

Delusions

Delusions are beliefs that guide one's interpretation of events and help make sense out of disorder. The delusions may be comforting or threatening, but they always form a structure for understanding situations that otherwise might seem unmanageable. A delusional disorder is one in which conceivable ideas, without foundation in fact, persist for more than 1 month. These beliefs are not always bizarre and do not originate in psychotic processes (APA, 1994). Common delusions are of being poisoned, of children taking their assets, of being held prisoner, or of being deceived by a spouse or lover. Delusional disorders in the absence of psychoses usually begin earlier in life but may continue into old age. In older adults, delusions often incorporate significant persons rather than the global grandiose or persecutory delusions of younger persons. When an individual becomes incapable of obtaining life's satisfactions or of maintaining function or adequate supplies, the delusions may allow the individual to avoid depression and maintain self-esteem by projecting blame onto others or society. One elderly woman persistently held onto the delusion that her son was a very important attorney and was coming to force the administration to discharge her from the nursing home. Her son, a factory worker, had been dead for 10 years. The events of her day, her hopes, and her status were all organized around this belief. It is clear that without her delusion she would have felt forlorn, lost, and abandoned. Many delusions related to family members and their actions or intentions occur among institutionalized older people. Some may aid in coping whereas others may be troubling to the person. One study found that 21% of 125 new nursing home residents had delusions (Grossberg, 2000).

The assessment dilemma is often one of determining the truth of the delusional belief and avoiding assumptions. It is never safe to conclude that someone is delusional unless you have thoroughly investigated his or her claims. In one case an 88-year-old man insisted that he must go and visit his mother. His thoughts seemed clear in other respects (often the case with people who are delusional), and one of the authors (P.E.) suspected that he had some unresolved conflicts about his dead mother or felt the need of comforting and caring. I did not argue with him about his dead mother, since arguing is never a useful approach to persons with delusions. Rather, I used the best techniques I could think of to assure him that I was interested in him as a person and recognized that he must feel very lonely sometimes. He continued to say that he must go and visit his mother. When I could delay his leaving no longer, I walked with him to the nurses' station and found that his 104-year-old mother did indeed live in another wing of the institution and that he visited her every day.

Frightening delusions, such as feeling that one is being poisoned, are usually in response to anxiety-provoking situations and are best managed by reducing situational stress, being available to the person, and attending to the fears more than the content of the delusion. Other suggestions are to avoid television, which can be confusing, especially if the person awakens and finds it on. In addition, reduce clutter in the person's room, eliminate large mirrors, and eliminate shadows that can appear threatening. Provide glasses and hearing aids to maximize sensory input and decrease misinterpretations.

Interventions for Delusions and Paranoia

Direct confrontation is likely to increase anxiety and agitation, the sense of vulnerability, and the need for the delusion; it also may disrupt the relationship. A more useful approach is to establish a trusting relationship that is nondemanding and not too intense. It is important to identify the client's strengths and build on them. This will reduce the alienation and feelings of insignificance that underlie paranoid ideation. Demonstrating respect and a willingness to listen to complaints and fears is important. It is important that the nurse be trustworthy, give clear information, and present clear choices. Do not pretend to agree with paranoid beliefs, but rather ask what is troubling to the person and provide reassurance of safety. When encountering suspicious elderly, the nurse's primary concern is first directed at establishing the reality of the feeling, but if the suspicions are not substantiated, the elder should not be challenged. Other strategies include not arguing with the person or giving false reassurance. Paranoia may act as an effective shield

Box 25-5	Guidelines for Nursing Care of Suspicious Patients

Remember that anger is pervasive and is not meant for the nurse per se.

Anger is a legitimate expression of feeling.

Suspicious persons will look for flaws or indications of injustice.

Attempt to accept criticism without resentment or defensiveness.

Arguing only increases the struggle for control.

The quality of nursing care may not be measurable by patient progress, particularly if the goals are unrealistic or not relevant to the patient. In other words, paranoia may lift slowly or not at all.

Nursing care should provide for the following needs:

1. Suspicious persons need to learn to trust themselves. Allow the patient to function independently in areas in which success can be achieved and identified.

2. Suspicious persons need to be able to trust others. Nurses should state what they are willing and able to do. Vague promises, such as "I'll be around whenever you need me," only increase opportunities for distrust and disappointment.

3. Suspicious persons need to test reality. When the larger reality is distorted, focus on smaller aspects of reality; for example:

    Mrs. J.: The whole world is against me.

    Nurse: What in this room gives you that feeling? Are there certain times when you feel that most strongly?

    Contact with the nurse and the nurse's accepting responses reassure the person and decrease the need for protective delusion.

4. Suspicious persons need outlets for their anger.

against intrusion into one's vulnerable state and as such may be a useful defensive posture. The presence of paranoid ideation is a problem only if it disturbs the patient or others in his or her environment. If symptoms are interfering with function, antipsychotic drugs may be needed for effective management (Beers, Berkow, 2000). The newer atypical antipsychotics (risperidone, olanzapine) are preferred. Careful monitoring for side effects is essential. Box 25-5 presents other guidelines for care.

Hallucinations

Hallucinations are best described as sensory perceptions of a nonexistent external stimulus and may be spurred by the internal stimulation of any of the five senses. Although not attributable to environmental stimuli, hallucinations may well occur because of the total environmental impact. Hallucinations arising out of psychological conflicts tend to be less predominant in old age, and those that are generated as security measures tend to increase. These hallucinations are thought to germinate in situations in which one is feeling alone, abandoned, isolated, or alienated. To compensate for insecurity, a hallucinatory experience, often in the form of a companion, is imagined.

Imagined companions may fill the intense void and provide some security, but they sometimes become accusing and disturbing.

The character and stages of hallucinatory experiences have not been adequately defined in late life. Many hallucinations are in response to physical disorders, such as dementia, Parkinson's disease, physiological and sensory disorders, and medications. Hallucinations of older adults most often seem mixed with disorientation, illusions, intense grief, and immersion in retrospection, the origins being difficult to separate. Most psychotic states in late life are associated predominantly with cognitive decline. Grossberg (2000) found that between 33% and 50% of elderly people with Alzheimer's disease or other dementias develop psychotic symptoms, and 63% to 67% develop delusions or hallucinations. Older people with severe vision and hearing deficits may also experience hearing voices or seeing people and objects that are not actually present (illusions). Some have explained this as the brain's attempt to create stimulation in the absence of adequate sensory input. If these illusions are not disturbing to the person, they do not need treatment.

Determining whether the hallucinations are the result of dementia, psychoses, deprivation, or overload is important because the treatment will vary. An isolated older person who is admitted to the hospital in a hallucinatory state must be carefully and thoroughly assessed physically and then gradually brought into socializing experiences. A subdued environment with staff continuity is important, and the person should be allowed peripheral participation and retreat when necessary. Individuals in the community who develop hallucinations must be assessed in terms of threats to security, severe physical or psychological disruptions, withdrawal symptoms, medications, and overload of stimuli. Antipsychotic medications are a significant aspect of management for hallucinations that impair function.

SCHIZOPHRENIA

The onset of schizophrenia usually occurs between adolescence and the mid-thirties, and the occurrence of schizophrenia is rare in older people. Older adults with late-onset schizophrenia show less formal thought disorder than younger people (Palmer et al, 2002). Theories suggest that many elderly people who are homeless may have chronic schizophrenia; discharged from state hospitals years ago after spending their young adulthood institutionalized, they were simply unable to develop satisfactory living situations. An estimated 43% of elderly schizophrenics now reside in nursing homes (Frampton, 2004). Individuals with severe persistent mental illnesses such as schizophrenia form a disenfranchised group whose access to medical care has been limited, leading to greater functional declines and mortality as demonstrated by statistics that individuals with schizophrenia have a life expectancy 20% lower than the general population (Davis, 2004).

Every patient presenting with psychosis should be evaluated for depression, dementia, suicidal and homicidal risk, extrapyramidal effects (if the patient has been taking antipsychotic drugs), and irreversible movement disorders, such as tardive dyskinesia (TD) (Antai-Otong, 2000). The abnormal involuntary movement scale (AIMS) is useful for evaluating early symptoms of TD (see Chapter 15). Environmental intervention is the most successful, least expensive, and safest form of treatment (Beers, Berkow, 2000). Behaviors that are appropriate should be supported, maintaining the

safety of the person. Physical activity is important to avoid emotional or physical outbursts and to promote sleep. Getting to know patients well helps the nursing staff know what kinds of cues the patient gives before a burst of agitation; sometimes pacing the floor is a precipitant to an outburst. Medications are used when the environmental changes are not enough to maintain a safe and tolerable milieu. OBRA guidelines for the use of antipsychotic medications in nursing homes provide the indications for use of these medications in schizophrenia. The newer atypical antipsychotics (risperidone, olanzapine, quetiapine), given in low doses, are less likely to cause the irreversible side effects of TD and seem to be very effective in late-onset schizophrenia (Frampton, 2004).

DEPRESSION

Prevalence

Depression is the most common mental health problem of late life and remains underdiagnosed and undertreated. Estimates of prevalence vary radically depending on the qualitative variables being considered and the definition being used. Although estimates suggest that 6% of older people meet the DSM-IV criteria for a major depressive disorder (NIMH, 2001), depression conditions of varying degrees are highly prevalent in older people. Single or widowed women have a higher prevalence of depression and seek treatment more often than men.

More than 15% of older adults with chronic physical conditions are depressed, and depression may be initiated or complicated by physical illness. Poststroke depression is very common, and administration of antidepressants within the first 3 months of stroke has been shown to prevent depression and improve performance in self-care activities (Frampton, 2004). The prevalence of depression in long-term care may be as high as 25% and has been attributed to stressors such as chronic illness and disability, dementia, chronic pain, preexisting depressive disorder, death of one's spouse, and relocation to an institution (Ugarriza, 2002; Frampton, 2004). Monitoring of depression, treatment, and response is part of the quality indicators for long-term care.

| Box 25-6 | Drugs That Can Cause Symptoms of Depression in Elderly Patients |

Antihypertensives
Reserpine
Methyldopa
Propranolol
Clonidine
Hydralazine
Guanethidine
Diuretics*

Analgesics
Narcotic
Morphine
Codeine
Meperidine
Pentazocine
Propoxyphene

Nonnarcotic
Indomethacin

Antiparkinsonian Agent
L-Dopa

Antimicrobials
Sulfonamides
Isoniazid

Cardiovascular Agents
Digitalis
Lidocaine†

Hypoglycemic Agents‡
Steroids
Corticosteroids
Estrogens

Others
Cimetidine
Cancer chemotherapeutic agents

From Kurlowicz LH, NICHE Faculty: Nursing standard of practice protocol: depression in elderly patients, *Geriatr Nurs* 18(5):192-200, 1997.
*By causing dehydration or electrolyte imbalance.
†Toxicity.
‡By causing hypoglycemia.

Many drugs and medical conditions common to the elderly are associated with depression (Boxes 25-6 and 25-7). In addition, the life situations of elders may result in depression. Depression may be considered a chronic illness in late life (like illnesses such as diabetes) with estimates that 30% of depressed older adults remain chronically depressed, take longer to recover from depression, and have shorter relapse times than do younger persons (Gallo, Coyne, 2000; Reynolds et al, 2002). Some experts express concern about the overdiagnosis of depression, particularly in long-term care, and caution us that a certain amount of what is called depression is a natural reaction to losses and is not necessarily unhealthy. It is important to determine how much of this thing we are calling depression is an expected reaction of sadness and grief and to determine when it requires intervention (Summary from the new directions in geriatric behavioral health for long-term care; accessed 8/8/04 from http://www.mhaging.org/info/improve_service.htm).

Minor Depression

A new class of disorders called subthreshold mental disorders (minor depression and subthreshold generalized anxiety disorders) is emerging as a significant concern. These disorders do not meet the full criteria for classification as specific mental disorders; however, they are associated with clinically significant distress and impairment and may progress to major depression. Minor depression is defined as the presence of at least two but fewer than five depressive symptoms, including depressed mood or loss of interest in normal daily activities, during the same 2-week period with no history of major depressive episode or dysthymic disorder but with clinically significant impairment or distress. A sense of hopelessness, sleep problems, memory problems, lethargy, and diminished appetite may be presenting symptoms. An estimated 10% of older adults in the community experience minor depression (Hegel et al, 2002).

| Box 25-7 | Physical Illnesses Associated with Depression in Elderly Patients |

Metabolical Disturbances
Dehydration
Azotemia, uremia
Acid-base disturbances
Hypoxia
Hyponatremia and hypernatremia
Hypoglycemia and hyperglycemia
Hypocalcemia and hypercalcemia

Endocrine Disorders
Hypothyroidism and hyperthyroidism
Hyperparathyroidism
Diabetes mellitus
Cushing's disease
Addison's disease

Infections
Viral
    Pneumonia
    Encephalitis
Bacterial
    Pneumonia
    Urinary tract
    Meningitis
    Endocarditis
Other
    Tuberculosis
    Brucellosis
    Fungal meningitis
    Neurosyphilis

Cardiovascular Disorders
Congestive heart failure
Myocardial infarction, angina

Pulmonary Disorders
Chronic obstructive lung disease
Malignancy

Gastrointestinal Disorders
Malignancy (especially pancreatic)
Irritable bowel
Other organic causes of chronic abdominal pain,
    ulcer, diverticulosis
Hepatitis

Genitourinary Disorders
Urinary incontinence

Musculoskeletal Disorders
Degenerative arthritis
Osteoporosis with vertebral compression or hip
    fractures
Polymyalgia rheumatica
Paget's disease

Neurological Disorders
Cerebrovascular disease
Transient ischemic attacks
Stroke
Dementia (all types)
Intracranial mass
    Primary or metastatic tumors
Parkinson's disease

Other Illnesses
Anemia (of any cause)
Vitamin deficiencies
Hematological or other systemic malignancy

From Kurlowicz LH, NICHE Faculty: Nursing standard of practice protocol: depression in elderly patients, *Geriatr Nurs* 18(5):192-200, 1997.

Bipolar Disorders

Bipolar disorders, characterized by periods of mania and depression, often level out in late life, and individuals tend to have longer periods of depression (NIMH, 2002). An individual with a bipolar disorder is afflicted with a chemical imbalance and must be treated as such. Lithium, the most commonly used substance for individuals with bipolar disorders, has neurological effects that make it difficult for older people to tolerate. Benzodiazepines, antipsychotics, antidepressants, and mood-stabilizing agents such as carbamazepine or valproic acid may be effective. Balancing the appropriate medication dosage and monitoring side effects are particularly precarious in elders and require very careful and consistent attention.

Differing Presentation of Depression in Elders

"Depression may be even more difficult to understand and diagnose than other illnesses and conditions because depression may take on different meanings when subjected to age and cultural variables" (Ugarriza, 2002, p 22). To understand depression, the nurse must understand the influences of late-life stressors and changes, culture, and the beliefs older people, society, and health professionals may have about depression and its treatment. Depressive symptoms may be seen as normal in older adults. Older people may not say they are depressed. The stigma associated with depression may be more prevalent in older people; and many, particularly those who have survived the depression, world wars, the Holocaust, and other tragedies, may see depression as shameful, evidence of flawed character, self-centered, a spiritual weakness, and sin or retribution (Whall, Hoes-Gurevich, 1999; Reynolds et al, 2002; Ugarriza, 2002).

Race and culture also affect perceptions of the meaning of depression as well as the likelihood of seeking treatment. In addition, assessment of depression in racial and ethnic minority populations is affected by cultural beliefs of the patient and the provider, as well as linguistic differences and the lack of culturally appropriate assessment tools. Further study of cultural and racial differences is needed, but estimates are that minor depression may affect as many as 10% of older African Americans, 15% of older Latinos, and 12% of older Asians (Hegel et al, 2002). Native Americans also have very high rates of depression (Kennedy-Malone et al, 2000).

Older people who are depressed report more somatic complaints, such as physical symptoms, insomnia, loss of appetite and weight loss, memory problems, or chronic pain. They are less likely to have feelings of guilt and worthlessness seen in younger depressed individuals. Hypochondriasis is also common, as are constant complaining and criticism, which may actually be expressions of depression. Decreased energy, motivation, and interest in activities, as well as a preoccupation with death or "giving up," are also signs of depression in older people. Agitated behavior in persons with dementia may be a symptom of depression. A summary of the symptoms of depression in late life and associated nursing care problems are presented in Table 25-1.

Etiology

Factors of health, gender, developmental needs, socioeconomics, environment, personality, losses,

---

Box 25-8	Common Risk Factors for Depression

Chronic medical illnesses (especially Parkinson's and certain stroke syndromes)
Alzheimer's disease and other dementias
Bereavement
Caregiving
Retirement
Smoking
Previous episode of depression
Family history of depression
Admission to long-term care or other change in environment
New stressful losses, including loss of autonomy, loss of privacy, loss of functional status, loss of body part, loss of family member, friend, roommate, or pet
Alcohol or substance abuse
Widowhood

---

functional decline, and awareness of time running out are all significant to the development of depression in later life. Depressive symptoms in an older adult are complex and may arise from several intersecting situations and conditions: biological changes of age, sleep cycle changes, neurotransmitter deficiency, and alterations in neuroendocrine substances. Some common risk factors for depression are presented in Box 25-8.

Assessment

Assessment involves a systematic and thorough evaluation using a depression screening tool (discussed in Chapter 14), interview, history and physical and laboratory tests, medication review, determination of iatrogenic or medical causes, family interview as indicated, and mutual decision making regarding treatment. It is most important that the nurse recognize suicidal potential in the depressed elder, inquire about suicidal thoughts, and provide necessary protection. For those suffering from iatrogenic or medical-induced depression, restoring basic function—sleep, nutrition, hydration, exercise, comfort, and pain control—will often help. Assessment of depression in elders is complicated by the fact that some somatic changes that occur normally in aging, such as tendencies toward constipation, early-morning waking, and slowed motor activity, which would

Table 25-1 Symptoms of Depression and Nursing Care Problems in Older Adults

Symptoms of Depression	Behavior
Decrease of energy, motivation, and interest	Decreased self-care ability: (1) refuses to do tasks requiring physical exertion; (2) asks staff to do total care when not medically indicated; (3) change in socialization patterns and attendance at activities
Frequent somatic complaints	Frequently rings call bell; numerous physical complaints that do not resolve with usual nursing measures
Decreased appetite	Takes inadequate nutrition or refuses food and fluids
Perceived cognitive deficits	Complains of being forgetful; loses familiar objects but performs well on mental status exam, poor on concentration; gives "I don't know" answers
Critical and envious of others	Complains about poor care, criticizes family and staff; may tell you others are getting better treatment
Decreased concentration and indecisiveness	Cannot keep his or her mind on what you are saying, especially patient teaching; has difficulty with decisions (e.g., "When would you like your bath?", "I don't know, I don't care, leave me alone.")
Loss of self-esteem and decreased sense of lifelong accomplishments	Ignores appearance; has no positive feelings about his or her life, hobbies, marriage, family, accomplishments; shares little about self
Combative or resistive behavior	May strike out at staff or be verbally abusive when being cared for or may lash out verbally or physically at other patients who he or she may consider a "bother"
"Model patient" who never uses call light	"Don't bother with me"; rarely complains or asks for anything, passive and apathetic

Adapted from Dreyfus JK: Depression assessment and interventions in medically frail elderly, *J Gerontol Nurs* 14(9):27-36, 38-39, 1988.

indicate depression in a young adult, may be the normal consequences of aging. If depression is diagnosed, treatment should begin as soon as possible and appropriate follow-up should be provided. Depressed people are usually unable to follow through on their own and may be candidates for deeper depression or suicide without appropriate treatment and monitoring (Whall, Hoes-Gurevich, 1999).

Treatment Considerations

In treating depression in the older adult, consider the following:
1. There are several types of depression. It is important that a comprehensive evaluation be made before a conclusion is reached.
2. Biochemical and hormonal changes of aging may intensify depression in the older adult (e.g., neurotransmitters change with aging;

most hormones, particularly thyroid hormones, are reduced.
3. Drugs that are used for medical problems may intensify depression (e.g., hypotensives, psychotropics, cardiotonics, hypnotics).
4. Antidepressant drugs may have idiosyncratic effects, toxic accumulation, and/or paradoxical effects. They should be used with expert knowledge, discrimination, and adequate observation (see Chapter 15).
5. Knowledge of the presence of depression may be helpful when assisting the older person to understand and cope with some of the unexplained symptoms that he or she is experiencing. Clients should be involved in assessment and discussion of depression. Having the individual assess the level of depression immediately engages the person actively in examining his or her own feelings. Tools that can be used in this manner are included in Chapter 14.

6. The importance of restoring a sense of control, choice, and mastery needs to be recognized.

7. Often, increased socialization and relief from physical discomfort and ailments will significantly lift depression.

8. One must be alert to early signs of recurrent depression because this is common in major depressions.

9. To decrease depression and raise self-esteem, defensive structures should be supported unless they are clearly detrimental to the client or family.

Interventions

Depression is often reversible with prompt and appropriate treatment; and 80% of older people will improve on appropriate medication, psychotherapy and psychosocial interventions, or a combination (NIMH, 2001b). Interventions are individual and are based on history, severity of symptoms, concomitant illnesses, and level of disability. Family and social support, grief management, exercise, humor, spirituality, cognitive-behavioral therapy, interpersonal therapy, reminiscence, life review therapy (discussed in Chapter 5), and problem-solving therapy have all been noted to be helpful in depression (Reuben et al, 2002; Jones, 2003). Electroconvulsive therapy may be useful in psychotic depression. Expert consensus guidelines for the management of depression in late life have been developed by Alexopoulos et al (2001) (http://www.psychguides.com). Other practice protocols and guidelines can be found in the Resources at the end of the chapter.

Medications

Drug therapies are very effective in managing depression. The newer selective serotonin reuptake inhibitors (SSRIs) are drugs of choice for most elders with depression. Choice of medications depends on co-morbidities, drug side effects, and type of effect desired. People with agitated depression and sleep disturbances may benefit from medications with a more sedating effect, whereas those who are not eating may do better taking medications that have an appetite-stimulating effect. If depression is immobilizing, psychostimulants may be used. Continuing treatment may be necessary since depression is considered a relapsing and chronic illness. If the person is in remission after a single lifetime episode of depression, 1 year of treatment may be necessary. If the person had two episodes, treatment may need to be continued for 2 years or longer (Reynolds et al, 2002). More severe depression complicated by psychosis or suicide intent may require lifetime medication therapy. The side effects of antidepressants need to be monitored closely, and several different medications may be tried before improvement is noted. Most medications take about 6 weeks to completely resolve symptoms, and inadequate dosing or duration of treatment is common (Kennedy, 2001). See additional discussion of antidepressant medications in Chapter 15.

Cognitive-behavioral Therapy

Cognitive-behavioral therapy is designed to modify thought patterns, improve skills, and alter the environmental states that contribute to the onset, or perpetuation, of emotional disorders. Cognitive-behavioral group therapy, focused visual imagery group therapy, and education and discussion groups on cognition, depression, and hopelessness have been used with moderate improvement in people with mild depression (Beers, Berkow, 2000). Cognitive-behavioral therapy focuses on negating cognitive errors that are common in mildly depressed elderly: (1) overgeneralizing, (2) "awfulizing," (3) exaggerating one's own importance, (4) demanding of others, (5) expecting mind reading, (6) self-blame, and (7) unrealistic expectations.

Interpersonal Support by Family and Professionals

The following interventions can help the person with depression:

- Provide structured, noncompetitive activities.
- Provide opportunities for decisions and to exercise control.
- Focus on spiritual renewal and rediscovery of meanings.
- Help the patient to write a guided autobiography.
- Engage the patient in self-analysis through journals and dreams.
- Reactivate latent interests, or develop new ones.
- Validate depressed feelings as aiding recovery; do not try to bolster the person's mood or deny his or her despair.

- Provide an accepting atmosphere and an empathic response.
- Share yourself.
- Demonstrate faith in the person's strengths.
- Praise any and all efforts at recovery, no matter how small.
- Assist in expressing and dealing with anger.
- Do not stifle the grief process; grief cannot be hurried.
- Create a hopeful environment where self-esteem is fostered and life is meaningful.
- Assist in dealing with guilt, real or neurotic.
- Foster development of connections with others.
- Create your own support system and care for yourself since working with elders who are depressed can be especially challenging.

SUICIDE

Although elders make up 13% of the population, they commit 20% of suicides (McAndrews, 2001). White men over the age of 85 years commit suicide at a rate approximately six times the national rate (NIMH, 2001). In most cases, depression and other mental health problems contribute significantly to suicide risk. Sixty percent of suicides are causally related to depression. One of the significant differences in suicidal behavior in the old and young is lethality of method. Eight of ten suicides of men over age 65 were with firearms, and most were successful. Elderly people rarely threaten to commit suicide; they just do it. Many studies have shown that, with few exceptions, a suicidal individual has seen a physician within 1 month before the suicide attempt. As with depression, physical complaints are the primary reason for seeking medical treatment. Consequently, it is very important to recognize warning signs and risk factors as well as assess for suicidal thoughts and ideas.

Common precipitants of suicide include physical or mental illness, death of one's spouse, substance abuse, and pathological relationships. Other behavioral clues and risk factors are presented in Box 25-9. Elderly widowers are thought to be most vulnerable because they have often depended on their wives to maintain the comforts of home and the social network of relatives and friends. Older white men may also suffer the most status loss because the American white male society is almost wholly devoted to occupational success, often to the neglect of other social roles. Women in all countries have much lower suicide rates, possibly because of greater flexibility in coping skills based on multiple roles that women fill throughout their lives. Suicide may also be less socially acceptable than for men. The more children a woman has, the lower her risk of suicide (Holkup, 2002).

Assessing the Suicidal Risk of an Elder

Older people with suicidal intent are encountered in many settings. It is our professional obligation to prevent whenever possible an impulsive destruction of life that may be a response to a crisis or a disintegrative reaction. The lethality potential of an elder must always be assessed when elements of depression, disease, and spousal loss are evident. However, any direct, indirect, or enigmatic references to the ending of life must be taken seriously and discussed with the elder. An excellent evidence-based protocol, *Elderly Suicide: Secondary Prevention* (Holkup, 2002), is available at http://www.guideline.gov.

The most important consideration is for the nurse to establish a trusting and respectful relationship with the person. Since many older people have grown up in an era when suicide bore stigma and even criminal implications, they may not discuss their feelings in this respect. It is also important to remember that in older people, typical behavioral clues such as putting personal affairs in order, giving away possessions, and making wills and funeral plans are indications of maturity and good judgment in late life and cannot be construed as indicative of suicidal intent. Even statements such as "I won't be around long" or "I'm ready to die" may be only a realistic appraisal of the situation in old age.

To increase communication and expression of feeling, depersonalizing the subject and discussing it on a more philosophical basis may be helpful; for example, "Suicide is a taboo subject that many people are uncomfortable discussing, but as a health professional I feel it is very important. Have you ever felt like you would be better off dead?" Use open-ended questions such as "Could you tell me how it is for you to feel so alone right now?"

Box 25-9   Suicide Risk and Recovery Factors

Risk Factors

Depression

Paranoia or a paranoid attitude

Rejection of help; a suspicious and hostile attitude toward helpers and society

Major loss, such as the death of a spouse

History of major losses

Recent suicide attempt

History of suicide attempts

Major mental, physical, or neurological illness

Major crises or transitions, such as retirement or imminent entry into a nursing home

Major crises or changes in others, especially among family members

Typical age-related blows to self-esteem, such as loss of income or loss of meaningful activities

Loss of independence, when dependency is unacceptable

Expressions of feeling unnecessary, useless, and devalued

Increased irritability and poor judgment, especially after a loss or some other crisis

Alcoholism or increased drinking

Social isolation: living alone; having few friends (The social isolation of the couple is also associated with suicide.)

Expression of the belief that one is in the way, a burden harmful to others or in a hopeless situation

Communication of suicidal intent: direct or indirect expression of suicidal ideation or impulses and symptomatic acts, such as giving away valued possessions, storing up medications, or buying a gun

Intractable, unremitting pain—mental or physical—that is not responding to treatment

Feelings of hopelessness and helplessness in the family and social network

Feelings of hopelessness in the therapist or other helpers; desire to be rid of the patient

Acceptance of suicide as a solution

Recovery Factors

A capacity for the following:

Understanding

Relating

Benefitting from experience

Benefitting from knowledge

Accepting help

Being loving

Expressing wisdom

Displaying a sense of humor

Having a social interest

Accepting a caring and available family

Accepting a caring and available social network

Accepting a caring, available, and knowledgeable professional and health network

From Richman J: A rational approach to rational suicide. In Leenars AA et al, editors: *Suicide and the older adult,* New York, 1992, The Guilford Press.

when asking people to describe their emotions and ask for clarification if needed. In evaluating lethality potential, the informed nurse will recognize the high-risk patient: male, old, widowed or divorced, white, in poor health, retired, alcoholic, and with a family history of unsatisfactory relationships and mental illness. A cluster of these factors should be a red flag of distress to all health professionals. Recent traumatic changes, mild dementia, depression, or cerebrovascular disease also increases the danger. Present relationships that are unsatisfactory, critical, or rejecting greatly enhance the potential for suicide.

If there is suspicion that the elder is suicidal, use direct and straightforward questions such as the following:

- Have you ever thought about killing yourself?
- How often have you had these thoughts?
- How would you kill yourself if you decided to do it?

The following must also be considered in assessing lethality potential:

- Internal resources (personality factors, coping strategies)
- External resources (money, family, friends, services)

• Communication skills (ability to ask for help and express feelings)

Crisis Intervention

If suicidal intent has been established, the following interventions, arranged in order of immediacy, are necessary:

1. Reduce immediate danger by removing hazardous articles.
2. Do not leave the person alone; evaluate the need for constant attendance; and arrange for family, friend, or professional to be present during the period of immediate danger.
3. Provide an honest expression of concern, such as "I do not want you to take your life. I will help you with this troubling situation."
4. Evaluate the need for consultation with a mental health professional and possible hospitalization.
5. Sometimes a no-suicide contract can be initiated. If the person demonstrates a high risk of suicide, a no-suicide contract cannot be relied on as a preventive measure.
6. Evaluate the need for medication.
7. Focus on the current hazard or crisis that gives the client the most present distress.
8. Mobilize internal and external resources by getting the person reinvolved with external supports and reconnected with internal capabilities. You or the family or caregiver may have to take the initiative to find activities, support systems, transportation, and other resources for the individual.
9. Implement a specific plan of action with an ongoing structured program. Develop a lifeline of individuals who can be called on at any hour of distress, and plan regular calls and follow-up for the individual.

Suicide is a taboo topic for most of us, and there is a lingering fear that the introduction of the topic will be suggestive to the patient and may incite suicidal action. Precisely the opposite is true. By introducing the topic, we demonstrate interest in the individual and open the door to honest human interaction and connection on the deep levels of psychological need. Superficial interest and mechanical questioning will not, of course, be meaningful. It is the nature of our concern and ability to connect with the alienation and desperation of the individual that will make a difference. Working with isolated, depressed, and suicidal elders challenges the depths of nurses' ingenuity, patience, and self-knowledge.

SUBSTANCE ABUSE

Substance abuse often arises in old age as a coping mechanism to deal with loss, anxiety, depression, or boredom. Alcohol and drug use are highly correlated with mental health problems. Alcohol-related problems in the elderly often go unrecognized, although the residual effects of alcohol abuse complicate the presentation and treatment of many chronic disorders of older people. Alcohol use significantly contributes to chronic diseases such as dementia, congestive heart failure, hypertension, cirrhosis, seizure disorders, neuropathies, and nutritional disorders. In the general population, abuse of alcohol is readily recognized because of social and work problems; however, elders may live alone and not come under scrutiny at work. They may easily hide their drinking.

The misuse and abuse of alcohol are prevalent among older adults and are a significant public health concern. Estimates suggest that between 2% and 17% of elders over the age of 60 have alcohol abuse and dependence (Blow et al, 2002), but prevalence is likely to increase with the aging of the baby boomers who had more access to drugs, alcohol, and other substances (Goodman, 2003). Surveys suggest that 10% to 21% of hospitalized elders and 11% of older persons residing in nursing homes have a severe alcohol addiction. In nursing homes, 28% have a past history of alcohol addiction (Goodman, 2003). Most severe alcohol abuse is seen in people ages 60 to 80, not in those over 80. Two thirds of elderly alcoholics are early-onset drinkers, and one third are late-onset drinkers (after age 60). Women comprise the majority of late-onset drinkers.

Little is known about substance abuse disorders other than alcohol. It is generally believed that most older adults who use or are dependent on illegal drugs have early-onset disorders and the current cohort of elders is less likely to use illicit drugs than younger people. Again, with the aging of the baby boomers, this may change (Blow et al, 2002). A more common concern seen among older adults is the inappropriate use of psychoactive prescription and over-the-counter medications, as well as nicotine. Some of the reasons for abuse of psychoactive prescription medications may be inappropriate prescribing and ineffective monitoring of response and follow-up. The misuse of these medications is particularly significant because of the older adults who use alcohol in combination with these medications. Blow et al (2002) note that increases in illness and mortality are associated with misusing prescription and nonprescription medications, although this is not considered a disorder by DSM-IV.

Assessment

Despite the high prevalence of alcohol problems, most of them go unidentified. Alcohol screening should be a part of the regular physical examination in people over age 60. Direct questions should be asked about drinking if a problem or use of psychoactive drugs is suspected. The Cage Alcohol Abuse Screener (CAGE) questionnaire is a commonly used screening tool. Other questions regarding abuse of alcohol are presented in Box 25-10. MacLean (2003) suggests that alcoholism is a disease of denial and not easy to diagnose, particularly in older people with psychosocial and functional decline from other conditions that may mask decline caused by alcohol. Further, alcohol users often reject or deny the diagnosis, or they may take offense at the suggestion of it. Health care providers may feel powerless over alcoholism or may approach the person in a judgmental manner. Elders are likely to feel excessively guilty and regretful about alcohol misuse, and it is important to reach out to them with understanding. It is productive to discuss the issue of substance abuse factually, avoiding judgmental overtones. For example, the nurse might say, "Many elders find that the stresses, loneliness, and losses of aging are very hard to bear. Some retreat into alcohol use as a way of coping. There are treatments and groups that assist individuals in these difficult adjustments. If this is a problem for you or if it becomes a problem, please let us know so that we may provide resources or referrals for you." Particularly in the case of substance abuse, nurses must search for the pain beneath the behavior.

Treatment

Acute alcoholic withdrawal in an elder is serious and sometimes life threatening. Recommended treatment includes frequent determination of vital signs, maintaining fluid balance without overhydrating, and the use of benzodiazepines during withdrawal. Treatment and intervention strategies include cognitive-behavioral approaches, individual and group counseling, medical and psychiatric approaches, referral to Alcoholics Anonymous, family therapy, case management and community and home care services, and formalized substance abuse treatment. Long-term self-help treatment programs for elders show high rates of success, especially when social outlets are emphasized and cohort supports are available.

An extensive protocol for developing a plan of care for the alcohol abuser is seen in Box 25-11. Additional information on late-life addictions can be found at http://www.samhsa.gov. Further research is needed to identify the most effective methods of treatment for alcohol and drug abuse in older people.

IMPLICATIONS FOR GERONTOLOGICAL NURSING AND HEALTHY AGING

The development of holistic and humanistic models of care for elders experiencing emotional health disturbances is critically important in gerontological nursing. Much of the distress associated with emotional illness in late life can

---

Box 25-10	**Questions Regarding Abuse of Alcohol**

Are you upset when people criticize your drinking? How do you handle that?

Do you believe that you sometimes drink too much? Are there particular occasions when that occurs?

Do you feel disturbed about your alcohol consumption?

Do you drink when you are feeling lonely?

Have you identified a pattern regarding your drinking?

Would you like to stop drinking?

The following potential diagnoses must be considered, as well as diagnoses unique to the particular individual:
Denial, ineffective
Knowledge, deficient
Poisoning, risk for
Sensory perception, disturbed
Sleep pattern, disturbed
Social interaction, impaired
Spiritual distress
Thought processes, disturbed

NURSING PROCESS

Etiologies and related factors
Stresses
  Environmental changes
  Losses
  Spousal illness
  Chronic illness
  Finances
Lack of purpose
Physiological changes (neurotransmitter depletion)
Physiovulnerability to depression

Defining characteristics
Denies alcohol use is a problem
Justifies use of alcohol
Argumentative with mate, friends, or authority
Unreasonable resentments
Paranoia
Impulsive judgment
Impatience
Incontinence
Coordination changes
Anxiety
Legal difficulties
Financial problems
Depression
Family problems
Poor nutrition, weight loss
Gastritis
Seizures
Daytime fatigue
Unsteady gait
Impaired memory
Apathy
Disorientation
Confusion
Slurred speech
Self-neglect
Social isolation
Blackouts
Falls, bruises, burns
Physical pathological conditions: myopathy, diarrhea, malnutrition, gout, decreased lower extremity sensation, tremors
Visual or tactile hallucinations

Knowledge
Alcohol abuse, alcoholism
Effects of alcohol on the older adult
Percentage of alcohol in various alcoholic beverages and over-the-counter medications
2 oz alcohol
  = 2 shots = 4 oz 100-proof whiskey
  = 4 glasses = 16 oz wine
  = 4 mugs = 48 oz beer
Physical and psychological assessment skills
Standard alcohol screening tests (e.g., CAGE alcohol abuse screener)
Signs and symptoms of withdrawal
Therapeutic communication skills
Crisis intervention skills
Group therapy
Coping strategies
Treatment of alcoholism
Community resources

Clinical judgment and related skills
Maintain a nonjudgmental approach.
Administer a standard alcohol screening tool and depression assessment.
Perform a physical and mental status examination.
Monitor nutritional status.
Teach the effects of alcohol on nutrition and sleep.
Help client to gain an understanding of alcoholism as an illness, its progressiveness, and its effects on the body and interpersonal relationships.
When there is suspected over-the-counter and prescription drug misuse, include specific information on interactive effects with alcohol.
Set realistic short-term goals.
Explore coping patterns that do not include alcohol.
Involve family (if there is one).
Conduct group sessions with recovering and recovered persons.
Educate family and community groups on the older adult and alcoholism.
Provide information on resources.
Make referrals as needed.

Evaluation
Admits is alcoholic
Abstains from alcohol use
States and recognizes need for continued treatment
Explains the physical and psychological effects of alcohol
Uses alternative coping mechanisms for stress
Takes pride in appearance
Reintegrates into social activities

be relieved through competent, caring, and compassionate gerontological nursing care. Awareness of appropriate assessment and treatment of the distressing reactions that can occur in late life as presented in this chapter is a very important component of best practice care. However, knowing and appreciating each elder's uniqueness, their past and present experiences, and how they color the present may contribute far more to healthy aging and emotional well-being than medications or therapy. Believing in and supporting the strength and wisdom of older people restores self-confidence and feelings of worth, an important component of emotional health. Appreciating the nature of loss and grief in old age means that gerontological nurses listen, really listen, and offer support to weather the storm. Our work needs to focus on the development of environments of care that enhance both physical and emotional functioning, create conditions of hope, and support elders in the often difficult journey in late life.

APPLICATION OF MASLOW'S HIERARCHY

Using Maslow's hierarchy of needs model, satisfaction of basic needs is a significant component of emotional health. Attention to basic needs of biological integrity, safety and security, belonging and attachment, self-esteem and self-efficacy in the daily lives of elders is essential to emotional well-being. The higher one rises in terms of needs met, the more likely one is to be emotionally healthy. Often, elders are not able to meet or receive assistance with basic needs. Illness, functional impairments, and losses of all kinds may make it difficult to create a life where one feels safe, connected, in control, and competent. This affects the ability of older people to move up the hierarchy toward finding meaning and fulfillment in life. However, the majority of elders face these challenges with grace, equanimity, good humor, and courage. To support them, as well as to assist those who do develop emotional distress, it is important to create relationships and environments of care that not only meet basic needs, but also contribute to health, happiness, and meaning throughout life, even at the end of life.

KEY CONCEPTS

- Emotional health in late life is difficult to determine because the accrual of life experiences makes for great variations. Emotional health in late life must be determined by the gratification and satisfaction that individuals feel in their particular situation.
- Emotional health is a fluctuating situation for most individuals, with peaks and valleys of happiness and pain.
- Elders are not well served within the mental health system as it exists today.
- Methods of assessing the impact of stressful events are inadequate if they do not consider chronic stressors that may exist over long periods of time, the particular population profile of the individual being assessed, the individual's personality, and the timing and frequency of events, as well as very early traumatic events that may have eroded the individual's sense of security.
- Reestablishing feelings of adequacy and control is the heart of crisis resolution and stress management.
- Psychological assessment of elders based on the common psychometric instruments will usually show deficits because these instruments, with few exceptions, have been designed for younger people and those who are not members of minority groups.
- Anxiety disorders are common in late life and are best managed by restoring some sense of control to the situation the individual perceives as out of control.
- Many psychological aberrations observed in the elderly are lifetime personality traits or coping strategies to deal with overwhelming anxiety and do not need treatment unless they interfere with function.
- Posttraumatic stress disorder is finally being recognized in older adults who have been subjected to extremely traumatic events. Programs are now available to provide support and insight for these individuals.
- The incidence of late-life onset of psychotic disorders is low among older people, but psychotic manifestations can occur as a secondary syndrome in a variety of disorders, the most common being Alzheimer's disease. Psychotic symptoms in Alzheimer's disease require dif-

NANDA and Wellness Diagnoses

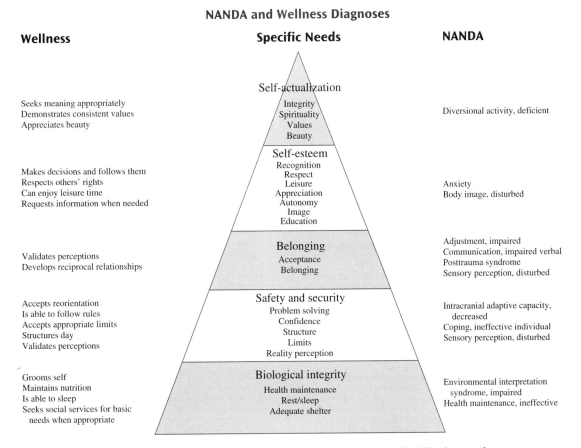

Wellness	Specific Needs	NANDA
	Self-actualization	
Seeks meaning appropriately Demonstrates consistent values Appreciates beauty	Integrity Spirituality Values Beauty	Diversional activity, deficient
	Self-esteem	
Makes decisions and follows them Respects others' rights Can enjoy leisure time Requests information when needed	Recognition Respect Leisure Appreciation Autonomy Image Education	Anxiety Body image, disturbed
	Belonging	Adjustment, impaired Communication, impaired verbal Posttrauma syndrome Sensory perception, disturbed
Validates perceptions Develops reciprocal relationships	Acceptance Belonging	
	Safety and security	
Accepts reorientation Is able to follow rules Accepts appropriate limits Structures day Validates perceptions	Problem solving Confidence Structure Limits Reality perception	Intracranial adaptive capacity, decreased Coping, ineffective individual Sensory perception, disturbed
	Biological integrity	

Grooms self
Maintains nutrition
Is able to sleep
Seeks social services for basic
  needs when appropriate
	Health maintenance
	Rest/sleep
	Adequate shelter
		Environmental interpretation
		  syndrome, impaired
		Health maintenance, ineffective

These are not all of the possible wellness or NANDA diagnoses that may be identified. The above are frequent examples of nursing diagnoses that should be considered when planning care for the older adult in whatever setting.

ferent assessment and treatment than long-standing psychotic disorders.

- Substance abuse and addictions may be distorted adaptational methods used by some older persons to cope with anxiety related to end-of-life concerns. These individuals have been successfully treated by being provided with supportive groups and relationships.
- Depression is the most common emotional disorder of aging and likewise the most treatable. Unfortunately, it is often neglected or assumed to be a condition of aging that one must learn to live with. Nurses may be instrumental in recognizing and properly assessing and treating depression in elders.

- Grief is a component of aging for most individuals as they confront various losses. Grief is not a mental illness, but it often requires grief counseling and support for resolution.
- Suicide is a significant problem among old men. Very old white men are highly suicidal and must be assessed for suicidal intent whenever they confront a trauma or catastrophe.

Activities and Discussion Questions

1. List the various crises you have encountered with older people you have taken care of, and then discuss what was done about them.

2. Discuss several of the unconscious defense mechanisms that serve to help people avoid anxiety states.
3. Discuss the three most common emotional disturbances that elders are likely to experience, and describe how these have appeared to you. How did you assess the problem, and what was done about it?
4. What is likely to be different in the appearance of depression in a person who is 70 years old versus the appearance in a person who is 20 years old?
5. What behaviors are indicative of suicidal intent in an elderly person? Discuss the methods of assessment and your reactions to these.
6. Discuss the various situations that may result in elder substance abuse and ways to effectively intervene.
7. Formulate strategies that may be used to promote emotional health in late life.

RESOURCES

Organizations

International Psychogeriatric Association
Suite 340
5215 Old Orchard Road
Skokie, IL 60077
(847) 663-0574
website: http://www.ipa-online.org
e-mail: ipa@ipa-online.org

Mental Health and Aging Network
American Society on Aging
833 Market Street, No. 511
San Francisco, CA 94103-1824
(800) 537-9728
website: http://www.asaging.org

National Association of States United for Action in Aging
Suite 350
1201 15th Street, NW
Washington, DC 20005
(202) 898-2583
website: http://www.nasua.org

National Coalition on Mental Health and Aging
3003 W. Touhy
Chicago, IL 60645
(773) 508-4745
website: http://www.ncmha.org

National Institute on Alcohol Abuse and Alcoholism
5635 Fishers Lane, MSC 9304
Bethesda, MD 20892
website: http://www.niaaa.nih.gov

National Institute of Mental Health
Office of Communications
6001 Executive Boulevard, Room 8184, MSC 9663
Bethesda, MD 20892-9663
(866) 615-6464
website: http://www.nimh.gov

Websites

Mental Health: A Report of the Surgeon General
Available at http://www.surgeongeneral.gov/library/mentalhealth/toc.html

National Guideline Clearinghouse (guidelines and protocols for management of depression in older adults and suicide prevention)
http://www.guideline.gov

Substance Abuse and Mental Health Services Administration
http://www.samhsa.gov

Video

Well Into Your Future (3-hour documentary)
Available from: Well Into Your Future
Suite B-200
4455 Connecticut Avenue
Washington, DC 20008
(202) 537-0818
website: wellme.stateart.com

REFERENCES

Alexopoulos GS et al: The Expert Consensus Guidelines Series: pharmacotherapy of depressive disorders in older patients, *Postgrad Med Special Rep 2001*.

American Psychiatric Association (APA): *Diagnostic and statistical manual of mental disorders (DSM-IV)*, ed 4, Washington, DC, 1994, The Association.

Antai-Otong D: Schizophrenia in the elderly, *Adv NP* 8(3):39, 2000.

Beck C, Doan R, Cody M: Nursing assistants as providers of mental health care in nursing homes, *Generations* 26(1):66-71, 2002.

Beers MH, Berkow R: *Merck manual of geriatrics*, ed 3, Whitehouse Station, NJ, 2000, Merck Research Laboratories.

Blow F, Oslin D, Barry K: Misuse and abuse of alcohol, illicit drugs, and psychoactive medications among older people, *Generations* 26(1):50-54, 2002.

Bludau J: Second institutionalization: Impact of personal history on patients with dementia, *Caring for the Ages*, 3(5):3-4, 2002.

Burnside IM: Listen to the aged, *Am J Nurs* 75(10):1800-1803, 1975.

Davis B: Assessing adults with mental disorders in primary care, the nurse practitioner, *Am J Primary Health Care* 29(5):19-27, 2004.

Frampton K: The state of geriatric mental health services in LTC, *Caring for the Ages* 5(4):47-51 2004.

Gallo JJ, Coyne JC: The challenge of depression in late life: bridging science and service in primary care, *JAMA* 284(12):1570-1572, 2000.

Goodman A: Update: geriatric psychiatry, *Caring for the Ages* 4(8):16-17, 2003. Available at http:www./amda.com/caring/august 2003/geropsych.htm.

Grossberg GT: Diagnosis and treatment of late-life psychosis in the elderly, *Long-Term Care Forum* 1(3):7, 2000.

Hegel M, Stanley M, Arean P: Minor depression and subthreshold anxiety symptoms in older adults: psychosocial therapies and special considerations, *Generations* 26(3):44-49, 2002.

Holkup P: *Evidence-based protocol. Elderly suicide: secondary prevention,* Iowa City, 2002, University of Iowa Gerontological Nursing Interventions Research Center, Research Dissemination Core.

Johnson B: Older adults' suggestions for health care providers regarding discussions of sex, *Geriatr Nurs* 18(2):65-66, 1997.

Jones ED: Reminiscence therapy for older women with depression: effects of nursing intervention classification in assisted-living long-term care, *J Gerontol Nurs* 29(7):26-33, 2003.

Kennedy GJ: Psychopharmacology of late-life depression, *Ann Long-Term* Care 9(3):35-40, 2001.

Kennedy-Malone L, Fletcher KR, Plank: L: *Management guidelines for gerontological nurse practitioners,* Philadelphia, 2000, FA Davis.

Kivnick HQ: Everyday mental health: a guide to assessing life's strengths. In Smyer MA, editor: *Mental health and aging,* New York, 1993, Springer.

MacLean D: Coming to terms with alcoholism in long-term care, *Caring for the Ages* 4(1), 2003. Available at http://www.amda.com/caring/january2003/alcoholism.htm, pp 16-17.

Maslow A: *Motivation and personality,* ed 2, New York, 1970, Harper & Row.

Moorhead SA, Brighton VA: Anxiety and fear: In Maas ML et al, editors: *Nursing care of older adults: diagnoses, outcomes, and interventions,* St. Louis, 2001, Mosby.

National Institutes of Mental Health (NIMH): *Older adults: depression and suicide facts,* 2001b. Available at http://www.nimh.nih.gov.

National Institutes of Mental Health (NIMH): A *story of bipolar disorder,* 2002. Available at http://www.nimh.gov/publicat/bipolstory08.cfm.

Palmer B, Folson D, Bartels S, Jeste D: Psychotic disorders in late life: implications for treatment and future directions for clinical services, *Generations* 26(1):39-39-42, 2002.

Qualls S: Defining mental health in later life, *Generations* 26(7):9-13, 2002.

Reuben DB et al: *Geriatrics at your fingertips,* 2002 ed, Malden, Mass, 2002, American Geriatrics Society-Blackwell.

Reynolds C, Alexopoulos G, Katz I: Geriatric depression: diagnosis and treatment, *Generations* 26(1):28-31, 2002.

Ugarriza DN: Elderly women's explanation of depression, *J Gerontol Nurs* 28(5):22-29, 2002.

Whall AL, Hoes-Gurevich ML: Missed depression in elderly individuals: why is this a problem? *J Gerontol Nurs* 25(6):44-46, 1999.

26

Loss, Grief, Dying, and Death in Late Life

> ## LEARNING OBJECTIVES

Upon completion of this chapter, the reader will be able to:

- Differentiate between loss and grief.
- Explain the different types of grief and the dynamics of the grieving process.
- Explain the characteristics required of the nurse to be able to effectively intervene in grief and bereavement.
- Identify and discuss the needs of the dying and appropriate interventions.
- Explain the role and responsibility of the nurse in advance directives.
- Explain the difference between passive and active euthanasia.

> ## GLOSSARY

Bereavement overload A number of grief situations in a short period of time (weeks, months, 1 year).
Euthanasia Death that is unrelated to the natural life processes.
Grief An emotional response to loss.

Mourning The process in which grief is experienced.
Physician-assisted suicide "When the physician facilitates a patient's death by providing the necessary means and/or information to enable the patient to end his or her life" (Minogue, 1996, p 80).

> ## THE LIVED EXPERIENCE

When we were in our sixties my friends and I met over cards, went on trips, and experienced all of the joys of retirement. We didn't have much time to worry about aches and pains. In our seventies we had less time to play because we were busy visiting one another in the hospital or in nursing homes. In our eighties we met frequently again, but it was usually at our friends' funerals, leaving little time for cards or travel. Now that I am in my nineties hardly any of my friends are still alive; you know it gets kind of lonely, so you just have to make new younger friends!

Theresa, age 93

Death is easy, it's the dying that is the hard part.

Author unknown

*L*oss, dying, and death are universal, incontestable events of the human experience that cannot be stopped or controlled. With age, the number of losses increases. Some of these are associated with the normal changes with aging, such as the loss of flexibility in the joints, and some are related to the normal changes in everyday life and life transitions, such as moving and retirement. Other losses are those of loved ones through death. Some deaths are considered normative and expected, such as older parents and friends. Other deaths are considered nonnormative and unexpected, such as the death of adult children or grandchildren.

Regardless of the type of loss, each one has the potential to trigger grief and a process we call bereavement or mourning. Grief and mourning are usually used synonymously. However, grief is an individual's response to a loss. Mourning is an active and evolving process (also called the grieving process and bereavement). Mourning includes those behaviors used to incorporate the loss experience into one's life after the loss. Mourning behaviors are strongly influenced by social and cultural norms that proscribe the appropriate ways of both reacting to the loss and coping with it (Spector, 2003). It is important to realize that there is no single way to grieve or respond to loss. Responses will vary widely among individuals and across cultures.

Although there are expected behaviors for grief related to loss through death, there are no guidelines for behavior when the loss is of another type (Shield, 1997). For example, an individual who is seriously ill, who moves to a nursing home (loses one's home), or who retires (willingly or unwillingly) may be very sad, irritable, and forgetful. The person may be suspected of developing dementia when he or she is actually grieving (Hegge, Fischer, 2000). When the losses accumulate in quick succession a state of bereavement overload may result. The griever may become incapacitated and require careful and skilled support and guidance.

The gerontological nurse needs to have basic knowledge of the grieving process and how to comfort and care for grievers, including one another. Additional knowledge and skills are needed of the dying process and care of the dying person and his or her survivors. In this chapter we hope to provide the baseline information needed to promote effective grieving, peaceful dying, and good and appropriate deaths.

GRIEF

Life is like a pinwheel, a thing of beauty and change. The wind, like loss, sets it in motion beginning the life-changing process of grieving. Throughout one's life the winds of loss will gently stir recurrent episodes of grief through sights, sounds, smells, anniversary dates, and other triggers. The arms of the pinwheel suggest movement by the bereaved, reaching out of the experience of grief by surrendering (i.e., resting, or the lowering of one's defenses toward life and being open to reality or the acceptance of the life event and reaching out to others and rejoining life through change). Each gust of wind may generate a resurgence of the grief experience, but the pinwheel will never lose its beauty.

The Grieving Process

Researchers have tried for years to understand the grieving process, resulting in a number of models that have been proposed to explain and predict the experience. The majority of these models evolved between the early 1900s and early 1980s and influence what caregivers and society in general have been taught about grief. Although intended to describe death-related grief, these same models can be applied to any of the losses in the lives of older adults that are considered significant or meaningful.

All models recognize similar physical and psychological manifestations of acute grief (when it is first felt), a middle period in which the manifestations of grief (e.g., despair, depression) affect the person's day-to-day functioning, and an ending phase where the person learns to adjust to life in a new way without that which has been lost. At the same time it is also recognized that the grieving process is not rigidly structured and a predictable pattern of responses does not always occur. Several models are described below.

Worden

Worden's (2002) model represents the grieving process as a series of evolving tasks, repeated for all losses or parts of losses. For example, the person diagnosed with Alzheimer's (and a loss of his or her former self, plans for the future, etc.) will, at some point, (1) accept the reality of the loss (diagnosis); (2) work through the physical and emotional pain (associated with the diagnosis and all of its implications, such as loss of driving ability); (3) adjust to a change in environment (may no longer be able to go to work); and (4) emotionally relocate the loss and move on with life (continuing to live with the new diagnosis). Doka (1993) added a fifth task, spiritual, to rebuild faith and philosophical systems that are challenged by the loss.

If this model is applied to someone who has lost a loved one, such as a life partner, the nurse may look for signs of the person accepting the reality of the death and loss as the person is referred to in the past tense rather than the present. Helen may speak of Chris as someone who "just loved to garden" rather than "just loves to garden."

Although working through the pain is an individual process, Helen has a support network of friends and church members. They encourage her to "tell her story" of not only Chris' life but also their life together and gently move her to thinking of her life without Chris. In working through acute grief, the grief-pain will not lessen if avoided with the regular use of medications such as tranquilizers, which are often prescribed. Although these may be necessary to enable the griever to accomplish some needed tasks, they are not recommended for everyday use.

Adjusting to a changed environment may take a considerable period of time, especially if the relationship with the deceased was a long and close one. Changes in the environment may be physical, emotional, or spiritual, such as rearrangement of furniture or a different seating pattern at the dinner table.

As Helen proceeds through the grieving process, her memories of life with Chris will be those of the past and she will be able to develop new memories of her life without Chris. Although the pain associated with the first birthday, anniversary, holiday, and so on, will never go away completely, it will lessen with subsequent years as the loss is relocated from the present to the past.

Bowlby

Bowlby (1961) suggests four phases of the grief: (1) numbness, anger, and distress; (2) yearning and searching for that which is lost; (3) disorganization and despair; and (4) reorganization. This model evolves as Worden's does. Its cycles or "revolutions" continue as each small part of the large loss is dealt with. For example, in the death of a spouse there may be loss of companionship, loss of income, loss of the role of husband or wife, and so forth. Not all of these losses are experienced or resolved at the same time, but the cycle continues (Figure 26-1).

A Loss Response Model

Nurse Barbara Giacquinta proposed a model of families facing the crisis of cancer (1977). Through modification and incorporation of a systems approach, the Loss Response Model (Jett, 2004) lends itself to an understandable and usable model of the grieving process from which nursing interventions are easily developed. In the Loss Response Model, the family and the person are viewed as a system that strives to maintain equilibrium.

When loss occurs within the system, the *impact* is experienced as acute grief. The system's equilibrium is in chaos and is seen as a *functional disruption*; that is, the system cannot perform its usual activities; either the person or the members are in a state of disequilibrium. The loss seems unreal. The family or individual then *searches for meaning*: why did this happen to them? How will they survive the loss? If an elder is responding to the loss of a child or a grandchild, thoughts of "why wasn't it me?" are common. The family then may become active in *informing others*. Each time the story is repeated, the loss becomes more real and the system moves toward a new steady state. Informing others involves *engaging emotions* that may have been previously withheld or subdued because of the shock of the impact. The expression of emotions can release energy that can be used to *reorganize* the family *structure*. As roles change, adaptation and accommodation are necessary. Someone else steps in to perform the roles of the person who is now absent or to complete the tasks no longer possible in the presence of the loss. For example, when the elder patriarch dies, the eldest son may step up and assume some of his father's roles and responsibilities. Finally, if the

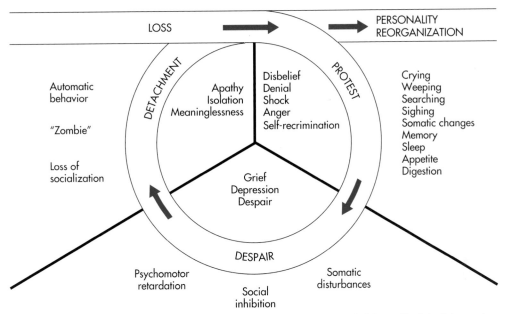

Figure 26-1   Illustration of John Bowlby's approach to loss. (From Beare PG, Myers JL: *Principles and practice of adult health nursing,* ed 2, St Louis, 1994, Mosby.)

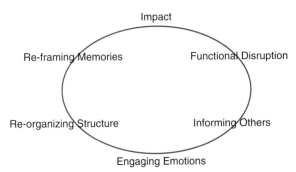

Figure 26-2   The loss response model. (From Jett KF: The loss response model, unpublished manuscript, 2004. Adapted from Giacquinta B: Helping families face the crisis of cancer, *Am J Nurs* 77(10):1585-1588, 1977.)

system is to survive, it will need to redefine itself. One of the ways that it does this is by *reframing its memories*; that is, families accept that portraits and reunions are still possible, just different than they were before the loss, or they accept that a person can still be vital, active, and important even after the loss of the ability to drive a car, to walk unassisted, or to live alone (Figure 26-2).

TYPES OF GRIEF

Grieving takes enormous amounts of physical and emotional energy. It is the hardest thing anyone can do and may be especially hard for older adults. The potential intensity of emotions may appear as confusion, depression, or preoccupation with thoughts of the deceased or loss and may be mistaken for other conditions, such as dementia, when it probably is a type of delirium, something that requires care. The gerontological nurse is most likely to work with elders who are experiencing anticipatory grief, acute grief, or chronic grief. A fourth type, disenfranchised grief, may be occurring and hidden but none the less significant.

Anticipatory Grief

Anticipatory grief is the response to a real or perceived loss before it occurs, a dress rehearsal, so to speak. One observes this grief in preparation for potential loss, such as loss of belongings (e.g., selling of a home), moving (e.g., into a nursing home), or knowing that a body part or function is going to change (e.g., a mastectomy), or in anticipation of the loss of a spouse or oneself either through dementia or through death. Behaviors that may signal anticipatory grief include preoccupation with the particular loss, unusually detailed planning, or a sudden change in attitude toward the thing or person to be lost.

The grieving process described by the models above will occur, with one significant difference: the loss has not yet occurred. If the loss is certain but no one can say when it will occur or if it does not occur when or as expected, those awaiting the actual loss or death may become irritable, hostile, or impatient, not because they want the loss to occur but in response to the emotional ups and downs of the waiting. Glaser and Strauss (1968) describe what they call an interruption in the sentimental order of a nursing unit when this occurs—no one quite knows how to behave. Professional grievers, such as nurses, as well as family and friends, usually deal much more easily with known losses at a known time or in a set manner (Glaser, Strauss, 1968).

Anticipatory grief can result in the phenomenon of premature detachment from an individual who is dying or detachment of the dying person from the environment. Pattison (1977) called the premature withdrawal of others sociological death, and the premature withdrawal of the person, psychological death. In either case, the person who is dying is no longer involved in day-to-day activities of living and essentially suffers a premature death.

Acute grief after anticipatory grief has not been found to be less painful but may help the griever develop some coping skills (Parks, Weiss, 1983). Dessonville and colleagues (1983) found that anticipatory grief not only did not lessen the eventual acute grief, but also in some cases may actually be associated with a poorer adjustment. Anticipatory grief, then, can be helpful or harmful to the griever but is recognized as a legitimate phenomenon.

Acute Grief

Acute grief is a crisis. It has a definite syndrome of somatic and psychological symptoms of distress that occur in waves lasting varying periods of time. These symptoms may occur every time the loss is acknowledged, others are informed, or another person offers condolences. Preoccupation with the loss is a phenomenon similar to daydreaming and is accompanied by a sense of unreality. Depending on the situation, feelings of self-blame or guilt may be present and manifest themselves as hostility or anger toward usual friends, depression, or withdrawal.

It is often difficult for persons who are acutely grieving to accomplish their usual activities of daily living or meet other responsibilities (functional disruption). Even if the tasks are accomplished, the person may complain of feeling distracted, restless, and "at loose ends." Common, simple activities such as dressing that normally takes a few minutes may take much longer; the decision making of which clothing to choose may seem too complex a task. Fortunately the signs and symptoms of acute grief do not last forever or else none of us could survive. Acute grief will be the most intense in the months immediately following the loss, with the intensity of feelings lessening over time. To follow Helen from above, in the first months she may cry any time her partner is mentioned. Later Helen will still be grieving but the tears are replaced with a surging sense of loss and sadness, and still later more fleeting emotions.

Chronic Grief

The normal grieving process or mourning takes time and sometimes takes much longer than anyone anticipates. Lund and colleagues (1986) and Arbuckle and de Vries (1995) found that it may take older widows and widowers much longer to reach the same level of adjustment than younger spouses. Horacek (1991) referred to this lingering grief as *shadow grief*. It may temporarily inhibit some activity but is considered a normal response. The intermittent pain of grief is often exacerbated on anniversary dates (birthdays, holidays, wedding anniversaries). For the survivors of tragedies, such as war, the Oklahoma City bombing, and the 9/11 attack, the "shadows" may never completely go away.

However, some chronic grief is more than that of shadow grief and crosses over the boundary to what we call impaired, pathological, abnormal, dysfunctional, or maladaptive grief. It has been thought that pathological chronic grief begins with normal grief responses, but obstacles interfere with its normal evolution toward adjustment, toward the reestablishment of equilibrium. The memories resist being reframed. Reactions are exaggerated, and memories are experienced as recurrent acute grief—over and over again, months and years later. Signs of possible pathological grief include excessive and irrational anger, outbursts in social settings, and insomnia that lingers for an extended time or surfaces months or years later, or a grief episode may trigger a major depressive episode. This type of grief requires the professional intervention of a grief counselor, a psychiatric nurse practitioner, or a psychologist who has skills at helping grieving elders.

Disenfranchised Grief

Disenfranchised grief is an experience of the person whose loss cannot be openly acknowledged or publicly mourned. The grief is socially disallowed or unsupported (Doka, 1989). The person does not have a socially recognized right to be perceived or function as a bereaved person. In other words, a relationship is not recognized; the loss is not sanctioned, or the griever is not recognized. Disenfranchised grief has frequently been associated with domestic partnerships in which the family of the deceased does not acknowledge the partner of the dead person or in secret relationships in which the involved party cannot tell others of the meaning or depth of the attachment. Disenfranchised grief can also occur in situations of family discord in which a member of the family is considered the "black sheep." The aged can experience this disenfranchisement when individuals associated and close to them do not understand the full meaning of a retiree's retirement, the impact of the death of a pet, or when gradual losses occur that are caused by chronic conditions that have great impact on the elder but are not seen as important to others. Families coping with a member who has Alzheimer's disease may also experience disenfranchised grief, particularly when others perceive death of the elder as a blessing and fail to support the griever or caregiver who has struggled for years with anticipatory grief and now must cope with the actual death.

Factors Affecting Coping with Loss

Coping as it relates to loss and grief is the ability of the individual or family to find ways to deal with the stress. In the language of the Loss Reaction Model (Jett, 2004), it is the ability to move from a state of chaos and disequilibrium to one of reorder, equilibrium, and peace. Many factors affect the ability to cope with loss and grief (Box 26-1).

Those at special risk for significantly adverse effects of grief are spouses (and likely same-gender partners). As far back as 1967, Rees and Lukin found that the mortality rate of an older surviving spouse was seven times greater than that of a younger surviving spouse. This was noted again in widowed men after the age of 75 (Bowling, 1989).

Those who are more likely to effectively deal with loss Weisman calls the "good copers" (1979, p 42). These are individuals or families who have experience with the successful management of crisis. They are resourceful, and they are able to draw on techniques that have worked in the past. Weisman (1979, pp 42-43; 1984) found persons who cope effectively with cancer as those who do the following:

Avoid avoidance
Confront realities, and take appropriate action
Focus on solutions
Redefine problems
Consider alternatives
Have good communication with loved ones
Seek and use constructive help
Accept support when offered
Can keep up their morale

In other words, the effective copers are those who can acknowledge the loss and try to make sense of it. They are able to maintain composure, use generally good judgment, and are able to remain optimistic without denying the loss. These good copers seek good guidance when they need it.

On the contrary, those who cope less effectively have few if any of these abilities. They tend to be more rigid and pessimistic, are demanding, and are given to emotional extremes. They are more likely to be dogmatic and expect perfection from themselves and others. Ineffective copers are also more likely to be individuals who live alone, socialize little, and have few close friends or have an ineffective support network. They may have a history of mental illness, or they may have guilt, anger, and ambivalence toward the individual who has died or that which has been lost. Those at risk for pathological grief will more likely have unresolved past conflicts or be facing the loss at the same time as other secondary stressors. They will have fewer opportunities as a result of the loss. They are the elders who are most in need of the expert interventions of grief counselors and skilled gerontological nurses.

Box 26-1	**Factors Influencing the Grieving Process**

Physical

Illness involves numerous losses

Each loss must be identified

Each loss prompts and requires its own grief response

Importance of the loss varies according to meaning by individual

Sedatives—deprive experience of reality of loss that must be faced

Nutritional state—if inadequate, leads to inability to cope or meet demands of daily living and numerous symptoms caused by grief

Rest—if inadequate, leads to mental and physical exhaustion, disease, unresolved grief

Exercise—if inadequate, limits emotional outlet, aggressive feelings, tension, anxiety, and leads to depression

Psychological

Unique nature and meaning of loss

Individual qualities of the relationship

Role that body part/self-image/aspect of self has to the individual and/or family

Individual coping behavior, personality, mental health

Individual level of maturity and intelligence

Past experience with loss or death

Social, cultural, ethnic, religious/philosophical background

Gender-role conditioning

Immediate circumstances surrounding loss

Timeliness of the loss

Perception of preventability (sudden versus expected)

Number, type, quality of secondary losses

Presence of concurrent stresses/crises

Specific to Dying/Death (in addition to above)

Role deceased occupied in family or social system

Amount of unfinished business

Perception of deceased's fulfillment in life

Immediate circumstances surrounding death

Length of illness before death

Anticipatory grief and involvement with dying patient

Social

Individual support systems and the acceptance of assistance of its members

Individual sociocultural, ethnic, religious/philosophical background

Educational, economic, occupational status

Ritual

From Hess PA: Loss, grief, and dying. In Beare PG, Myers JL, editors: *Principles and practice of adult health nursing*, ed 2, St Louis, 1994, Mosby.

IMPLICATIONS FOR GERONTOLOGICAL NURSING AND HEALTHY AGING

The goal of the nurse is not to prevent grief but to support those who are grieving. Although the loss will never change, the potential long-term detrimental effects can be ameliorated. Working with grieving elders is part of the normal workday of the gerontological nurse and a very special privilege. It is one of the few areas in nursing where small actions can make a large difference in the quality of life for the person to whom we provide care.

Assessment

The goal of the grief assessment is to differentiate those who are likely to cope effectively with those who are risk for ineffective coping, so that appro-

priate interventions can be planned. A grief assessment is based on knowledge of the grieving process and the subsequent mourning. Data are obtained through observation of behavior of the individual, keeping cultural context in mind. Behaviors may range from the stoic response of a person from a German or English heritage to the highly vocal expressions typical of persons from some Hispanic groups (Lipson et al, 1996).

A thorough grief assessment includes questions about recent significant life events, life or religious values, and relationship to that which has been lost. How many other stressful or demanding events or circumstances are going on in the griever's life? Information about these concurrent life stresses will help determine who may be at more risk for impaired grieving. The more concurrent stressors the person is dealing with the more he or she will need the nurse or other grief specialists. What stress management techniques are normally used, and are they potentially helpful (e.g., talking) or potentially harmful ones (e.g., substance use or abuse)? Was the griever's identity closely tied to that which is lost, such as a lifelong athlete who is faced with never walking again? If the loss is of a partner, how was the relationship? The loss of an abusive or controlling partner may liberate the survivor, who may feel guilty for not feeling the amount of grief that is expected. For many older women who have been dependent financially on their spouses, death may leave them impoverished, significantly complicating their grief. Knowing more about the loss and the effect of the loss on the elder's life will enable the nurse to construct and implement appropriate and caring responses.

Interventions

One goal of intervention is to assist the individual (or family) in attaining a healthy adjustment to the loss experience and reestablishing equilibrium. Actions that can meet this goal are basic and simple; however, the emotional overlay makes the simple often difficult. For the new nurse who is confronted with a person's grief for the first time, there may be discomfort, fear, and insecurity. The tendency is to be sympathetic rather than empathetic. Questions arise in one's mind: What do I say? Should I be cheerful or serious? Should I talk about or even mention the dead person's name?

Nursing interventions, especially when elders are in crisis, begin with the gentle establishment of rapport. Nurses introduce themselves, explain the nature of their roles (e.g., charge nurse, staff nurse, medication nurse) and the time they will be available to the elder. If it is the time of impact (e.g., just after a new serious diagnosis, at the death of a family member, or as a new but resistant resident of a long-term care facility), the most we can do is to provide support and a safe environment and ensure that basic needs, such as meals, are met. The nurse can soften the despair by fostering reasonable hope, such as, "You will survive this time, one moment at a time, and I will be here to help."

Nurses observe for functional disruption and offer support and direction. They may have to help the family figure out what needs to be done immediately and find ways to do it—either the nurse offers to complete the task or find a friend or family member who can step in so the disruption does not have any deleterious effects.

As grievers search for meaning they may need help finding what they are looking for. Sometimes it is information about a disease, a situation, or a person. Sometimes it is a spiritual search and help in finding a resource or a place of peace, such as the chapel. Often what is needed the most is someone to listen to the "whys" and "hows"—which cannot always be answered.

Sometime nurses offer to inform others for the grievers, thinking that this is something that will help. Since it is usually quite therapeutic for grievers to talk to others about the losses, nurses should refrain from helping in this way. Instead, the nurse can offer to find a phone number or hold the griever's hand during the conversation or just "be there" when the news is being shared. In this way the nurse can be available to provide support when the griever's emotions engage.

As the elder moves forward in adjusting to the loss, such as a move from home to a nursing home, the nurse can help the person reorganize this new life. The nurse talks with the elder about what was most valued about living at home and what habits were comforting and finds ways to incorporate these in a new way to the new environment. If the elder does not have access to a kitchen and always had a cup of tea before bed, this can become part of the individualized plan of care.

In order for the cycle of grieving to be completed, at least according to the Loss Reaction Model, new memories are needed. The grandmother who had always hosted her eldest daughter's birthday party can still do that even if she is now a resident in a long-term care facility. When the nurse has the information about this important ritual, she or he can help the person reserve a private space, send out invitations, and have the birthday party as always but now reframed as it is catered by the facility in the elder's new "home."

Countercoping

Avery Weisman (1979) described the work of health care professionals related to grief as "countercoping." Although he was speaking of working with people with cancer, it is equally applicable to working with people who are grieving. "Counter-coping is like counterpoint in music, which blends melodies together into a basic harmony. The patient copes; the therapist [nurse] countercopes; together they work out a better fit" (Weisman, 1979, p 109). Weisman suggests four very specific types of interventions or countercoping strategies: (1) clarification and control, (2) collaboration, (3) directed relief, and (4) cooling off.

Clarification and control. The nurse helps elders cope with dying by helping them confront the loss by getting or receiving information, considering alternatives, and finding a way to make the grief manageable. The nurse helps persons resume control by encouraging them to avoid acting on impulse.

Collaboration. The nurse collaborates by encouraging the griever to share stories with others and repeat the stories as often as is necessary as he or she "talks it out." The nurse as a collaborator is more directive than usual; it may be acceptable to say, "No, this is not a good time to make any major decisions."

Directed relief. Some temporary directed relief may be necessary, especially during acute grief. Catharsis may be helpful. In many instances it is the nurse who encourages the griever to cry or otherwise express feelings such as hurt or anger. The nurse may have to say something like, "Expressing your feelings is important." Activity may also be recommended as a natural extension of feelings. Intense physical activity gives one some control over emotions. In some cultures people may tear their clothes or cut their hair. Today, there are numerous ways of acting out feelings—from throwing things, to taking a walk, to busying oneself with tasks, to expressing feelings through creative works.

Cooling off. From time to time the griever might be encouraged to temporarily avoid processing the grief through diversions that worked in the past during times of stress, especially when things need to be done or decisions need to be made. The nurse may need to suggest new tactics that may prove helpful. Cooling off also means encouraging the person to modulate emotional extremes and to think about ways to make sense of the loss, to build a new sense of self-esteem after the loss and help him or her reestablish life patterns.

In all interventions related to grief, the nurse must have skills in therapeutic communication. Active listening is greatly preferable to giving advice. When listening, the nurse soon discovers that it is not the actual loss that is of utmost concern but, rather, the fear associated with the loss. If the nurse listens carefully to both the stated and the implied, what will be heard may be expressions such as the following: "How will I go on?" "What will I do now?" "What will become of me?" "I don't know what to do." "How could he (she) do this to me?" Because the nurse knows there is resolution, such comments may seem exaggerated or melodramatic, but to the one who is grieving there seems to be no resolution. The person who is actively grieving cannot yet look ahead and know that the despair and other feelings will resolve.

Like good copers, good gerontological nurses must be flexible, practical, resourceful, and abundantly optimistic.

DEATH AND DYING

Many people have said that death is not the problem, it is the dying that takes the work. This is true for all involved: the person, the loved ones, and the professional caregivers, such as the nurses and, in long-term care facilities, the nursing assistants.

Death and Dying in the United States

Before the 1900s most women died at home during childbirth. Men also died at home of unknown causes or on the battlefield. Now most women live well after menopause, and both men and women die most often from heart disease and too often in acute care settings. Life expectancy has gone from about 49 in the late 1800s to 74 for men and 79 for women by the end of the 1900s with variation by race and ethnicity (Federal Interagency Forum on Aging-Related Statistics, 2002). At this time persons most often die in acute care settings.

Dying is both a challenging life experience and a private one. How one deals with dying is often a reflection of the way the person has handled earlier losses and stressors. Most people probably do die as they have lived. Although not all older adults have had fulfilling lives or have a sense of completion, transcendence, or self-actualization, their deaths at the age or after that of their parents are considered normative. If the dying process is particularly long or the death occurs after a painful illness, we may rationalize it or view it as relief, at least in part. Death at a younger age or as the result of trauma or catastrophe is viewed as tragic and sometimes incomprehensible. After 9/11 no one rationalized the deaths of the older victims as a relief; all deaths were considered an unacceptable loss of human potential.

Conceptual Models

As models have been proposed to explain the grieving process, so have they been proposed for the process of dying. One of the most well known has been that of Dr. Elizabeth Kübler-Ross. In her book *On Death and Dying* (1969) she reported on observations of predominately middle-aged inpatients on the psychiatric ward where she did her psychiatry residency. She proposed the stages of dying as denial, anger, bargaining, depression, and acceptance. Nurses and many others have tried to help the dying work through denial to achieve acceptance before their deaths. However, we have come to realize that the "stages" are actually types of emotional reactions to dying that people experience and not a model at all. An alternative model that has been very useful is presented below.

The Living-Dying Interval

Whereas physically we may begin dying early in life as proposed by the theories of aging (see Chapter 7), in personal terms dying begins at a moment called the "crisis knowledge of death" (Pattison, 1977, p 44) and ends at the moment of physiological death. Pattison (1977) calls the time between these two points the living-dying interval, made up of the acute, chronic, and terminal phases. The chronological time of the living-dying interval is accordion-like because of remissions and exacerbations in the terminal diagnosis; it may last days, weeks, months, or years. The manner in which one faces dying is an expression of personality, circumstances, illness, and culture.

The "crisis knowledge of death" occurs when someone receives the information that he or she will not live as long as previously anticipated.

Certainly it would appear that the more the discrepancy between the previously believed length of life and the newly projected length of life, the more the adjustment and perhaps the intensity of the grief experienced.

The point of crisis is a moment in time that is followed by an acute phase. It is usually the peak time of stress and anxiety as the life and future of the individual and the family are thrown into disequilibrium. Crisis intervention is most effective here because the individual, family, and caregivers are struggling to come to terms with the knowledge. A significant amount of anticipatory grieving may be observed.

Since no one can withstand a crisis indefinitely, most of the dying time is spent in the chronic phase. During this time the dying and those about them are forced to resume some sense of normalcy. Bills still need to be paid, dishes still need to be done, and life can still be lived. The challenge for persons with terminal diagnoses and their families is to work toward living while dying and not dying while still living. Entertainment, work, and relationships can be maintained as normally as the individual's condition permits. Life goes on despite the anticipation of its end.

The terminal phase is reached when the speed of the physical dying is accelerated and the dying person no longer has the energy to maintain the activities of everyday life. The person may withdraw or turn away from the outside world; or the person may engage in coded communication, such as saying "good-bye" instead of the usual "good night," giving away cherished possessions as gifts, or urgently contacting friends and relatives with whom the person has not communicated for a long time. The focus then turns to preserving energy and completing life's journey. In some cultures this period of time is called the "death watch" and is associated with proscribed rituals.

The living-dying interval can reflect an integrated or disintegrated experience (Pattison, 1977). The interval is integrated when each new crisis occurs, is dealt with effectively, and the quality of life while dying is preserved. The interval is disintegrated if one crisis tumbles on to the next one without any effective resolution and the quality of life while dying is compromised (Figure 26-3).

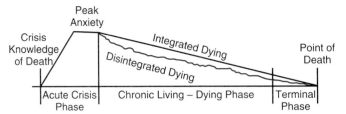

Figure 26-3 The living-dying interval. (From Pattison EM: *The experience of dying*, Englewood Cliffs, NJ, 1977, Prentice-Hall.)

The Needs of the Dying and Their Families and Implications for Gerontological Nursing

The needs of the dying are like threads in a piece of cloth. Each thread is individual but necessary to the integrity and completeness of the fabric. If one thread is pulled, it touches the other threads, affecting the material's appearance, the thread placement, and the stability of the piece. When one need is unmet it will affect all others because they are both building and interwoven.

The responsibility of the nurse is to provide safe conduct as the dying and their families navigate through unknown waters to a good and appropriate death. A good and appropriate death is one that a person would choose if choosing were possible. A good and appropriate death is one in which one's needs are met to the extent possible. There are several ways to approach an understanding of the needs of persons who are dying and the responsibilities of the nurse. The approaches discussed here include a task orientation and what can be called the 6 C's approach.

Task-Based Approach

A task-based approach attempts to address coping with dying from an individual's own perspective and with coping tasks grounded in situational tasks that are fundamental markers of human living (Corr, 1995). The dimensions of coping are physical, psychological, social, and spiritual. Each has a specific function in the person's life and has associated implications for the development of nursing interventions.

The **physical dimension** addresses the satisfaction of basic body needs and the minimization of physical distress in ways that are consistent with the person's values. Correlating closely to Maslow's level of biological integrity, these needs include nutrition, hydration, elimination, and shelter. Pain, nausea, vomiting, and constipation are among the common causes of physical distresses in dying persons that the nurse can respond to. The development of the field of palliative care nursing has contributed much to our skills in effectively helping persons with needs in the physical dimension. See Chapter 17 for details on how we might intervene regarding pain and discomfort (Table 26-1).

The **psychological dimension** deals with three aspects of the common desires of dying persons: freedom from anxiety, fear, and apprehension; autonomy and security; and self-governance or control of one's life, especially for that which makes it satisfying, such as serenity, activity, and creativity.

The **social dimension** addresses one's relationships with others and with society. Relationships with others—individuals or groups—sustain and enhance interpersonal attachments. Some significant ties continue while one is dying; others fall by the wayside as death nears. We focus on the relationships that the dying person feels are important, not those that others think are important. No matter how much individuals think that they are alone, they are connected to society as a whole through family, culture, congregations, and governmental entities.

The **spiritual dimension** is that from which one draws meaning for both life and death and connection to some force outside of oneself. Spirituality is the manner in which one integrates one's knowledge or belief system, inner life experiences, and exterior life and institutional activities in support of these beliefs (Thibault et al,

Table 26-1 Physical Signs and Symptoms Associated with the Final Stages of Dying, Rationale, and Interventions

Physical Signs and Symptoms	Rationale	Intervention (if any)
Coolness, color, and temperature change in hands, arms, feet, and legs; perspiration may be present	Peripheral circulation diminished to facilitate increased circulation to vital organs	Place socks on feet; cover with light cotton blankets; keep warm blankets on person, but *do not use electric blanket.*
Increased sleeping	Conservation of energy	Spend time with the patient; hold the hand; speak normally to the patient even though there may be a lack of response.
Disorientation; confusion of time, place, person	Metabolic changes	Identify self by name before speaking to patient; speak softly, clearly, and truthfully.
Incontinence of urine and/or bowel	Increased muscle relaxation and decreased consciousness	Maintain vigilance; change bedding as appropriate; utilize bed pads; try not to use an indwelling catheter.
Congestion	Poor circulation of body fluids, immobilization, and inability to expectorate secretions cause gurgling, rattles, bubbling	Elevate the head with pillows or raise the head of the bed; gently turn the head to the side to drain secretions.
Restlessness	Metabolic changes and decrease in oxygen to the brain	Calm the patient by speech and action; reduce light; gently rub back, stroke arms, or read aloud; play soothing music; *do not use restraints.*
Decreased intake of food and fluids	Body conservation of energy for function	Do not force patient to eat or drink; give ice chips, soft drinks, juice, Popsicles as possible; apply petroleum jelly to dry lips; if patient is a mouth breather, apply protective jelly more frequently as necessary.
Decreased urine output	Decreased fluid intake and decreased circulation to kidney	None.
Altered breathing pattern	Metabolic and oxygen changes of respiratory system	Elevate the head of bed; hold hand, speak gently to patient.
		ADDITIONAL GENERAL INTERVENTIONS Learn to be "with person" without talking; a moist washcloth on the forehead may be soothing; eye drops may help soothe the eyes.

From Hess PA: Loss, grief, and dying. In Beare PG, Myers JL, editors: *Principles and practice of adult health nursing*, ed 2, St Louis, 1994, Mosby.

Table 26-2 Emotional/Spiritual Symptoms of Approaching Death, Rationale, and Interventions

Emotional/Spiritual Symptoms	Rationale	Intervention
Withdrawal	Prepares the patient for release and detachment and letting go of relationships and surroundings	Continue communicating in a normal manner using a normal voice tone; identify self by name; hold hand, say what person wants to hear from you.
Vision-like experiences (dead friends or family, religious vision)	Preparation for transition	Do not contradict or argue regarding whether this is or is not a real experience; if the patient is frightened, reassure him or her that it is normal.
Restlessness	Tension, fear, unfinished business	Listen to patient express his or her fears, sadness, and anger associated with dying; give permission to go.
Decreased socialization	As energy diminishes, the patient begins making his or her transition	Express support; give permission to die.
Unusual communication: out of character statements, gestures, requests	Signals readiness to let go	Say what needs to be said to the dying patient; kiss, hug, cry with him or her.

From Hess PA: Loss, grief, and dying. In Beare PG, Myers JL, editors: *Principles and practice of adult health nursing,* ed 2, St Louis, 1994, Mosby.

1991, p 29). The spiritual dimension deals with the transcendental relationship between the dying person and another: between persons and their God or the person and significant others. Spirituality may be met through religious acts or through human caring relationships. A person's internal beliefs, personal experiences, and religion are expressions of spirituality. This leads to self-discovery, affirmation of self-love, and a connection with all others that are brought about by loving the most unlovable aspects of self and others (Table 26-2).

Nurses can tend to the spiritual needs of dying elders in the following ways:

• Ask the individual his or her source of strength and hope.
• Ask if the individual sees any connection between physical health and spiritual beliefs.
• Discuss sources of spiritual strength throughout life.

Signs of spiritual distress include doubt, despair, guilt, boredom, and anger at God (Box 26-2). Interventions may involve calling clergy;

sharing spiritual readings, poems, and music; obtaining religious articles such as a Bible or rosary; or praying. The nurse is cautioned that these interventions must be consistent with the culture and wishes of the patient and not as expressions of the nurse's belief system.

Spirituality is the basic human capacity for hope. Hope empowers, generates courage, motivates action and achievement, and can strengthen physiological and psychological functioning. Hope involves faith and trust. Hope can be classified as desirable or expectational (Pattison, 1977). Expectational hope sounds like "I hope to get better" or "I hope my children get here in time." If this hope is a reflection of expectations that are not realistic, they can increase stress for the person and caregiver. However, this hope can be modified without being lost. In desirable hope the wishes are something that would be appreciated if it were to occur without the expectation that it will or must occur. The nurse can respond to the comment "I hope I get better" from someone who is rapidly declining with "That would be really great; in the meantime

Box 26-2   Assessing and Intervening in Spiritual Distress

Assessment

Brief history:
  Losses
  Challenged belief or value system
  Separation from religious and cultural ties
  Death
  Personal and family disasters
Symptoms (defining characteristics), such as the
    following:
  Unmet needs
  Threats to self
  Change in environment, health status,
    self-concept, etc.
  Seeking spiritual assistance
  Questioning meaning of own existence
  Depression
  Feelings of hopelessness, abandonment, fear
Assessment of etiology of spiritual distress:
  Depletion anxiety
  Helplessness and hopelessness
  Perceived powerlessness

Medication reactions
Hormonal imbalances

Interventions

Create a therapeutic environment.
Assess support system.
Assess past methods of decreasing distress
    (i.e., prayer, imagery, healing, memories
    and reminiscence therapy, medication,
    relaxation).
Determine environmental changes needed to
    enhance functioning.
Assess and assist implementation of coping
    mechanisms.
Refer to clergy.
Evaluate effects of nursing interventions.
Evaluate medications and their interactions.
Activate and evaluate appropriate community
    referrals.
Use techniques to assist client and family in
    reducing spiritual distress.

there is so much we can do for you (i.e., comfort)." Hope may be related to a cure, a holiday, the birth of a grandchild, or reconciliation.

Nurses seldom recognize the small things they do, routinely and unconsciously, to impart hope. The act of helping with grooming conveys a quiet belief that the person matters. Pain relief and comfort measures reinforce the recognition of an individual's needs and reinforce the value of the person. Several approaches that may help the nurse to more clearly foster and sustain hope in the physically failing elder are to (1) confirm the value of life, (2) establish a support system, (3) incorporate humor, (4) incorporate the person's religion, and (5) set realistic goals (Hickey, 1986).

Like Weisman's countercoping, Sister Rosemary Donley defines the nursing role in the spiritual search of suffering persons as compassionate accompaniment—entering into another's reality and quietly, attentively sharing the experience. "Nurses need to be with people who suffer, to give meaning to the reality of suffering, and insofar as possible, to remove suffering and its causes. Here lies the spiritual dimension of health care" (Donley, 1991, p 180).

Based on task analysis, Corr (1993, 1995), Doka (1993), and Coolican et al (1994) focused on living with life-threatening illness and developed tasks that are needed at the time of the initial diagnosis, the living-dying interval, recovery or death, and the aftermath. These tasks confront general issues and acute, chronic, and terminal phases of the life-death cycle. Some of them are outlined in Table 26-3 from which nursing care plans can be developed.

The 6 C's Approach

Weisman (1979) identified six needs of the dying: care, control, composure, communication, continuity, and closure.

Care. The dying should have the best care possible; this means expert management of symptoms and support at all times. Care means the adequate treatment of pain. Uncontrolled pain can occupy the patient's whole attention, isolating him or her from the world. Care also goes beyond the physical to psychological pain, induced by depression, anxiety, fear, and other unresolved emotional concerns that are just as strong and just as real. When emotional needs are not met, the

Table 26-3 Tasks in Life-Threatening Illness

General	Acute Phase	Chronic Phase	Terminal Phase
1. Responding to the physical fact of disease	1. Understanding the disease	1. Managing symptoms and side effects	1. Dealing with symptoms, discomfort, pain, and incapacitation
2. Taking steps to cope with the reality of disease	2. Maximizing health and lifestyle	2. Carrying out health regimens	2. Managing health procedures and institutional stress
3. Preserving self-concept and relationships with others in the face of disease	3. Maximizing one's coping strengths and limiting weaknesses	3. Preventing and managing health crisis	3. Managing stress and examining coping
4. Dealing with effective and existential/spiritual issues created or reactivated by the disease	4. Developing strategies to deal with the issues created by the disease	4. Managing stress and examining coping	4. Dealing effectively with caregivers
	5. Exploring the effect of the diagnosis on a sense of self and others	5. Maximizing social support and minimizing isolation	5. Preparing for death and saying good-bye
	6. Ventilating feelings and fears	6. Normalizing life in the face of the disease	6. Preserving self-concept
	7. Incorporating the present reality of diagnosis into one's sense of past and future	7. Dealing with financial concerns	7. Preserving appropriate relationships with family and friends
		8. Preserving self-concept	8. Ventilating feelings and fears
		9. Redefining relationships with others throughout the course of the disease	9. Finding meaning in life and death
		10. Ventilating feelings and fears	
		11. Finding meaning in suffering, chronicity, uncertainty, and decline	

From Coolican MB et al: Education about death, dying, and bereavement in nursing programs, *Nurs Educ* 19(6):35-40, 1994.

total pain experience, physical and psychosocial, may be exacerbated or intensified. Medication alone cannot relieve this pain. Instead, empathetic listening and allowing the dying person to verbalize what is on his or her mind are important interventions that must be based on the energy level of the one who is dying. If tears and sadness are present, silence and touch are worth more than words could ever convey. Gentleness of touch, closeness, and sitting near the person may be appropriate. As an advocate, the gerontological nurse also makes sure that the medical care that is needed is received.

Care also means helping the patient conserve energy. Dying requires great amounts of energy to cope with the physical assault of illness on the body and the emotional unrest that dying initiates. How much can the individual do without becoming physically and emotionally taxed? What activities of daily living are most important for the person to do independently? How much energy is needed for the patient to be able to talk with visitors or staff without becoming exhausted? Only the person who is dying can answer these questions, and the nurse can advocate for the person to be given the opportunity to do so; and in doing so, the patient is able to remain in better control and maintain composure.

Control.   As one proceeds along the living-dying interval it often feels that control over one's life has been lost. The person is in the process of losing everything he or she has every known or would ever know. The potential loss of identity, independence, and control over body functions can lead to a sense of loss of control and self-esteem. The person may begin to feel ashamed, humiliated, and like a "burden." Control is the need to remain in a collaborative role relating to one's own living and dying and as active a participant in the care as desired. The nurse can help the person meet these needs by taking every opportunity to return the control to the person and in doing so bolster the patient's self-esteem. Whenever possible the nurse can have the person decide when to groom, eat, wake, sleep, etc. The nurse never has the right to determine the activities of the individual, especially relating to visitors and how time is spent.

Composure.   Dying is usually an emotional activity—for the dying and for those around them. The need for composure is that which enables the person to modulate emotional extremes within cultural norms as is appropriate. This is not to avoid the sadness; this is to have moments of relief. The nurse may use many of the counter-coping techniques discussed to help persons meet this need.

Communication.   The need for communication is broad, from the need for information to make decisions to the need to share information. Although the type and content of communication that is acceptable to the person vary by culture, the nurse has a responsibility to make sure that the dying person has an opportunity for the communication he or she desires.

In a study of communication about terminal illness and among the patient, family, and hospital staff, Glaser and Strauss (1963) identified four types: closed awareness, suspected awareness, mutual pretense, and open awareness. Each of these influenced the work on the hospital unit. *Closed awareness* is described as "keeping the secret." Hospital staff and the family and friends know that the patient is dying, but the patient does not know it or knows and keeps the secret as well. Generally, caregivers invent a fictitious future for the patient to believe in, in hopes that it will boost the patient's morale. Although this happens less today with the legislation related to patients' rights, it still occurs. In *suspected awareness,* the patient suspects that he or she is going to die. Hints are bandied back and forth, and a contest ensues for control of the information. *Mutual pretense* is a situation of "let's pretend." Everyone knows the patient has a terminal illness and may be dying, but the patient, family, friends, nurses, and physicians do not talk about it—real feelings are kept hidden. *Open awareness* acknowledges the reality of approaching death. The patient, family, friends, nurses, and physicians openly acknowledge the eventual death of the patient. The patient may ask, "Will I die?" and "How and when will I die?" The patient becomes resigned to dying, and the family grieves with the patient rather than for the patient. The nurse can encourage open awareness whenever possible while at the same time respecting the patient's culture. In some cultures talking about an anticipated death is deemed helpful. In others, one can be aware of the dying but talking about it openly may be taboo (Irish et al, 1993).

Continuity.   The need for continuity is that of the preservation of as normal a life as possible while dying and the need to transcend the present, leaving a legacy for the future. Too often a dying patient can feel shut off from the rest of the world at a time when he or she is still capable of being involved and active in some way. Loneliness is the result of a loss of continuity with one's life. The nurse may ask about the person's life and those things most valued and work with the family and the patient or resident on a plan to remain engaged in as many of the activities and past roles as possible. A father who watches a certain ballgame with his son every Sunday can continue to do this regardless of the need to be in a hospital, a nursing home, or an inpatient hospice unit. If the person is at home and is bed bound, it may make more sense to have the bed in a central area rather than in a distant room. Treating the dying aged person as an intelligent adult, holding a hand, or putting an arm around a shoulder if culturally acceptable says, "I care" and "You're not alone" and "You are important."

Legacies can take many different forms and may range from memories that will live on in the minds of others to bequeathed fortunes. A grandmother who is likely to die before a favorite grandchild's wedding can be asked to participate in anticipatory planning, regardless of the age of the grandchild, thereby leaving an enduring and special legacy. The nurse can assist older adults in meeting continuity needs by helping them think about a possible legacy, by doing the following:
- Find out lifestyle interests.
- Establish a method of recording.
- Identify recipients (either generally or specifically).
- Help to record the legacy.

Box 26-3 lists examples of legacies that are as diverse as individual contributions to humanity.

Closure.   The need for closure is the need for the opportunity for reconciliation and transcendence, the highest of Maslow's Hierarchy. Reminiscence is one way of putting one's life in order, to evaluate the pluses and minuses of life. It is a means of resolving conflicts, giving up possessions, and making final good-byes. Learning to say "good-bye" today leaves open the possibility of many more "hellos." Pain and other symptoms that are not well cared for may interfere with this reconciliation, making appropriate interventions by the nurse especially important.

Box 26-3	Examples of Legacies

Oral histories
Autobiographies
Shared memories
Taught skills
Works of art and music
Publications
Human organ donations
Endowments
Objects of significance
Written histories
Tangible or intangible assets
Personal characteristics, such as courage or integrity
Bestowed talents
Traditions and myths perpetuated
Philanthropical causes
Progeny: children and grandchildren
Methods of coping
Unique thought: Darwin, Einstein, Freud, and others

For some, closure means coming to terms with their spiritual selves, with Jesus, God, Allah, or Buddha. If the expressions of the patient have spiritual overtones, arranging for pastoral care may be offered but should never be done without the person's permission. The nurse can foster transcendence by providing patients with the time and privacy for self-reflection as well as an opportunity to talk about whatever they need to talk about, especially about the meanings of their lives and the meanings of their deaths.

Care, control, composure, communication, continuity, and closure create the borders necessary to complete the fabric of needs of the dying aged. Their influence is omnipresent in the other needs. Without them, the cloth can fray, and attempts to meet the needs will be limited.

The Family

The nurse is often present and supporting the family at the moment of death and in the moments preceding it. Regardless of the age of the surviving family members, as spouse, partner, children, or friends, they too have needs and nurses have a responsibility to care for them. Newly bereaved persons were asked what they had found most helpful (Richter, 1987). They most appreciated nurses who did the following:

- Kept me informed
- Asked how I was doing and offered support
- Put an arm around me when I cried
- Brought me food
- Knew my name
- Cried with me
- Brought a bed and encouraged me to stay in the room with my dying husband
- Told me to hold my husband's hand while he was dying
- Held my hand
- Got the chaplain for me
- Let me take care of my husband
- Stayed with me after their shift was over

Although these will not provide comfort to all, nor are all these behaviors always possible, they can be used as starting points. See Table 26-4 for sample care plans for survivors.

DYING AND THE NURSE

Nurses are professional grievers. We invest time and caring, and if working with older adults, especially those who are frail and in acute and long-term care settings, we experience the death of patients and residents over and over again. Some consider the death of a patient as a failure, that they have "lost" the person they cared for; yet, when they are good deaths, they can be viewed as professional successes each time we share the special and very personal experience of providing safe conduct for elders while dying and gentle caring for their survivors. We can use the reminders of our own mortality as motivation to live the best we can with what we have. Nurses can seek support and give it to one another. As grievers, we too may need to tell the story of the dying, or the person, to those professionals around us, either in formal or informal support groups; and we need to listen to those stories of our colleagues.

Caring for older adults requires knowledge of the grieving and dying processes as well as skills in providing relief of symptoms or palliative care. However, it is also acknowledged that working with the grieving or dying day in and day out is an art. The development of the art necessitates inner strength. The nurse needs to have spiritual strength, strength from within. This does not mean that the nurse must have a specific religious orientation or affiliation but, rather, that the nurse must have a positive belief in self and a belief that there is meaning to life. The effective nurse has developed a personal philosophy of life and of death. Although this can and does change over time, and cannot be assumed to be held by anyone else, one's beliefs about life and death will help the nurse through difficult times. Emotional maturity allows the nurse to deal with disappointment and postponement of immediate wants or desires. Maturity means that the nurse can reach out for help for self when needed. Finally, in order to provide comfort to grieving persons, nurses must be comfortable with their own lives or at least be able to set aside their own sadness and grief while working with the sadness and grief of others.

Palliative Care

Nurses routinely care for elders who have irreversible and progressive conditions, such as Alzheimer's disease or Parkinson's disease. Other elders have exhausted all treatment options or have decided that they want no further treatment for conditions such as cancer or end-stage heart or renal disease. A nursing home resident may elect to remain at the facility rather than return (ever) to a hospital, even if faced with an acute event, such as a myocardial infarction (MI) or stroke. These persons are receiving a type of care called palliative care, or that which focuses on comfort rather than care, on the treatment of symptoms rather than disease, on quality of life left rather than quantity of life lived. Palliative care is much of what is done in gerontological nursing and may indeed be the heart of caring. Palliative care can be provided anywhere by anyone sharing these goals and skills (see Box 26-4 for Core Competencies for Palliative/End-of-Life Care).

The scope and specialty of this knowledge base have grown considerable over the years; research has been conducted, professional organizations have been formed, and most recently standardized curricula have been developed. With the support of the American Association of Colleges of Nursing and City of Hope Medical Center, a broad initiative was established to train nurses through the End of Life Nursing Consortium (ANA-ELNEC).

Table 26-4 Nursing Care Plan for Survivors

Nursing Diagnosis	Expected Outcomes	Interventions
DEPRESSION, LONELINESS, SOCIAL ISOLATION RELATED TO LOSS OF SPOUSE, SEXUAL PARTNER, FRIEND, COMPANION, OR CONFIDANT		
Manifestations: teariness, crying, sleep disturbance, weight gain, compulsive eating, weight loss, anorexia, fatigue, confusion, forgetfulness, withdrawal, disinterest, indecisiveness, inability to concentrate, guilt feelings; displays feelings of detachment, inferiority, rejection, alienation, emptiness, isolation; unable to initiate social contacts; seeks attention	*Short-term/intermediate goals:* The survivor will do the following: Develop or use immediate support systems Express feelings of security Exhibit meaningful social relationships Show decreasing signs of depression *Long-term goal:* The survivor will demonstrate readiness to build a new life as a single person.	Attempt to develop a therapeutic relationship through touch, empathy, and listening. Listen to perceived feelings. Help person realize that grief is a painful but normal transitional process. Encourage use of other women, daughters, widows, men, and friends as support systems. Encourage balance between linking phenomena (mementos, photographs, clothes, furniture) associated with the deceased and the bridging phenomena (new driving skills, evening classes, new job). Establish contact with Widow to Widow Program for counseling if appropriate. Refer to appropriate agencies.
ANXIETY RELATED TO INCREASED LEGAL, FINANCIAL, AND DECISION-MAKING RESPONSIBILITIES		
Manifestations: anger, nervousness, palpitations, increased perspiration, face flushing, dyspnea, urinary frequency, nausea, vomiting, restlessness, apprehension, panic, fear, headache	*Short-term/intermediate goals:* The survivor will demonstrate adequate decision-making skills in financial and legal matters as evidenced by the following: Seeking legal aid Writing or calling appropriate agencies Formulating a realistic budget *Long-term goals:* The survivor will do the following: Cope with legal, financial, and decision-making responsibilities with only a moderate degree of anxiety Make rational decisions about single life	Assist in obtaining attorney if necessary. Encourage to contact Social Security and/or spouse's employer to ensure receipt of all benefits. Encourage to contact insurance agencies if applicable. Discourage immediate decision making regarding assets (e.g., home, stocks). Encourage to seek advice from individuals who are trusted. Contact proper social agencies if indigent or in need. Assist in seeking employment if health permits and client so desires. Offer alternatives for decision making. Refer to any other proper community agencies that offer needed assistance.

From Alexander J, Kiely A: Working with the bereaved, *Geriatr Nurs* 7(2):85-86, 1986.

Box 26-4	Core Competencies for Palliative/End-of-Life Care

The nurse should be able to do the following:

Talk to patients and families about dying.

Be knowledgeable about pain control and pain-control techniques (opioid dosing and other pharmacological interventions).

Provide comfort-oriented nursing interventions.

Provide palliative treatments.

Recognize physical changes that precede eminent death.

Deal with own feelings.

Deal with angry patients and families.

Be knowledgeable and deal with the ethical issues in administering end-of-life palliative therapies.

Be knowledgeable, and inform patients about advance directives.

Be knowledgeable of the legal issues in administering end-of-life palliative care.

Be adaptable and sensitive to religious and cultural perspectives.

Explain the meaning of hospice.

Modified from White KR, Coyne PJ, Patel UB: Are nurses adequately prepared for end-of-life care? *Image J Nurs Sch* 33(2):147-151, 2001.

It is hoped that by training nurses and faculty, nursing as a profession can provide the highest level of palliative care (Matzo, Sherman, 2004).

Whereas initially palliative care was the specialty of community-based hospices, specialized units and staff are now seen in long-term care and acute care facilities across the United States. Palliative care was once not a well-reimbursed service, but since a hospice benefit was added to Medicare Part A in the 1980s, the number of private insurance companies and health maintenance organizations (HMOs) offering a hospice option has increased and programs have grown considerably (Matzo, Sherman, 2004).

Hospice

Hospice is described as the link among the needs of the terminally ill, their families, and the staff; it employs the medieval concept of hospitality in which a community assists the traveler at dangerous points along his or her journey. It returns nursing to its roots—as humane compassionate care, an ideal that has been the basis of nursing for centuries. The dying are indeed travelers—travelers along the continuum of life—and the community consists of friends, family, and specially prepared people to care—the hospice team. The philosophy of hospice care is that "the last stages of life should not be seen as defeat, but rather as life's fulfillment. It is not merely a time of negation, rather an opportunity for positive achievement . . ." (Ulrich, 1978, p 20). It is a reorientation in health care for the patient and family.

The concept of the contemporary hospice was made famous by Dr. Cicely Saunders, founder of Saint Christopher's Hospice in London more than 30 years ago. Hospice organizations, some non-profit and others for-profit, are now all over the United States and provide comprehensive and interdisciplinary care to persons in the last 6 months of life. Under Medicare, hospice provides, at a minimum, medical, nursing, nursing assistant, chaplain, social work, and volunteer support available 24 hours per day. Potential services may also include music, art, and pet therapy and others. Hospices provide care not only to the dying but also to their families and friends through support groups before and after the deaths.

The majority of hospice care is provided in people's homes to support the informal caregiver. The home becomes the primary center of care, and care is provided by family members or friends who are taught basic nursing care, including diet, exercise, and medication needed to care for the dying individual. However, a limited number of in-patient hospice facilities exist as well. Hospice staff may also see patients who are residents in long-term care facilities, working with the staff to supplement care and provide expertise. Long-term care facilities may also provide services from their own staff that are consistent with the hospice principles derived from the work of the American Geriatrics Society (Box 26-5) or from those established by the American Nurses Association and the National Hospice and Palliative Care Organization (see Resources at the end of this chapter).

The unprecedented contribution of hospice continues to be reestablishment of control for the dying person. Through polypharmaceutical means, control of distressful symptoms and pain

Box 26-5	Principles for Measuring the Quality of Care at the End of Life

1. Physical and emotional symptoms

Pain, shortness of breath, fatigue, depression, fear, anxiety, nausea, skin breakdown, and other physical and emotional problems often destroy the quality of life at its end. The focus should be on these needs and ensuring that people can count on a comfortable and meaningful end to their lives.

2. Support of function and autonomy

Maintaining a patient's personal dignity and self-respect is extremely important.

3. Advance care planning

Planning ahead allows for decisions to be made that reflect the patient's preferences and circumstances rather than only a response to crises.

4. Aggressive care near death—site of death, CPR, and hospitalization

Although aggressive care is often justified, most patients would prefer to have avoided it when the short-term outcome is death.

5. Patient and family satisfaction

Both patient and family satisfaction should be measured by the following elements: the

decision-making process, the care given, and the outcomes achieved.

6. Global quality of life

Overall well-being can be good, despite declining physical health. Care systems that achieve this goal should be valued.

7. Family burden

When possible, serious financial and emotional effects from the costs of care and the challenges of direct caregiving should be reduced.

8. Survival time

That death may be too readily accepted is reason to worry. Purchasers and patients need to know that survival times vary across plans and provider systems.

9. Provider continuity and skill

Providers must have relevant skills, including rehabilitation, symptom control, and psychological support. Care systems must demonstrate competent performance on continuity and provider skill.

10. Bereavement

Survivors may benefit from relatively modest interventions, when immediately available.

Modified from American Geriatrics Society: Measuring quality of care at the end of life: a statement of principles, *AGS Newsletter* 25(3), 1996.

CPR, Cardiopulmonary resuscitation.

can be accomplished without denying the patient full alertness and the ability to communicate with others. This gift, so to speak, allows normality for the patient. The crux of accomplishing this end is the anticipation of symptoms and intervention by the caregiver before problems occur.

Pain control and the opportunity to die at home are the key ideas and activities that people associate with hospice. In actuality, hospice represents much more. It supports and guides the family in patient care and ensures that the patient will not die alone and that the family will not be abandoned. Bereavement services for the family extend for a period of time on an emergency and regular basis after the death of the patient. Life is made as meaningful as possible.

Nurse's role in hospice care. Nursing practice and hospice incorporate the mind-body continuum. Nursing is considered to be the cornerstone of hospice care. The nurse provides much of the direct care and functions in a variety of roles: as staff nurse giving direct care, as coordinator implementing the plan of the interdisciplinary team or as executive officer responsible for research and educational activities, and as an advocate for the patient and hospice in the clinical and political arena.

The American Nurses Association's *Standards and Scope of Hospice and Palliative Nursing Practice* (2002) enumerates the special skills, knowledge, and abilities needed by a nurse who provides end of life care:

1. Thorough knowledge of anatomy and physiology and considerable familiarity with pathophysiological causes of numerous diseases
2. Well-grounded skill in physical assessment and in various nursing procedures, such as catheterization, colostomy, and traction care
3. Above-average knowledge of pharmacology, especially of analgesics, narcotics, antiemetics, tranquilizers, antibiotics, hormone therapy, steroids, cardiotonic agents, and cancer chemotherapy
4. Skill in using psychological principles in individual and group situations
5. Great sensitivity in human relationships
6. Personal characteristics such as stamina, emotional stability, flexibility, cooperativeness, and a life philosophy or faith
7. Knowledge of measures to comfort the dying in the last hours

The Hospice and Palliative Care Nurses Association provides guidance in end-of-life care. These guidelines bring gerontological theory, nursing concepts, and knowledge of medical management of acute and chronic conditions of elders together to provide the most sensitive and comprehensive care possible.

DECISION MAKING AT END OF LIFE

Decision making regarding life-prolonging procedures when death is inevitable have become legal, ethical, medical, and professional issues today. The blurring of the lines between living and dying results from technological advances, the ambivalence of whether death is to be fought or accepted, and the dilemma brought about by medical technologies. Decision making at the end of life has become increasingly complex because most people die in advanced age from chronic illnesses—dying over a period of years and slowly declining from degenerative conditions, including Alzheimer's disease and Parkinson's disease.

Who makes end-of-life decisions has been the subject of research, debate, and federal legislation. The individual adult is generally recognized as the decision maker; however, this assumption is based on a very Euro-American or Western perspective. Persons who are from non-Western traditions place less emphasis on the individual and more on the needs of the family or community (Blackhall et al, 1995; Mazanec, Tyler, 2003).

The nurse has an obligation to know legal expectations and then work with the elder and the family in how these will fit with their cultural patterns and needs related to end-of-life decisions.

Advance Directives

Whereas people have always had opinions about their wishes, their right to refuse medical treatment was legislated in the Patient Self-Determination Act (PSDA) enacted by Congress in October 1990 and implemented in all states in December 1991. Under the PSDA, the adult was recognized as the ultimate authority in the decisions to forego life-sustaining treatment for himself or herself, rather than a physician or a health care agency. In other words, through the PSDA, adults were granted the legal authority to complete what are known as advance directives—or statements about their wishes, or directions to others, before the need for decisions. These directives may be as detailed or as vague as desired, from "no treatment if I am terminally ill" to a breakdown of decisions about dialysis, antibiotics, tube feedings, cardiopulmonary resuscitation (CPR), and so on. Through the PSDA any adult may also appoint any other adult (not necessarily next of kin or relative) to speak for him or her and make decisions if the patient is unable to do so.

Two common forms of advance directives are known as living wills and durable power of attorney for health care (DPAHC), also called advanced health care directive (AHCD). A living will is restricted to represent a person's wishes specific to the condition of a terminal illness. In most states a proxy may be appointed in a living will to speak on behalf of the person if he or she is unable to do so. In contrast, a DPAHC appoints a person, called a health care surrogate, to speak for the other in all matters of health care. However, in some cases the DPAHC cannot make decisions related to withdrawal of life support. Both the proxy and the health care surrogate are expected to make the decisions for the person that he or she would make if able to do so using what is known as substituted judgement. Advance directives are legally binding documents that nurses, physicians, and health care institutions are required to respect.

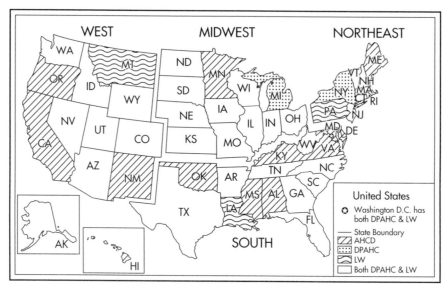

Figure 26-4   Advance directive documents officially sanctioned by states and Washington, DC. *DPAHC,* Durable power of attorney for health care; *LW,* living will; *AHCD,* advance health care directive. (From Gunter-Hunt G, Mahoney JE, Sieger CE: A comparison of state advance directive documents, *Gerontologist* 42[1]:51-60, 2002.)

All agencies that receive Medicare and Medicaid funds are mandated to disseminate PSDA information to their clients and inquiry as the existence of living wills (Mezey et al, 1994; Berrio, Levesque, 1996; Mezey, 1996). Hospitals and long-term care facilities are responsible for providing written information at the time of admission about the individual's rights under law to refuse medical and surgical care and the right to initiate this in a written advance directive. HMOs are required to do the same at the time of membership enrollment, and home health agencies are required to do it before the patient comes under the care of the agency. Hospices are obliged to inform patients of their self-determination rights on the initial visit (Berrio, Levesque, 1996; Mezey, 1996; Parkman, 1996). Providers (physicians and nurse practitioners) are encouraged but not under obligation to provide this same information to their patients.

Although the exact format and signature (e.g., notary) requirements vary from state to state, the PSDA is a federal mandate and applies to persons in all jurisdictions (Figure 26-4). There are several clearinghouses of related information, including www.fivewishes.com, wherein persons can obtain information relevant to their state and forms can be ordered or downloaded.

Although the nurse cannot provide legal information, she or he does serve as a resource person ready to answer many of the questions people have about end-of-life decision making. The nurse may be called not only to inquire about the presence of an existing advance directive, but also to ensure that the directive still reflects the person's wishes and advocate that the wishes are followed. The nurse also has the responsibility to make sure that existing or newly created advance directives are available in the appropriate locations in the medical record.

The nurse can help the elder understand treatments that are available to sustain life and the implications of interventions such as resuscitation efforts (CPR), intubation, and artificial nutrition, as well as the technical terms associated with them. However, in providing this information the nurse must avoid injecting personal bias into the discussion.

Advocacy

The gerontological nurse is an advocate for the patient regardless of the setting but is particularly important in the long-term care setting (Kayser-Jones, 2002). There, the nurse advocates for the self-determination of all patients, even those with questionable cognitive functioning.

In a small study of elderly patients who were diagnosed with dementia using standard measures, 30% were found to possess the cognitive ability to understand the nature of a health care proxy and to designate a relative as their decision maker. Twenty-seven percent of the group were able to express their preference for or against a do-not-resuscitate (DNR) option; 21% could do both a DNR and a health care proxy (Schmitt, 1996). Although this is a limited study, it suggests that decision-making capacity is not always accurately predicted by the standard testing procedures. The implication for elders in long-term care facilities is that these elders should not be excluded from participating in executing an advance directive.

The nurse may also be a patient advocate by bringing family members and the elder together to discuss the difficult issues addressed in making a directive or just to discuss the elder's wishes. It may be the nurse who brings the patient and the physician together to ensure that the patient and the physician agree on the meaning of the directive and whether the physician can honor the patient's wishes. It may also be the nurse who obtains the appropriate advance directive form for the elder who is well or ill. Counseling of patients by hospital representatives, nurses, and others has been shown to be an effective and generalizable way of improving recognition and execution of advance directives (Meier et al, 1996).

No one can think of all possible contingencies that might require decisions with serious illness or a current condition. The use of values assessment may help clarify what the elder holds important in his or her life and how this relates to his or her desires for health care and quality of life. Does the elder want measures to be taken to prolong life at all costs, or does he or she wish for a natural death if the alternative may mean prolonged maintenance on machines? Are there any persons the elder feels comfortable with who can act as a proxy to ensure that the elder's wishes will be carried out? Answers to these questions are helpful when discussing the elder's wishes. The discussion should include the family and perhaps the clergy and friends, before a directive is completed, to identify if those who are to be involved are comfortable with the decisions and will adhere to the

directive. For elders without family, the nurse may become a sounding board.

Euthanasia

The recognition of a patient's right to refuse life-sustaining medical measures renewed age-old questions over the patient's right to make decisions about the continuation of life. Some people, especially those who are suffering at the end of life, have ended their lives. Others have asked for assistance in accomplishing this in the most painless way possible.

In May 1992 the *Journal of the American Medical Association* reported that 73% of the general public in a large sample approved of some form of euthanasia. Physician-assisted death, physician-assisted suicide, physician aid in dying, and passive and active euthanasia are all terms that are heard. An example of physician-assisted suicide might be the physician providing the patient with sleeping pills and instructions about a lethal dose. This form is considered passive euthanasia because the physician has not withheld or withdrawn life-sustaining treatment. The person who injects lethal poison into a patient who voluntarily requested to be helped to die would be practicing active euthanasia.

In 1994 and again in 1997 voters in the state of Oregon passed the Death with Dignity Law, and Oregon became the only state in the United States to legalize physician-assisted suicide in the form of passive euthanasia. This law enables an Oregon resident who (1) is a terminally ill adult, (2) has less than 6 months to live, and (3) is judged to be mentally competent, to obtain the assistance of a physician for the purpose of a dignified death at a time and manner of his or her choosing. The additional criteria required before the request can be granted are stringent and include one written and two oral requests at 15-day intervals followed by a 15-day waiting period to certify the person's desire to end his or her life. Two physicians must certify the diagnosis, prognosis, competency, and voluntary nature of the request. The individual must be counseled on alternatives and also receives counseling from a pharmacist. If these criteria are met, the patient's request is granted, and he or she may receive a prescription of a lethal dose of a medication from the physician. The

Table 26-5 Arguments For and Against Physician-Assisted Suicide

For	Against
Physicians have a duty to alleviate uncontrollable pain and suffering, including the obligation to provide an assisted death at a competent patient's request.	Society runs the risk of sliding into a practice of involuntary euthanasia and subtle coercion of vulnerable and disenfranchised patients.
Patients have the right to autonomy, which presently includes the right to forego or have withdrawn life-sustaining therapy.	There is a potential for abuse. Involuntary euthanasia has a higher priority in permissive environments where euthanasia is legal.
It allows the terminally ill to preserve their autonomy and exert final control.	The healing ethos of medical practice may be adversely affected, and public trust in physicians may be eroded.

Data from Morrison RS, Meier DE: Physician-assisted dying: fashioning public policy with an absence of data, *Generations* 18(4):48, 1994.

person then decides if and when the dose is taken and it cannot be in the presence of the prescribing physician. Lethal injection or active euthanasia is not allowed. In 1998 the U.S. Attorney General tried various ways of preventing the enactment of this law; however, the voters' rights to make this decision have been upheld.

The impact of this law on the public has been an improvement in end-of-life care. Oregon has gone from eleventh place to the second highest per capita distribution of morphine in the United States, implying more attention to pain control; 33% of Oregonians now die in hospice care—this is a 70% increase in Oregonians who die in hospice (national average is 17%) (Lee, 1999). From 1997 to 2001, 141 prescriptions were issued with only 91 terminally ill persons taking advantage of the opportunity, the majority of whom had cancer (Lee, Brody, 2002; Chronicle News Services, 2002).

Nurses have had strong opinions pro and con on the topic. The American Nurses Association's position statement on assisted suicide was developed to provide nurses with a point of reference for discussion and understanding of the many difficulties involved in the issue of a patient's request to terminate his or her life. The American Nurses Association advises nurses not to participate in assisted suicide, citing such action as a "violation of the Code for Nurses with Interpretive Statements and the ethical traditions of the profession"

(Canavan, 1996, p 8). The nurse is involved in many end-of-life care situations because she or he is the primary care provider who implements decisions of others around end-of-life care. Such advice should not mean patients who want their life terminated should be abandoned.

Considerable confusion exists regarding terminology and interpretation of what effects the nurse's role may have. Many nurses believe that turning off the ventilator, turning off tube feedings, stopping intravenous fluids, or giving as much pain medication as is needed, even if the side effect is death, constitutes assisted suicide. Nurses must understand that withdrawal of devices such as feeding tubes and ventilators is allowing natural death to occur, which is very different from actively doing something to cause death (Murphy, 1996; Huang, Ahronheim, 2000; Kuebler, McKinnon, 2002).

The general trend in American law is toward greater freedom for the individual to choose when and how to die. Many people believe that broader physician-assisted suicide might soon be reality based on constitutional grounds of the right to privacy (Messinger, 1993) or the due process clause of the Fourteenth Amendment to the U.S. Constitution (Sedler, 1993; Carter, 1996; Wilkes, 1996). Morrison and Meier (1994) presented some intriguing points both for and against physician-assisted suicide and may help the nurse thinking about this topic (Table 26-5). Nurses individually

NANDA and Wellness Diagnoses

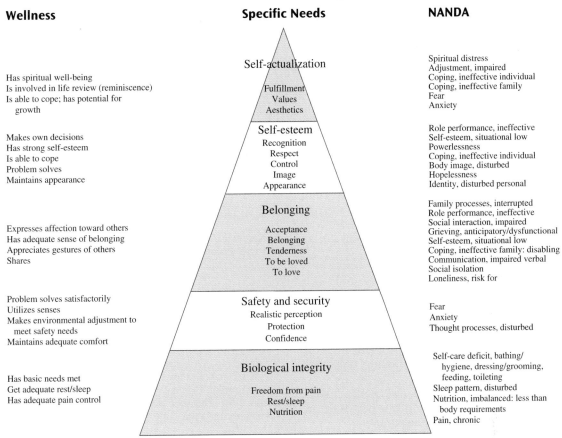

Wellness

Has spiritual well-being
Is involved in life review (reminiscence)
Is able to cope; has potential for
    growth

Makes own decisions
Has strong self-esteem
Is able to cope
Problem solves
Maintains appearance

Expresses affection toward others
Has adequate sense of belonging
Appreciates gestures of others
Shares

Problem solves satisfactorily
Utilizes senses
Makes environmental adjustment to
    meet safety needs
Maintains adequate comfort

Has basic needs met
Get adequate rest/sleep
Has adequate pain control

Specific Needs

Self-actualization

Fulfillment
Values
Aesthetics

Self-esteem
Recognition
Respect
Control
Image
Appearance

Belonging

Acceptance
Belonging
Tenderness
To be loved
To love

Safety and security
Realistic perception
Protection
Confidence

Biological integrity

Freedom from pain
Rest/sleep
Nutrition

NANDA

Spiritual distress
Adjustment, impaired
Coping, ineffective individual
Coping, ineffective family
Fear
Anxiety

Role performance, ineffective
Self-esteem, situational low
Powerlessness
Coping, ineffective individual
Body image, disturbed
Hopelessness
Identity, disturbed personal

Family processes, interrupted
Role performance, ineffective
Social interaction, impaired
Grieving, anticipatory/dysfunctional
Self-esteem, situational low
Coping, ineffective family: disabling
Communication, impaired verbal
Social isolation
Loneliness, risk for

Fear
Anxiety
Thought processes, disturbed

Self-care deficit, bathing/
    hygiene, dressing/grooming,
    feeding, toileting
Sleep pattern, disturbed
Nutrition, imbalanced: less than
    body requirements
Pain, chronic

These are not all of the possible wellness or NANDA diagnoses that may be identified. The above are frequent examples of nursing diagnoses that should be considered when planning care for the older adult in whatever setting.

and collectively must consider the implication of this for themselves and our profession.

▶ **KEY CONCEPTS**

- Grief is an emotional and behavioral response to loss. Grief responses are individual; what is appropriate for a person from one ethnic group may be considered inappropriate by another.
- One never completely resolves grief. Instead, the individual incorporates the loss as a part of his or her life.

- Dying is a multifaceted active process. It affects all involved: the one who is dying, the family, and the professional caregivers.
- The stages or phases of dying and the type of coping are not obligatory or prescriptive of the way one should die. Such expectations place an added burden on the one who is dying.
- The dying older adult is a living person with all the same needs for good and natural relationships with people as the rest of us.
- Hope is empowering. It generates courage and motivates action and achievement. The degree

of hope that a dying individual possesses depends on a caring relationship with others.

- The health professional who is interested in caring for the dying should have outside interests and support systems before considering this nursing specialty.
- For some persons, living can be more painful than dying and they may elect suicide.
- Hospice is a process or unique ideology that links the needs of the terminally ill, the family, and staff to fulfill the remainder of the dying individual's life by enabling or returning control to the dying person.
- Advance directives allow an individual control over life and death decisions by written communication and allow (in some instances) an appointed person (a proxy) to be the individual's advocate when he or she is not able to communicate desires personally.

Activities and Discussion Questions

1. Explore your response to being given a terminal diagnosis. What coping mechanisms work for you? With which awareness approach would you be comfortable?
2. Describe how you would deal with a dying person and his or her family when they are especially protective of one another.
3. Describe and strategize how you would bring up the topic of advance directives.
4. What advance directive is legally recognized in your state?
5. Describe how you would introduce the topic of dying with a patient who is critically ill and not expected to live.

RESOURCES

Websites

Americans for Better Care of the Dying
www.abcd-caring.org

Association for Death Education and Counseling
www.adec.org

Dying Well
www.dyingwell.org

End-of-Life Nursing Education Consortium
www.aacn.nche.edu/elnec

Five Wishes (source for advance directives information)
www.fivewishes.org

Last Acts
www.lastacts.org

National Consensus Project for Quality Palliative Care
www.nationalconsensusproject.org

National Effort to Improve End of Life Nursing Care
www.aacn.nche.edu

National Hospice and Palliative Care Nurses Association
www.hpna.org*

National Hospice and Palliative Care Organization
www.nho.org

REFERENCES

American Nurses Association: *Standards and scope of hospice and palliative nursing practice,* Kansas City, Mo, 1987, The Association. Available at www.ana.org.

Arbuckle NW, de Vries B: The long-term effects of late life spousal and parental bereavement on personal functioning, *Gerontologist* 35(5):637-647, 1995.

Berrio MW, Levesque ME: Advance directives: most patients don't have one. Do yours? *Am J Nurs* 96(8):24-28, 1996.

Blackhall LJ et al: Ethnicity and attitude toward patient autonomy, *JAMA* 274(10):820-825, 1995.

Bowlby J: Process of mourning, *Int J Psychoanal* 42:317-340, 1961.

Bowling A: Who dies after widow(er)hood? A discriminate analysis, *Omega J Death Dying* 19:135, 1989.

Canavan K: ANA advises nurses not to participate in assisted suicide: RNs should consider implications of possible legalization, *Am Nurse* 28(4):8, 1996.

Carter SL: Rush to lethal judgment, *New York Times Magazine,* July 2, 1996, p. 28.

Chronicle News Services: Judge reins in Ashcroft on assisted suicide, *San Francisco Chronicle,* April 18, 2002.

Coolican MB et al: Education about death, dying, and bereavement in nursing programs, *Nurs Educ* 19(6):35-40, 1994.

Corr CA: Coping with dying: lessons that we should and should not learn from the work of Elizabeth Kübler-Ross, *Death Stud* 17(1):69, 1993.

*Contains very useful list of links.

Corr CA: A task-based approach to coping with dying. In DeSpelder LA, Strickland AL, editors: *The pathway ahead,* Mountainview, Calif, 1995, Mayfield.

Dessonville CL, Thompson LW, Gallagher D: The role of anticipatory bereavement in the adjustment to widowhood in the elderly, *Gerontologist* 23(special issue):309, 1983.

Doka KJ: Disenfranchised grief. In Doka KJ, editor: *Disenfranchised grief: recognizing hidden sorrow,* Lexington, Mass, 1989, Lexington Books.

Doka KJ: The spiritual crisis of bereavement. In Doka KJ, Morgan JD, editors: *Death and spirituality,* Amityville, NY, 1993, Baywood.

Donley R: Spiritual dimensions of health care: nursing's mission, *Nurs Health Care* 12(4):178-183, 1991.

Federal Interagency Forum on Aging-Related Statistics: *Older Americans 2000: key indicators of well-being,* Washington, DC, 2002. Administration on Aging. Available at wwww.aoa.gov.

Giacquinta B: Helping families face the crisis of cancer, *Am J Nurs* 77(10):1585-1588, 1977.

Glaser BG, Strauss AL: *Awareness of dying,* Chicago, 1963, Aldine.

Glaser BG, Strauss AL: *Time for dying,* Chicago, 1968, Aldine.

Godow S: Death and dying: a natural connection? *Generations* 11:15, 1987.

Hegge M, Fischer C: Grief responses of senior and elderly widows: practice implications, *J Gerontol Nurs* 26(2):25-43, 2000.

Hickey SS: Enabling hope, *Cancer Nurs* 9(3):133-137, 1986.

Horacek BJ: Toward a more viable model of grieving and consequences for older persons, *Death Stud* 15(5):459, 1991.

Huang ZB, Ahronheim JC: Nutrition and hydration in terminally ill patients: an update, *Clin Geriatr Med* 16(2):313-325, 2000.

Irish DP, Lundquist KF, Nelson VJ: *Ethnic variations in dying, death, and grief: diversity in universality,* Philadelphia, 1993, Taylor & Francis.

Jett KF: The loss reaction model, Unpublished manuscript, 2004.

Kayser-Jones J: The experience of dying: an ethnographic nursing home study, *Gerontologist* 42(special no. 3):11-19, 2002.

Kübler-Ross E: *On death and dying,* New York, 1969, Macmillan.

Kuebler S, McKinnon S: Dehydration. In Kuebler KK, Berry PH, Heidrich DE, editors: *End-of-life care: clinical practice guidelines,* Philadelphia, 2002, WB Saunders.

Lee BC: In Oregon's assisted suicide law scrutinized after first year, *Clinician News* 3(7):1, 1999.

Lee BC, Brody R: *Compassion in dying, presentation at Commonwealth Club,* San Francisco, March 6, 2002.

Lipson JG, Dibble SL, Minarik PA: Culture *and nursing care: a pocket guide,* San Francisco, 1996, UCSF Nursing Press.

Lund DA, Caserta MD, Dimond MF: Gender differences through two years of bereavement among the elderly, *Gerontologist* 26(3):314-320, 1986.

Matzo ML, Sherman DW: *Gerontologic palliative care nursing,* St. Louis, 2004, Mosby.

Mazanec P, Tyler MK: Cultural considerations in end-of-life care: how ethnicity, age & spirituality affect decisions when death is imminent, *Am J Nurs* 103(3):50-59, 2003.

Meier DE et al: Marked improvement in recognition and completion of health care proxies: a randomized controlled trial of counseling by hospital patient representatives, *Arch Intern Med* 156(11):1227-1232, 1996.

Messinger TJ: A gentle and easy death: from ancient Greece to beyond Cruzan—toward a reasoned legal response to the societal dilemma of euthanasia, *Denver Univ Law Rev* 71(1):175-251, 1993.

Mezey M: Advance directives protocol: nurses helping to protect patient rights, the NICHE faculty, *Geriatr Nurs* 17(5):204-209, 1996.

Mezey M, Ramsey GC, Mitty E: Making the PDA work for the elderly, *Generations* 18(4):13, 1994.

Minogue B: *Bioethics: A committee approach,* Boston, 1996, Jones & Bartlett.

Morrison RS, Meier DE: Physician-assisted dying: fashioning public policy with an absence of data, *Generations* 18(4):48, 1994.

Murphy P. In Canavan K: ANA advises nurses not to participate in assisted suicide: RNs should consider implications of possible legalization, *Am Nurs* 28(4):8, 1996.

Parkman C: Using advance directives: part 2, *NURSEweek* 9(12):10, 1996.

Parks CM, Weiss RS: *Recovery from bereavement,* New York, 1983, Basic Books.

Pattison EM: The experience of dying. In Pattison EM, editor: *The experience of dying,* Englewood Cliffs, NJ, 1977, Prentice-Hall, pp 43-60.

Rees WD, Lukin SG: The mortality of bereavement, *BMJ* 4:13, 1967.

Richter JM: Support: a resource during crisis of mate loss, *J Gerontol Nurs* 13(11):18-22, 1987.

Schmitt L: *The right to choose: capacity study of demented residents in nursing homes (executive summary),* Chicago, 1996, Franciscan Sisters of the Poor Hospital Systems.

Sedler RA: The constitution and hastening inevitable death, *Hastings Center Report* 23(5): 20, 1993.

Shield RR: Liminality in an American nursing home: The endless transition. In Sokolovsky J, editor: *The cultural context of aging: worldwide perspectives,* Westport, Conn, 1997, Bergin & Garvey.

Spector R: *Cultural diversity in health and illness*, ed 6, Upper Saddle River, NJ, 2003, Prentice-Hall.

Thibault JM, Ellor JW, Netting FE: Conceptual framework for assessing spiritual functioning and fulfillment of older adults in long-term care settings, *J Relig Gerontol* 7(4):29, 1991.

Ulrich LK: The challenge of hospice care, *Bull Am Protestant Hosp Assoc* 41(3):20-21, 1978.

Weisman A: *Coping with cancer*, New York, 1979, McGraw-Hill.

Weisman A: *The coping capacity: on the nature of being mortal*, New York, 1984, Human Sciences Press.

Worden JW: *Grief counseling and grief therapy: a handbook for mental health practitioners*, ed 3, New York, 2002, Springer.

Life Space Options for Elders

Upon completion of this chapter, the reader will be able to:

- Explain the significance of personal space to adaptation in late life.
- Identify factors in the environment that contribute to the safety and security of older adults.
- Compare the major features, advantages, and disadvantages of several housing situations available to the older adult.
- Name several aspects of relocation stress.
- Describe a desirable long-term care living situation.
- Discuss changes in the environment and the effects on individual function.
- Assist an elder in making an informed choice when planning a move to a protected setting.

Cognizant Being observant and aware of happenings.
Equitable Just and fair.

Iatrogenic A disorder or condition caused by medical treatments or diagnostic procedures.
Nosocomial Hospital-acquired infection.

"This is my home. We are all like a family, and I will die here. The girls that help me during the day, we treat one another like family members. We have some days when we are grumpy, some days we are happy, and we don't hold our feelings back, like you would do with your own family at home."

An 85-year-old resident of a skilled nursing facility

"We are their family now, and that is how we have to treat them. I think we do a pretty good job here because a lot of patients say when they leave and come back, 'Oh, I am so glad to be home.' Our philosophy here is that we don't work at this facility, we are guests in these people's home."

A 50-year-old director of nursing in a skilled nursing facility

A mobile, youth-oriented society may find it difficult to fully comprehend the insecurity that elders feel when moving from one site to another in their later years. In addition to the stress of relocation and the initial anxiety of adapting to a new setting, elders typically move to ever more restrictive environments, often in times of crisis. This chapter considers the various options along the continuum of care and living environments. The major issues are the choice and control elders have about relocation, assistance provided to the elder in making personally appropriate choices, the stress of relocation, and the anxiety surrounding institutionalization. Nursing care is focused on providing orientation, information, resources, advocacy, safety, comfort, and creation of as home-

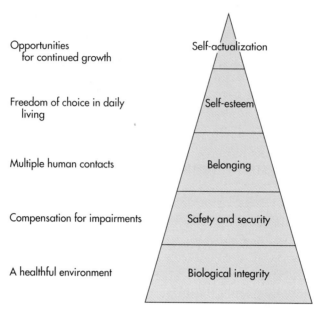

Figure 27-1   Environmental needs of older Americans. (Modified from Herreth J, Orr P, Jones B: *Environmental needs of older Americans,* Atlanta, 1984, The Exchange.)

like an environment as possible in whatever situation the elder is encountering. All of these are considered in this chapter in terms of maintaining personal space and life space in a safe and satisfactory manner. Figure 27-1 addresses the basic environmental supports that elders require to function maximally at each level of need.

PERSONAL SPACE

Each person needs a private space for solitude, intimacy, anonymity, and centering oneself. The amount of time needed and the boundaries of this private space are individually and culturally variable. An older adult with no opportunity for privacy may erect psychological walls for self-protection from personal invasion and will no longer care about seeking enlargement in life space.

Personalized boundaries define one's space and reflect the personality and interests of the inhabitant. Older people characteristically maintain a sense of personal space by saving small items and arranging environmental props (significant personal items) in a particular manner. A thoughtful

nurse will respect these territorial boundaries, will not move into private space too rapidly, and will bring together health and illness behavioral needs to establish a secure place for the elder. For example, one elderly woman saved her paper napkins, cups, and drinking straws. She had grown up in an era of deprivation and needed the security of saving.

Problems such as sensory overload (related to loss of environmental control), medication haze, isolation from significant persons, pain, and biological disorders all affect one's sense of personal space. These are all discussed in various other chapters throughout this text. Suggestions and nursing interventions throughout this chapter are designed to restore pattern and order and environmental competence, resulting in a sense of safety and security.

LIFE SPACE

Beyond immediate personal space, each person has a defined life space that may diminish as one ages. A person's life space includes the arena in which the individual functions in the neighborhood, community, and world at large. It is dictated by mobility, economics, energy, and status. It is geographically and perceptually defined and subject to enlargement, constriction, and energy exchanges. Although one's personally significant geographical space may be limited to a 5- × 10-foot cubicle, perceptual life space is limited only to the creativity and capacity of the individual. In this chapter we consider older individuals and their personal and geographical life space.

Personal territories and life space are the fabric of human existence. How people cluster together, where they establish their roots, and how they personally define the limits of their range influence all other aspects of adaptation. When one reaches old age, environmental response is strongly rooted in experiences and the emotional impact of certain houses, areas, and events connecting them. When relocation is essential, the environment should be matched as carefully as possible to previous desirable aspects. The most positive outcomes are seen when the individual has a sense of control and transitional supports. We will be much more effective in dealing with environmental issues if we remember the strong instinctive nature of territorial occupancy.

REMAINING AT HOME

"Home" provides basic shelter, is a place to establish security, and is the place where one "belongs." It should provide the highest possible level of independence, function, and comfort. Most older people prefer to remain in their own homes rather than relocate, particularly to institutional living. A survey by the American Association of Retired Persons (AARP) completed in 2001 found that at least 88% of seniors want to age in place. The ability to age in place requires helping the older person to stay where he or she wants with appropriate support for changing needs. Older people want to remain independent and not become a burden on their families, although this varies by ethnic group. Americans are a mobile society, and families often do not all live in the same place. Many younger families have two-worker situations, making it difficult to help with older members of the family who may be living alone and perhaps not in close proximity. Even though families may not live near their older relative, a

great deal of caregiving goes on from a distance. The emergence of gerontological care managers, many of whom are nurses, assists families to ensure the needs of their elderly relative are met. Chapter 23 discusses the relationships between older people and their families.

Although many older people are staying in single-family homes, some are looking for smaller or more convenient housing such as town houses or condominiums where maintenance needs, particularly outdoor needs, are eliminated or minimized. Many seniors do not want to continue to care for a large home. The baby boomer generation is changing the housing market of the future, which is likely to be "empty nester" type housing, smaller but not necessarily lower in quality. It is also important to remember that many current seniors who wish to change housing arrangements are caught in a situation where organized senior housing is too expensive for middle class and lower–middle class citizens, but the seniors may have too much income and assets to qualify for subsidized housing.

There are some seniors who by choice or need wish to move into some type of senior housing. Such housing ranges from independent living where people live much as they did in their single-family homes, only with many optional services available and little or no maintenance requirements, through assisted living in its various forms, to skilled nursing facilities. For some older people, remaining at home increases isolation and loneliness. Choosing to relocate to an environment such as a continuing care community or retirement home often provides safety, security, and increased opportunities for socialization. Often, the older person may become more independent when relieved of the burden of caring for a home. The following quote from a resident interviewed in a study of residents' perspectives on their first year in a long-term care facility after relocation from home offers insight: *"I decided that I couldn't look after a 5-bedroom house any longer and it was an actual burden as well . . . I did my own cooking, got my own meals, looked after myself. Then you get to the point where you can't do that anymore"* (Iwasiw et al, 2003, p. 49)

There are many different models of senior housing, and older people may seek assistance from gerontological nurses in choosing what kind of living situation will be best for them.

Programs to Help Elders Remain at Home

Recognizing the needs of the growing number of older people, many states and local communities have begun efforts to become "elder friendly" through environmental modifications and services to assist older people to remain in their own homes. A good example is Hope House in New Jersey, a not-for-profit service organization that provides free or low-cost light housekeeping, minor home repair, help with shopping, and other services (Bruno, 2002). The Program of All-Inclusive Care for the Elderly (PACE) in several sites nationwide also provides models for keeping individuals in their own homes with sufficient supports. Local Area Agencies on Aging are good resources for obtaining information about these kinds of programs.

A new concept receiving attention across the United States is naturally occurring retirement communities (NORCs). The term *NORC* was coined in the 1990s and is basically a concentration of people 55 and over who organize to provide supportive services to enable them to age in place. The first NORC was begun in New York City with funding from the city, state, and local philanthropies and in-kind contributions from housing corporations and health care providers. There are now 27 NORCs that serve more than 46,000 seniors in New York City (Dionne, 2004). In 2001, the U.S. Congress, through the Administration on Aging (AOA), began providing grants to Jewish Federation agencies to develop NORCs in cities across the United States.

NORCs are partnerships that unite housing entities and their residents, health and social service providers, government agencies, and philanthropical organizations to provide a wide range of services, early intervention, and activities for seniors in communities where they already live. Key to NORCs is the active involvement of the residents themselves in the planning and implementation of the program. Programs are designed to engage older residents before a crisis and respond to their changing needs over time and are designed to augment existing services and fill in the gaps (Dionne, 2004). Each community will identify its own unique needs and work with partners to develop needed services. Such services might include care coordination, medical management, referrals, home repair, security and surveillance, emergency response systems, transportation, wellness and health education, homemaker and home-health services, and outreach. Eligibility for services is based on age and residence in the NORC rather than on medical needs or economic status, a major drawback of the current long-term care system. NORCs may be likened to assisted living or continuing care retirement communities without the price tag and the stress of relocation. This new model holds promise for aging in place for millions of seniors.

Considerations for Providing Care in the Home

Although staying in one's home is the desired option for many older people, those who need 24 hr/day or high-tech and palliative care often face many challenges. In some instances, the hospital has been brought to the home in the form of equipment needed for this type of care. Some refer to this as the *hypermedicalization* of the home (Arras, Dubler, 1994). Even more difficult, the client and family requiring specialized home care must forego the security of the hospital and take on responsibilities that they may not feel capable of or willing to manage. For some people, this may not be a reasonable expectation or one that they can accept. In many instances, relocation to a nursing facility will be the best option. In helping older adults and their families make decisions about the best care options, gerontological nurses can discuss the benefits and burdens of such care and the alternatives. The following factors are some of the things to be considered for remaining at home when specialized care is needed:

1. Assistance in arranging medical equipment comfortably and instruction in safety issues
2. Explanations of rationale and demonstrations of appropriate use of equipment, medication administration, and disposal of potentially contaminated or toxic materials
3. Acknowledgment that home care brings intrusions into the client's surroundings and assistance with lifestyle modification to produce the most acceptable ambience
4. Information about alternatives that may be more feasible for the client than those typically recommended

5. Discussion of any modifications needed to ensure safety
6. Availability and affordability of assistance, particularly around the clock, as well as support and relief for family caregivers
7. Ready access to assistance when needed and emergency responses for necessary services

Home Modifications and Home Safety

Minor repairs may present a major problem for older adult homeowners. Those who do not have the strength or skills to make needed repairs often rely on friends and relatives, but many elders have no one to assist them if they cannot afford to purchase services. Some communities have organized a home repair service particularly for the low-income older adult and disabled. Home maintenance service can be managed by retired workers with special skills, and the work can be done by youths who need jobs. The retirees can teach badly needed job skills to youths while providing an inexpensive service to elders in the home.

Elders who have planned ahead and have adequate resources often modify their home or buy a more convenient home long before they become frail. Some of the features they seek are absence of stairs, roomy bathrooms with grab bars strategically placed, closets and shelves that are easily accessible without reaching, security systems, lights that may be dimmed at night, and other convenience features. Chapter 22 discussed home modifications and resources to make the home safe.

Safety in the Community

In many communities special programs such as escort services, victim counseling, and safety information have been initiated. AARP conducted a national search to identify programs in crime prevention that have proved effective (Leach, 1996). One of the model programs is in Broomfield, Colorado, where a specially assigned police officer presents crime education at senior and community centers within the city, as well as advising individual isolated elders on ways to reduce vulnerability to crime. Another program in Chicago involves low-rent housing occupants who act as representatives of their units to work

directly with police to improve building safety. In Dana Point, California, older persons are recruited as volunteers to work with police. They are issued special uniforms and canvas their neighborhoods, performing vacation and neighborhood checks; serve to control crowds and traffic at special neighborhood events; and perform foot patrols in business and shopping areas. Several other creative methods of involving elders and the police in cooperative programs to reduce crime are reported in an AARP Consumer Fact Sheet authored by Leach (1996) (also see Resources at the end of this chapter). Nurses need to learn about programs in crime protection and prevention, how to obtain assistance, and how to obtain legal redress for victims.

Goods and Services

Senior centers, nutrition sites, senior discounts on numerous goods and services, surplus foods, food stamps, Meals on Wheels, homemakers, and family caregiving are only a few of the items that increase the possibility of elders remaining in their own homes regardless of failing health and chronic disorders. Basic services that may keep older people in their homes longer than would otherwise be feasible include the following: (1) home health maintenance; (2) rehabilitation and medical services when necessary; (3) home household help; (4) mobile meals; (5) transportation services; and (6) counseling, crisis intervention, and advocacy (case management).

Keeping the Home

Often a home that has increased immensely in value is the major asset of an elder. However, taxes and maintenance costs have likewise risen. If monthly income is low, a deprived state of existence may be chosen over selling the home. If the elder does choose to sell, some exemptions from the capital gains tax are allowed. If you have lived in your house for the last 5 years, you can sell your house and not pay capital gains tax up to $250,000 per person. The Internal Revenue Service (IRS) information regarding this is available through www.irs.gov.

To address the need for liquidity in assets for older adults who need cash more than they need equity, certain financial vehicles have been established in law to assist them to remain in their homes and have money to provide for their needs. The reverse mortgage is a mechanism for converting the equity in a house to cash. To be eligible for a reverse mortgage, an individual must be at least 62 years old, occupy at least one unit in the residence subject to the reverse mortgage, be able to service the mortgage, receive appropriate and adequate counseling concerning the transaction, and have a very low to no mortgage balance (Nacev, Rettig, 2002). Elders should be advised to seek information from several major home loan lenders and counsel from senior legal services before making a decision.

RELOCATION

In light of the strong instinctual nature of territorial needs, it is not surprising that much attention has been given to the crisis of relocation. Regardless of the type of move and its desirability or undesirability, some degree of stress will be experienced. Relocation to a long-term care facility is identified as one of the most stressful. With each move, if the adaptation is to be satisfying, one must begin to claim personal space by in some way placing one's stamp of individuality on the new surroundings. Because the older adult is particularly likely to move or be moved, the subject of relocation is significant. The first issue to address in any move is whether it is necessary and whether it will provide the least restrictive lifestyle appropriate for the individual. Questions that must be asked to assess the impact on the individual after a move include the following:

- Are significant persons as accessible in the new location as they were before the move?
- Is the individual developing new and reciprocal relationships in the new setting?
- Is the individual functioning as well, better, or not as well in the new location? This determination cannot be made immediately but must be assessed at least 6 weeks after the move.
- Was the individual given options before the move?
- Was the individual given the opportunity to assess the new environment before making a decision to move?

- Has the individual been able to move important items of furniture and memorabilia to the new setting?
- Has a particular individual who is familiar with the environment been available to assist with orientation?
- Was the decision to move made hastily or with inadequate information?
- Does the new situation provide adequately for basic needs (food, shelter, physical maintenance)?
- Are individual idiosyncratic needs recognized, and is there an opportunity to actualize them?
- Does the new situation decrease the possibility of privacy and autonomy?
- Is the new living situation an improvement over the previous situation, similar, or worse?

Nurses' concerns are with assessing the impact of relocation and determining methods to mitigate any negative reactions. The growing numbers of persons who will spend some of their later years in institutions have made this an urgent issue.

Relocation Stress Syndrome

Relocation stress syndrome is a nursing diagnosis describing the confusion resulting from a move to a new environment. Characteristics of relocation stress syndrome include anxiety, insecurity, altered mental status, depression, insecurity, loss of control, as well as physical problems (Iwasiw et al, 2003). An abrupt and poorly prepared transfer actually increases illness and disorientation. An individual who has functioned quite well before a major move may show previously unrecognized signs of dementia when in an unfamiliar environment. An accurate assessment of mental status before the move must be obtained from family or significant others. If this is not possible, it must be temporarily assumed that the changes in cognitive functioning are a transient response. An elder who has been transferred to an institution from a residence in which considerable autonomy was possible may react more intensely than one whose change in lifestyle has not been so severe. Some, of course, move to a much more comfortable and supportive situation and adapt well.

To avoid some of the effects of relocation stress syndrome, the individual must have some control over the environment, prior preparation regarding new situations, and maintenance of familiar situations to the greatest degree possible. Nurses must carefully assess and monitor older people for relocation stress syndrome effects. Working with families to help them plan relocations, understand the effects of relocation, and implement effective approaches is also necessary. It is important that some familiar and some treasured items accompany the transfer. Too often, elders arrive at long-term care institutions via ambulance stretcher from the hospital with nothing but a hospital gown. Everything familiar and necessary in their lives remains at the home they have left when they became ill. Even more distressing is when families or responsible parties sell the home to finance long-term care stays without the input of the elder. It is no wonder so many residents with dementia in nursing homes wander the hallways looking for home and for something familiar and comforting. Family members will need considerable support when an elder is moved into an institution. No matter what the circumstances are, the family invariably feels that they have in some way failed the elder. These issues are discussed in more depth in Chapter 23.

Cognitive Maps

One's state of security depends greatly on perceived environmental order or disorder and how it is visualized. People in unfamiliar settings often need assistance developing cognitive maps. Some of the following suggestions may be useful:

1. Maps of buildings and surroundings need to be displayed in centrally accessible areas.
2. Individuals feel more secure with directional orientations (north, south, east, west). These should be given.
3. The locations of important services must be emphasized and color coded.
4. A person familiar with the environment can be asked to orient a newcomer.
5. Discussion of visual points of reference may help (e.g., "Did you notice the large red painting?").
6. Important reference points or services should not be arbitrarily moved without prior information. In a public building a women's restroom was temporarily assigned to men. Several women automatically wandered in and left looking rather bewildered.

7. Preparation should be made before relocation of a familiar item or service.
8. Orientation to new surroundings should be delayed until persons have become settled in their individual space. They need time to establish some security and reduce anxiety. Poorly timed orientation tours are of little help.
9. The nurse should recap and ask for questions at the end of an orientation tour.
10. In a large facility or complex, orientation sessions should be spread out over several days.

A summary of relocation stress syndrome and nursing actions to prevent relocation stress are noted in Box 27-1.

CONTINUUM OF HOUSING OPTIONS FOR THE OLDER ADULT

There are currently approximately 32 million people over 65 years of age in the United States who are living in numerous types of independent, partially dependent, or fully dependent situations. This portion of the chapter examines the continuum of housing options available to older adults, from those who are fully independent to those requiring long-term sheltered care (Figure 27-2). As Medicare health maintenance organizations (HMOs) continue to expand, managed care providers will find it necessary to establish more networks with housing providers, because the living site of elders will ultimately also be the site where most economical and preventive health services will be dispensed.

Housed with Family Members

The factors most likely to result in shared housing among adult children and dependent elders are widowhood, a small support network, and low economic status. However, strong cultural influences predict the frequency of multigenerational residences. Among Asians, South Americans, and African Americans, it is often an expectation, although increasing industrialization in any country changes these traditional patterns. There are many cultural variations, but the important issue is for social policy and supports to provide choices for the individual and the family.

Box 27-1   Relocation Stress Syndrome

Relocation stress syndrome is a physiological and/or psychosocial disturbance as a result of transfer from one environment to another.

Defining Characteristics

Major
Change in environment or location
Anxiety
Apprehension
Increased confusion
Depression
Loneliness

Minor
Verbalization of unwillingness to relocate
Sleep disturbance
Change in eating habits
Dependency
Gastrointestinal disturbances
Increased verbalization of needs
Insecurity
Lack of trust
Restlessness
Sad affect
Unfavorable comparison of posttransfer and pretransfer staff
Verbalization of being concerned or upset about transfer
Vigilance
Weight change
Withdrawal

Related Factors

Past, concurrent, and recent losses
Losses involved with the decision to move
Feeling of powerlessness
Lack of adequate support system
Little or no preparation for the impending move
Moderate to high degree of environmental change
History and types of previous transfers
Impaired psychosocial health status
Decreased physical health status

Sample Diagnostic Statement

Relocation stress syndrome related to admission to long-term care setting as evidenced by anxiety, insecurity, and disorientation

Expected outcomes
1. The resident will socialize with family members, staff, and/or other residents.

2. Preadmission weight, appetite, and sleep patterns will remain stable. If previous patterns were dysfunctional, more appropriate health patterns will develop.
3. The resident will verbalize feelings, expectations, and disappointments openly with members of the staff and/or family.
4. Inappropriate behaviors (i.e., "acting out," refusing to take medicines) will not occur.

Expected short-term goals
1. The resident will become independent in moving to and from areas within the facility during the next 3 months.
2. The resident will react in a positive manner to staff effort to assist in adjusting to nursing home placement in the next 3 months.
3. The resident will express his or her thoughts or concerns about placement when encouraged to do so during individual contacts in the next 3 months.
4. During the next 3 months the resident will not develop physical or psychosocial disturbances indicative of translocation syndrome as a result of the change in living environment.

Expected long-term goals
1. The resident will verbalize acceptance of nursing home placement within the next 6 months.
2. The resident will indicate acceptance of nursing home placement through positive body language within the next 6 months.

Specific nursing interventions
1. Identify previous coping patterns during admission assessment. Clearly document these, and share the information with other staff members.
2. Include the resident in assessing problems and developing the care plan on admission.
3. Adjust for limitations in sensory/perceptual disturbances when planning care for residents. Visual disturbances need special intervention to assist residents in finding their way around.
4. Staff members will introduce themselves when entering the resident's room, indicating the nature of their relationship with the resident. Example: "Hello, Mr. S. My name is Nancy. I'll be your nurse attendant today, helping you with your meals and your bath."

Box 27-1	Relocation Stress Syndrome—*cont'd*

5. Each staff member providing care for the resident should make it a point to spend at least 5 minutes each day with new admissions to "just visit."
6. Allow the resident as many opportunities to make independent choices as possible.
7. Identify previous routines for activities of daily living (ADLs). Try to maintain as much continuity with the resident's previous schedule as possible. Example: If Mr. S. has taken a bath before bed all of his life, adjust his schedule to continue that practice.
8. Familiarize the resident with unit schedules.
9. Encourage family participation through frequent visits, phone calls, and activity sessions. Be sure to let the family know schedules.

10. Establish familiar landmarks for the resident when leaving his or her room so that he or she can recognize areas more quickly.
11. Encourage family members to bring familiar belongings from home for the resident's room decorations.
12. Provide reorientation cues frequently. Example: "You are in the dining room. Your room is down the hall three doors just past the window."
13. Encourage the resident to talk about expectations, anger, and/or disappointments and the recent life changes that he or she has experienced.
14. Review the patient's medication list with the physician to verify the need for medications that might promote disorientation.
15. Provide for constructive activities. Initiate activity therapy consultation.

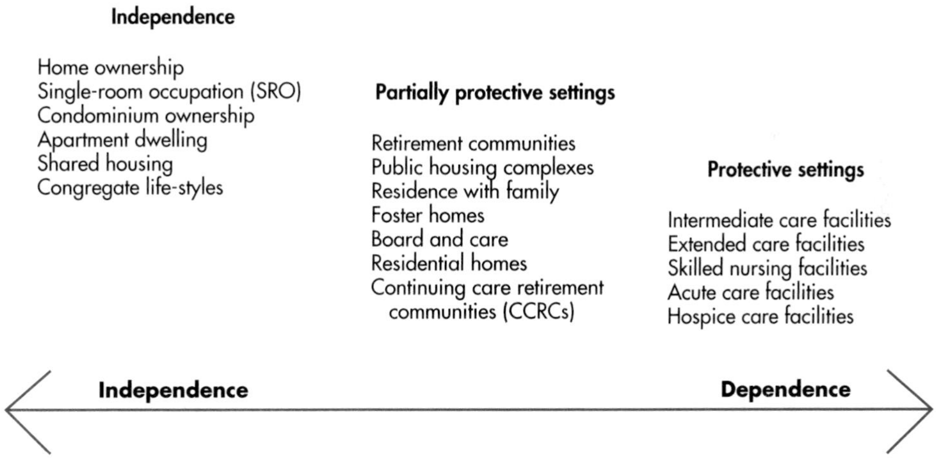

Independence

Home ownership
Single-room occupation (SRO)
Condominium ownership
Apartment dwelling
Shared housing
Congregate life-styles

Partially protective settings

Retirement communities
Public housing complexes
Residence with family
Foster homes
Board and care
Residential homes
Continuing care retirement
  communities (CCRCs)

Protective settings

Intermediate care facilities
Extended care facilities
Skilled nursing facilities
Acute care facilities
Hospice care facilities

⟨————— **Independence**   **Dependence** —————⟩

Figure 27-2   Continuum of housing security.

"Granny Flat" Solution

Almost 30 years ago the "granny flat" was developed in Australia as a model for providing independent housing for elders with prefabricated small housing units constructed on family property. These units allow families to be close enough to be of assistance if needed but remain separate. They are practical and economical, and their pro-duction has continually expanded in Australia. In the United States there has been little indication of this model being used, although existing "mother-in-law" cottages and apartments have served a similar purpose for many families. An additional model that has great popularity in certain areas is the use of mobile homes. These may in fact be mobile and moved onto family property or may in reality be quite immobile and set in established mobile home parks that cater to older people and their needs.

Senior Retirement Communities

Communities designed for elders are proliferating. There are numerous combinations of cottages, apartments, activities, optional services, meals in the home, cafeterias, restaurants, housekeeping, golf, tennis, security, and emergency services and clinics. Some have sections designed especially for assisted living. These are all designed to make independent living feasible with the least effort on the part of the elder. They are usually expensive, and services are purchased outright. The various names for such communities include "retirement community," "independent living centers," and "life care." Box 27-2 presents considerations important to an older adult contemplating entering one of these communities.

Life Care Retirement Communities

These organizations, also called *continuing care retirement communities,* are residential communities for retired people that provide long-term access to different levels of health care and other services in a single location. Levels of care available include independent living, assisted living, and several degrees of skilled nursing care. Most of these communities provide access to these levels of care for a community member's entire remaining lifetime. Having all levels of care in one location allows community members to make the transition between levels without life-disrupting moves. For married couples in which one spouse needs more care than the other, life care communities allow them to live nearby in a different part of the same community. More than 200 such communities are accredited by the Continuing Care Accreditation Commission (CCAC), a national, private nonprofit organization founded in 1985 and sponsored by the American Association of Homes and Services for the Aging (*Life Care Guide,* 2000). Most life care communities charge an entrance fee, which can range from $75,000 to more than $400,000 that covers and reflects the cost of the residence in which the person will live and the possible future care needed. There are also monthly payments. Important to remember about these types of com-

---

Box 27-2 | Considerations for Moving to Retirement Communities

- Plan far ahead, and anticipate needs. Good facilities have long waiting lists.
- Meals, activities, health care, and housekeeping must be readily available and affordable if desired or needed.
- Examine the compatibility of the residents; look for evidence of interaction and involvement in activities and committees.
- Study the effectiveness of the staff from administrator to maintenance personnel.
- Determine the community's compliance with standards in terms of licenses or certificates or by other evidence.
- Inquire about the availability of financial statements and marketing projections.
- Contracts should include fixed increases over time or amounts directly related to the inflation index; costs and limits of nursing care should be clearly stated. What amount of the fee is refundable if the client dies or moves?
- Does the resident have a voice in management?
- If a complex is not yet in operation, request a financial incentive before signing up, and put up only a nominal, fully refundable deposit before operation begins.

---

munities is the fact that the residence purchased belongs to the community or company after the death of the owner. More information about life care communities is available from the American Association of Homes and Services for the Aging (http://www.ahasa.org) and the CCAC.

Federally Assisted Housing

There are several federally subsidized rental options; most older adults benefiting from this option are assisted through HUD-subsidized rental housing. These are not specific to older people, but nearly 45% of the units are occupied by elders. Section 202 of the Housing Act, U.S. Department of Housing and Urban Development, approved the construction of low-rent housing units especially for elders. These units also have provisions for health, recreation, and transportation. More than 91% of these apartment units have waiting lists of eight or more applicants for each vacancy that occurs. Under Section 8 of the Housing Act of 1983, tenants locate their own unit. Usually, the tenant pays 30% of his or her adjusted gross income toward the rent, and HUD assists with supplementary vouchers ranging from 30% to 120% of the tenant's contribution to meet the fair market value of the rental.

An ideal public housing complex for low-income older people will provide modern facilities, security, accessible services, privacy, and some entertainment and activities. An important consideration in planning low-cost housing units for older adults is the potential for evolution of services. Residents rarely move out, and as they age, their ability and independence are likely to decrease. Retirement communities often solve this dilemma by building semidependent units. For those less affluent people currently in subsidized public housing, the only alternatives may be residential care facilities or nursing homes.

Shared Housing

Since so many older adults own their homes, house sharing has been proposed as a feasible way to keep one's home. Older people often live in houses with ample space geared to family life, purchased in their young adult years. It is estimated that one half the space is underused. Sharing a house can be easily implemented by locating, screening, and matching older people looking for houses to share with those who have them. The National Shared Housing Resource Center (NSHRC) has established subgroups nationally to assist individuals interested in home sharing. Those who have done so report feeling safer and less lonely. Studies on home sharing need to focus on the effects on well-being, finances, health, social life, and daily satisfaction. Most successful is the intergenerational model, in which an elder with a home locates a younger person to share the home (Bergman, 1994). In each situation the individuals must consider the following:

- Should men and women live together?
- Should the house include older peers only or people of all ages?
- Should there be equal or reciprocal exchange?
- Should the house provide temporary or permanent residence?
- Should residents sign an agreement form?

- Will residents respect privacy?
- What is the motivation for moving into a shared house: financial need, companionship, or services and assistance?

Shared housing as a method of providing for the needs of several frail older adults in one renovated home has been used with varying degrees of success. Problems arise from long-standing patterns of living, as well as privacy and interpersonal needs. However, small groups of older adults living under the same roof are a growing trend. The following are characteristics of successful group homes:

- They usually have a nonprofit sponsor.
- Services include housekeeping, cooking, maintenance, and social services.
- Spontaneity and interaction are encouraged but not forced.

Foster Care

Adult foster care is meant to provide assistive care in a homelike setting that will enhance function and the quality of life and allow the elder to remain in a community-based setting. The operational definition of *adult foster care* is as follows: adult foster care offers a community-based living arrangement to adults who are unable to live independently because of physical or mental impairment or disabilities and are in need of supervision or personal care.

Homes providing adult foster care offer 24-hour supervision, protection, and personal care in addition to room and board. They may also provide additional services. Adult foster care serves a designated, small number of individuals (generally from one to six) in a homelike and family-like environment; one of the primary caregivers often resides in the home (Folkemer et al, 1996). A growing number of homes are under corporate ownership, and in these situations the homelike atmosphere tends to be lost. However, with state-regulated, outcome-oriented quality assurance strategies focused on achieving maximal function, autonomy, and social integration, adult foster care may fill a real need.

Residential Care Facilities

Residential care facility is the broad term for a range of nonmedical community-based residential settings that house two or more unrelated adults and provide services such as meals, medication supervision or reminders, activities, transportation, or assistance with ADLs. These kinds of facilities are for elders who cannot live independently, but do not need nursing home care. Residential care facilities are known by more than 30 different names across the country, including adult congregate living facilities, group homes, personal care homes, homes for the aged, domiciliary care homes, board and care homes, sheltered housing, rest homes, family care homes, retirement homes, assisted living facilities, among other names (Hawes, 1999).

Residential care facilities are the fastest growing housing option available for older adults in the United States. This kind of care is viewed as more cost-effective than nursing homes while providing more privacy and home-like environments. Medicare does not cover the cost of care in these types of facilities. In some cases, costs may be covered by private and long-term care insurance and some other types of assistance programs. There is a growing trend for states to establish waiver programs to extend Medicaid services to this type of housing, but most residents of these types of facilities pay privately for their care. The rates charged and what services those rates include vary considerably as do regulations and licensing.

Hawes (1999) raises three major concerns related to residential care facilities: the considerable variability among places known as residential care in terms of services; insufficient or inaccurate information provided about whether the facility can meet the consumer's needs, for how long, and under what circumstances; and quality of care in light of limited regulations, supervision, and licensing standards. Because of the wide variation in types of services provided, it is important to advise older people and their families to identify exactly what is provided and the costs associated with the services. Particularly important is how much assistance will be provided and the associated costs if the older person develops physical and cognitive decline.

Gerontological nurses need to be knowledgeable about the range of options and are often involved in assisting older people and their families in making appropriate housing choices. Elders and their families should be advised to ask about and carefully consider the following:

What services are offered?
What is the out-of-pocket cost?
What levels of assistance are provided?
Is the staff trained in care of older people?
Are there licensed nurses available?
Is the staffing adequate at all times during the day?
What safety factors are in place?
Are individual preferences respected?
What range of physical and cognitive impairments can be accommodated?
What are the security measures?
What agencies, if any, are responsible for monitoring quality?
What are the special features for the frail or disabled?
What is the process for reporting abuse, neglect, or exploitation?

Assisted Living Facility

A popular type of residential care facility is an assisted living facility (ALF). An ALF is defined as a "special combination of housing, personalized supportive services, and health care designed to meet the needs, both scheduled and unscheduled, of those who need help with activities of daily living" (Munroe, 2003, p 100). Assisted living is a residential long-term care choice for seniors who need more than an independent living environment can offer but do not need the 24 hr/day skilled nursing care and the constant monitoring of a skilled nursing facility. Assisted living generally provides single-occupancy units with private baths, kitchenettes, meals, and some support services (Munroe, 2003). There are often several levels of assisted living, or one can purchase the care needed and live relatively independently otherwise. Assisted living provides security with independence and privacy, and it supports physical and social well-being with the health care supervision it provides.

The mean age of ALF residents is 80, but almost one half are 85 years of age or older. According to Munroe (2003), 25% had moderate to severe cognitive impairment, 33% experienced urinary incontinence, 51% received assistance with bathing, and 77% received assistance with medications. More than two thirds of assisted living residents are women.

Assisted living is more expensive than independent living and less costly than skilled nursing home care, but it is not inexpensive. Costs vary by geographical region, size of a unit, and relative luxury. Costs can range from a low of $1200 per month to a high of $5000 per month. Most ALFs offer two or three meals each day, light weekly housekeeping, and laundry services, as well as optional social activities at various times of the day. Some states provide Medicaid reimbursement for a limited number of low-income seniors who live in ALFs, but generally the cost is borne by the older person.

Many seniors and their families prefer ALFs to nursing homes because they are lower in cost, are more homelike, and offer more opportunities for control, independence, and privacy. However, many residents of ALFs have chronic care needs and over time may require more care than the facility is able to provide. Services (e.g., home health, hospice, homemakers) can be brought into the facility, but some question whether or not this replaces the need for 24-hour supervision by registered nurses (RNs). Not every ALF has an RN or licensed practical nurse (LPN), and in most states, there is not a requirement to provide skilled nursing in ALFs. Medication administration and delegation to unlicensed assistive personnel are of concern, especially for residents with cognitive impairment. Although we do not advocate the strict and stifling regulations seen in skilled nursing facilities, we do worry that these often frail older people receive little to no nursing assessment and supervision. Wallace (2003) noted that there are increasing cases of litigation in ALFs related to understaffing, inability to meet resident needs, inadequate staff training, inappropriate use of medications, lack of monitoring and medical supervision, and lack of communication with family about changes in resident status.

The Joint Commission on Accreditation of Healthcare Organizations (JCAHO) and the Commission for Accreditation of Rehabilitation Facilities have published standards for accreditation of ALFs, but many persons are advocating for more comprehensive federal and state standards and regulations. Advanced-practice gerontological nurses are well suited to the role of primary care provider in ALFs, and many have assumed this role. Certainly more research is needed on care outcomes of residents in ALFs and the role of unlicensed assistive personnel, as well as RNs, in these facilities. However, the nonmedical nature of ALFs

is the primary factor in keeping costs down. Consumers are well advised to inquire as to exactly what services will be provided and by whom if an ALF resident becomes more frail and needs more intensive care.

Subacute Care and Rehabilitation Units

As the acute care hospital has become the site of surgical, emergency, and intensive care, the traditional nursing home has been transformed into a center for the coordination of the continuum of care. After spending a few days in an acute care hospital, the elder is often moved to either a rehabilitation hospital for specific therapies expected to increase the elder's function or to a subacute (sometimes called *postacute*) care unit that functions much like the general medical-surgical hospital units of the past, although they are presently most often located in nursing homes. Subacute care is more intensive than traditional nursing facility care and several times more costly, but it is far less costly than similar care in an acute care hospital. Medicare usually covers most of the cost for subacute care if the person has skilled needs. The expectation is that the patient will be discharged home or to a less intensive setting. The stay in a subacute care unit is likely to be less than 1 month and is largely reimbursed by Medicare. Patients in subacute care facilities are usually younger and less likely to be cognitively impaired than those in traditional nursing home care. Generally, higher levels of professional nurse staffing are found in this setting. The definition of *subacute care* is provided in Box 27-3.

Acute Care: Special Concerns for Older Adults

Acute care settings largely comprise intensive care special units, extensive surgeries, and day surgeries. Length of stay is shorter and shorter, and as soon as a person is stabilized, he or she is discharged to home or a subacute or skilled nursing facility. Approximately 40% of all hospitalized patients are over the age of 65, and this figure rises to 60% in critical care units (Fulmer et al, 2002). Hospitals are dangerous places for elders: 34% to

Box 27-3	Subacute Care as Defined by the American Health Care Association and the Joint Commission on Accreditation of Healthcare Organizations

Subacute care is comprehensive inpatient care designed for someone who has an acute illness, injury, or exacerbation of a disease process. It is goal-oriented treatment rendered immediately after, or instead of, acute hospitalization to treat one or more specific active complex medical conditions or to administer one or more technically complex treatments, in the context of a person's underlying long-term conditions and overall situation.

Generally, the individual's condition is such that the care does not depend heavily on high-technology monitoring or complex diagnostic procedures. Subacute care requires the coordinated services of an interdisciplinary team including physicians, nurses, and other relevant professional disciplines who are trained and knowledgeable to assess and manage these specific conditions and perform the necessary procedures. Subacute care is given as part of a specifically defined program, regardless of the site.

Subacute care is generally more intensive than traditional nursing facility care and less than acute care. It requires frequent (daily to weekly) recurrent patient assessment and review of the clinical course and treatment plan for a limited (several days to several months) time period, until the condition is stabilized or a predetermined treatment course is completed.

From American Health Care Association, Washington, DC.

50% of older hospitalized patients experience functional decline, and iatrogenic complications occur in as many as 29% to 38%, a rate three to five times higher than in younger patients (Inouye et al, 2000). Functional declines and iatrogenic complications are associated with longer hospital stays, higher costs, and increased risk of institutionalization (Lyons, Landefeld, 2001). As discussed in Chapter 21, elders frequently experience delirium in acute care settings. Common iatrogenic complications include functional decline, new-onset incontinence, malnutrition, pressure ulcers, medication reactions, falls, and functional decline. Several classic articles on iatrogenesis in the elderly (Gorbien et al, 1992; Creditor, 1993) document the hazards of hospitalization for older people.

The Nurses Improving Care for Healthsystem Elders (NICHE) program of the Hartford Geriatric Nursing Institute (Fulmer et al, 2002) has developed several models of nursing care practice to prevent iatrogenesis and improve outcomes. More than 105 hospitals nationwide have participated in the development of NICHE units of various types, including the geriatric resource nurse (GRN) model, the acute care of the elderly (ACE) unit, and the syndrome specific model. Any acute care hospital interested in improving care for hospitalized elderly can seek out the resources of the NICHE program (Mezey et al, 2004). Geriatric evaluation and management (GEM) and postacute gerontological units are examples of other successful models (Lyons, Landefeld, 2001). Models utilizing gerontological nurse practitioners (GNPs) are described by Smyth et al (2001). The Nurse Competence in Aging project described in Chapter 2 is another important initiative in enhancing knowledge of nurses in care of older adults.

Transfers Between Acute and Long-Term Care

Older adults who are residents of nursing homes are at particularly high risk of experiencing the negative consequences of hospitalization. It is preferable to treat acute problems in the nursing home setting rather than transferring residents to the hospital, but problems outside the scope of care often require transfer. The transitions between acute care and long-term care are cause for concern. Inadequate communication, medical errors, service duplication, inappropriate care and service utilization, lack of expertise in gerontological care, and missing critical care plan elements have all been cited as problems associated with transitions (Vance, 2004). Both hospitals and nursing homes need to improve in communication of accurate and complete information during transfers to ensure the best care outcomes for the patient. The American Geriatrics Association's position statement *Improving the Quality of Transitional Care for Persons with Complex Care Needs* (http://www.americangeriatrics.org/products/positionpapers/complex_care.pf.shtml) and the American Medical Directors Association's *Acute Change of Condition Guideline* (http://www.amda.com) are valuable resources for understanding and improving transfers between acute and long-term care. Nurses play an important role in ensuring that needed information is communicated effectively when transfers are necessary to and from either setting. Box 27-4 presents suggestions about transfers.

Nursing Homes

Nursing homes provide around-the-clock care for those needing subacute, chronic, rehabilitative, and palliative care. Nursing homes are complex health care settings that are a mix of hospital, rehabilitation facility, hospice, dementia-specific units, and for many elders, a final home. Although the current trend is to use the term *skilled nursing facility*, the authors prefer the word *nursing home* since it truly is a place where nurses create a home for chronically ill older people who need nursing care. Nursing homes range in size from 10 to more than 1000 beds with the average size 107 beds. Approximately 66% of nursing homes are for-profit facilities; 27% are not-for-profit, and 7% are government owned (Nursing Home Statistics, American Health Care Association [AHCA], http://www.efmoody.com/longterm/nursingstatistics.html). Box 27-5 presents the differing care orientations of acute and long-term care.

Resident Characteristics

There are approximately 1.5 to 2 million nursing home residents (4% to 5% of the older adult population), but predictions are that there will be 5.3 million Americans residing in nursing homes by 2030, representing more than a threefold increase

---

Box 27-4	Suggestions for Transfer Between Acute and Long-Term Care

Older people need:
- Preparation for what to expect at next care site
- Opportunity to give input about their values and preferences regarding care
- Advice on management of their conditions
- Glasses, hearing aids, dentures, clothing
- Input into arrangements for the next level of care (e.g., subacute, home)
- Explanation of all actions
- Notification and involvement of family or decision makers
- Professionals with gerontological care competencies to prevent iatrogenesis

Health care professionals require:
- An accessible record with current problem list, medication regimen, allergies, advance directives, baseline physical and cognitive function, contact information for all care providers (family and professional)
- Record of medication administration
- Recent laboratory, x-ray reports
- History of illness and treatment
- Input from care providers who know the older person (e.g., nursing home staff)
- Information about the person's patterns
- Person's past functional and cognitive status
- Activity or mobility orders and special precautions or needs
- Diet orders and special nutritional requirements
- Safety precautions or needs
- Contact information for care providers, family, decision makers
- Copy of DPA
- Copy of latest H&P
- Copy of last two progress notes pages

Adapted from Meiner S: Physician's orders and nurses' notes: when time is pressing, details can be lost, *Geriatr Nurs* 19(5):291, 1998; The American Geriatric Society: *Improving the quality of transitional care for persons with complex care needs* (http://www.americangeriatrics.org/products/positionpapers/complex_carePF.shtml.
DPA, Durable power of attorney; *H&P,* history and physical.

Box 27-5	Focus of Acute and Long-Term Care

Acute Care Orientation
- Illness
- High technology
- Short term
- Episodic
- One dimensional
- Professional
- Medical model
- Cure

Long-Term Care Orientation
- Function
- High touch
- Extended
- Interdisciplinary model
- Ongoing
- Multidimensional
- Paraprofessional and family
- Care

Adapted from Ouslander J, Osterweil D, Morley J: *Medical care in the nursing home,* New York, 1997, McGraw-Hill.

in the next 25 years (Burggraf, 2004). Clearly this calls for increased education and recruitment of gerontological nurses to this setting as well as creation of new models of care.

Residents of nursing homes are predominantly women, 80 years or older, Caucasian, widowed, and dependent in activities of daily living (ADLs) and instrumental activities of daily living (IADLs). More than 60% are cognitively impaired. Nursing home residents represent the most frail of the older adult population. In many cases, their needs for 24-hour care were not able to be met in the home or residential care setting, or their needs may have exceeded the family's ability to provide required care.

Costs of Care

Costs for nursing homes vary significantly with the location but average $54,900 annually. In the 10 most expensive areas of the United States, annual costs can be approximately $80,000 or more (Nursing Home Statistics [AHCA], http://www.efmoody.com/longterm/nursingstatistics.

html). Fees are usually obtained through a combination of Medicare (11.9%), Medicaid (66%), and private pay and long-term care insurance (22%) (American Health Care Association, 2004, http://www.ahca.org/research/oscar_patient.htm). The purchase of long-term care insurance is becoming a popular option for many Americans. Estimates are that this trend will continue, and by the year 2020, financing of long-term care by private insurance will increase to 6.6% (Lueckenotte, 2000). For younger people, the cost of long-term care insurance is less prohibitive than for older people. (See Chapter 24 for discussion on long-term care insurance.)

The limited reimbursement by Medicare of nursing home costs shifts the burden of payment to the individual resident or to the federal and state governments (Medicaid). For many older people, the costs are excessive. For those who can afford care, many have spent down all their savings paying for that care. There is growing concern nationwide related to the financing of long-term care and the ability of states and the federal government to continue to support costs through the Medicaid programs. Reimbursement levels now do not cover actual costs, and there is fear that if further cuts are made, the often precarious quality of care in these settings will be further compromised.

Regulations and Quality of Care

Nursing homes are one of the most highly regulated industries in the United States. Although nursing homes recognize the need to enact legislation to ensure quality, the lack of additional funding for legislated initiatives has left many nursing homes struggling to maintain quality and meet standards with few resources. Criteria and standards often create a bureaucratic structure and a punitive environment that challenges those caring for nursing home residents. Federal and state regulations have become more onerous and time consuming than the care. The Omnibus Budget Reconciliation Act (OBRA) of 1987 and the frequent revisions and updates are designed to impact the actual quality of resident care and have had a positive impact. Some of the requirements of OBRA and subsequent legislation include the following: comprehensive resident assessments, increased training requirements for nursing assistants, elimination of the use of medications and

Box 27-6	Goals of Long-Term Care

1. Provide a safe and supportive environment for chronically ill and functionally dependent people
2. Restore and maintain highest practicable level of functional independence
3. Preserve individual autonomy
4. Maximize quality of life, well-being, and satisfaction with care
5. Provide comfort and dignity at the end of life for residents and their families
6. Provide coordinated interdisciplinary care to subacutely ill residents who plan to return to home or a less restrictive level of care
7. Stabilize and delay progression, when possible, of chronic medical conditions
8. Prevent acute medical and iatrogenic illnesses and identify and treat rapidly when they do occur
9. Create a homelike environment that respects dignity of each resident

Adapted from Ouslander J, Osterweil D, Morley J: *Medical care in the nursing home*, New York, 1997, McGraw-Hill.

restraints for discipline or convenience, higher staffing requirements for nursing, social work staff, standards for nursing home administrators, protection of resident rights, and quality assurance activities. Goals of nursing home care are presented in Box 27-6.

Staffing and Role of Professional Nursing

A growing concern is the lack of adequate staffing, particularly professional nurses, in nursing homes. Current federal standards require only one RN in the nursing home for 8 hours per day—a figure quite shocking considering the ratio of RNs to patients in acute care, even with shortages in that setting. Despite increases in the acuity level of nursing home patients, and the well-documented positive relationship between nurse staffing and quality of nursing home care, care continues to be provided in U.S. nursing homes almost devoid of professional providers. The bulk of care is provided by unlicensed nursing personnel, and shortages are acute at this level as well. Results of a 2000 report by the Health Care Financing Administration revealed that fewer than one half of the nation's nursing homes had enough licensed nurses to provide adequate planning, direct care, and supervision (http: www.nccnhr.org/govpolicy/51_162_701.cfm).

An expert panel on nursing home care convened by the John Hartford Institute for Geriatric Nursing (Harrington et al, 2000) confirmed that poor quality of care in nursing homes is related to inadequate levels of staff. Adding to the problem of limited staff are the substantially lower levels of education of nursing home nurses when compared with nurses in hospitals. "Caregiving, the central feature of a nursing home, needs to be improved to ensure high quality of care to residents" (Harrington et al, 2000, p 14). These nursing experts made comprehensive recommendations for improved RN staffing, increased gerontological nursing education requirements for all staff (including a bachelor of science in nursing [BSN] degree for directors of nursing), and increased staffing ratios for RNs, LPNs, and nursing assistants. Additional recommendations were that most nursing homes should have a full-time gerontological clinical nurse specialist (CNS) or gerontological nurse practitioner (GNP) on staff.

Estimates of the cost of implementing higher staffing standards would equate to approximately a 2% to 7% increase in total nursing home expenditures over what was spent in 1996 on U.S. nursing homes, although savings may occur as a result of improved care, staff morale, and decreased turnover (Harrington et al, 2000). Many aging advocacy groups as well as the American Nurses Association have supported the critical need for adequate staffing in nursing homes, but to date, the federal government has not acted to mandate increases in minimum staffing requirements (http://www.nccnhr.org/govpolicy/51_162_701.cfm). The full report to Congress on the appropriateness of minimum nurse staffing ratios in nursing homes (2002) can be downloaded from the following site: http://www.cms.hhs.gov/medicaid/reports/rp1201home.asp.

For those of us committed to quality care for the most frail of our elders, the lack of professional nurse staffing in nursing homes is reason for grave concern. Millions of dedicated caregivers are daily providing competent and compassionate care to very sick elders in nursing homes against great odds, for example, a lack of support, inadequate salaries and staff, and lack of respect. It is time for their stories of care to be told, and it is time to recognize their needs for adequate staff to do this very important work:

> Care of the frail elderly and seriously ill persons is labor intensive and costly. . . in many nursing homes staff is assigned to more residents than they can properly care for. In situations where unrealistic workloads exist, resident needs are often unmet, raising the risk of harmful and costly complications. This frustrates those who feel responsible for the care of residents. . . Reasonable workloads are a necessary condition for quality care (National Coalition for Nursing Home Reform, 2002, http://www.nccnhr.org).

We urge our readers to join with the professional nursing organizations and consumer advocacy groups to lobby for adequate nurse staffing with funding to support it, improved education in gerontological nursing, and an increasing presence of professional nurses in nursing homes. The positive outcomes of GNPs in nursing homes are reason for encouragement, and projections are that they will assume maximum responsibility for care of the elderly in this setting. The nursing home provides professional nurses the opportunity to practice from a nursing model of care in a variety of roles ranging from administrative (directors of nursing, supervisors, educators, Minimum Data Set [MDS] coordinator, quality improvement coordinator) to direct care provider. We agree with Eliopoulos (2001, pp 533, 537) when she says: "The increased demands and complexities of long-term care facilities necessitate that highly competent nurses be employed in this setting . . . gerontological nurses can cast a new vision for long-term care that can enable residents of nursing facilities to experience the highest possible quality of life for the time remaining in their lives." See Chapter 2 for additional discussion of some of these issues.

NEW MODELS OF CARE: CULTURE CHANGE IN NURSING HOMES

The public, as well as many health care professionals, hold a very negative view of nursing homes. Many older adults express that they would rather die than have to be "put into" a nursing home. If a move to a nursing home is necessary, families experience guilt and anxiety. Caregivers in nursing homes are held in low esteem by health care professionals, paid little, and rarely recognized for the important work they do. Nursing homes are often blamed for all of the societal problems associated with the aging of our population. Older adults who live in nursing homes are thought to be depressed, helpless, waiting to die. Although there are continued challenges and opportunities to improve care in nursing homes, and in the very fabric of the long-term care system, many nursing homes provide an environment that truly represents the best of caring and quality of life. The commitment and dedication of staff need to be honored and supported. They have much to teach us about aging, nursing, and caring. See Box 2-5 in Chapter 2 for a description of caring themes expressed by nursing home caregivers in a recent study.

Across the United States, the movement to transform typical medical model nursing homes into "homes" that fully support and nurture quality of life for older people is changing the face of long-term care. Begun by the Pioneer Network, a national not-for-profit organization that serves the culture change movement, many facilities are changing from a rigid institutional approach to one that is person centered. "The Pioneer Network works to promote a new vision: a culture of aging that is life-affirming, humane and meaningful in whatever setting that takes place—home, assisted living, or nursing home" (Pioneer Network, 2004, http://www.pioneernetwork.net). The Eden Alternative, founded by Dr. Bill Thomas (www.edenalt.com), and the Wellspring Model developed by Wellspring Innovative Solutions in Seymour, Wisconsin (www.wellspringis.org) are examples of philosophies and programs of culture change. The Eden Alternative is best known for the addition of animals, plants, and children to nursing homes. However, cats and dogs are not the heart of culture change. Truly transforming a nursing home requires involvement of all levels of staff and changes in values, attitudes, structures, and management practices. Staff empowerment, resident involvement in decision making, individualized rather than routine task-oriented care, relationship building, a sense of community and belonging, meaningful activities, and a homelike environment are some of the principles of culture

---

Box 27-7   **Institution-Centered Versus Person-Centered Culture**

Institution-Centered Culture

- Schedules and routines are designed by the institution and staff, and residents must comply.
- Focus is on tasks to be accomplished.
- Rotation of staff from unit to unit occurs.
- Decision making is centralized with little involvement of staff or residents and families.
- There is a hospital environment.
- Structured activities are provided to all residents.
- There is little opportunity for socialization.
- Organization exists for employees rather than residents.
- There is little respect for privacy or individual routines.

Person-Centered Culture

- Emphasis is on relationships between staff and residents.
- Individualized plans of care are based on residents' needs, usual patterns, and desires.
- Staff members have consistent assignments and know the residents' preferences and uniqueness.
- Decision making is as close to the resident as possible.
- Staff members are involved in decisions and plans of care.
- Environment is homelike.
- Meaningful activities and opportunities for socialization are available around the clock.
- There is a sense of community and belonging—"like family."
- There is involvement of the community—children, pets, plants, outings.

Adapted from The Pioneer Network: http://www.pioneernetwork.net.

---

change activities. Box 27-7 presents some of the differences between an institution-centered culture and a person-centered culture.

Much more research is needed on the effect of culture change on resident and staff outcomes, but anecdotal reports and qualitative observations include positive outcomes, such as decreased staff turnover and increased resident and family satisfaction (Coleman et al, 2002). According to the Pioneer Network, "culture change has been shown to transform demoralized, dispirited staff into productive teams and dispirited elders into active members of engaged communities" (http://www.pioneernetwork.net). Barbara Haight, a gerontological nursing leader, and colleagues (Haight et al, 2002) offer a nursing model in an article entitled "Thriving: a Life Span Theory" that guides nurses in understanding how care practices and environments of care support the full development (thriving not merely surviving) of older adults. In an issue of the *Journal of Gerontological Nursing* devoted to these ideas, Barba et al (2002) fully discuss thriving in nursing homes using the Eden Alternative as well as research related to care outcomes. Gerontological nurses have known these things for years, and from the past to the present, they have been the leaders in

the provision of person-centered care in all settings. It is an exciting time to be a gerontological nurse.

MAKING NURSING HOME DECISIONS

Gerontological nurses are frequently asked for assistance in helping older adults and their families make decisions about choosing a nursing home. Many sources are available to assist in decision making including a Care Planner available from Medicare (http://www.careplanner.org) (see also Resources at the end of the chapter). Gerontological nurse Marilyn Rantz and her colleagues have done extensive research and writing on quality of care in nursing homes. *The New Nursing Homes: a 20-Minute Way to Find Great Long-Term Care* (Rantz et al, 2001) is an excellent resource to share with older people and their families. *Person Centered Care: a Model for Nursing Homes* (Rantz, Flesner, 2004), published by the American Nurses Association, is another resource that will also be helpful. Box 27-8 presents a guide to selecting a nursing home. The Centers for Medicare and Medicaid Services (CMS) have a website, NH

Box 27-8	Selecting a Nursing Home

Central Focus
- Residents and families are the central focus of the facility

Interaction
- Staff members attentive and caring
- Staff members listen to what residents say
- Staff members and residents smile at one another
- Prompt response to resident and family needs
- Meaningful activities provided on all shifts to meet individual preferences
- Residents engage in activities with enjoyment
- Staff members talk to cognitively impaired residents; cognitively impaired residents involved in activities designed to meet their needs
- Staff members do not talk down to residents, talk as if they are not present, ignore yelling or calling out
- Families involved in care decisions and daily life in facility

Milieu
- Calm, active, friendly
- Presence of community, volunteers, children, plants, animals

Environment
- No odor, clean and well maintained
- Rooms personalized
- Private areas

- Protected outside areas
- Equipment in good repair

Individualized Care
- Restorative programs for ambulation, ADLs
- Residents well dressed and groomed
- Resident and family councils
- Pleasant mealtimes, good food, residents have choices
- Adequate staff to serve meals and assist residents
- Flexible meal schedules, food available 24 hours per day
- Ethnic food preferences

Staff
- Well trained, professional
- Professional in appearance and demeanor
- RNs involved in care decisions and care delivery
- Active staff development programs
- Physicians and advanced-practice nurses involved in care planning and staff training
- Adequate staff (more than the minimum required) on each shift
- Low staff turnover

Safety
- Safe walking areas indoors and outdoors
- Monitoring of residents at risk for injury
- Restraint-appropriate care, adequate safety equipment and training on its use

Adapted from Rantz MJ et al: Nursing home care quality: a multidimensional theoretical model, *J Nurs Care Qual* 12(3):30-46, 1998.

ADLs, Activities of daily living; *RNs*, registered nurses.

Compare (www.medicare.gov/NHCompare), that posts nursing home quality indicators for nursing homes across the United States as well as a nursing home checklist with tips to use when visiting nursing homes. Although these may be helpful for consumers, they are basically derived from yearly nursing home survey data and measures of quality improvement, and they may need considerable interpretation by health care professionals to be useful for consumers. The data may or may not be representative of the quality of the nursing home. The most appropriate way of choosing a nursing

home is to personally visit the facility, meet with the director of nursing, observe care routines, discuss the potential resident's needs, and use a format such as the one presented in Box 27-8 to ask questions.

FAMILY AND COMMUNITY INVOLVEMENT IN NURSING HOMES

A good nursing home views families as essential care partners and actively seeks their input and encourages their involvement in all aspects of care for their family member. Nursing homes provide family councils and offer many other ways for families to provide input, voice concerns, and receive information. Families often need a great deal of support to deal with feelings of guilt associated with placing a loved one in the nursing home. Nursing home staff must appreciate families' experiences and feelings, hear their stories of care, help them participate in care if they choose, and inspire trust that the care the nursing home provides will honor and respect the family member who resides in the facility.

Family members too must come to know the staff in the nursing home and appreciate and support their work. In the nursing homes that one of the authors (TT) worked in, many family members often came to feel that they were now part of a new family. They would frequently bring treats for the staff and residents, assist other residents and family members, plan and participate in activities, and offer a great deal of assistance in care for their family member, working as a team with facility caregivers. Staff members in nursing homes often describe their relationship with residents as "like family," and often families feel this way as well. Listening, offering emotional support, including families in planning care, and helping families plan ahead and prepare for changes in the resident's health status are important staff interventions.

ADVOCACY FOR OLDER ADULTS

Advocacy consists of acting on behalf of, supporting, and defending a client in his or her cause. The advocate can be any person, including family members, professional nurses, attorneys, physicians, and other health care personnel. Nurses act as advocates of their clients when they act to support the person as a free agent who has autonomy in the health care situation (Rini, 1998).

Advocacy for Institutionalized Elders

Advocacy organizations for nursing home residents are active throughout the United States. They are engaged in complaint resolution, confrontation and/or negotiation with nursing homes, community education, legal intervention, and legislative reform. Professional nurses must remain alert to their advocacy role in institutions. Nurses need to be aware of the procedure for filing a complaint against a nursing home. Some may wish to do so and will need the support of the legal system and other nurses in the advocacy of humane care for clients. A complaint about practices, procedures, physical conditions, or quality of care in a nursing home is initially a request to the state health department to inspect a particular home and determine if a violation exists. Any person may file such a request. Toll-free numbers are available in each state and are to be posted in the nursing home.

Ombudsman is a term used to denote the nursing home advocate prepared to deal squarely but sensitively with the realities of a nursing home resident's life. An ombudsman must view the resident's problem as impartially as possible and act as advocate but not in an adversarial role with the nursing home administration. Issues brought to the attention of ombudsmen include abuse, neglect, poor care, poorly trained staff, understaffing, inadequate laundry procedures, roommate conflicts, denial of rights, violation of privacy, and lack of grievance procedures. In addition to acting as advocate, the ombudsman often locates appropriate resources and links residents to them, trains friendly visitors, provides a clearinghouse for problems or complaints, gives legislative updates, and provides assistance in conducting family councils and resident councils. The ombudsman must also assist families in transferring or discharging patients from a nursing home to another setting.

The long-term care ombudsman program is mandated by the Older Americans Act (OAA). Each state must have an Office of the State Ombudsman to which all substate programs report. Models may vary to reflect the needs and conditions within the state. Nursing home and board-and-care residents must have direct and immediate access to an ombudsman when necessary for protection and advocacy. The ombudsman is concerned about maintaining good relationships with nursing home personnel. Many nurses function in the ombudsman role. Ways that a nursing home can ensure a more collaborative relationship with the ombudsman are summarized in Box 27-9.

Box 27-9	Working Effectively with an Ombudsman

1. The administrator should become acquainted with the ombudsman.
2. The administrator should introduce the ombudsman to the entire staff.
3. The ombudsman should be invited to the facility on a routine basis and on special occasions to become a part of the facility resources rather than an adversary.
4. The ombudsman and administrator should share perceptions and facts openly with one another while maintaining confidentiality.
5. The administrator should discuss some of his or her concerns and legislative issues that need attention.
6. The administrator should inform the residents' council that an ombudsman is available.
7. The administrator should likewise inform the family council about the ombudsman.

Rights of Residents

Patients' rights in facilities and institutions of all types are mandated by federal and state laws and the U.S. Constitution, as are the rights of the general population. Legal rights vary according to the setting and individual competency. Rights in institutions are to be posted in a place visible to all and are to be reviewed with the individual soon after admission to a facility. For the older adult who resides in a nursing home, the following are additional important activities to meet the resident rights requirements: public display of annual CMS survey results (also available at public libraries and on the individual state government websites); display of ombudsman information; provisions for residents to participate in public elections; resident council participation; use of informed consent for use of side rails, chemical and physical restraints, and withdrawal or withholding of life-sustaining treatments; opportunities for competent residents to self-administer their medications; and establishment of a grievance process for residents and families regarding care provision (Lueckenotte, 2000).

Nursing responsibilities are (1) to ensure that the patient has seen, read, and/or understands the rights; (2) to document explicitly when and why any rights may be temporarily suspended; (3) to observe and record observations attesting to the individual's ability or inability to manage daily affairs; and (4) to be sure that the patient's status is reviewed at appropriate time intervals (these vary from one state to another) and that he or she obtains legal assistance in presenting his or her defense. The rights of patients are enforced largely because of the integrity of nurses and our willingness to act as patient advocates.

Consent

Consent is a concept that arises out of the idea of human self-determination and autonomy. In the health care situation, consent is related to accepting or refusing care and treatments and is expressed in the legal doctrine of informed consent. Informed consent requires the disclosure of information about a proposed treatment that might be material to a client's decisions about consenting to the treatment. State law generally specifies the extent of information to be disclosed. Most courts have upheld providing information that a reasonable health care provider would disclose in the same or similar circumstances or that a reasonable client would consider material to his or her decision.

Consent for treatment is based on the decision-making capacity of the client. Such capacity is determined by the provider or providers proposing the care or treatment and intending to carry it out. It means that the client is able to understand the nature and purpose of the procedure and appreciate its possible risks and benefits. There is a presumption of decisional capacity in adults, elderly persons, and others unless there is a reason to believe the person cannot understand the provided information or is unable to make an informed decision. Providers then need to seek consent from guardians, attorneys-in-fact, or family members acting as health care surrogates (Rini, 1998). With regard to consent, it is important for nurses to remember that all actions should be explained to clients, even those with dementia. When working with patients with dementia, refusal to participate as indicated by words or behavior should be respected in most circumstances.

MacLean (2001, p 8) discusses the "sliding scale of competence" and reminds us "that impairment

NANDA and Wellness Diagnoses

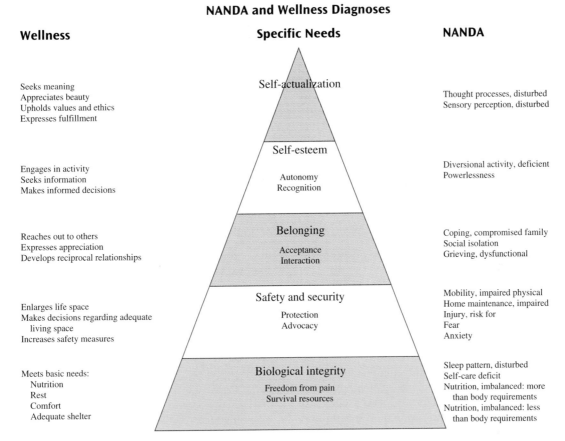

Wellness	Specific Needs	NANDA
Seeks meaning Appreciates beauty Upholds values and ethics Expresses fulfillment	**Self-actualization**	Thought processes, disturbed Sensory perception, disturbed
Engages in activity Seeks information Makes informed decisions	Self-esteem Autonomy Recognition	Diversional activity, deficient Powerlessness
Reaches out to others Expresses appreciation Develops reciprocal relationships	Belonging Acceptance Interaction	Coping, compromised family Social isolation Grieving, dysfunctional
Enlarges life space Makes decisions regarding adequate living space Increases safety measures	Safety and security Protection Advocacy	Mobility, impaired physical Home maintenance, impaired Injury, risk for Fear Anxiety

Meets basic needs:
    Nutrition
    Rest
    Comfort
    Adequate shelter
	Biological integrity
	Freedom from pain
	Survival resources
		Sleep pattern, disturbed
		Self-care deficit
		Nutrition, imbalanced: more
		    than body requirements
		Nutrition, imbalanced: less
		    than body requirements

These are not all of the possible wellness or NANDA diagnoses that may be identified. The above are frequent examples of nursing diagnoses that should be considered when planning care for the older adult in whatever setting.

of decision making capacity needed for a particular decision depends on the difficulty (complexity, ambiguity, and multiplicity of options) of the decision. A person may be able to make a decision in one domain but not another, and partially impaired persons may retain full capacity to make some difficult decisions even when unable to make simpler ones." Competency, capacity, and decision making about life prolonging treatment and advance directives are extremely complex issues with regard to consent and patient rights and have been discussed in other sections of this book.

Consent for research participation is a more detailed and extensive process, because treatments provided in such circumstances may not necessarily directly benefit the client. However, research

is an important tool in directing evidence-based practice, and there are many concerns that need further study. For those readers who wish to learn more about research with older adults, there are several excellent resources (West et al, 1991; Phillips, Van Ort, 1995; Burnside et al, 1998; White, 2000).

IMPLICATIONS FOR GERONTOLOGICAL NURSING AND HEALTHY AGING

Throughout this chapter and the book we have offered many implications for gerontological nursing and healthy aging. Nurses with competence in care of older people will be in great demand as the population ages. Gerontological nurses have always assumed a leadership role in improving care for elders, ensuring fulfillment of all levels of needs on Maslow's hierarchy, and promoting healthy aging. Through their expertise, commitment, dedication, advocacy, and compassion, gerontological nurses who work with older adults in all settings will continue to be leaders in creation of models that truly change the culture of existing systems. Perhaps our words in this book will provide you with the knowledge you need to fulfill this vision. Our hope is that you find as much joy and fulfillment as we have in our nursing of older adults. Irene Burnside (1980, p 32) quoted Martin Buber when she wrote: "No one can say thank you the way an old person can." May you hear many thank you's in your practice.

KEY CONCEPTS

- A familiar and comfortable environment allows an elder to function at his or her highest capacity.
- Relocation has variable effects, depending on the individual's personality, health, cognitive capacities, self-esteem, and preferred lifestyle.
- Environmental cues such as wall maps, clear directive labels, calendars, and clocks will assist individuals in adjusting to a new setting and remaining oriented.
- Nurses must be knowledgeable about the range of housing options for older people so that they can assist the elder and the family to make appropriate decisions.
- There is a great need for professional nursing in assisted living and nursing home settings.
- Nurses must take the lead in creating cultures of caring for older adults in all settings.

Activities and Discussion Questions

1. Identify three objects in your living space that are important to you, and explain why these are significant. Will you take these with you whenever you relocate?
2. Ask an older relative about the items or conditions in his or her home that make him or her feel secure and comfortable.
3. Discuss with this elder various moves he or she has made and how he or she felt about them.

4. How might the care needs of an older adult in assisted living, subacute care, and a nursing home differ? What is the role of the professional nurse in each of these settings?
5. Select three places listed in your phone book as retirement communities, and make inquiries regarding possible placement of an older adult parent. What questions did you ask? What is the cost? What are the provisions for health care? What types of activities and assistance are available? Which would you select for your grandmother and why?
6. If you were the director of nursing, what would your nursing home be like (design, staffing, quality of care, training)?

RESOURCES

Organizations

American Association of Homes and Services for the Aging
2519 Connecticut Avenue, NW
Washington, DC 20008
(202) 783-2242
website: http://www.aasha.org

American Association of Retired Persons
601 E Street NW
Washington, DC 20049
website: www.aarp.org

American Health Care Association
1201 L Street NW
Washington, DC 20005
(202) 833-2050
website: http://www.ahca.org

Assisted Living Federation of America
11200 Waples Mill Road, Suite 150
Fairfax, VA 22030
(703) 691-8900
website: http://www.alfa.org

Continuing Care Accreditation Commission
2519 Connecticut Avenue, NW
Washington, DC 20008
(202) 783-2286
website: http://www.ccaonline.org

The Eden Alternative
742 Turnpike Road
Sherburne, NY 13460
(907) 247-1997
website: http://www.edenalt.com

National Center for Assisted Living
American Health Care Association
1201 L Street NW
Washington, DC 20005-4014
(202) 842-4444

National Center for Home Equity Conversion
(NCHEC)
110 E. Main, Room 1010
Madison, WI 53703

Public Policy Institute, Research Group
Consumer Fact Sheets
National Citizens Coalition for Nursing Home
Reform
1424 16th Street, NW
Washington, DC 20036
(202) 339-2275
website: http://www.nccnhr.org

Retirement Living
9302 Lee Highway, Suite 750
Fairfax, VA 22031
(800) 394-9990
website: http://www.retirement-living.com

Wellspring Innovative Solutions, Inc.
2149 Velp Avenue, Suite 500
Green Bay, WI 54303
(920) 434-0123
website: http://wellspringis.org

The Wellspring Program
Pioneer Network
PO Box 18648
Rochester, NY 14618
(585) 271-7570
website: http://www.pioneernetwork.net

Websites

Care Planner from Medicare (care options)
Available from http://www.careplanner.org

Centers for Medicare and Medicaid Services
http://www.cms.hhs.gov

REFERENCES

Arras JD, Dubler NN: Bringing the hospital home: ethical and social implications of high-tech home care, *Hastings Cent Rep* 24(5, suppl):S19-S28, 1994.

Barba BE, Tesh AS, Courts NF: Promoting thriving in nursing homes: the Eden Alternative, *J Gerontol Nurs* 28(3):7-13, 2002.

Bergman G: Shared housing—not only for the rent, *Aging Today* 15(1):1, 1994.

Bruno L: Senior living can be lonely, *Daily Record,* March 24, 2002, Morris County, NJ. Available at www.dailyrecord.com/news/wherewelive/series1/32402seniorliving.htm.

Burggraf V: Promoting education: improving quality in long-term care, *J Gerontol Nurs* 30(3):3, 2004.

Burnside I: Why work with the aged? *Geriatr Nurs* 2(3):29-33, 1980.

Burnside I, Preski S, Hertz JE: Research instrumentation and elderly subjects, *Image J Nurs Sch* 30(2):185-190, 1998.

Coleman M et al: The Eden alternative: findings after 1 year of implementation, *Gerontologist* 57A(7):M422-M427, 2002.

Creditor MC: Hazards of hospitalization of the elderly, *Ann Intern Med* 118(3):219-223, 1993.

Dionne B: Super service providers, *Caring for the Ages* 5(4):44-45, 2004.

Edelstein S: *Fair housing laws for group residences for frail older persons,* Washington, DC, 1995, American Association of Retired Persons.

Eliopoulos C: *Gerontological nursing,* Philadelphia, 2001, Lippincott Williams & Wilkins.

Folkemer D et al: *Adult foster care for the older adult: a review of state regulatory and funding strategies,* Washington, DC, 1996, American Association of Retired Persons.

Fulmer T et al: Nurses improving care for health system elders (NICHE): using outcomes and benchmarks for evidenced-based practice, *Geriatr Nurs* 23(3):121-127, 2002.

Gorbien M et al: Iatrogenic illness in hospitalized elderly people, *J Am Geriatr Soc* 40(10):1031-1042, 1992.

Haight BK et al: Thriving: a life span theory, *J Gerontol Nurs* 28(3):14-22, 2002.

Harrington C et al: Experts recommend minimum nurse staffing standards for nursing facilities in the United States, *Gerontologist* 40(1):5-15, 2000.

Hawes C: A key piece of the integration puzzle: Managing the chronic care needs of the frail elderly in residential care facilities, *Generations* 23(2):51-55, 1999.

Inouye S et al: The hospital elder life progress: A model of care to prevent cognitive and functional decline in older hospitalized patients, *J Am Geriatr Soc* 48(12):1657-1706, 2000.

Iwasiw C et al: Resident and family perspectives: the first year in a long-term care facility, *J Gerontol Nurs* 29(1):45-54, 2003.

Leach D: *Making your community livable: programs that work,* Washington, DC, 1996, AARP Public Policy Institute.

Leisure world at Laguna Hills, press release, Laguna Hills, Calif, May 1996.

Life care guide, 2000. Available at www.lifecareguide.com.

Lueckenotte A: *Gerontological nursing,* ed 2, St Louis, 2000, Mosby.

Lyons W, Landefeld S: Improving care for hospitalized elders, *Ann Long-Term Care* 9(4):35-40, 2001.

MacLean D: Managing decision-making capacity: how to draw the line? *Caring for the Ages* 2(5):8,11, 2001.

Maddox G: *Encyclopedia of aging,* New York, 1995, Springer.

Mezey M et al: Nurses improving care to health system elders (niche): Implementation of best practice models, *Journal of Nursing Administration* 34(10):451-457, 2004.

Munroe D: Assisted living issues for nursing practice, *Geriatr Nurs* 24(2):99-105, 2003.

Nacev AN, Rettig J: A survey of key issues in Kentucky elder law, *North KY Law Rev* 29(1):139, 2002.

Omnibus Budget Reconciliation Act (OBRA) of 1987 (Public Law No. 100-203): Amendments 1990, 1991, 1992, 1993, and 1994, Rockville, Md, US Department of Health and Human Services, Health Care Financing Administration.

Phillips LR, Van Ort S: Issues in conducting intervention research in long-term care settings, *Nurs Outlook* 43(6):249-253, 1995.

Pynoos J: Strategies for home modification and repair, *Generations* 16(2):21, 1992.

Rantz M, Flesner M: *Person centered care: a model for nursing homes,* Washington, DC, 2004, American Nurses Association.

Rantz M, Popejoy L, Zwygart-Stauffacher M: *The new nursing homes: a 20-minute way to find great long-term care,* Lanham, Md, 2001, National Book Network.

Rantz M et al: Nursing home care quality: a multidimensional theoretical model, *J Nurs Care Qual* 12(3):30-46, 1998.

Rini AG: Legal and ethical issues, section VIII. In Luggen AS, Travis SS, Meiner S: *NGNA core curriculum for gerontological advanced practice nurses,* Thousand Oaks, Calif, 1998, Sage Publications.

Smyth C et al: Creating order out of chaos: models of GNP practice with hospitalized older adults, *Clin Excell Nurse Pract* 5(2):88-95, 2001.

Vance J: LTC bridges the gap, *Caring for the Ages* 5(6):9-10, 2004.

Wallace M: Is there a nurse in the house? The role of nurses in assisted living: past, present and future, *Geriatr Nurs* 24(4):218-221, 235, 2003.

West M, Bondy E, Hutchinson S: Interviewing institutionalized elders: threats to validity, *Image J Nurs Sch* 23(3):171-176, 1991.

White H: Alzheimer's disease research in the nursing home setting, *J Am Med Directors Assoc* 1:29-33, 2000.

Index

Page numbers with "t" denote tables; those with "f" denote figures; and those with "b" denote boxes